New and Emerging Entities in Dermatology and Dermatopathology

Franco Rongioletti • Bruce R. Smoller
Editors

New and Emerging Entities in Dermatology and Dermatopathology

Springer

Editors
Franco Rongioletti
Unit of Clinical Dermatology
Vita-Salute S.Raffaele University
Milan, Italy

Bruce R. Smoller
Department of Pathology
University of Rochester
Rochester, NY
USA

ISBN 978-3-030-80026-0 ISBN 978-3-030-80027-7 (eBook)
https://doi.org/10.1007/978-3-030-80027-7

This Springer imprint is published by the registered company Springer Nature Switzerland AG
The registered company address is: Gewerbestrasse 11, 6330 Cham, Switzerland

Foreword

Among the more appealing aspects of dermatology and dermatopathology are the frequent discovery of new entities and the investigations that provide better understanding of established entities. There are several codicils to this statement: (1) experience teaches that you can never tell when a patient with a new or unusual disorder will present in your clinic, or when a biopsy of such a disorder will come across your desk and appear under the objective of your microscope, and (2) the disease you read about for the first time today is likely to present itself in your office very soon thereafter.

With this in mind, I am delighted that my friends and colleagues, Franco Rongioletti and Bruce R. Smoller, have prepared this volume *New and Emerging, Entities in Dermatology and Dermatopathology.* A group of distinguished contributors have lent their expertise to this work, which considers a spectrum of disorders ranging from entities with little or no systemic involvement, such as pediatric cutaneous mucinoses and terra firma-forme dermatosis, to those with systemic implications, including immunoglobulin G4-related disease and lymphocytic thrombophilic arteritis. The chapter on COVID-19 related cutaneous manifestations is especially timely, providing the latest information about chilblain-like lesions, acro-ischemic-necrotic lesions, the varicella-like vesicular eruption, and other skin lesions that may accompany infection with the virus responsible for the worldwide pandemic that is still with us.

I hope that all those who have an interest in cutaneous diseases and wish to be up to date on the latest advances in the specialty will purchase this volume, read it, and keep it in an accessible spot in their offices and clinics, where they will be sure to find it useful. I will be one of them!

Charlottesville, VA, USA — James W. Patterson, M.D.

Preface

As is the case throughout medicine, dermatology and dermatopathology are rapidly evolving fields. As investigators learn more about immunologic reaction patterns and as new therapeutic interventions are developed, a plethora of truly new diseases and other newly described eruptions and explanations threaten to overwhelm practitioners. As the specialty develops more sensitive and specific methods of observation and association, new patterns emerge. Large, comprehensive textbooks in both dermatology and dermatopathology generally take years to complete and thus cannot possibly keep up with the pace of change. The panoply of journal articles that appear each month makes it nearly impossible for even the most diligent physician to keep abreast of the changing landscape. It is for this reason that the editors decided to invite a panel of internationally renowned leaders in the field to provide state-of-the-art descriptions and insights into new and emerging areas within the specialty. In some cases, the authors have written the seminal papers describing these entities, and in other situations, the chosen authors are well-known for their contributions to the literature across the discipline. The editors hope is that each chapter will provide the reader with an organized and concise introduction to the latest scholarship regarding each of the presented entities. As is the case with any such project, it is impossible to include every entity; even with the shorter production time for a thinner volume such as the present one, new entities have been described and others more fully understood since the inception of the project. It is also the case that any selection process is likely to omit certain entities that others might have chosen to include and to include diseases that might have been left out by other editors. Ultimately, the editors hope that practicing dermatologists, dermatopathologists, and general pathologists in the field have been provided with an update that covers many of the rapidly developing aspects of the dermatology and dermatopathology. The systemic implications of some of these entities can be of strong interest for internists, immunologists, hematologists, pediatricians, infettivologists, and general practitioners to improve their skill in the differential diagnosis and management of skin diseases, if one considers the skin as a window to internal imbalances.

The editors would like to thank sincerely each of the contributing authors for their adherence to a rapid timeline and strict formatting guidelines. Most importantly, the editors would like to thank them for contributing their expertise, without which this endeavor would have been impossible. As has been the case throughout his career, Dr. Smoller would like to thank, again, his wife Laura for enduring the trials and tribulations inherent in an academic career. Without her undying support and love, none of these efforts would seem worthwhile. He would also like to thank his students (some of whom have participated in this project) for the inspiration that they provide to him in all facets of his career, and Dr. Rongioletti for his longstanding friendship and continued vote of confidence. Dr. Rongioletti wishes to thank Valentina, his mother Rosanna and his daughter Francesca for their support, inspiration, and love. He wants to thank Bruce for their long and solid friendship over time and for the fruitful scientific partnership.

Milan, Italy Franco Rongioletti
Rochester, NY, USA Bruce R. Smoller

Contents

Contributors

Masashi Akiyama, MD, PhD Department of Dermatology, Nagoya University Graduate School of Medicine, Nagoya, Japan

Sarah M. Al-Naqshabandi, MD Departments of Pathology and Dermatology, Wake Forest University School of Medicine, Winston-Salem, NC, USA

Patricia J. Alvarez, MD Universidad de Piura, Peru

James Anderson-Vildósola, MD Departments of Dermatology and Pathology, Hospital Infantil Universitario Niño Jesús, Madrid, Spain

Laura Atzori, MD Dermatology Clinic, Department of Medical Sciences and Public Health, University of Cagliari, Cagliari, Italy

Maxime Battistella, MD Pathology Department, Hôpital Saint-Louis, AP-HP, Université de Paris, INSERM U976, Paris, France

Francisco G. Bravo, MD Universidad Peruana Cayetano Heredia, Peru

Luis Requena Caballero, MD Department of Dermatology, Fundacion Jimenez Diaz, Madrid, Spain

Eduardo Calonje, MD DipRCPath Dermatopathology Department, St John's Institute of Dermatology, St Thomas' Hospital, London, UK

Serafinella Patrizia Cannavò, MD Department of Clinical and Experimental Medicine, University of Messina, Messina, Italy

Avrom Caplan, MD The Ronald O. Perelman Department of Dermatology, NYU Grossman School of Medicine, New York, NY, USA

Valentina Caputo, MD Unit of Surgical Pathology, ASST Grande Ospedale Metropolitano Niguarda, Milan, Italy

WenChieh Chen, MD Department of Dermatology and Allergy, Technical University of Munich, Munich, Bavaria, Germany

Catherine G. Chung, MD The Ohio State University Wexner Medical Center, Columbus, OH, USA

Giulia Ciccarese, MD, PhD Department of Specialized Medicine, Dermatology Unit, Ospedale Policlinico San Martino, Genoa, Italy

Chiara Colato, MD Section of Pathology, Department of Diagnostics and Public Health, University of Verona, Verona, Italy

Isabel Colmenero, MD Departments of Dermatology and Pathology, Hospital Infantil Universitario Niño Jesús, Madrid, Spain

Bernard Cribier, MD Clinique Dermatologique, Hôpitaux Universitaires de Strasbourg, Strasbourg, France

Francesco Drago, MD Department of Specialized Medicine, Dermatology Unit, Ospedale Policlinico San Martino, Genoa, Italy

Joseph C. English 3rd, MD University of Pittsburgh Medical Center, Pittsburgh, PA, USA

Alberto Fernández, MD Departments of Dermatology and Pathology, Hospital Infantil Universitario Niño Jesús, Madrid, Spain

Maria-Teresa Fernández-Figueras, MD, PhD Anatomic Pathology, Hospital Universitari General de Catalunya. Grupo Quironsalud and Universitat Internacional de Catalunya, Sant Cugat del Vallés (Barcelona), Spain

Caterina Ferreli, MD Dermatology Clinic, Department of Medical Sciences and Public Health, University of Cagliari, Cagliari, Italy

Gabriel Quintero-Bustos, MD Pathology Department, National Institute of Medical Sciences and Nutrition Salvador Zubirán, Mexico City, Mexico

T. Gambichler, MD Department of Dermatology, Ruhr-University Bochum, Bochum, Germany

Giovanni Genovese, MD, PhD Dermatology Unit, Department of Pathophysiology and Transplantation, Università degli Studi di Milano, Milan, Italy

Giampiero Girolomoni, MD Section of Dermatology and Venereology, Department of Medicine, University of Verona, Verona, Italy

Claudio Guarneri, MD Department of Biomedical and Dental Sciences and Morpho Functional Imaging, University of Messina, Messina, Italy

Fabrizio Guarneri, MD Department of Clinical and Experimental Medicine, University of Messina, Messina, Italy

Lucie Heinzerling, MD Department of Dermatology, Ludwig-Maximilian University Hospital of Munich, Munich, Germany

Saskia Ingen-Housz-Oro, MD Department of Dermatology, Hopital Henri Mondor, Assistance-Publique – Hopitaux de Paris, Creteil, France

Camila Jaramillo, MD Nova Southeastern University, Dr. Kiran C. Patel College of Medicine, Ft. Lauderdale, FL, USA

Jacqueline M. Junkins-Hopkins, MD Consultant, Cutaneous Lymphoma, Geisinger Medical Center, Danville, PA, USA

Jean Kanitakis, MD Department of Dermatology, Edouard Herriot Hospital, Lyon, France

Roula Katerji, MD Department of Pathology and Laboratory Medicine, University of Rochester School of Medicine and Dentistry, Rochester, NY, USA

Werner Kempf, MD Kempf und Pfaltz Histologische Diagnostik, Zürich, Switzerland

Department of Dermatology, University Hospital Zürich, Zürich, Switzerland

Helmut Kerl, MD Department of Dermatology, University of Graz, Medical School, Graz, Austria

Katrin Kerl, MD Department of Dermatology, Ludwig-Maximilian University Hospital of Munich, Munich, Germany

Steven Kossard, FACD, PhD Kossard Dermatopathologists, Laverty Pathology, Macquarie Park, NSW, Australia

Konstantinos-Antonios Kostopoulos-Kanitakis, MD Department of Medicine, European Uiversity Cyprus, School of Medicine, Nicosia, Cyprus

Cynthia M. Magro, MD Weill Cornell Medicine, Department of Laboratory Medicine, New York, NY, USA

Marcela Saeb-Lima, MD Pathology Department, National Institute of Medical Sciences and Nutrition Salvador Zubirán, Mexico City, Mexico

Zlatko Marušić, MD, PhD Clinical Department of Pathology and Cytology, University Hospital Centre Zagreb, Zagreb, Croatia

Angelo Valerio Marzano, MD Dermatology Unit, Department of Pathophysiology and Transplantation, Università degli Studi di Milano, Milan, Italy

Martina Maurelli, MD Section of Dermatology and Venereology, Department of Medicine, University of Verona, Verona, Italy

Bodo Melnik, MD Department of Dermatology, Environmental Medicine and Health Theory, University of Osnabrueck, Osnabrueck, Lower Saxony, Germany

Mary Gail Mercurio, MD University of Rochester Medical Center, Rochester, NY, USA

Mariya Miteva, MD Miller School of Medicine, Dr. Phillip Frost Department of Dermatology and Cutaneous Surgery University of Miami, Miami, FL, USA

Christina Mitteldorf, MD University Medical Center Göttingen, Department of Dermatology, Venereology and Allergology, Göttingen, Germany

Josh H. Mo, MD Weill Cornell Medicine, Department of Laboratory Medicine, New York, NY, USA

Chiara Moltrasio, MRes, PhD Dermatology Unit, Department of Pathophysiology and Transplantation, Università degli Studi di Milano, Milan, Italy

Nicolas Ortonne, MD, PhD Department of Pathology, Hopital Henri Mondor, Assistance-Publique – Hopitaux de Paris, Creteil, France

Gerd Plewig, MD Department of Dermatology and Allergy, University of Munich, Munich, Bavaria, Germany

Shital Poojary, MD KJ Somaiya Medical College, Mumbai, India

Lluís Puig, MD, PhD Dermatology, Hospital de la Santa Creu i Sant Pau, Barcelona, Spain

Tatsiana Pukhalskaya, MD Department of Pathology and Laboratory Medicine, University of Rochester Medical Center (URMC), Rochester, NY, USA

Leslie Robinson-Bostom, MD Division of Dermatopathology, Department of Dermatology, The Warren Alpert Medical School of Brown University, Providence, RI, USA

Paolo Romanelli, MD Miller School of Medicine, Dr. Phillip Frost Department of Dermatology and Cutaneous Surgery University of Miami, Miami, FL, USA

Franco Rongioletti, MD Unit of Dermatology, IRCCS San Raffaele Hospital Vita Salute San Raffaele University, Milan, Italy

Unit of Dermatology, Department of Medical Sciences and Public Health, University of Cagliari, Cagliari, Italy

Dermatology Clinic, Vita-Salute S.Raffaele University, Milan, Italy

University Vita-Salute S.Raffaele, Milan, Italy

Section of Dermatology of the Department of Medical Science and Public Health, University of Cagliari, Cagliari, Italy

Vita-Salute S.Raffaele University, Milan, Italy

Misha Rosenbach, MD Perelman School of Medicine, University of Pennsylvania, Philadelphia, PA, USA

Omar P. Sangueza, MD Departments of Pathology and Dermatology, Wake Forest University School of Medicine, Winston-Salem, NC, USA

Bruce R. Smoller, MD Department of Pathology and Laboratory Medicine, University of Rochester Medical Center (URMC), Rochester, NY, USA

Department of Pathology and Laboratory Medicine, University of Rochester School of Medicine and Dentistry, Rochester, NY, USA

Takuya Takeichi, MD, PhD Department of Dermatology, Nagoya University Graduate School of Medicine, Nagoya, Japan

Antonio Torrelo, MD Departments of Dermatology and Pathology, Hospital Infantil Universitario Niño Jesús, Madrid, Spain

Karolyn A. Wanat, MD Medical College of Wisconsin, Milwaukee, WI, USA

Hatice B. Zengin, MD Department of Pathology and Laboratory Medicine, University of Rochester Medical Center (URMC), Rochester, NY, USA

Part I
Entities Without or Little Systemic Implications

Autoinflammatory Keratinization Diseases

Takuya Takeichi and Masashi Akiyama

Abbreviation

AiKDs	Autoinflammatory keratinization diseases
ER	Endoplasmic reticulum
GPP	Generalized pustular psoriasis
HS	Hidradenitis suppurativa
KLC	Keratosis lichenoides chronica
KLICK	Keratosis linearis with ichthyosis congenita and sclerosing keratoderma
PRP	Pityriasis rubra pilaris

Introduction

In 2017, we proposed the new umbrella term "autoinflammatory keratinization diseases" (AiKDs) to cover inflammatory keratinization diseases with autoinflammatory mechanisms [1]. We suggested the following definition for AiKDs. (i) The primary and main inflammation sites are the epidermis and the upper dermis. (ii) The inflammation at these sites leads to hyperkeratosis, which is the main and characteristic phenotype of AiKDs. iii) AiKDs have primary genetic causative factors associated with the hyperactivation of innate immunity (autoinflammation), mainly in the epidermis and upper dermis. iv) The concept of AiKDs encompasses diseases with mixed pathomechanisms of autoinflammation and autoimmunity [1]. AiKDs are genetically heterogeneous and their distinct subtypes have variable disease

T. Takeichi · M. Akiyama (✉)
Department of Dermatology, Nagoya University Graduate School of Medicine, Nagoya, Japan
e-mail: takeichi@med.nagoya-u.ac.jp; makiyama@med.nagoya-u.ac.jp

F. Rongioletti, B. R. Smoller (eds.), *New and Emerging Entities in Dermatology and Dermatopathology*, https://doi.org/10.1007/978-3-030-80027-7_1

Table 1 Clinical entities categorized as AiKDs

Disease	Genetic causative factor	Pathogenic inflammatory mechanisms and pathways in keratinocytes
Pustular psoriasis and related disorders	*IL36RN* mutations	IL-36 → MyD88 → NFκB/MAPK →TNF, IL-1, IL-8, IL-17, IL-36, CXCL1, CXCL2, CCL20
Pustular psoriasis and pityriasis rubra pilaris	*CARD14* variants/ mutations	CARD14 → NFκB→IL-36, IL-8, CXCL1, CXCL2, CCL20
Keratosis lichenoides chronica	*NLRP1* mutations	NLRP1 → inflammasome →caspase-1 → IL-1 →TNF, GM-CSF, IL-36
Hidradenitis suppurativa	*NCSTN* mutations *PSENEN* mutations *PSEN1* mutations	γ-Secretase complex↓ →Notch signaling↓ →IL-1β↑?, IL-17↑, IL-18↑
	Variants in *MEFV, NOD2, LPIN2, NLRP3, NLRP12, PSMB8, MVK, IL1RN*	Various inflammatory pathways
Porokeratosis	*MVK* mutations *MVD* mutations *PMVK* mutations *FDPS* mutations	5-Phosphomevalonate↓ →5-Pyrophosphomevalonate↓ →Geranylgeranyl pyrophosphate↓ →Cholesterol↓, small GTPase↓ → IL-1β↑?
Keratosis linearis with ichthyosis congenita and sclerosing keratoderma (KLICK) syndrome	Specific *POMP* mutations (1-bp deletion in the 5′ UTR)	Pomp↓ →Proteasome insufficiency →ER stress↑↑ →UPR activation↑ →Disturbance of terminal differentiation, autoinflammation↑?

associations, complications, and prognoses, although they share the clinical characteristic of hyperkeratotic lesions with inflammation. A number of clinical subtypes/ syndromes involving a multitude of biologic pathways and processes have been categorized as AiKDs (Table 1).

Pustular Psoriasis and Related Disorders

Clinical Features

Pustular psoriasis includes a group of serious inflammatory cutaneous diseases that show recurrent, repeated skin lesions with pustules. Generalized pustular psoriasis (GPP) is typically classified as the most severe of the pustular psoriases, although several reports have proposed that GPP without psoriatic plaque lesions be treated as having a distinct etiology, because it obviously differs from psoriasis vulgaris in terms of clinical, histological, and genetic backgrounds [2]. GPP is a chronic, systemic inflammatory disorder that is accompanied by high fever and general malaise [2]. Clinical cutaneous features are diffuse erythema of the trunk and extremities accompanied by multiple sterile pustules over the entire body (Fig. 1). GPP that occurs with pregnancy as a trigger is termed impetigo herpetiformis. Palmoplantar pustular psoriasis (or palmoplantar pustulosis) is a chronic pustular psoriasis that affects the palms and soles, and acrodermatitis continua of Hallopeau is a chronic form of pustular psoriasis that is restricted to the tips of the fingers and toes.

Histopathologic Features

Hyperkeratosis and neutrophilic microabscesses in the epidermis are seen (Fig. 2). Subcorneal pustules and spongiform pustules of Kogoj are features of pustular psoriasis. Additionally, neutrophilic and lymphocytic infiltration is often noticed in the upper dermis [2].

Differential Diagnosis

For the accurate diagnosis of pustular psoriasis, several inflammatory disorders should be clinically excluded. Diagnoses for differentiating pustular psoriasis include infectious diseases such as acute generalized pustular bacteroid, impetigo (bullous or non-bullous), and multiple sweat gland abscesses in infants arising from

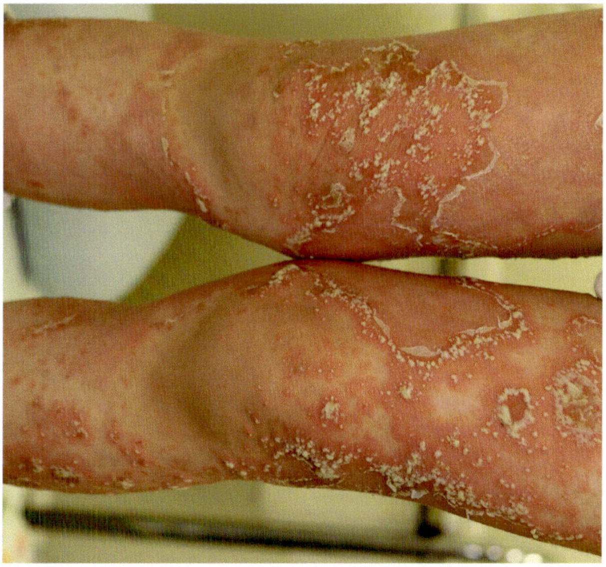

Fig. 1 Generalized pustular psoriasis: a three-year-old male carrying an *IL36RN* mutation shows pustular erythema on the legs

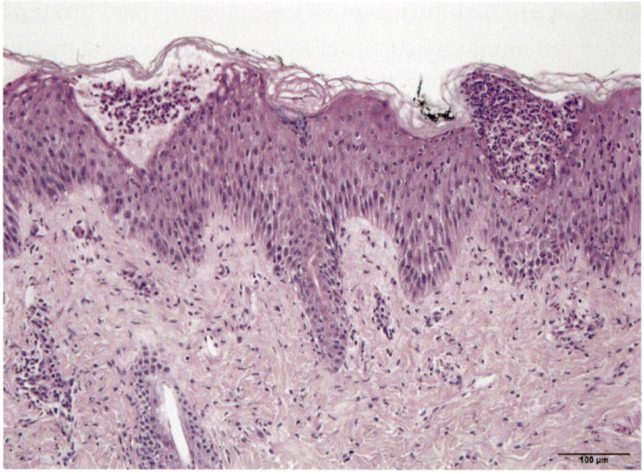

Fig. 2 Generalized pustular psoriasis: a skin biopsy specimen from the pustule shows acanthosis. Neutrophilic infiltration is observed in the upper epidermis. Scale bar = 100 µm

bacterial infections and subcorneal pustular dermatosis [2]. In addition, various types of systemic autoinflammatory diseases have features that overlap with GPP features, although the existence of pustulosis is the specific differential characteristic of pustular psoriasis [3]. Moreover, differential diagnoses from other drug-induced eruptions (e.g., pustular drug eruptions or acute generalized exanthematous pustulosis) are important [4, 5].

Etiopathogenesis

Various reports indicate that the GPP pathogenesis involves a combination of autoinflammation and T-cell-associated mechanisms, although these pathomechanisms might tend to seem unrelated or even contradictory [2]. In 2011, several GPP cases were shown to result from loss-of-function mutations in the *IL36RN* gene, suggesting defects of the IL-36 receptor antagonist [6, 7]. Furthermore, *CARD14* mutations/variants associated with GPP were reported [8–10]. Mutations/variants in *IL36RN*, *CARD14*, and *AP1S3* underlie acrodermatitis continua of Hallopeau and palmoplantar pustular psoriasis, although their frequencies vary depending on the type of pustular psoriasis [11]. NF-κB activation was shown to be boosted by pro-inflammatory genetic variants in the *CARD14* and *AP1S3* genes found in GPP [12].

Therapies

The proper management of medications and of the systemic condition is crucial to GPP therapy, because death can occur, frequently from cardiorespiratory failure [13]. Effective treatments consist of the management of cardiorespiratory failure and of infectious diseases and the discontinuation of aggravating drugs along with the systemic administration of corticosteroids [13]. Various other systemic treatments have been reported as effective: etretinate, cyclosporin, methotrexate or biologics administration, and granulocyte and monocyte adsorption apheresis [2]. The literature has described the efficacy and safety of various biologics (IL-1 receptor antagonist, anti-human TNF-α antibody, antibodies against Th17-IL-12/IL-23 axis cytokines, etc.) for GPP patients [2, 14]. From the viewpoint of considering pustular psoriasis to be an AiKD, new therapies for GPP that use biologics targeting pro-inflammatory pathways, including the IL-36 axis, are in various stages of drug development [2, 15]. However, controlling the disease severity of pustular psoriasis, especially of GPP, remains challenging.

Prognosis and Course

Pustular psoriasis including GPP often relapses over the whole life, and fatal outcomes have been described [2]. Mortality data from the cohort studies of GPP patients are limited, but rates of less than 7% have been reported [15].

Pityriasis Rubra Pilaris

Clinical Features

Pityriasis rubra pilaris (PRP) is an inflammatory keratinization disorder that is characterized by scaly hyperkeratotic follicular inflammatory papules on the extensor surface of the extremities and the trunk (Fig. 3). Of note, additional pityriasis capitis and palmoplantar keratoderma have been seen in PRP individuals [16].

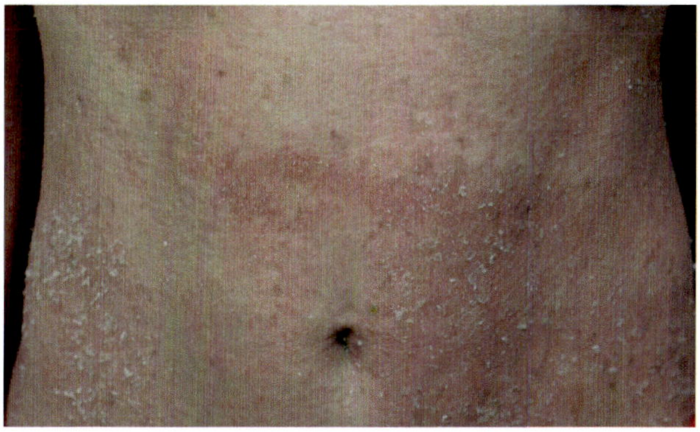

Fig. 3 Pityriasis rubra pilaris: a 20-year-old woman with a *CARD14* mutation shows diffuse scaly erythema on the abdomen

Histopathologic Features

Acanthosis and hyperkeratosis are seen in the epidermis of the lesional skin. A "checkerboard pattern" of alternating orthokeratosis and parakeratosis in the epidermis is a characteristic feature [17]. Perivascular lymphohistiocytic infiltration is seen in the dermis [17].

Differential Diagnosis

Differential diagnoses for PRP include psoriasis vulgaris, contact dermatitis, eczema, and spongiotic dermatitis [17]. For type V PRP, congenital ichthyosiform erythroderma might be potentially included as a differential diagnosis.

Etiopathogenesis

Linkage analysis was used in combination with targeted whole-exome sequencing and candidate-gene screening for four families with PRP to identify autosomal dominant mutations in *CARD14* [18]. If the patient has a gain-of-function mutation in *CARD14*, the mutant CARD14 hyperactivates NF-κB in the keratinocytes of the epidermis [18]. Then, several chemokines are released by the patient's keratinocytes, leading to autoinflammation that results in hyperkeratosis and inflammation in the skin lesions of PRP. Familial and sporadic type V PRP have been reported to be caused by *CARD14* mutations [19]. Rare variants in *CARD14* have also been implicated in the pathophysiology of some cases of other forms of PRP.

Therapies

Systemic retinoids and methotrexate are often effective in patients with definitive PRP, as are TNF-α inhibitors, although such inhibitors have been used only in a limited number of such patients [17]. Ross et al. reported that only 1 in 15 patients (8%) who had been treated with phototherapy found it helpful [17]. Thus, no topical or systemic treatment has been established sufficiently to uniformly improve most of the patients with PRP. Very recently, Craiglow et al. reported that PRP patients with *CARD14* mutations (PRP patients categorized as having an AiKD) may benefit from treatment with ustekinumab, which is a monoclonal antibody to the p40 subunit of interleukins 12 and 23 [20].

Prognosis and Course

Griffiths [16] categorized PRP into the five types of classic adult type (type I), atypical adult type (type II), classic juvenile type (type III), circumscribed juvenile type (type IV), and atypical juvenile type (type V), according to the age at onset, the disease course, and associated underlying conditions. A sixth type was later added: human immunodeficiency virus-associated PRP (type VI) [21]. About half of all patients remit completely within three years [16]. However, PRP type II (atypical adult-onset PRP) has an atypically long duration of often 20 years or more and shows atypical morphological features [16]. Furthermore, PRP type V is a distinct form of PRP which is associated with mutations in *CARD14* [19]. Of note, the cutaneous findings in PRP type V first are noticed in infancy or early childhood and persist throughout life without sustained clearance of the skin.

Keratosis Lichenoides Chronica

Clinical Features

Keratosis lichenoides chronica (KLC), which is extremely rare, is characterized by keratotic papules arranged along parallel lines that are symmetrically distributed on the dorsal aspects of the extremities and on the buttocks [22, 23]. These eruptions have a chronic course and are usually asymptomatic [22]. Pediatric-onset KLC may represent a distinct disease, or it may be a subset of adult-onset KLC with special genetic and clinical characteristics [22]. Pediatric-onset KLC has several characteristic features: familial occurrence; likely autosomal recessive inheritance; congenital or early onset with erythematous purpuric facial macules; alopecia of the forehead, eyebrows, and eyelashes; pruritus; and a low frequency of other cutaneous or systemic abnormalities [22].

Histopathologic Features

Histopathologically, the features include a pattern of lichenoid tissue reaction with marked hyperkeratosis, as well as focal parakeratosis, and predominant acanthosis with areas of atrophy [24]. In addition, there are dense, band-like, mononuclear-cell infiltrates in the upper dermis, with liquefaction degeneration of the basal cells, colloid bodies, and pigmentary incontinence [22].

Differential Diagnosis

The differential diagnosis of KLC includes lichen striatus, linear porokeratosis with a lichenoid tissue reaction, PRP, psoriasis vulgaris, lichenoid drug reaction, keratosis follicularis, and Kyrle's disease [25].

Etiopathogenesis

In 2016, Zhong et al. reported that the overlapping skin disorders of multiple self-healing palmoplantar carcinoma and familial KLC were caused by germline mutations in *NLRP1*, which encodes the inflammasome sensor NLRP1 [26]. In human skin, NLRP1 is the most important inflammasome sensor, and pathogenic *NLRP1* mutations result in gain-of-function alleles that lead to the hyperactivation of inflammasomes [26]. In this context, KLC, at least familial KLC, is considered to be an AiKD-caused autoinflammation due to inflammasome hyperactivation.

Therapies

It is difficult to assess the therapeutic efficacy of treatments based on reports of just several KLC cases. The use of natural, ultraviolet A [27] and ultraviolet B lights, other phototherapies and photochemotherapies, as well as the use of oral retinoids such as acitretin or isotretinoin in conjunction with phototherapy may improve the appearance of the skin [22, 28].

Prognosis and Course

KLC has a course that is chronic and usually progressive, with a mean follow-up of 14 years in adults [24]. Rarely, the spontaneous resolution or remission of KLC occurs [25].

Hidradenitis Suppurativa

Clinical Features

Hidradenitis suppurativa (HS) is a chronic inflammatory disorder of the follicles in which painful, recurrent, deep-seated, inflamed eruptions affect apocrine gland-bearing areas (i.e., the axillary, inguinal, and anogenital regions) (Fig. 4) [29]. The

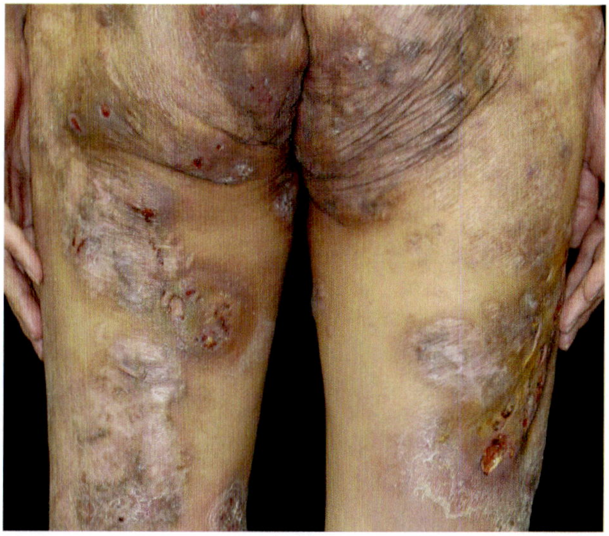

Fig. 4 Hidradenitis suppurativa: a 42-year-old male with an *NCSTN* mutation shows many scars, crusts, comedones, and ulcers on the buttocks and back of the thighs

three diagnostic criteria are the characteristic lesions, a predilection for flexural sites, and the recurrence of the lesions [30, 31].

Histopathologic Features

Skin biopsy may show follicular occlusion due to infundibular hyperkeratosis and hyperplasia of the follicular epithelium. Psoriasiform hyperplasia of the interfollicular epidermis is regarded as the initial event in HS, followed by follicular dilatation and rupture [32, 33]. Immunohistochemical investigations show the perifollicular and subepidermal infiltration of CD3-, CD4-, CD68-, CD79-, and CD8-positive cells [32]. A striking selective epidermotropism has been seen in the interfollicular regions [32].

Differential Diagnosis

Differential diagnoses of HS include staphylococcal infection, cutaneous Crohn's disease, simple abscesses, primary or secondary neoplasm, lymphogranuloma venereum, acne, cat scratch disease, steatocystoma multiplex, cutaneous actinomycosis, and scrofuloderma (cutaneous tuberculosis) [34, 35]. Lesions from staphylococcal infections spread randomly and are more pustular than those of HS. Mostly, cutaneous Crohn's disease is related to intestinal Crohn's disease. Simple abscesses are usually seen as a single lesion. Primary and secondary neoplasms are diagnosed from systemic symptoms and histological examinations. Cutaneous actinomycosis frequently presents with sinus tract disease [34, 35].

Etiopathogenesis

Some cases of HS result from heterozygous mutations in genes encoding γ-secretase subunits (*NCSTN*, *PSENEN*, and *PSEN1*) [36]. The frequency of HS patients with pathogenic variants in these genes is low even in familial HS cases (~5% of overall HS cases) [34, 37]. No significant genotype/phenotype correlation has been described [38]. γ-Secretase plays essential roles in normal immune system functioning and in the maturation of hair follicle cells [31]. In families with these mutations, HS is inherited autosomal dominantly, with incomplete penetrance, and the patients tend to have more severe eruptions than those of patients without any mutations [39]. HS immunopathogenesis is complex and is still being elucidated, but several cytokines (e.g., TNF-α and IL-17) appear to be particularly relevant [31]. The disease severity has been reported to correlate with TNF-α levels in HS lesional skin and with IL-17 serum levels [31].

In addition, variants in the autoinflammation-associated genes *IL1RN, LPIN2, MEFV, MVK, NLRP3, NLRP12, NOD2, PSMB8*, and *PSTPIP1* are related to HS [40]. The variants are thought to bring about autoinflammation resulting in follicular hyperkeratosis in the pathogenesis of HS. The fact that several biologics, including adalimumab, are effective against HS suggests that HS should be included in AiKDs.

Therapies

Anti-inflammatories, surgery, and antibiotics are established treatments for HS. Based on the concept of HS as an AiKD, biologics against cytokines in the autoinflammatory pathways are promising treatments. TNF-α inhibitors are safe, effective treatments for HS [41]. Several clinical trials for novel biologics targeting various cytokines are ongoing [42]. Surgery is still beneficial treatment for HS, and wide excision is the only known curative procedure [42]. To reduce inflammation and to treat secondary infection, antibiotics are useful [42]. Systemic retinoids, weight loss, and smoking cessation counseling also should be considered as other therapeutic options.

Prognosis and Course

HS most frequently occurs in young adults and tends to recur over time. HS significantly decreases the patient's quality of life [31]. In a cross-sectional study on HS, 39.4% of patients reported remission [43]. Worse prognoses and poorer treatment outcomes were reported for smokers [42, 43]. Notably, squamous cell carcinoma occasionally occurs in chronic HS lesions [44]. Squamous cell carcinoma in association with HS has a prevalence of approximately 4.6% [44].

Porokeratosis

Clinical Features

Porokeratosis is a keratinization disorder that is traditionally classified into five main subgroups based on the clinical appearance: porokeratosis of Mibelli, disseminated superficial actinic porokeratosis, disseminated superficial porokeratosis (Fig. 5), porokeratosis plantaris palmaris et disseminata, and linear porokeratosis [45, 46]. Porokeratosis is a cutaneous autoinflammatory disease that is often inherited and is linked to immunosuppression and ultraviolet light exposure [47].

Histopathologic Features

A cornoid lamella, which is a vertical "column" of parakeratosis, is a histological hallmark, and the lamellar pattern relates to acanthosis and dermal inflammation [48]. However, a cornoid lamella is not a unique feature of porokeratosis because it

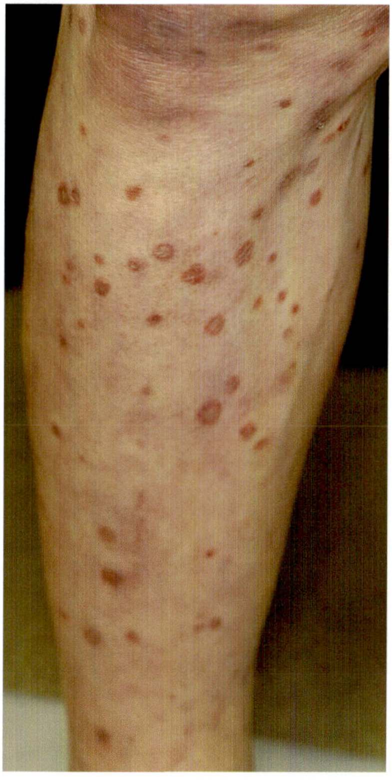

Fig. 5 Porokeratosis: a 78-year-old man harboring an *MVD* mutation presents small round plaques with well-defined boundaries on the right lower leg

can be seen in certain inflammatory and inherited cutaneous disorders and as an incidental finding [49].

Differential Diagnosis

The differential diagnosis of porokeratosis includes allergic contact dermatitis, Bowen disease, candidiasis, hypertrophic lichen planus, irritant dermatitis, lichen simplex chronicus, psoriasis, and cutaneous tuberculosis [50].

Etiopathogenesis

Germline mutations in the mevalonate pathway (*MVK*, *MVD*, *PMVK*, and *FDPS*) or in *SLC17A9* encoding solute carrier family 17 member 9 are able to cause porokeratosis [51, 52]. Recently, second-hit somatic mutations were identified in disseminated superficial actinic porokeratosis and linear porokeratosis [46, 53]. In isoprenoid biosynthesis, the mevalonate pathway provides precursors of terpenoids, also known as isoprenoids, which are ubiquitous in plants and animals and have diverse biological functions, such as serving as precursors of cholesterol, heme A, ubiquinones, dolichol, and isoprenylated proteins [47]. The above suggests that the individual eruptions of various porokeratosis variants arise in regions that are affected by second-hit mutations in genes encoding key components of the mevalonate pathway [54]. Moreover, the isoprenylated proteins regulate cell growth, division, and differentiation, and they are probably associated with nuclear retention in the stratum corneum [47]. Aberrant activation of the small GTPase Rac1 and inflammasome activation are preceded by shortages of geranylgeranyl pyrophosphate, which is a non-sterol terpenoid product of the mevalonate pathway [55]. Therefore, defective mevalonate metabolism might lead to both autoinflammation and hyperkeratosis in porokeratosis [48].

Therapies

Treatments for porokeratosis primarily focus on the destruction of the lesions by cryotherapy, photodynamic therapy, carbon dioxide laser treatments, topical 5-fluorouracil ointments, or a combination of these [56]. The administration of acitretin, topical corticosteroids, and vitamin D analogs are other conventional strategies for reducing the scaling and inflammation that are associated with the lesions [56]. Very recently, topical cholesterol/lovastatin was reported to be effective as a treatment for porokeratosis [54].

Prognosis and Course

Porokeratotic lesions, especially those that are large and linear, may be associated with malignant transformation, with a transformation incidence of 7.5–11% in patients with these lesions [51, 54]. Patients should receive regular checkups and be advised to use sun protection and to avoid excessive sunlight [57]. Upon suspicion of malignancy changes, the lesions should be biopsied [57].

KLICK Syndrome

Clinical Features

Pujol RM et al. reported four individuals with ichthyosis in a consanguineous family in 1989 [58]. The four patients shared six features: (i) generalized ichthyosiform dermatosis, (ii) diffuse palmoplantar keratoderma with sclerosis, deformities, pseudoainhum, and functional impairment, (iii) multiple keratotic papules arranged in a symmetrical cordlike line involving the flexures and showing peculiar acrosyringeal keratoses, (iv) possible autosomal recessive inheritance, (v) inconsistent dental abnormalities, and (vi) no systemic involvement (e.g., neurologic or ophthalmologic) [58]. Later, the term KLICK (keratosis linearis with ichthyosis congenita and sclerosing keratoderma) was proposed by Vahlquist et al. to describe this disease [59].

Histopathologic Features

Histologically, the thickening of the spinous, granular, and horny layers in the epidermis is observed [58–60]. Additionally, in the upper dermis, mild, sparse lymphohistiocytic infiltration is seen [58, 59].

Differential Diagnosis

The skin manifestations of KLICK syndrome resemble those of erythrokeratoderma or loricrin keratoderma, in which there is also hyperkeratosis and occasionally inflammatory infiltration in the dermis [60].

Etiopathogenesis

A single-nucleotide deletion in the 5′UTR (c.-95delC) of *POMP* was identified in 12 patients with KLICK syndrome [61]. The c.-95delC deletion in KLICK patients causes a negative switch in transcription start sites for *POMP*, which is predicted to decrease the protein expression levels of proteasome maturation protein (POMP) in terminally differentiated keratinocytes [61]. POMP is a ubiquitously expressed protein that functions as a chaperone for proteasome maturation [61]. KLICK syndrome is caused by a decrease in POMP levels that leads to proteasome insufficiency in differentiating keratinocytes. Proteasome inhibition is known to cause elevated endoplasmic reticulum (ER) stress [62]. The increased expression of two ER stress markers (BiP and/or CHOP) has been shown in KLICK patients, and prolonged ER stress has been reported to induce inflammation and to be responsible for many chronic inflammatory disorders [63, 64]. In addition, inflammation in many chronic inflammatory skin diseases is caused by prolonged ER stress [65]. The chronic ER stress present in the epidermis of patients with KLICK syndrome might eventually trigger autoinflammation [64].

Therapies

Remarkable improvements of the skin eruptions with oral etretinate treatments have been reported in some patients with KLICK syndrome [60, 66, 67].

Prognosis and Course

KLICK syndrome due to *POMP* mutations usually persists throughout life. The symptoms of KLICK syndrome are limited to the skin and its appendages; thus, the patient's vital prognosis is good.

Conclusions

Recent genetic and clinical investigations have revealed that multiple inflammatory keratinization diseases including pustular psoriasis and related disorders, pityriasis rubra pilaris, keratosis lichenoides chronica, hidradenitis suppurativa, porokeratosis, and KLICK syndrome are AiKDs. The pathogenesis of each AiKD has been intensively studied. Chronic and recurrent itching, desquamation, fissures, pustules, scars, and occasional systemic symptoms from continuous cutaneous inflammation are known to significantly affect quality of life in patients with AiKDs. The establishment of safe, effective therapies is hoped for in patients with AiKDs, based on an advanced understanding of the molecular pathogeneses of these diseases.

References

1. Akiyama M, Takeichi T, McGrath JA, Sugiura K. Autoinflammatory keratinization diseases. J Allergy Clin Immunol. 2017;140(6):1545–7.
2. Takeichi T, Akiyama M. Generalized pustular psoriasis: clinical management and update on autoinflammatory aspects. Am J Clin Dermatol. 2020;21(2):227–36.
3. Tripathi SV, Leslie KS. Autoinflammatory diseases in dermatology: CAPS, TRAPS, HIDS, FMF, Blau, CANDLE. Dermatol Clin. 2013;31(3):387–404.
4. Kardaun SH, Kuiper H, Fidler V, Jonkman MF. The histopathological spectrum of acute generalized exanthematous pustulosis (AGEP) and its differentiation from generalized pustular psoriasis. J Cutan Pathol. 2010;37(12):1220–9.
5. Navarini AA, Simpson MA, Borradori L, Yawalkar N, Schlapbach C. Homozygous missense mutation in IL36RN in generalized pustular dermatosis with intraoral involvement compatible with both AGEP and generalized pustular psoriasis. JAMA Dermatol. 2015;151(4):452–3.
6. Marrakchi S, Guigue P, Renshaw BR, Puel A, Pei XY, Fraitag S, et al. Interleukin-36-receptor antagonist deficiency and generalized pustular psoriasis. N Engl J Med. 2011;365(7):620–8.
7. Onoufriadis A, Simpson MA, Pink AE, Di Meglio P, Smith CH, Pullabhatla V, et al. Mutations in IL36RN/IL1F5 are associated with the severe episodic inflammatory skin disease known as generalized pustular psoriasis. Am J Hum Genet. 2011;89(3):432–7.
8. Sugiura K, Muto M, Akiyama M. CARD14 c.526G>C (p.Asp176His) is a significant risk factor for generalized pustular psoriasis with psoriasis vulgaris in the Japanese cohort. J Invest Dermatol. 2014;134(6):1755–7.
9. Berki DM, Liu L, Choon SE, David Burden A, Griffiths CEM, Navarini AA, et al. Activating CARD14 mutations are associated with generalized pustular psoriasis but rarely account for familial recurrence in psoriasis vulgaris. J Invest Dermatol. 2015;135(12):2964–70.
10. Takeichi T, Kobayashi A, Ogawa E, Okuno Y, Kataoka S, Kono M, et al. Autosomal dominant familial generalized pustular psoriasis caused by a CARD14 mutation. Br J Dermatol. 2017;177(4):e133–e5.
11. Twelves S, Mostafa A, Dand N, Burri E, Farkas K, Wilson R, et al. Clinical and genetic differences between pustular psoriasis subtypes. J Allergy Clin Immunol. 2019;143(3):1021–6.
12. Setta-Kaffetzi N, Simpson MA, Navarini AA, Patel VM, Lu HC, Allen MH, et al. AP1S3 mutations are associated with pustular psoriasis and impaired Toll-like receptor 3 trafficking. Am J Hum Genet. 2014;94(5):790–7.
13. Fujita H, Terui T, Hayama K, Akiyama M, Ikeda S, Mabuchi T, et al. Japanese guidelines for the management and treatment of generalized pustular psoriasis: the new pathogenesis and treatment of GPP. J Dermatol. 2018;45(11):1235–70.
14. Akiyama M, Takeichi T, McGrath JA, Sugiura K. Autoinflammatory keratinization diseases: an emerging concept encompassing various inflammatory keratinization disorders of the skin. J Dermatol Sci. 2018;90(2):105–11.
15. Gooderham MJ, Van Voorhees AS, Lebwohl MG. An update on generalized pustular psoriasis. Expert Rev Clin Immunol. 2019;15(9):907–19.
16. Griffiths WA. Pityriasis rubra pilaris. Clin Exp Dermatol. 1980;5(1):105–12.
17. Ross NA, Chung HJ, Li Q, Andrews JP, Keller MS, Uitto J. Epidemiologic, clinicopathologic, diagnostic, and management challenges of Pityriasis Rubra Pilaris: a case series of 100 patients. JAMA Dermatol. 2016;152(6):670–5.
18. Fuchs-Telem D, Sarig O, van Steensel MA, Isakov O, Israeli S, Nousbeck J, et al. Familial pityriasis rubra pilaris is caused by mutations in CARD14. Am J Hum Genet. 2012;91(1):163–70.
19. Takeichi T, Sugiura K, Nomura T, Sakamoto T, Ogawa Y, Oiso N, et al. Pityriasis Rubra Pilaris Type V as an autoinflammatory disease by CARD14 mutations. JAMA Dermatol. 2017;153(1):66–70.

20. Craiglow BG, Boyden LM, Hu R, Virtanen M, Su J, Rodriguez G, et al. CARD14-associated papulosquamous eruption: a spectrum including features of psoriasis and pityriasis rubra pilaris. J Am Acad Dermatol. 2018;79(3):487–94.
21. Misery I, Faure M, Claidy A. Pityriasis rubra pilaris and human immunodeficiency virus infection--type 6 pityriasis rubra pilaris? Br J Dermatol. 1996;135(6):1008–9.
22. Ruiz-Maldonado R, Duran-McKinster C, Orozco-Covarrubias L, Saez-de-Ocariz M, Palacios-Lopez C. Keratosis lichenoides chronica in pediatric patients: a different disease? J Am Acad Dermatol. 2007;56(2 Suppl):S1–5.
23. Margolis MH, Cooper GA, Johnson SA. Keratosis lichenoides chronica. Arch Dermatol. 1972;105(5):739–43.
24. Masouye I, Saurat JH. Keratosis lichenoides chronica: the centenary of another Kaposi's disease. Dermatology. 1995;191(3):188–92.
25. Grammatikopoulou E, Wilson BB, Cordoro K, Patterson JW. Keratosis lichenoides chronica: a case report. Cutis. 2010;86(5):245–8.
26. Zhong FL, Mamai O, Sborgi L, Boussofara L, Hopkins R, Robinson K, et al. Germline NLRP1 mutations cause skin inflammatory and cancer susceptibility syndromes via inflammasome activation. Cell. 2016;167(1):187–202. e17
27. Lang PG Jr. Keratosis lichenoides chronica. Successful treatment with psoralen-ultraviolet-A therapy. Arch Dermatol. 1981;117(2):105–8.
28. Redondo P, Solano T. Keratosis lichenoides chronica in childhood. Clin Exp Dermatol. 2002;27(4):283–5.
29. Shavit E, Alavi A, Bechara FG, Bennett RG, Bourcier M, Cibotti R, et al. Proceeding report of the second symposium on hidradenitis suppurativa advances (SHSA) 2017. Exp Dermatol. 2019;28(1):94–103.
30. Vekic DA, Frew J, Cains GD. Hidradenitis suppurativa, a review of pathogenesis, associations and management. Part 1. Australas J Dermatol. 2018;59(4):267–77.
31. Goldburg SR, Strober BE, Payette MJ. Hidradenitis suppurativa: epidemiology, clinical presentation, and pathogenesis. J Am Acad Dermatol. 2020;82(5):1045–58.
32. von Laffert M, Helmbold P, Wohlrab J, Fiedler E, Stadie V, Marsch WC. Hidradenitis suppurativa (acne inversa): early inflammatory events at terminal follicles and at interfollicular epidermis. Exp Dermatol. 2010;19(6):533–7.
33. von Laffert M, Stadie V, Wohlrab J, Marsch WC. Hidradenitis suppurativa/acne inversa: bilocated epithelial hyperplasia with very different sequelae. Br J Dermatol. 2011;164(2):367–71.
34. Zouboulis CC, Desai N, Emtestam L, Hunger RE, Ioannides D, Juhasz I, et al. European S1 guideline for the treatment of hidradenitis suppurativa/acne inversa. J Eur Acad Dermatol Venereol. 2015;29(4):619–44.
35. Saunte DML, Jemec GBE. Hidradenitis suppurativa: advances in diagnosis and treatment. JAMA. 2017;318(20):2019–32.
36. Wang B, Yang W, Wen W, Sun J, Su B, Liu B, et al. Gamma-secretase gene mutations in familial acne inversa. Science. 2010;330(6007):1065.
37. Nomura T. Hidradenitis suppurativa as a potential subtype of autoinflammatory keratinization disease. Front Immunol. 2020;11:847.
38. Frew JW, Hawkes JE, Sullivan-Whalen M, Gilleaudeau P, Krueger JG. Inter-rater reliability of phenotypes and exploratory genotype-phenotype analysis in inherited hidradenitis suppurativa. Br J Dermatol. 2019;181(3):566–71.
39. Pink AE, Simpson MA, Desai N, Dafou D, Hills A, Mortimer P, et al. Mutations in the gamma-secretase genes NCSTN, PSENEN, and PSEN1 underlie rare forms of hidradenitis suppurativa (acne inversa). J Invest Dermatol. 2012;132(10):2459–61.
40. Vural S, Gundogdu M, Gokpinar Ili E, Durmaz CD, Vural A, Steinmuller-Magin L, et al. Association of pyrin mutations and autoinflammation with complex phenotype hidradenitis suppurativa: a case-control study. Br J Dermatol. 2019;180(6):1459–67.
41. Kimball AB, Okun MM, Williams DA, Gottlieb AB, Papp KA, Zouboulis CC, et al. Two phase 3 trials of adalimumab for hidradenitis suppurativa. N Engl J Med. 2016;375(5):422–34.

42. Goldburg SR, Strober BE, Payette MJ. Hidradenitis suppurativa: current and emerging treatments. J Am Acad Dermatol. 2020;82(5):1061–82.
43. Kromann CB, Deckers IE, Esmann S, Boer J, Prens EP, Jemec GB. Risk factors, clinical course and long-term prognosis in hidradenitis suppurativa: a cross-sectional study. Br J Dermatol. 2014;171(4):819–24.
44. Chapman S, Delgadillo D III, Barber C, Khachemoune A. Cutaneous squamous cell carcinoma complicating hidradenitis suppurativa: a review of the prevalence, pathogenesis, and treatment of this dreaded complication. Acta Dermatovenerol Alp Pannonica Adriat. 2018;27(1):25–8.
45. Chernosky ME. Porokeratosis. Arch Dermatol. 1986;122(8):869–70.
46. Atzmony L, Khan HM, Lim YH, Paller AS, Levinsohn JL, Holland KE, et al. Second-hit, postzygotic PMVK and MVD mutations in linear porokeratosis. JAMA Dermatol. 2019;155(5):548–55.
47. Zhang Z, Li C, Wu F, Ma R, Luan J, Yang F, et al. Correction: genomic variations of the mevalonate pathway in porokeratosis. elife. 2016;5:e14383.
48. Takeichi T, Akiyama M. Familial or sporadic porokeratosis as an autoinflammatory keratinization disease. J Dermatol. 2019;46(4):e125–e6.
49. Biswas A. Cornoid lamellation revisited: apropos of porokeratosis with emphasis on unusual clinicopathological variants. Am J Dermatopathol. 2015;37(2):145–55.
50. Joshi R, Minni K. Genitogluteal porokeratosis: a clinical review. Clin Cosmet Investig Dermatol. 2018;11:219–29.
51. Zhang SQ, Jiang T, Li M, Zhang X, Ren YQ, Wei SC, et al. Exome sequencing identifies MVK mutations in disseminated superficial actinic porokeratosis. Nat Genet. 2012;44(10):1156–60.
52. Cui H, Li L, Wang W, Shen J, Yue Z, Zheng X, et al. Exome sequencing identifies SLC17A9 pathogenic gene in two Chinese pedigrees with disseminated superficial actinic porokeratosis. J Med Genet. 2014;51(10):699–704.
53. Kubo A, Sasaki T, Suzuki H, Shiohama A, Aoki S, Sato S, et al. Clonal expansion of second-hit cells with somatic recombinations or C>T transitions form porokeratosis in MVD or MVK mutant heterozygotes. J Invest Dermatol. 2019;139(12):2458–66 e9.
54. Atzmony L, Lim YH, Hamilton C, Leventhal JS, Wagner A, Paller AS, et al. Topical cholesterol/lovastatin for the treatment of porokeratosis: a pathogenesis-directed therapy. J Am Acad Dermatol. 2020;82(1):123–31.
55. van der Burgh R, Ter Haar NM, Boes ML, Frenkel J. Mevalonate kinase deficiency, a metabolic autoinflammatory disease. Clin Immunol. 2013;147(3):197–206.
56. Weidner T, Illing T, Miguel D, Elsner P. Treatment of porokeratosis: a systematic review. Am J Clin Dermatol. 2017;18(4):435–49.
57. Schierbeck J, Vestergaard T, Bygum A. Skin cancer associated genodermatoses: a literature review. Acta Derm Venereol. 2019;99(4):360–9.
58. Pujol RM, Moreno A, Alomar A, de Moragas JM. Congenital ichthyosiform dermatosis with linear keratotic flexural papules and sclerosing palmoplantar keratoderma. Arch Dermatol. 1989;125(1):103–6.
59. Vahlquist A, Ponten F, Pettersson A. Keratosis linearis with ichthyosis congenita and sclerosing keratoderma (KLICK-syndrome): a rare, autosomal recessive disorder of keratohyaline formation? Acta Derm Venereol. 1997;77(3):225–7.
60. Onnis G, Bourrat E, Jonca N, Dreyfus I, Severino-Freire M, Pichery M, et al. KLICK syndrome: an unusual phenotype. Br J Dermatol. 2018;178(6):1445–6.
61. Dahlqvist J, Klar J, Tiwari N, Schuster J, Torma H, Badhai J, et al. A single-nucleotide deletion in the POMP 5' UTR causes a transcriptional switch and altered epidermal proteasome distribution in KLICK genodermatosis. Am J Hum Genet. 2010;86(4):596–603.
62. Ding WX, Yin XM. Sorting, recognition and activation of the misfolded protein degradation pathways through macroautophagy and the proteasome. Autophagy. 2008;4(2):141–50.
63. Dahlqvist J, Torma H, Badhai J, Dahl N. siRNA silencing of proteasome maturation protein (POMP) activates the unfolded protein response and constitutes a model for KLICK genodermatosis. PLoS One. 2012;7(1):e29471.

64. Poli MC, Ebstein F, Nicholas SK, de Guzman MM, Forbes LR, Chinn IK, et al. Heterozygous truncating variants in POMP escape nonsense-mediated decay and cause a unique immune dysregulatory syndrome. Am J Hum Genet. 2018;102(6):1126–42.
65. Park K, Lee SE, Shin KO, Uchida Y. Insights into the role of endoplasmic reticulum stress in skin function and associated diseases. FEBS J. 2019;286(2):413–25.
66. Morice-Picard F, Jonca N, Pichery M, Mermin D, Leaute-Labreze C, Taieb A, et al. KLICK syndrome: recognizable phenotype and hot-spot POMP mutation. J Eur Acad Dermatol Venereol. 2017;31(3):e154–e6.
67. Pujol RM, Alomar A, De Moragas JM. A new type of erythrokeratoderma, or KLICK syndrome? Br J Dermatol. 2005;153(2):461; author reply 2.

Adult Mucinoses: New and Revisited Variants

Franco Rongioletti, Laura Atzori, and Caterina Ferreli

Introduction

The cutaneous mucinoses are a heterogeneous group of disorders in which an abnormal amount of mucin (acid glycosaminoglycans) accumulates in the skin, especially in the dermis (dermal mucinoses) and also in the follicles (follicular mucinoses) [1]. The cutaneous mucinoses may be classified as primary in which the mucin deposit is the main histologic finding resulting in clinically distinctive lesions and secondary mucinoses in which histologic mucin deposition is only an additional finding (Table 1). The former is associated with systemic disorders such as monoclonal gammopathies, autoimmune diseases, diabetes mellitus, or altered thyroid function. In the last years, several new presentations of cutaneous mucinoses in adults have been described. They include (a) obesity-associated lymphedematous mucinosis and pretibial stasis mucinosis, (b) cutaneous mucinosis associated with drug exposure including biologic therapy, anti-colony-stimulating factor 1 receptor (CSF1R) and subcutaneous intralesional interferons, (c) cutaneous mucinosis after physical and mechanical traumas, (d) cutaneous mucinosis after knee replacement, and (e) nodular mucinosis of the breast.

F. Rongioletti
Dermatology Clinic, Department of Medical Sciences and Public Health, University of Cagliari, Cagliari, Italy

Vita-Salute S.Raffaele University, Milan, Italy
e-mail: rongioletti@unica.it

L. Atzori (✉) · C. Ferreli
Dermatology Clinic, Department of Medical Sciences and Public Health, University of Cagliari, Cagliari, Italy
e-mail: atzoril@unica.it; ferreli@unica.it

F. Rongioletti, B. R. Smoller (eds.), *New and Emerging Entities in Dermatology and Dermatopathology*, https://doi.org/10.1007/978-3-030-80027-7_2

Table 1 Classification of the cutaneous mucinoses

Primary mucinosies: mucin deposition is pathognomonic of the disease		
Dermal	**Follicular**	**Hamartomatous neoplastic**
Scleromyxedema or generalized and sclerodermoid lichen myxedematosus Localized lichen myxedematosus (syn. Papular mucinosis) • Discrete papular form • Acral persistent papular mucinosis • Cutaneous mucinosis of infancy • Nodular form Self-healing cutaneous mucinosis • Juvenile type • Adult type Scleredema Mucinoses associated with altered thyroid function • Pretibial myxedema • Generalized myxedema Reticular erythematous mucinosis Papulonodular mucinosis associated with autoimmune connective tissue diseases Cutaneous focal mucinosis Digital mucous (myxoid) cyst Miscellaneous mucinoses	Follicular mucinosis (Pinkus) Urticaria-like follicular mucinosis	Mucinous nevus (Angio)myxoma Nodular mucinosis of the breast
Secondary mucinosies: mucin deposition is an epiphenomenon of the disease		
Dermal	**Follicular**	**Epithelial**
Granuloma annulare Lupus erythematosus Dermatomyositis Systemic sclerosis Degos disease Hypertrophic scars Chronic graft-versus-host disease Hereditary progressive mucinous histiocytosis Drug-induced mucinosis Obesity-associated mucinosis and pretibial stasis mucinosis Cutaneous mucinosis after physical and mechanical traumas Cutaneous mucinosis after knee replacement	Lymphoma Pseudolymphoma Leukemic skin infiltrates Spongiotic dermatitis Lupus erythematosus Insect bites	Mycosis fungoides Spongiotic dermatitis Basal cell carcinomas Keratoacanthomas Squamous cell carcinomas Vulgar warts

Obesity-Associated Cutaneous Mucinosis and Pretibial Stasis Mucinosis

In 1993 Somach et al. described pretibial mucin deposition in euthyroid patients with associated features of stasis dermatitis [2]. Additional cases of euthyroid pretibial mucinosis have been since found with chronic venous insufficiency, lymphedema, and trauma [3]. These reports suggest that pretibial mucinosis may occur not only in patients with hyperthyroidism but also in patients with typical findings of leg stasis. Subsequently, increased mucin deposition has been described in obese patients with lymphedema of the legs, being called "obesity-associated lymphedematous mucinosis" (OALM) [4].

Clinical Features

The clinical manifestations of OALM are characterized by asymptomatic, skin-colored to erythematous-yellowish semi-translucent papules and nodules progressing to plaques and arising on the legs being associated with erythema, edema, and lymphostasis on the pretibial areas in a bilateral way (Fig. 1a). The thighs are rarely involved as well as the foot or ankles [4]. Occasionally, when lymphedema is marked, vesicles may appear. Stasis mucinosis may present with blue-violet, smooth, pebbly and partially blanchable nodules and plaques, sometimes painful. In addition, there may be overlying telangiectasias on the pretibial area associated with signs of chronic venous insufficiency [5].

Histopathology

OALM is characterized by basket wave hyperkeratosis, thinning of the epidermis with flattening of the rete ridges, and mucin deposits in the superficial dermis and around the blood vessels (Fig. 1b). A characteristic clue is dermal angioplasia with vertically running vessels in the edematous superficial and mid-dermis. Colloidal iron or Alcian blue at pH 2.5 enhances the visibility of mucin (Fig. 1c). In the reticular dermis, there is also a variable fibrosis with increased, activated fibroblasts [3]. Occasionally, edema of the papillary dermis can lead to the formation of subepidermal blisters. D2–40 staining can highlight lymphatic dilation. In venous-insufficiency-associated dermal mucinosis, mucin deposition is located in the superficial portion of the dermis, as in OALM; however, the deposit distinctively surrounds the eccrine glands and the pilosebaceous follicles [5]. It may be associated with a small increase in small blood vessel density, slightly thickened vessel walls, and no inflammatory infiltrate. Both conditions may have deposits of hemosiderin in the papillary dermis [4, 5].

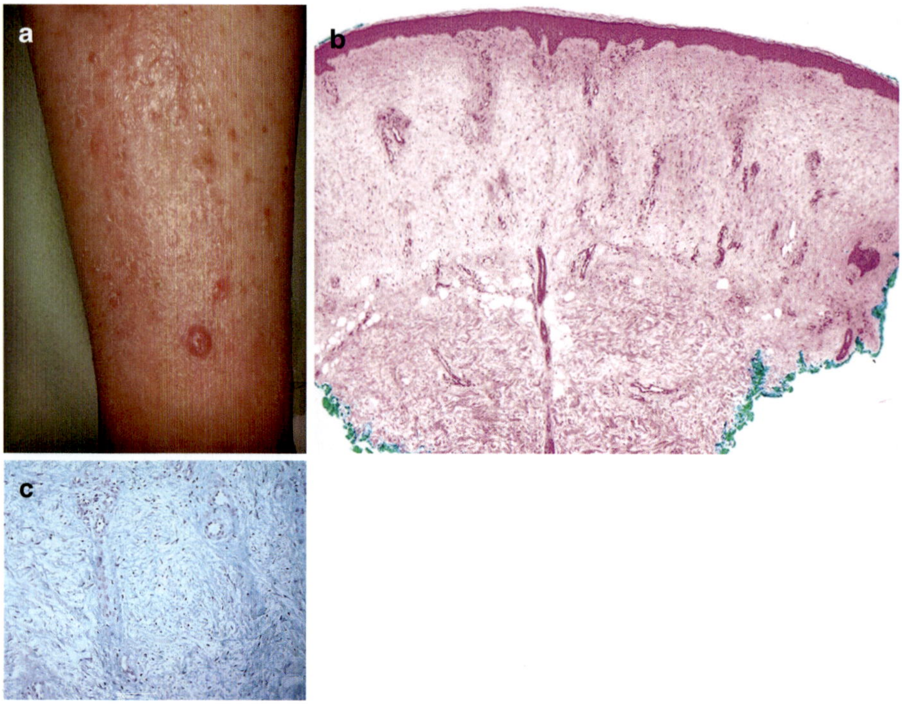

Fig. 1 (**a**) Obesity-associated lymphedematous mucinosis. Skin-colored to erythematous-yellowish semi-translucent papules arising in an erythematous edematous lymphostatic skin of the pretibial area. (**b**) Obesity-associated lymphedematous mucinosis. Histopathology of a papule showing hyperkeratosis, flattening of the rete ridges, dermal angioplasia with vertically running vessels, and edematous mucinosis in the superficial and mid-dermis. (**c**) Obesity-associated lymphedematous mucinosis. Mucin deposition with increased fibroblasts highlighted by Alcian blue stain at pH 2.5

Workup

When mucin is found on the shins, thyroid function should be tested. Duplex ultrasonography is the study of choice for the evaluation of venous insufficiency syndromes.

Differential Diagnosis

The main differential diagnosis of stasis mucinosis and OALM is pretibial myxedema that represents a manifestation of hyperthyroidism, in particular of Graves' disease. In addition to the shins, pretibial myxedema may spread to the ankle and dorsum of the foot and rarely involves the elbows, knees, back, or neck [1].

Histologically, in pretibial myxedema, there are hyperorthokeratosis, acanthosis, follicular hyperkeratosis, abundant mucin deposition throughout all the reticular dermis, and sometimes the subcutaneous tissue with an occasional presence of mast cells [4]. Although the terms pretibial myxedema and pretibial mucinosis have been used as synonyms, pretibial myxedema should be reserved only for patients with associated thyroid disease.

Pathogenesis

Although pathogenesis is unclear, in OALM the lymphatic stasis due to obesity causes a local hypoxia with subsequent increased production of mucin from fibroblasts in response to reduced oxygen tension [4]. The interstitial deposition of plasmatic proteins, such as fibrinogen, albumin, and coagulation factors, due to a defect of the lymphatic drainage and the associated venous insufficiency worsens edema, decreasing local oxygen delivery and stimulating fibroblasts to further synthesize and deposit glycosaminoglycans [5].

Prognosis and Treatment

OALM has a benign course causing mainly a cosmetic disfigurement. Strong dietary restriction for weight reduction is the mainstay of management [4]. Pressure bandages with gradual compression have been recommended for improving lymphostasis and venous insufficiency [4]. When vascular insufficiency is severe, a surgical procedure can be considered [5, 6] While topical corticosteroids under occlusion and compression therapy are the mainstay of treatment in true pretibial myxedema, these measures are not helpful in OLAM without the benefit of weight reduction.

Cutaneous Mucinoses Associated with Drug Exposure (Toxic Dermal Mucinoses)

In 1989, eosinophilia-myalgia syndrome after taking medicines containing tryptophan for depression or sleep disorders was reported in the United States [7]. This syndrome resembled toxic oil syndrome, described in Spain in 1981, due to the ingestion of rapeseed oil intended for industrial use that had been denatured and subsequently sold fraudulently as olive oil. In the acute phase, a toxic dermal mucinosis consisting of a generalized eruption of flesh-colored papules was associated with both syndromes. Finally, a characteristic sclerodermatous condition may develop. The lesions tended to improve and slowly regress after L-tryptophan was discontinued. Recently, the development of cutaneous mucinosis has been related to the therapy with biologics (i.e., anti TNF-alpha drugs and anti IL12/23) [8–11] or to a new class of immune-modulatory drugs, anti-colony-stimulating factor 1 receptor (CSF1R), that have been investigated in clinical trials in different malignant neoplasms [12]. Mucinous skin lesions were also triggered by subcutaneous injections of interferons [13–15].

Clinical Findings and Histopathology

Table 2 includes the main characteristics of reported cases.

Workup

Laboratory studies were normal including thyroid function and immunoelectrophoresis.

Pathogenesis

TNF-alpha inhibitors may indirectly activate fibroblastic mucin production by blocking active TNF-alpha. In fact, this block allows skin dendritic cells to produce elevated amounts of IFN-α, which likely activates lymphocytes, thereby stimulating fibroblasts to produce mucin. Another theory is that there is less of an inhibitory effect of TNF on dermal dendrocytes, which could be a source of the abundant hyaluronic acid production. As for ustekinumab, this biologic drug decreasing IL-23 and consequently T-helper 17 cell-induced TNF-a levels could also stimulate mucin production by fibroblasts through a paradoxical increase of IFN- α.

As for local reaction triggered by type I IFNs, these cytokines can increase the inflammatory potential of dermal fibroblasts stimulating the production of mucin [16]. A reduced degradation of the components of extracellular matrix by macrophages secondary to CSF1 pathway inhibition has been suggested.

Differential Diagnosis

Clinical-pathologic correlation is mandatory. Cutaneous mucinosis at the inoculation site of interferon should be differentiated from similar lesions presenting with a microscopic lupus erythematosus-like pattern. The latter, in addition to dermal mucin deposits, shows a dense superficial and deep periadnexal and perivascular lymphocytic infiltrate with hydropic degeneration of the basal layer [17]. The

Table 2 Main characteristics of cases of cutaneous mucinosis induced by drugs (toxic dermal mucinoses)

Authors	Age/sex	Clinical presentation	Histopathology	Diagnosis	Triggering drug	Time from start of treatment to onset of lesions	Course
Benito-León et al. [13]	36 F	Erythematous lesions with telangiectasias at injection sites on thighs and buttocks	Dermal mucin with inflammatory infiltrate	"Cutaneous mucinosis"	Subcutaneous interferon beta-1b for multiple sclerosis	Within first month of treatment	Spontaneous healing. Long persistence between 6 and 9 months
Siewert et al. [14]	59 M	Painful erythematous thickened skin with ulceration	Dermal mucin	"Cutaneous mucinosis"	Subcutaneous injection of interferon alfa-1 for HCV	After 10 weeks	Healing with scarring after 3–6 months
Wells et al. [15]	46 F	Reticulate erythema with ulceration	Prominent interstitial mucinosis, superficial thrombosed vessels with focal epidermal necrosis	"Mucinosis"	Subcutaneous interferon beta-1 injection for multiple sclerosis	Few injections	Slow healing with low-molecular-weight heparin
Duparc et al. [9]	44 M	Papulonodules on scalp, forearms	Polypoid lesion with dermal accumulation of mucin. Elastic tissue absent	Multiple focal mucinosis	Anti-TNF-α (etanercept, infliximab) for plaque psoriasis	Not well defined, starting after etanercept and relapsing after infliximab	Excision, cryosurgery
Lesiak et al. [8]	66F	Yellow-brown, papulonodular lesions on back	Dermal mucin	Cutaneous focal mucinosis	Anti-TNF-α (infliximab/adalimumab) + ustekinumab for plaque psoriasis	After 2 years of anti-TNF-α and 2 months of ustekinumab	Topical steroids with little improvement after 2 months

(continued)

Table 2 (continued)

Authors	Age/sex	Clinical presentation	Histopathology	Diagnosis	Triggering drug	Time from start of treatment to onset of lesions	Course
Garber et al. [10]	57F	Flesh-colored non-pruritic, non-tender, dome-shaped papules on the upper lip	Dermal mucin with ectatic vessels	Localized lichen myxedematosus of discrete type	Ustekinumab and methotrexate for palmoplantar psoriasis	8 weeks	Topical tacrolimus without benefit. No resolution
Montero et al. [11]	44 M	Multiple firm, erythematous, slightly elevated nodules of 10–20 mm in diameter on both upper extremities	Mucin deposits in periadnexal dermis and hypodermis without fibrosis	Nodular lichen myxedematosus	Ustekinumab for Crohn's disease	4 months	Topical steroids. Lesions disappeared after 6 months decreasing ustekinumab
Olmos-Alpiste et al. [12]	63 M	Multiple skin-colored to whitish papules in a cobblestone pattern preceded by eczematous eruption on trunk	Mucin deposits in the papillary and reticular dermis with a discrete lymphoid perivascular infiltrate. Neither fibroblast proliferation nor sclerosis. Fragmented elastic fibers	Diffuse dermal mucinosis	Colony-stimulating factor 1 receptor monoclonal antibody treatment for lung adenocarcinoma	16 weeks	Complete regression after 10 months of withdrawal
	72 M	Multiple skin-colored to whitish papules in a cobblestone pattern preceded by lichenoid eruption on trunk	Same to case 1	Diffuse dermal mucinosis	Colony-stimulating factor 1 receptor monoclonal antibody treatment for small cell lung carcinoma	13 weeks	Patient died 6 months later without clinical clearance of the lesions

	60 F	Multiple skin-colored to whitish papules in a cobblestone pattern on the trunk and extremities. Facial and palpebral edema	Same to case 1	Diffuse dermal mucinosis	Colony-stimulating factor 1 receptor monoclonal antibody treatment for melanoma	14 weeks	Treatment was withdrawn with clear-cut improvement 8 months later
	52 M	Multiple skin-colored to whitish papules in a cobblestone pattern on the trunk and extremities. Facial and palpebral edema	Same to case 1	Diffuse dermal mucinosis	Colony-stimulating factor 1 receptor monoclonal antibody treatment for melanoma	26 weeks	Lost to follow up

possibility of a spectrum going from simple mucin deposition to inflammatory lupus erythematosus-like lesion induced by IFNs cannot be ruled out.

Prognosis and Therapy

In four cases under biologics, lesions persist in spite of topical steroids or calcineurin-inhibitor treatment while biologic therapies were continued. Cryosurgery healed some lesions. In the nodular variant, healing of the lesions occurred after stopping ustekinumab. Cutaneous mucinosis induced by interferons resolved spontaneously, sometimes with scar, after discontinuation of interferon, and the same occurred for lesions with a lupus-like histology. When ulceration occurred, treatment with low-molecular-weight heparin resulted in healing of the lesion and also allowed the interferon injections to be continued. Complete regression after 8 and 10 months occurred in two patients after withdrawal of anti-CSF1R monoclonal antibodies [12].

Cutaneous Mucinoses After Physical and Mechanical Traumas

Although UV radiation has been implicated in exacerbating some types of mucinosis [1], the role of physical and mechanical traumas in the development of cutaneous mucinosis has been recently outlined [18, 19]. The clinical presentation is polymorphous, and while some lesions could be classified as well-known entities such as cutaneous focal mucinosis, other lesions could not fit a precise nosology and have been simply called "cutaneous mucinosis," mainly due to histopathologic findings [18, 19]. The microscopic features were either those of a dermal mucinosis or those of a follicular mucinosis [20, 21]. In a broad sense, cutaneous mucinosis after knee replacement could also be considered a form of trauma-induced cutaneous mucinosis, while primary cutaneous dermal mucinosis arising on herpes zoster scars can be considered more a postherpetic isotopic response rather than a post-traumatic mucinosis [22].

Clinical Features

The diagnosis of trauma-induced cutaneous mucinosis is based upon the history and the clinical-pathologic correlation. In two patients, cutaneous focal mucinosis developed on the mammary areola (Fig. 2a), respectively, after a laser-based epilation of hairs and a piercing procedure, while blunt trauma was a trigger in another case [18, 19]. Localized papular mucinosis (lichen myxedematosus) and follicular mucinosis may develop also after radiation therapy for the management of neoplasms [20, 21].

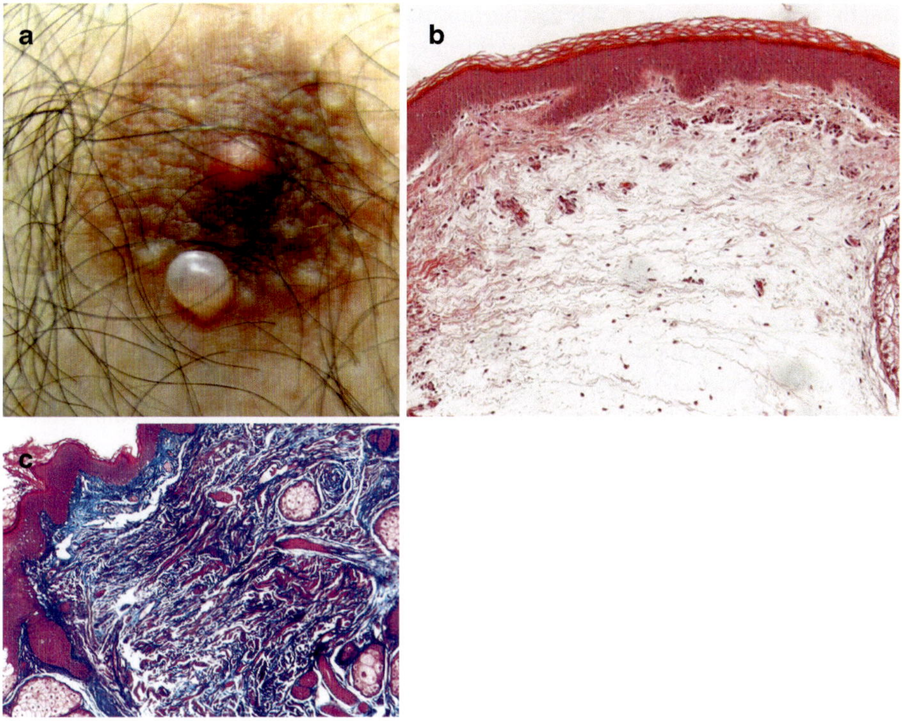

Fig. 2 (**a**) Trauma-induced cutaneous focal mucinosis. Translucent, whitish exophytic nodule with a bluish hue on the mammary areola after piercing. (**b**) Histopathology showing a slightly dome-shaped papule with abundant mucin filling the dermis with attenuation of collagen, normal fibroblast number, and absence of inflammatory infiltrate. (**c**) Colloidal iron stain highlights mucin dermal deposition

Pathogenesis

Why trauma can trigger mucin skin deposition is unclear, but it is thought to be a reactive process arising as a result of the dysfunction of fibroblasts in a circumscribed area. Chronic antigenic stimulation, inflammation, and viral infections could account for the observed features [18].

Histopathology

Histology is essential for the diagnosis showing a circumscribed abundant dermal mucin deposits with a normal or slightly increased number of fibroblasts and absence of inflammatory infiltrate (Fig. 2b). Alcian blue stain at pH 2.5 or colloidal iron stain highlights the mucin deposits (Fig. 2c). In cutaneous focal mucinosis, mucin deposition involves only the dermis, elastic fibers are absent, and there is no increased vascularity. Spindle-shaped fibroblasts are the predominant cell type, with occasional admixed factor XIIIa+ dendritic cells without any reactivity for CD34, smooth muscle actin, desmin, CD68, and S-100. The epidermis may be normal or hyperplastic [18]. Follicular mucinosis is an epithelial reaction pattern that has been associated with various inflammatory and neoplastic cutaneous disorders [21].

Differential Diagnosis

Cutaneous focal mucinosis should be differentiated from benign neoplasms with myxoid stroma, such as angiomyxoma, neurothekeoma, and nerve sheath myxoma. In particular, angiomyxoma (syn. myxoma) is a benign neoplasm, presenting with a multinodular growth of myxoid areas that contains scattered fibroblasts of variable size and shape, multinucleated histiocytic giant cells, as well as an increased number of small capillary vessels. In contrast to CFM, angiomyxoma is a larger lesion involving also the subcutis, displays a higher vascularity and expression of SMA by the fibroblastic stromal cells, and may be a marker of Carney complex. Follicular mucinosis is generally divided into a primary benign idiopathic form and a secondary form usually occurring in association with cutaneous lymphomas (especially mycosis fungoides) [23].

Prognosis and Therapy

Surgical excision is the treatment of choice for solitary lesion, resulting in complete remission without recurrence.

Cutaneous Mucinosis After Knee Replacement

In addition to the ground substance of the skin, mucin is important also for the homeostasis of joint fluid where it is usually produced by synovial cells. Resorption of intra-articular fluid typically occurs through uptake by lymphatics, blood vessels, and perineural spaces. There are four cases of cutaneous mucinosis developing adjacent to replaced joints.

Clinical Features

Two patients presented with clinical features consistent with localized lichen myxedematosus, the third one showed feature of plaque-like cutaneous mucinosis (belonging to the spectrum of reticular erythematous mucinosis), while in the last patients, the lesions showed features similar to small myxoid cysts [24–26]. A monoclonal gammopathy was present in one patient. The prosthesis itself was not compromised and was fully functional in spite of cutaneous mucinosis.

Histopathology

Mucin deposition involved the upper dermis in all patients in the absence of increased fibroblast or fibrosis, reminiscent of localized lichen myxedematosus. A cystic-like appearance with well-demarcated space filled with mucin and a pseudocapsule made by circumscribed fibrous wall without epithelial line was observed in one patient, while a plaque-like cutaneous mucinosis pattern including enlarged interstitial spaces filled with mucin, marked vascular dilation, and a dense lymphocytic perivascular infiltrate was observed in the last patient.

Workup

Magnetic resonance imaging with contrast is useful to evaluate the presence of skin–joint communication.

Pathogenesis

The pathogenesis of cutaneous mucin deposition after joint replacement surgery is unclear, although several mechanisms have been suggested: traumatic damage of the lymphatic system responsible for the drainage and absorption of the synovial fluid, accidental implantation of the synovial cells at the surgical site, local reactive process to foreign body antigens from prosthesis, and increased secretion of hyaluronic acid from osteoarthritic joints.

Prognosis and Therapy

The cystic-like lesions have been aspirated and injected with polidocanol 1% solution leaving a minimal residual post-inflammatory dyschromia. Skin lesions were not associated with prosthesis dysfunction.

Nodular Mucinosis of the Breast

Nodular mucinosis of the breast (NMB) is an extremely rare stromal lesion described as a nerve sheath myxoma by Wee et al. in 1989. The term has been coined by Michal et al. [25] in 1998 to name a myxoid lesion located in the nipple and areola that usually occurs in young women. Twelve cases of NMB have been reported in the English literature, all involving the nipple/areolar regions of the breast (Table 3) [27–36].

Clinical Features

Nodular mucinosis of the breast is predominantly found on the nipple, areola, or supernumerary nipple of young, healthy women with a mean age of 25 years [27]. The only patient with a more advanced age is a 72-year-old woman presenting with a

Table 3 Reported cases of nodular mucinosis of breast (NMB)

Reference	Age (years)	Sex	Location	Size (cm)	Presentation	Follow-up	Prognosis
Michal et al. [27]	40	M	Left nipple	2 × 1.5	Soft nodule	6 years	No recurrence
	28	F	Right nipple	1.5 × 1.5	Nodule	3 years	No recurrence
	29	F	Right nipple	2.5 × 2.5	Nodule	6 months	No recurrence
Koide et al. [28]	30	F	Right upper outer to nipple	2.9 × 2.1	Well-demarcated, mobile hard nodule	NA	NA
Sanati et al. [29]	21	F	Left nipple	1.5 × 0.9	Rubbery mass	NA	NA
Chisholm and Greene [30]	72	F	Right subareolar	0.9 × 0.8	Nodule on the same breast affected with previous carcinoma	4 mo	No recurrence
Manglik et al. [31]	15	F	Right subareolar (supernumerary nipple)	2 × 2	Non-tender tumor	NA	NA
Bulut et al. [33]	37	F	Right subareolar	3.2 × 2.5	Nodule	29 months	No relapse
Koh et al. [34]	22	F	Right subareolar	1.1 × 0.6	Well-demarcated, protruding, and movable cystic nodule	3 years	No relapse
Fernandez-Figueras et al. [32]	46	M	Left nipple	3.2 × 2.4	Nodule	3 years	No relapse
Feng et al. [35]	40	F	Right nipple	1.1 × 1.1	Nodule	NA	No relapse
Weil Lara et al. [36]	33	F	Left subareolar	3 × 3	Asymptomatic nodule	8 years	No relapse

previous history of mucinous carcinoma of the same breast [30]. Fernandez-Figueiras disputed the real nature of this case, suggesting that it represents a reactive form of mucinosis, probably of traumatic origin [32]. The lesion has been described also in men [32]. The typical clinical manifestation is a gradually enlarging, asymptomatic, soft or cystic nodular mass ranging from 0.9 to 3.2 cm in diameter under the nipple or in the subareolar region that occasionally presents with nipple discharge or pain. Nodular mucinosis of the breast does not have an established link with Carney complex which is an autosomal dominant syndrome characterized by cutaneous myxomas at various sites, endocrine tumors, and lentiginosis related to genetic defects.

Histopathology

The lesion is located in the dermis and subcutaneous tissue and is characterized by an abundant myxoid tissue with a few scattered spindle cells and a multi-lobular appearance with fibrocollagenous stroma [30–32] (Fig. 3a, b). Capillaries and thin-walled vessels are present within the nodule. A slight inflammatory infiltrate made by rare histiocytes, lymphocytes, and plasma cells is seen. Neither mammary ducts nor epithelial elements were observed. A cellular component of spindle cells with bland-looking nuclei and elongated amphiphilic cytoplasm is typically present without atypia or mitosis (Fig. 3c). The myxoid tissue stains positively with Alcian blue at pH 2.5 and is negative with periodic acid-Schiff (PAS), indicating the presence of acidic glycosaminoglycans. The spindle cells are reactive to vimentin, calponin, and variably reactive to smooth muscle actin (Fig. 3d) or CD34, while are negative for cytokeratin, smooth muscle myosin, and S-100. Mammary ducts and breast stroma tissue are usually either absent or located in the periphery; in particular, no epithelial cells are present inside the lake of mucin.

Workup

Ultrasonography shows a well-circumscribed, lobulated, homogenous, hypoechoic lesion, and mammography shows a round lobular, radiopaque mass without microcalcifications. Fine needle aspiration typically reveals mucin without epithelial cells or sign of malignancy [29].

Pathogenesis

The controversy if NMB is a reactive lesion of a benign stromal neoplasm or a true neoplasm remains open. In fact, the immunohistochemical coexpression of CD34, actin, and calponin in some cases would favor the existence of a link between NMB

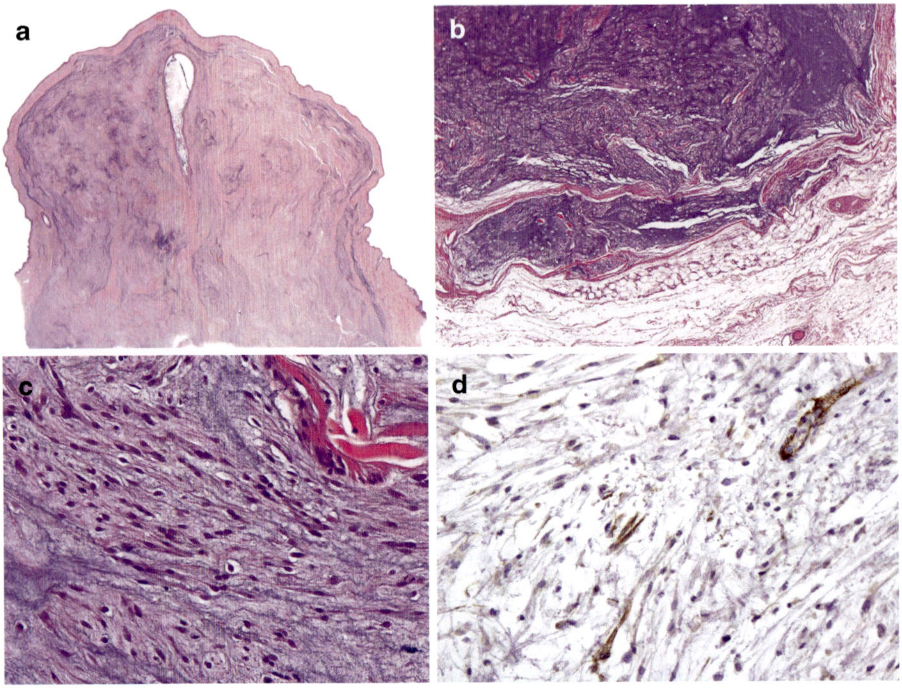

Fig. 3 (**a**) Nodular mucinosis of the breast. Abundant myxoid tissue with a few scattered spindle cells and a multilobular appearance with fibrocollagenous stroma. Neither mammary ducts nor epithelial elements were observed (Courtesy of Maria Teresa Fernández Figueras, Barcelona, Spain). (**b**) Large pools of mucinous material with well-demarcated base involving deep dermis and subcutaneous tissue (Courtesy of Maria Teresa Fernández Figueras, Barcelona, Spain). (**c**) Loosely arranged fascicle of spindle cells with slender cytoplasms in a myxoid background (Courtesy of Maria Teresa Fernández Figueras, Barcelona, Spain). (**d**) Spindle cells show a weak-to-moderate expression of actin (Courtesy of Maria Teresa Fernández Figueras, Barcelona, Spain)

and myofibroblastoma of the breast. It has also been suggested that NMB may be related to spindle cell lipoma, which typically expresses CD34, and may rarely be positive for S-100 protein [32].

Differential Diagnosis

NMB exhibits mucin deposition without epithelial cells or sign of malignancy on histopathology and should be differentiated from other myxoid lesions such as mucinous carcinoma, micropapillary carcinoma in situ with excessive mucin, fibroadenoma with myxomatous stroma. and mucocele-like lesions described by Rosen [37]. The latter are benign mucin-filled cysts lined by uniform flat or cuboidal epithelium without nuclear atypia frequently associated with rupture and mucin extravasation into the adjacent stroma and microcalcifications. Moreover, mucin in mucocele-like lesions is stained with PAS but appears negative on Alcian blue.

Prognosis and Therapy

The treatment of choice is surgical excision, which usually leads to a successful outcome without residual disease.

Conclusions

OALM and pretibial stasis mucinosis are uncommon and newly recognized disorders occurring in obese patients or in patients with venous insufficiency. They are not different entities but belong to a spectrum of mucinoses secondary to an increased body mass index, chronic lymphedema, and/or chronic venous insufficiency. Diet restriction and compression are usually of benefit. Cutaneous mucinosis consistent with localized papular or nodular lichen myxedematosus has been related to the therapy with biologics (i.e., anti TNF-alpha drugs and anti-IL12/23). Mucinous lesions were also triggered by subcutaneous injections of interferons. The role of physical and mechanical traumas such as epilation, piercing, blunt trauma, and radiation therapy in the development of cutaneous mucinosis has been recently outlined with a polymorphous clinical-pathologic presentation ranging from cutaneous focal mucinosis to localized lichen myxedematosus or follicular mucinosis. Cutaneous mucinosis may develop adjacent to replaced joints, possibly due to a skin–joint communication. Clinically and histopathologically, skin lesions were variably consistent with localized lichen myxedematosus, multiple myxoid cyst, and also plaque-like cutaneous mucinosis. Skin lesions were not associated with prosthesis dysfunction. Finally, nodular mucinosis of the breast is a controversial benign entity in young women that has been considered both a reactive lesion and a true neoplasm. In any case, it is imperative to distinguish it from other lesions that occur near the nipple, especially mucinous carcinoma, via pathologic examination after surgical excision.

References

1. Rongioletti F. Mucinoses. In: Rongioletti F, Smoller BR, editors. Clinical and pathological aspects of skin diseases in endocrine, metabolic, nutritional and deposition disease. New York: Springer; 2010. p. 139–52.
2. Somach SC, Helm TN, Lawlor KB, Bergfeld WF, Bass J. Pretibial mucin. Histologic patterns and clinical correlation. Arch Dermatol. 1993;129:1152–6.
3. Milman Lde M, Grill AB, Müller GP, De Villa D, Souza PR. Pretibial mucinosis in an euthyroid patient. An Bras Dermatol. 2016;91:100–2.
4. Ferreli C, Pinna AL, Pilloni L, Corbeddu M, Rongioletti F. Obesity-associated lymphedematous mucinosis: two further cases and review of the literature. Dermatopathology (Basel). 2018;5:16–20.

5. Pugashetti R, Zedek DC, Seiverling EV, Rajendran P, Berger T. Dermal mucinosis as a sign of venous insufficiency. J Cutan Pathol. 2010;37:292–6.
6. Hirt PA, MacQuhae FE, Cho-Vega JH, Kirsner RS. Stasis mucinosis: insights into euthyroid localized mucinosis. Wounds. 2019;31:E58–E560.
7. Valicenti JM, Fleming MG, Pearson RW, Budz JP, Gendleman MD. Papular mucinosis in L-tryptophan-induced eosinophilia-myalgia syndrome. J Am Acad Dermatol. 1991;25:54–8.
8. Lesiak A, Włodarczyk M, Sobolewska A, et al. Can biologic treatment induce cutaneous focal mucinosis? Postepy Dermatol Alergol. 2014;31:413–6.
9. Duparc A, Gosset P, Lasek A, Modiano P. Mucinose cutanée focale multiple : rôle des anti-TNF alpha ? [Multiple lesions of focal cutaneous mucinosis: a side-effect of anti-TNF alpha therapy?]. Ann Dermatol Venereol. 2010;137:140–2.
10. Garber C, Rosmarin D, Nguyen B, et al. Cutaneous mucinosis in a patient taking ustekinumab for palmoplantar psoriasis. Dermatol Online J. 2017;23:13030/qt2s2128vw.
11. Montero-Vilchez T, Martinez-Lopez A, Cuenca-Barrales C, et al. Nodular lichen myxoedematous: a new adverse event associated with ustekinumab. Australas J Dermatol. 2020;61:e344–5.
12. Olmos-Alpiste F, Segura S, Tomás-Velázquez A, et al. Diffuse dermal mucinosis secondary to colony-stimulating factor 1 receptor monoclonal antibody treatment: a novel and peculiar drug-induced diffuse cutaneous mucinosis. J Dermatol. 2020; https://doi.org/10.1111/1346-8138.15662. Epub ahead of print.
13. Benito-León J, Borbujo J, Cortés L. Cutaneous mucinoses complicating interferon beta-1b therapy. Eur Neurol. 2002;47:123–4.
14. Siewert E, Weyers W, Dietrich CG, Geier A, Lammert F, Matern S. Cutaneous mucinosis and skin necrosis complicates interferon alfacon-1 (consensus interferon) treatment of chronic hepatitis C. Eur J Med Res. 2005;10:63–7.
15. Wells J, Kossard S, McGrath M. Abdominal wall ulceration and mucinosis secondary to recombinant human interferon-beta-1b. Australas J Dermatol. 2005;46:202–4.
16. Agarwal SK, Wu M, Livingston CK, et al. Toll-like receptor 3 upregulation by type I interferon in healthy and scleroderma dermal fibroblasts. Arthritis Res Ther. 2011;11(13):R3.
17. Arrue I, Saiz A, Ortiz-Romero PL, Rodríguez-Peralto JL. Lupus-like reaction to interferon at the injection site: report of five cases. J Cutan Pathol. 2007;34:18–21.
18. Kempf W, von Stumberg B, Denisjuk N, Bode B, Rongioletti F. Trauma-induced cutaneous focal mucinosis of the mammary areola: an unusual presentation. Dermatopathology. 2014;1:24–8.
19. Verma G, Mrig PA, Gautam RK, Malhotra P. Trauma-induced focal nodular mucinoses: a rare entity. Indian Dermatol Online J. 2018;9:50–2.
20. Fernandez-Flores A, Barja-Lopez JM, Saeb-Lima M. Papular mucinosis of the breast after radiation therapy. J Cutan Pathol. 2014;41:969–71.
21. Takeda H, Nakajima K, Kaneko T, Harada K, Matsuzaki Y, Sawamura D. Follicular mucinosis associated with radiation therapy. J Dermatol. 2011;38:1116.
22. Camacho D, Feltes F, Machán S, et al. Primary cutaneous dermal mucinosis on herpes zoster scars. Cutis. 2016;98:E19–23.
23. Rongioletti F, Rebora A. Cutaneous mucinoses: microscopic criteria for diagnosis. Am J Dermatopathol. 2001;23:257–67.
24. Haught JM, Serrao R, English JC 3rd. Localized cutaneous mucinosis after joint replacement. Arch Dermatol. 2008;144:1399–400.
25. Gómez-Bernal S, Ruiz-González I, Delgado-Vicente S, Alonso-Alonso T, Rodríguez-Prieto MÁ. Plaque-like cutaneous mucinosis after joint replacement. J Cutan Pathol. 2012;39:562–4.
26. Juhl ME, Sidiropoulos M, Antonijevic S, Lyon M, Krunic A. Focal cutaneous mucinosis after knee replacement: a rare entity successfully treated with intralesional polidocanol. JAAD Case Rep. 2016;24(3):16–8.
27. Michal M, Ludvíková M, Zámecník M. Nodular mucinosis of the breast: report of three cases. Pathol Int. 1998;48:542–4.

28. Koide N, Akashi-Tanaka S, Fukutomi T, Nanasawa T, Hasegawa T. Nodular mucinosis of the breast: a case report with clinical and imaging findings. Breast Cancer. 2002;9:261–4.
29. Sanati S, Leonard M, Khamapirad T, Eltorky MA. Nodular mucinosis of the breast: a case report with pathologic, ultrasonographic, and clinical findings and review of the literature. Arch Pathol Lab Med. 2005;129:e58–61.
30. Chisholm C, Greene JF Jr. Nodular mucinosis of the breast: expanding our understanding with an unusual case. Am J Dermatopathol. 2010;32:187–9.
31. Manglik N, Berlingeri-Ramos AC, Boroumand N, Eltorky M. Nodular mucinosis of the breast in a supernumerary nipple: case report and review of the literature. J Cutan Pathol. 2010;37:1178–81.
32. Fernández-Figueras MT, Kazakov DV, López Martos R, Ojanguren I, Vila J, Ariza A. Nodular mucinosis of the breast in a male: reassessment of diagnostic criteria and proposal for its classification as a soft tissue tumor in the myofibroblastoma and spindle cell lipoma spectrum. Dermatopathology (Basel). 2014;1:47–54.
33. Bulut T, Celik B, Nassar A, Yalcin AD. Nodular mucinosis of breast: a case report. J Med Cases. 2015;6:457–9.
34. Koh HM, Maeng YH, Jang BG, Choi JH, Hyun CL. A rare case of nodular mucinosis of the breast. J Pathol Transl Med. 2017;51:332–4.
35. Feng TT, Oh HB, Pang YH, Tan CC. A rare case of nodular mucinosis of the breast away from the nipple-areola complex. Breast J. 2019;25:1280–1.
36. Weil Lara B, Pérez Martínez D, Romero Madrid B. Mucinosis nodular de la mama [Nodular mucinosis of the breast]. Rev Esp Patol. 2020;53:42–7. Spanish.
37. Ginter PS, Tang X, Shin SJ. A review of mucinous lesions of the breast. Breast J. 2020;26:1168–78.

Pediatric Cutaneous Mucinoses

Franco Rongioletti and Valentina Caputo

Introduction

Primary cutaneous mucinoses are a heterogeneous group of diseases characterized by the abnormal deposition of glycosaminoglycans (mucin) in the skin, both in the dermis and in the follicular unit [1]. Cutaneous mucinoses usually affect adults and are uncommon in children, in whom the diagnosis and management are a difficult task. In particular, the classification of primary cutaneous mucinoses occurring in childhood is confusing. A classification is proposed in which the pediatric cutaneous mucinoses are divided into two groups: primary (idiopathic) cutaneous mucinoses and secondary mucinoses, in which histological mucin deposition is only an additional finding [2] (Table 1). Some examples of secondary cutaneous mucinoses that can be seen in pediatric patients are granuloma annulare or neonatal lupus mucinosis. Primary pediatric cutaneous mucinoses can be further divided into degenerative/inflammatory and hamartomatous/neoplastic, both dermal and follicular.

Cutaneous Mucinosis of Infancy (CMI)

CMI is one of the subtypes of localized lichen myxedematosus (also known as papular mucinosis) and is considered the pediatric variant of the discrete papular form or of acral persistent papular mucinosis [3].

F. Rongioletti (✉)
Unit of Dermatology, IRCCS San Raffaele Hospital Vita Salute San Raffaele University, Milan, Italy

Unit of Dermatology, Department of Medical Sciences and Public Health, University of Cagliari, Cagliari, Italy

V. Caputo
Unit of Surgical Pathology, ASST Grande Ospedale Metropolitano Niguarda, Milan, Italy

F. Rongioletti, B. R. Smoller (eds.), *New and Emerging Entities in Dermatology and Dermatopathology*, https://doi.org/10.1007/978-3-030-80027-7_3

Table 1 Pediatric cutaneous mucinoses

I. Degenerative/inflammatory
A. Dermal/subcutaneous
1. Cutaneous mucinosis of infancy (localized lichen myxedematosus)
Yellowish, erythematous or skin-coloured asymptomatic papules, nodules or plaques arranged into different clinical patterns on the neck, trunk and extremities
2. Self-healing juvenile cutaneous mucinosis
Acute eruption of papules on the hand, head, trunk and extremities and subcutaneous nodules on the face and periarticular areas with fever, arthralgia, weakness and muscle tenderness sometimes preceded by upper-airway infection
3. Atypical papular mucinosis of infancy
Isolated or confluent papules with absent or variable accompanying symptoms or cutaneous mucinosis of infancy/self-healing cutaneous mucinosis overlap
4. Scleredema (postinfectious)
Firm, non-pitting, indurated oedema on the neck and upper back sparing the hands and feet after febrile illness
B. Follicular
5. Pinkus' follicular mucinosis
Solitary or just a few alopecic plaques, follicular-based papules and nodules, follicular spines, acneiform eruptions on the head and neck area
II. Hamartomatous/neoplastic
A. Dermal
6. Mucinous naevus
Brownish/yellowish or skin-coloured papules or plaques, in a linear, zosteriform or group distribution on the back
Connective tissue naevus of proteoglycan type
Combined epidermal-connective tissue naevus of proteoglycan type
Perifollicular type
7. Mucinous eccrine naevus
Unilateral, solitary, erythematous or brownish nodule or plaque on the legs or multiple lesions in a linear configuration or following Blaschko's lines or with a bilateral pattern. Hyperhidrosis
8. Superficial angiomyxoma (cutaneous myxoma)
Solitary nodules on the trunk, head and lower limbs
In Carney complex multiple lesions located on external ears or eyelids
B. Follicular
9. Nevoid follicular mucinosis
Multiple linear flesh-coloured coalescent papules similar to epidermal naevus, distributed along Blaschko's lines on the face, trunk and arms

Clinical Features

CMI is an idiopathic, benign condition, characterized by an eruption of multiple, 2–5-mm, yellowish, erythematous or skin-coloured, asymptomatic papules that may be arranged into different clinical patterns such as grouped (Fig. 1a), dispersed (Fig. 1b), linear, confluent into plaques, bilateral and generalized. Rarely, nodular lesions are the main pattern of presentation. There is no sex predominance and the onset occurs at birth or in the first months or years of life. The most common areas of involvement are the neck, trunk and extremities [4]. The cases that have been reported as plaque-like cutaneous mucinosis are in fact more consistent with a form of CMI in plaque rather than as a variant of reticular erythematous mucinosis [5].

Histopathologic Features

Histopathology shows a focal well-circumscribed deposit of mucin filling only the papillary dermis or involving more deeply the reticular dermis with no or few fibroblast proliferation (Fig.1c). A superficial perivascular mononuclear cell infiltrate is also present. Mucin is stained with Alcian blue at pH 2·5 and with colloidal iron.

Work-Up

No exam is needed.

Differential Diagnosis

Histologic examination helps to distinguish CMI from several papular eruptions that have a similar appearance, such as granuloma annulare, lichen planus and other lichenoid eruptions and eruptive collagenoma.

Etiopathogenesis

The pathogenesis is unclear. A genetic background is suggested by some familial cases.

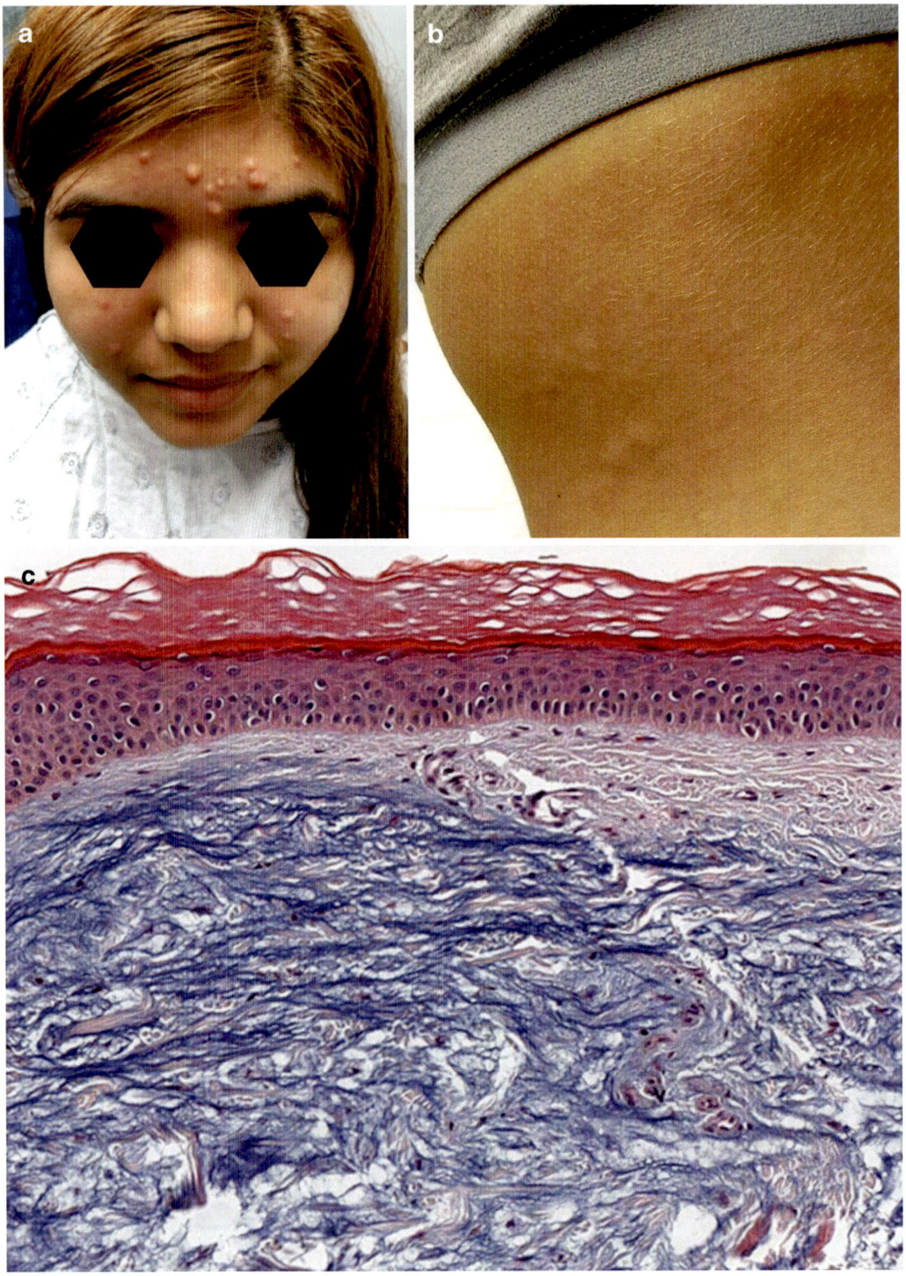

Fig. 1 Cutaneous mucinosis of infancy. (**a**) Grouped papules and nodules on the face. (**b**) Dispersed and grouped papules and nodules on the thigh. (**c**) Mucin is deposited in the upper dermis (colloidal iron stain)

Therapy

No treatment is required. Topical corticosteroids and calcineurin inhibitors can be tried with variable results.

Prognosis and Course

The prognosis is benign. CMI is a persistent condition, although dynamic changes in its course have been reported, including spontaneous healing of some papules with the development of new lesions.

Self-Healing Juvenile Cutaneous Mucinosis

Self-healing juvenile cutaneous mucinosis (SHJCM) is a rare pediatric condition that is actually considered an entity *sui generis* [6].

Clinical Features

SHJCM presents with a constellation of acute-onset, characteristic skin symptoms including the following: (1) an eruption of multiple papules (Fig. 2a) on the head, trunk and extremities, sometimes arranged in a linear fashion, (2) the development of subcutaneous nodules on the face and the extensor surface of periarticular areas (Fig. 2b) and (3) oedema of the face and particularly of the periorbital area. The condition is sometimes preceded by upper-airway infection symptoms. SHJCM occurs in childhood or adolescence, with an age at onset between 13 months and 15 years. Patients exhibit systemic symptoms such as fever, weakness, arthralgia (involving the elbows, hands and knees) and muscle tenderness. Coincidental findings described in single cases include nephroblastoma, myositis and bilateral carpal tunnel syndrome. A few cases of SHJCM have been described in adults [7].

Histopathologic Features

The histopathology of papules and nodules demonstrates some differences. The papules are characterized by mucin deposition in the upper and reticular dermis (Fig. 3a) with a moderate fibroblast proliferation and a slight perivascular lymphocytic infiltrate. The nodules show a deeper proliferative fasciitis-like findings (Fig. 3b) with subcutaneous and/or fascial prominent plump spindle-cell infiltrate, and large epithelioid ganglion-like cells embedded in a myxoid stroma. Sometimes, a lobular panniculitis is also seen (Fig. 3c) [5].

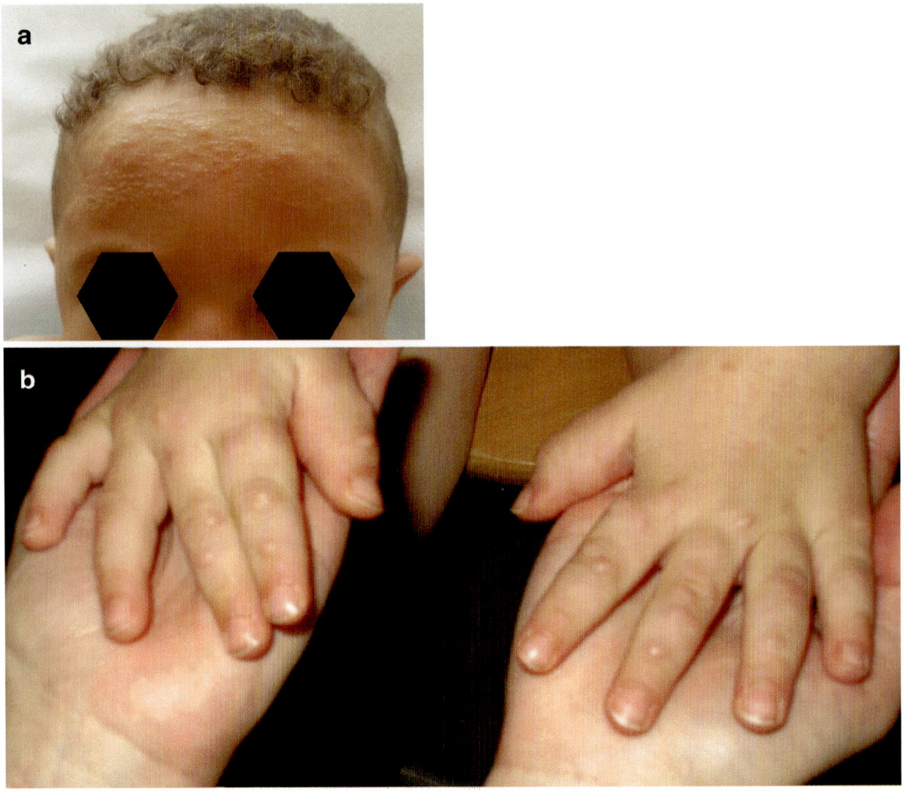

Fig. 2 Self-healing juvenile cutaneous mucinosis. (**a**) Acute eruption of multiple papules affecting the forehead. (**b**) Subcutaneous nodules on the periarticular areas of the hands

Work-Up

Blood exams may reveal an elevation of markers of inflammation such as erythrocyte sedimentation rate and C-reactive protein, leucocytosis, thrombocytosis, hypoalbuminaemia and hyper-alpha-2-globulinaemia.

Differential Diagnosis

The differential diagnoses of SHJCM include juvenile dermatomyositis, scleromyxedema, erythema elevatum diutinum, multicentric reticulohistiocytosis, rheumatoid nodules, subcutaneous panniculitis and eosinophilic fasciitis. Scleromyxedema is an adult disease that has not been reported in infants and children. The definitive diagnosis relies on clinical-pathologic correlation.

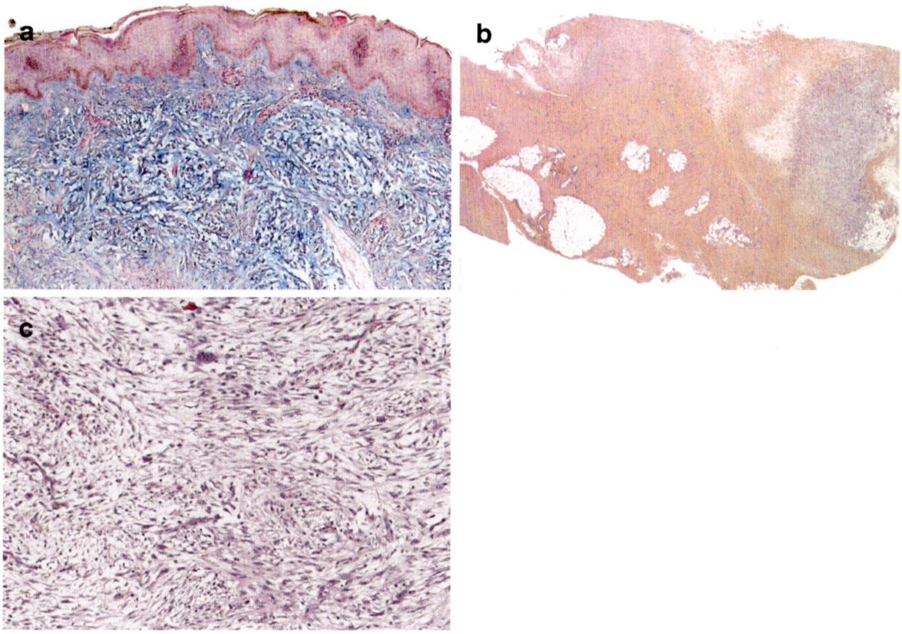

Fig. 3 Histopathology of self-healing juvenile cutaneous mucinosis. (**a**) Histopathology of a papule is characterized by mucin deposition in the upper dermis with mild fibroblast proliferation (Alcian blue stain). (**b**) Histopathology of a nodule shows a proliferative fasciitis-like pattern with focal areas of myxoid stroma (haematoxylin–eosin stain). (**c**) Plump spindle-cell infiltrate and large epithelioid ganglion-like cells in a myxoid stroma (haematoxylin–eosin stain)

Etiopathogenesis

The exact cause of mucin deposition in SHJCM is unclear. An immunologic reaction to an infectious condition has been hypothesized, as signs of an active viral disease due to human herpesvirus 6 and rotavirus or a bacterial disease due to *Bartonella* have been discovered in a few anecdotal cases.

Therapy

The disease may create great concern for parents and treating doctors, but the course is benign with spontaneous resolution in a period ranging from a few weeks to several months (usually 2–8 months).

Prognosis and Course

Although a benign and autoresolutive prognosis is expected, a transition from SHJCM to fibroblastic rheumatism in one patient and to an unspecified autoinflammatory rheumatological condition in another case has been described. Thus, an accurate follow-up for these patients is recommended.

Atypical or Intermediate Forms of Papular Mucinosis of Infancy (Cutaneous Mucinosis of Infancy/Self-Healing Cutaneous Mucinosis Overlap)

The nomenclature and classification of cutaneous mucinosis presenting with papules and nodules in pediatric patients is quite complex. Sometimes there are unusual or atypical conditions that do not fit well with the clinicopathological presentation of the two more classical entities (i.e. CMI and SHJCM) or show overlapping features of the two conditions. These atypical forms have been reported only as single anecdotal case reports [2].

Scleredema

Scleredema is a primary cutaneous fibromucinosis that can be divided into a diabetic and nondiabetic form [8]. The nondiabetic form includes an idiopathic type, a postinfectious type that predominates in the pediatric age range, and a type associated with different pathologies, the most common of which include monoclonal gammopathies.

Clinical Features

Scleredema is characterized by poorly defined woody, non-pitting induration of the skin, with inconstant overlying erythema or hyperpigmentation. It starts on the posterior neck and then spreads to the shoulders, the upper trunk and the arms symmetrically, sparing the hands and feet. Rarely, the face and lower extremities are involved. The affected skin has a '*peau d'orange*' appearance when pinched. In children, scleredema is of the postinfectious type with an acute onset, usually following a streptococcal upper respiratory infection, but also influenza, measles, mumps, chickenpox, cytomegalovirus, diphtheria or encephalitis. It is more common in female patients and is seen in patients of all races. About one third of patients with postinfectious scleredema were between the ages of 11 and 20 years [2].

Congenital scleredema may also occur. Patients may experience significant physical and functional impairment. Extracutaneous complications (in all forms) include serositis, dysarthria, dysphagia, myositis, parotitis, hepatosplenomegaly and ocular and cardiac manifestations.

Histopathologic Features

The dermis is up to four times thicker than normal (Fig. 4a). The collagen fibres appear swollen and are separated by fenestrations in which abnormal deposits of mucin are seen in the reticular dermis (Fig. 4b). The subcutaneous tissue is also involved, with replacement of fat by coarse collagen fibres. Fibroblast proliferation and inflammatory infiltrate are usually lacking [9]. Mucin also accumulates in skeletal muscle and the heart, but systemic involvement is not common.

Work-Up

There are no specific laboratory abnormalities, but the diagnostic workup in children should include analysis of anti-streptolysin O titre, a throat culture to exclude group A streptococcal infection and additional tests for viral infections.

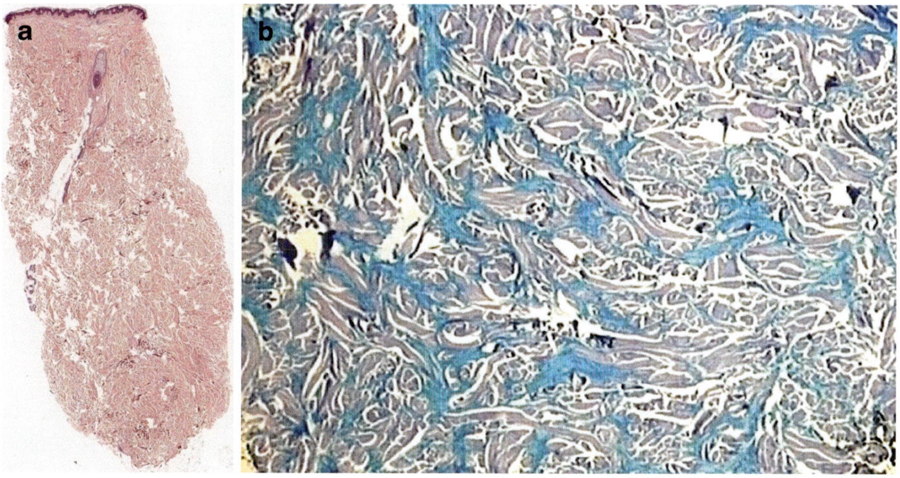

Fig. 4 Postinfectious scleredema. (**a**) Under a spared epidermis, the dermis is four times thicker than normal. Fibroblast proliferation and inflammatory infiltrate are lacking (haematoxylin–eosin stain). (**b**) Fenestrations of collagen bundles with abnormal deposits of mucin in the reticular dermis (Alcian blue stain)

Differential Diagnosis

The differential diagnosis of scleredema in pediatric patients may include sclerema neonatorum, subcutaneous fat necrosis of the newborn and cold panniculitis. Sclerema neonatorum is an uncommon fatal panniculitis occurring in the first week of life, mostly in premature and low-birth-weight infants. On histopathology, sclerema neonatorum shows a lobular panniculitis with needle-shaped clefts in adipocytes without significant or a little inflammatory infiltrate. Subcutaneous fat necrosis of the newborn typically presents around 1 to 4 weeks of life as localized hardened areas of erythematous-brownish skin in healthy-term or post-term neonates. Different from sclerema neonatorum, lesions of subcutaneous fat necrosis develop later and tend to remain circumscribed, and the skin freely moves over the underlying tissue. Hypoxia, obstetrical distress and hypothermia are risk factors. On histopathology, subcutaneous fat necrosis of the newborn reveals a panniculitis with crystal clefts spaces similar to those in sclerema neonatorum but with a more prominent inflammatory infiltrate of lymphocytes, histiocytes and multinucleated cells and foci of calcification. Moreover, subcutaneous fat necrosis of the newborn is a more limited process with a favourable prognosis compared to sclerema neonatorum which is associated with a high mortality rate. Cold panniculitis is characterized by erythematous, firm, well-demarcated plaques that appear within hours to a few days after cold exposure and resolve spontaneously in older infants. Whereas the clinical findings may be similar to those of subcutaneous fat necrosis of the newborn, its histopathology lacks the characteristic needle-shaped clefts and microcystic spaces, while adipocyte necrosis and sometimes mucin are often apparent [10].

Etiopathogenesis

The pathogenesis of scleredema is unclear. Increased synthesis of type 1 collagen by dysfunctional fibroblasts in the affected skin has been suggested. Streptococcal hypersensitivity and injury to lymphatics can play a role.

Therapy

Postinfectious scleredema is usually self-healing and no therapy is needed. Patients with motion or respiratory disability should be referred for physiotherapy. A course of antibiotics could be considered if there is evidence of a recent streptococcal infection.

Prognosis and Course

Postinfectious scleredema, which predominantly affects children and young adults, usually resolves within several months up to 1–2 years.

Pinkus Primary Follicular Mucinosis (Alopecia Mucinosa/ Follicular Mucinosis)

Follicular mucinosis (FM) is a rare condition characterized by mucin deposition within hair follicles and sebaceous glands. After the initial reports, two forms have been recognized: a primary, benign idiopathic form (Pinkus primary FM, alopecia mucinosa/FM or type I FM) that occurs mostly in children and young adults, with a tendency to resolve spontaneously, and a secondary form (type II FM) occurring in older patients, which associates with cutaneous lymphoma, mainly mycosis fungoides or Sézary syndrome [2, 11].

Clinical Features

FM is rare in the pediatric population, presenting with a solitary lesion or just a few scaly alopecic patches and plaques (Fig. 5a, b), follicular-based papules or a combination of both types of lesions. Nodules, annular plaques, folliculitis, follicular spines, acneiform eruptions and alopecia areata-like patterns have also been described. The face, neck and scalp are the most frequently affected sites, although lesions may occur on any site of the body. A congenital case of FM in a neonate has been reported only once [12].

Histopathologic Features

Histopathology shows mucin deposits in the outer root sheath of the hair follicle and sometimes sebaceous glands, in addition to a perifollicular inflammatory infiltrate consisting of lymphocytes, macrophages and eosinophils (Fig. 5c). The primary, benign form is characterized by the presence of eosinophils and significant mucinous alterations in the follicular epithelium [5]. The presence of epidermotropic lymphocytes and dense perifollicular infiltrate of atypical cells suggest a malignant form of the condition. However, there are no strict single specific clinical or histopathological criteria to distinguish cases of primary FM from cases associated with mycosis fungoides. Clonal T-cell rearrangement is not always useful to differentiate the two forms.

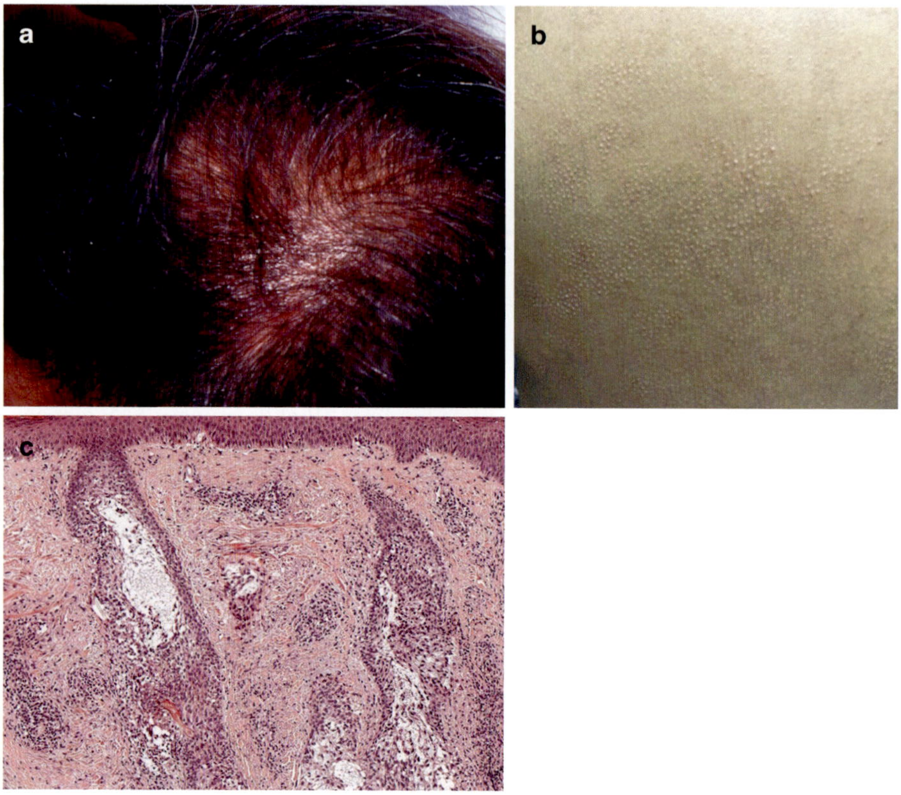

Fig. 5 Pinkus primary follicular mucinosis. (**a**) A solitary patch of alopecia with follicular hyperkeratosis on the scalp. (**b**) Follicular mucinosis on the trunk. (**c**) Deposits of mucin accumulate within the follicular epithelia causing keratinocytes to disconnect and forming cystic spaces. A perifollicular infiltrate is seen (haematoxylin–eosin stain)

Work-Up

Histopathology is essential for diagnosis. A 10% potassium hydroxide (KOH) examination of skin scrapings rules out the presence of fungi.

Differential Diagnosis

FM involving the head may be misdiagnosed as seborrheic dermatitis, psoriasis or tinea capitis. In the absence of scarring, alopecia areata may also be considered, whereas in the presence of scarring, discoid lupus erythematosus and lichen planopilaris may be considered. FM in children may also mimic lichen spinulosus and keratosis pilaris both of which show different microscopic features. Urticaria-like FM is a benign dermatosis characterized by an itchy and cyclical eruption of urticarial scaly papules and plaques in a seborrheic distribution or on a background of rosacea. A real challenge is to distinguish the primary benign form of FM from FM associated with T-cell lymphoma. The main clues in favour of a primary form are the young age of the patient, a solitary lesion on the head or neck with tendency to spontaneous resolution and the absence of histological features of epidermotropism and atypical lymphocytes. Although the real existence of a primary FM has been questioned as it has been considered an 'indolent' localized form of cutaneous T-cell lymphoma, two studies in pediatric populations concluded that FM in children is not generally indicative of mycosis fungoides. Nevertheless, FM in children is not always self-limiting or benign but can also be associated with lymphoproliferative diseases such as Hodgkin disease.

Etiopathogenesis

It is unclear why mucin is deposited selectively within a follicular structure. Although follicular keratinocytes have been considered to be the source of the mucin, an etiological role for cell-mediated immune mechanisms has been proposed. A reaction to persistent antigens such as *Staphylococcus aureus* or *Malassezia* has also been hypothesized. Familial cases suggest a genetic predisposition.

Therapy

No standard treatment regimens have been established. Many therapies have been tried with varying results including corticosteroids (topical, intralesional and systemic), phototherapy, dapsone, antimalarial agents, oral retinoids and interferon alfa-2b. A wait-and-follow approach can be considered as many cases heal spontaneously in 2–24 months.

Prognosis and Course

Although most of the cases in pediatric patients have shown a benign course, long-term follow-up of children with primary FM is nevertheless warranted, especially in case of chronic, persistent lesions [13].

Mucinous Naevus

Mucinous naevus (MN) is a rare, benign form of connective tissue naevus of proteoglycan type, although there has been debate about its nosological classification. About one-half of the reported cases have been described in Asiatic patients [14].

Clinical Features

MN is characterized by a collection of brownish–yellowish or skin-coloured papules or plaques in a linear, Blaschko's linear or group distribution, most commonly on the back (Fig. 6a). Single lesions have been described as well, presenting with

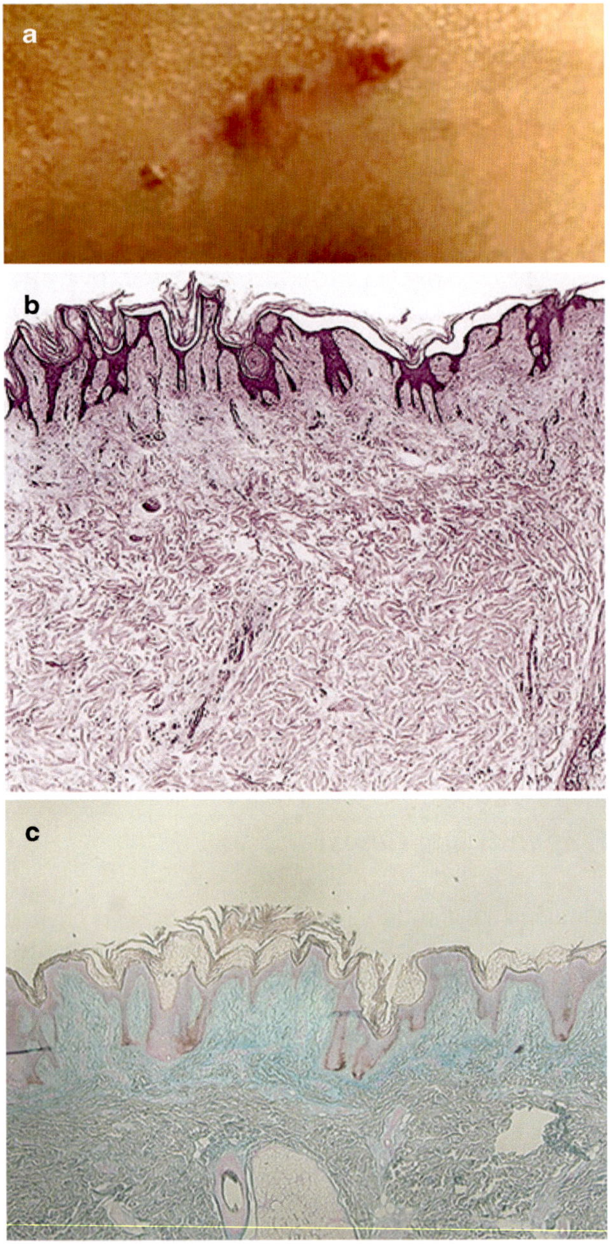

Fig. 6 Mucinous naevus. (**a**) Brownish–yellowish papules arranged into a linear plaque on the back. (**b**) A diffuse deposit of mucin is evident in the upper papillary dermis with epidermal naevus-like changes (combined type) (haematoxylin–eosin stain). (**c**) Mucin fills the papillary dermis (Alcian blue stain)

pedunculated, soft nodules or verrucous plaques. There is a predominance of male to female patients (3·5: 1). Most lesions are congenital or may occur in adolescence, or more rarely in adulthood, and tend to grow slowly. Rarely, patients complain of itching by friction from clothes. Although most cases are sporadic, the possibility of familial association has been suggested.

Histopathologic Features

Histologically, MN is characterized by an accumulation of mucin in the papillary dermis, with a relative reduction or loss of collagen and elastic fibres within the mucinous area (Fig. 6b,c). Rarely, mucin fills the upper reticular dermis. Two histological subtypes have been described: pure mucinous dermal naevus (connective tissue naevus of the proteoglycan type) and combined mucinous naevus associating epidermal naevus with dermal mucin deposits [15]. A third type, characterized by mucin deposits in the perifollicular dermis with dilation of the hair follicles, has been reported as follicular mucinous naevus [16]. Some cases with mature fat cells in the upper dermis similar to naevus lipomatosus superficialis have been reported. The cellular component of the mucinous naevus consists of CD34-positive fibroblasts and a few factor XIIIa-positive dendritic cells.

Work-Up

No laboratory investigations are needed.

Differential Diagnosis

Both a naevus lipomatosus superficialis and an epidermal naevus show nevoid features similar to those of a MN. Histological data are necessary.

Etiopathogenesis

Mucinous naevus is a hamartomatous condition that may be congenital or acquired.

Therapy

Treatment is not necessary except for cosmetic purposes. Surgical operation, carbon dioxide laser and topical therapy, including keratolytic, corticosteroid ointments and retinoids, have been tried. In particular, combined mucinous naevus, associating epidermal naevus with dermal mucin, has been considered suitable for laser ablation with carbon dioxide laser, while pure mucinous dermal naevus is not for the risk of hypertrophic scarring [17].

Prognosis and Course

Prognosis is good due the benign nature of MN but there is no spontaneous regression.

Mucinous Eccrine Naevus

Mucinous eccrine naevus (MEN) is an extremely rare variant of eccrine naevus [18].

Clinical Features

In most cases, MEN presented before puberty as a unilateral, solitary, erythematous or brownish nodule or plaque occurring on the legs. However, onset at birth or after the age of 40 years has been described. Patients with multiple lesions in a linear configuration or following Blaschko's lines, or with a bilateral pattern of distribution, have been reported. Localized hyperhidrosis may be a feature. There is no sex predilection.

Histopathology

An increased number of lobulated eccrine glands and ducts are seen within the reticular dermis surrounded by an abundant mucinous deposit. The small vessels close to the glands are thicker than in normal glands. The dermal stroma shows mild fibroblastic hyperplasia.

Etiopathogenesis

MEN is a hamartomatous benign lesion. A role for mechanical stress and trauma has been suggested, or for some cytokines such as growth factors that stimulate the fibroblasts to synthesize more mucin.

Therapy

Surgical excision should be considered in case of tenderness, swelling and/or hyperhidrosis; otherwise, a wait-and-see approach is suggested. Hyperhidrosis is treatable with topical aluminium chloride, systemic anticholinergic agents, iontophoresis and botulinum toxin. Monthly intralesional injections of steroids were reported to flatten and improve the lesion.

Prognosis and Course

Lesion is benign, but there is no spontaneous regression.

Superficial Angiomyxoma (Cutaneous Myxoma)

Superficial angiomyxoma is an acquired benign neoplasm [19]. There is a known association of angiomyxomas with Carney complex, a rare endocrine tumour syndrome caused by LOF mutations in the *PRKAR1A* tumour suppressor gene [20].

Clinical Features

This tumour can be solitary or multiple presenting as a nodular or polypoid, skin-coloured, soft lesion of 1–5 cm in size involving the trunk, head, neck and lower limbs. Although it has a predilection for men in their fourth decade, the occurrence of multiple angiomyxomas located on the external ear canal or eyelids in youngsters could be a manifestation of Carney complex. However, multiple lesions in children without any other component of Carney complex have been described. Congenital cases have also been reported [2]. Dermoscopy describes superficial angiomyxoma as a red, translucent, globular exophytic lesion with arborizing vessels that looks like a blood moon.

Histological Features

Superficial angiomyxoma is a poorly circumscribed tumour with a multilobular pattern of growth. The component cells suspended within a myxoid stroma include scattered, bland, spindle-shaped cells that may be positive for CD34 and negative for S100, smooth muscle actin and muscle-specific actin. Prominent vascularization with arborizing thin-walled vessels is a characteristic feature. An inflammatory infiltrate of neutrophils may be present.

Differential Diagnosis

Cutaneous focal mucinosis is a benign reactive lesion involving only the dermis that should be distinguished histologically from other myxoid neoplasms. In particular, superficial angiomyxoma should be distinguished from aggressive angiomyxoma that occurs commonly in the pelvic and peritoneal region of females.

Etiopathogenesis

The pathogenesis is unclear, although it is thought that angiomyxoma arises from dysfunctional mesenchymal cells with genetic abnormalities.

Therapy

Treatment is surgical and the excision is curative.

Prognosis and Course

The prognosis is good, but local recurrence is possible if excision is incomplete.

Nevoid Follicular Mucinosis

This is a type of hamartomatous epidermal or hair-follicle naevus exhibiting typical histopathologic features of follicular mucinosis [21]. Clinically it presents with congenital multiple linear flesh-coloured coalescent papules similar to an epidermal naevus, which follows the Blaschko's lines on the face, trunk and arms. Histopathologically, follicular epithelia show spongiosis with cystic spaces filled with mucin.

Conclusions

Primary cutaneous pediatric mucinoses are uncommon diseases of pediatric age. Very recently, a classification has been proposed in which they are divided into degenerative/inflammatory and hamartomatous/neoplastic conditions, both dermal and follicular. The diagnosis is not easy and requires a good clinical-pathologic correlation in addition to be aware of these entities. Most of these conditions are benign or resolve spontaneously. Knowledge of these entities may indeed prevent unnecessary diagnostic testing and aggressive treatment in pediatric patients.

References

1. Rongioletti F. Mucinoses. In: Rongioletti F, Smoller BR, editors. Clinical and pathological aspects of skin diseases in endocrine, metabolic, nutritional and deposition disease. New York, NY: Springer; 2010. p. 139–52.
2. Rongioletti F. Primary pediatric cutaneous mucinoses. Br J Dermatol. 2020;182(1):29–38.
3. Rongioletti F. Lichen myxedematosus, ed. UpToDate. Waltham, MA: UpToDate Inc http://www.uptodate.com. Accessed on 02 Jan 2017.
4. Pita da Veiga G, Pérez-Feal P, Fernández-Redondo V, et al. Cutaneous mucinosis of infancy: a rare entity in pediatrics. Int J Dermatol. 2020;59(12):e464–5.
5. Álvarez-Salafranca M, Colmenero I, Torrecilla Idoipe N, Torrelo A, Ara-Martín M. Plaque-like cutaneous mucinosis of childhood. Pediatr Dermatol. 2020; https://doi.org/10.1111/pde.14381. Epub ahead of print.
6. Luchsinger I, Coulombe J, Rongioletti F, Haspeslagh M, Dompmartin A, Melki I, et al. Self-healing juvenile cutaneous mucinosis: Clinical and histopathologic findings of 9 patients: The relevance of long-term follow-up. J Am Acad Dermatol. 2018;78:1164–70.
7. Lecanu P, Haidar D, Lafargue O, et al. Mucinose cutanée « juvénile » auto-involutive chez l'adulte [A case of "juvenile" self-healing cutaneous mucinosis in an adult]. Ann Dermatol Venereol. 2020;147(11):769–74. French.
8. Rongioletti F, Kaiser F, Cinotti E, et al. Scleredema. A multicentre study of characteristics, comorbidities, course and therapy in 44 patients. J Eur Acad Dermatol Venereol. 2015;29:2399–404.
9. Rongioletti F, Rebora A. Cutaneous mucinoses: microscopic criteria for diagnosis. Am J Dermatopathol. 2001;23:257–67.
10. Grassi S, Borroni RG, Brazzelli V. Panniculitis in children. G Ital Dermatol Venereol. 2013;148(4):371–85.
11. Rongioletti F, De Lucchi S, Meyes D, Mora M, Rebora A, Zupo S, Cerruti G, Patterson JW. Follicular mucinosis: a clinicopathologic, histochemical, immunohistochemical and molecular study comparing the primary benign form and the mycosis fungoides-associated follicular mucinosis. J Cutan Pathol. 2010;37:15–9.
12. Valdivielso-Ramos M, Alonso S, Sanchez B, Carrascosa R, Galiano S, Silvente C, de la Cueva P. Primary follicular mucinosis in childhood. Int J Dermatol. 2020; https://doi.org/10.1111/ijd.15309. Epub ahead of print.
13. Khalil J, Kurban M, Abbas O. Follicular mucinosis: a review. Int J Dermatol. 2020; https://doi.org/10.1111/ijd.15165. Epub ahead of print.
14. Rongioletti F, Rebora A. Mucinous nevus. Arch Dermatol. 1996;132:1522–3.
15. Chi CC, Wang SH, Lin PY. Combined epidermal-connective tissue nevus of proteoglycan (a type of mucinous nevus): a case report and literature review. J Cutan Pathol. 2009;36:808–11.
16. Fischer AS, Pei S, McMahon P, Taylor JA, Elenitsas R, Rubin AI. Cutaneous follicular mucinous nevus presenting with congenital grouped papules and plaques initially misdiagnosed as a cutaneous myxoma. J Cutan Pathol. 2021;48(1):1–5.
17. Mulcahy A, Shumack S, Lim A, Cheung K. Mucinous Naevus: a case of suboptimal response to laser treatment. Australas J Dermatol. 2017;58:e261–2.

18. Lee SH, Cho YJ, Han M, Bae JW, Park JW, Oh SR, Kim S. Superficial angiomyxoma of the vulva in a postmenopausal woman: a case report and review of literature. J Menopausal Med. 2016;22(3):180–3.
19. Ladd R, Davis M, Dyer JA. Genodermatoses with malignant potential. Clin Dermatol. 2020;38(4):432–54. https://doi.org/10.1016/j.clindermatol.2020.03.007. Epub 2020 Mar 30.
20. Rodríguez-Villa Lario A, Gómez-Zubiaur A, Trasobares-Marugán L, Medina-Montalvo S, Quesada-Cortés A, Medina-Expósito I. Eccrine mucinous nevus: clinical and histopathological description in an adult Nevus mucinoso ecrino en el adulto: descripción clínicohistológica. Dermatol Online J. 2020;26(7):13030/qt3m22r261.
21. Tadini G, Boldrini MP, Brena M, Pezzani L, Marchesi L, Rongioletti F. Nevoid follicular mucinosis: a new type of hair follicle nevus. J Cutan Pathol. 2013;40:844–7.

Circumscribed Palmoplantar Hypokeratosis

Jean Kanitakis

Introduction

Circumscribed palmoplantar hypokeratosis (CPH) is a peculiar, rare dermatosis of the palms and soles with characteristic clinical and histopathological features, first reported in 2002 [1]. CPH still remains poorly known and is probably underreported. A Medline-based search of the international literature (until September 27, 2020) revealed 68 articles reporting a total of 114 patients with CPH [1–69]. One case was published as a 'dermatopathology quiz' but provided no clinical data [70]. CPH is probably underreported as it was recognized rather recently and because it is as a rule asymptomatic, so that patients do not always seek medical care. The majority of cases reported were from the USA [4, 5, 10, 17, 20, 23, 24, 32, 35, 36, 41, 43, 48, 59, 67], Japan [13, 14, 18, 21, 26, 28, 33, 34, 42, 46, 47, 51, 56, 62, 66] and Spain [1, 3, 6, 25, 27, 37, 38, 44, 55, 60, 61, 63, 65, 69], but CPH has been also diagnosed in patients from other European, American, Asian and Pacific countries, including Austria [2], Brazil [39], France [22, 29, 52], Germany [1, 6, 8, 11, 19, 31] Italy [30, 57, 64, 68], Korea [7, 12, 54], Malta [16], Mexico [50, 53], New Zealand [15], Peru [9], Poland [49], Serbia [40], Turkey [45] and the UK [58]. Of the 114 patients reported, 85 (74.6%) were women (female:male ratio 2.9:1). All but three cases were acquired and were diagnosed at a mean age of 62 years (range 17–84 years) [38, 39]. At the time of diagnosis, CPH had been present for several months, years or even decades, up to 40 years [15, 17]. Remarkably, three congenital cases have been reported [35, 44, 64].

J. Kanitakis (✉)
Department of Dermatology, Edouard Herriot Hospital, Lyon, France
e-mail: jean.kanitakis@univ-lyon1.fr

F. Rongioletti, B. R. Smoller (eds.), *New and Emerging Entities in Dermatology and Dermatopathology*, https://doi.org/10.1007/978-3-030-80027-7_4

Clinical Features

CPH manifests with well-circumscribed annular, erosion-like plaques with an erythematous, slightly depressed surface (corresponding to the area of hypokeratosis), rimmed by a slightly hyperkeratotic border (corresponding to the surrounding normal-thickness horny layer) (Figs. 1 and 2). The lesions usually measure 5–15 mm in diameter, the largest reported lesion measuring 7 cm [50]. They are single in most cases (87%); 2, 3 or 4 lesions were present in the same patient in 7%, 1% and 3% of cases, respectively. The maximum number of lesions reported is 14, and in this particular patient, they had a linear arrangement [17]. The lesions are almost invariably restricted to the palmoplantar skin. A unique case of non-palmoplantar (chest) localization of CPH has been reported [41]. In 80 cases (70%), the lesions were present on palmar skin, especially the thenar (50%) and hypothenar (14%) eminences. The lesions affected the fingers (palmar or more rarely dorsal aspects) in 18 patients (17%) [1, 10, 22, 24, 28, 29, 31, 32, 37, 47, 50, 52, 53, 55]. The right hand was slightly more often affected than the left one (52 vs 41). Bilateral palmar lesions were present in five patients [10, 28, 31, 39]. The lesions affected the soles in 17% of patients [1, 6, 17, 20–22, 29, 35, 38, 44, 48, 50, 57, 60], more often the left (n:11) than the right (n:6) one. Only one patient had both palmar and plantar lesions [17]. The lesions are in the majority of cases asymptomatic; mild pruritus [60], slight tenderness [67], burning sensation [4, 68], irritation [23] or pain [38] have been occasionally reported. In one case decreased sweating was evidenced in the diseased epidermis [62].

Dermatoscopic examination shows a homogeneous erythematous area with scattered white and red spots, representing acrosyringia and dermal vessels, respectively, surrounded by a peripheral keratotic collarette [33, 47, 52, 55, 57, 60, 61, 69]. This collarette is not double-edged as in porokeratosis, allowing distinction of these

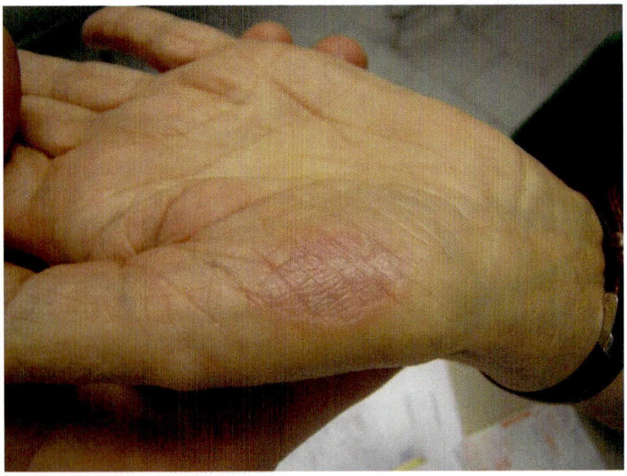

Fig. 1 Circumscribed palmar hypokeratosis presenting as a well-circumscribed, depressed, reddish lesion with a scaly border on the thenar eminence of a palm

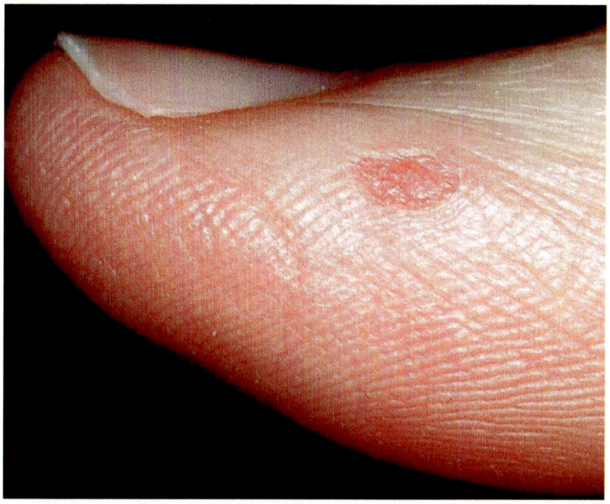

Fig. 2 Circumscribed palmar hypokeratosis presenting on a finger as a small annular, well-circumscribed plaque with an erythematous, slightly depressed surface bordered by a keratotic rim

two conditions which bear some clinical similarity [66]. The vessels [67] and acrosyringia [68] were poorly visible in two patients. High-frequency ultrasound examination has shown an abrupt change of double to single entrance echo in the transition zone of the lesion, highlighting the decrease of the thickness of the hyperechoic horny layer [51, 64, 68]. Optical coherence tomography, performed in four patients, identified the typical sharp step-off from the thick horny layer to the thin stratum corneum over the diseased epidermis [58, 68] and was able to detect also preclinical lesions in one patient [58]. In vivo confocal laser microscopy also can show the decrease of the horny layer thickness [68].

Some patients with CPH had associated diseases, including diabetes mellitus [3, 9, 45, 60], hypercholesterolaemia/dyslipidaemia [4, 9, 15], osteoarthritis [4, 24, 59], coronary artery disease [15, 45], hay fever [4, 15], arterial hypertension [17, 45], carcinoma of the stomach [12], breast [31] or the colon [45], periarteritis nodosa [3], depression [9], hypothyroidism [4], otosclerosis [3], tremor [17] and asthma [24]. These associations are likely fortuitous, explained by the age of the patients. Regarding skin diseases, CPH has been diagnosed in the setting of generalized atrophic benign epidermolysis bullosa [29], in patients with actinic keratoses [17, 29], chronic lupus erythematosus [25], squamous- and basal-cell cutaneous carcinomas [17], palmoplantar keratoderma of the Unna-Thost type [51] and disseminated superficial actinic porokeratosis [27]; this latter association was tentatively explained by the presence of abnormal clones of keratinocytes in genetically predisposed patients.

As CPH is almost invariably found on the extremities, the term ‘circumscribed acral hypokeratosis’ has been used [6, 17, 22, 24, 32, 35, 43–45, 52, 67, 69]; however, this has been considered less appropriate as other (non-palmoplantar) acral sites (such as the nose or ears) are not affected by CPH [71].

Histopathological Features

The microscopic aspect of CPH is characteristic and diagnostic, provided the biopsy includes the edge of the lesion. The characteristic finding is an abrupt and markedly decreased thickness of the horny layer overlaying the lesion, compared with the adjacent normal epidermis. The border between the decreased thickness and adjacent normal horny layer is usually sharp, often showing a stair-like configuration from the normal to diseased skin (Figs. 3 and 4); its border has sometimes a frayed appearance [1, 10, 18, 50]. This 'hypokeratosis' may affect also the acrosyringia present in the lesion [1], although these are often unaffected [21, 43, 45]. The decreased thickness horny layer may contain foci of parakeratosis [8, 10, 11, 19, 27, 31, 43, 45, 47, 50, 60]. The underlying granular layer is also often slightly thinned [12, 15, 16, 18, 19, 20–22, 25, 29, 32, 35, 37, 39, 42–44, 50–52, 54, 57, 59, 61, 63] but may be normal or more rarely slightly thickened [10, 17, 29, 60] and is very rarely vacuolated [50]. The underlying viable epidermis is usually unremarkable; it may be slightly acanthotic and/or papillomatous [17, 19, 22, 26, 29, 39, 44, 45, 47, 62], more rarely thinned [29, 63] or spongiotic [47]. PAS stain shows no fungi [1, 8, 22, 29, 45], in keeping with negative mycological examinations [30, 39]; it may disclose a scale crust defining the beginning of hypokeratosis [53]. No cornoid lamella is present, allowing differentiation from porokeratosis, which may also affect the palms [1]. The epidermis underneath the horny layer as a rule lacks atypia; however, two cases have been reported where the epidermis showed features of actinic keratosis (termed 'premalignant CPH', by analogy to premalignant/actinic keratosis) [72] or of Bowen disease/squamous cell carcinoma in situ ('malignant CPH') [67]. The dermis is usually unremarkable or shows minimal inflammation [18, 19, 30, 47, 50, 54, 55] and elastosis [1]. Dilatation of the dermal capillary vessels can be seen [22, 30, 33, 42, 50, 52, 55, 57, 63] accounting, along with the decreased thickness of the horny layer, for the erythematous appearance of the lesions.

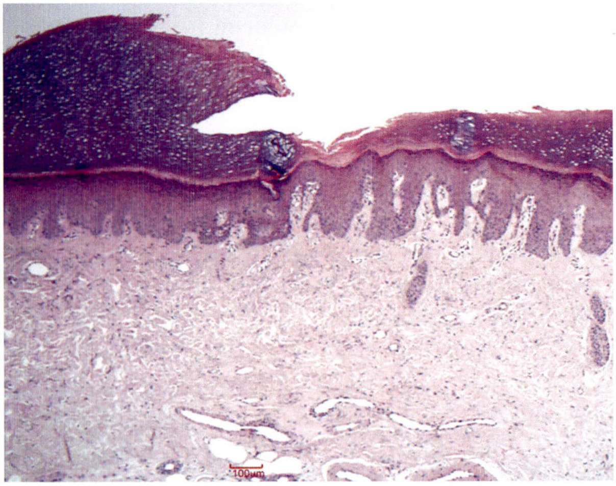

Fig. 3 Microscopic aspect of circumscribed palmar hypokeratosis showing an abrupt, well-demarcated decrease in the thickness of the stratum corneum (haematoxylin-eosin stain)

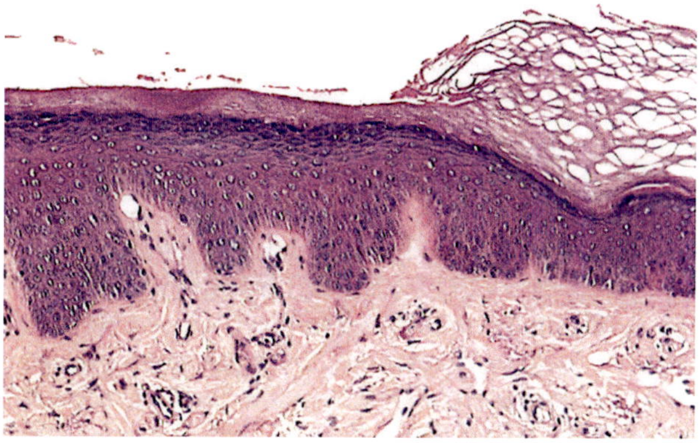

Fig. 4 Microscopic aspect of circumscribed palmar hypokeratosis: a stair-like thinning of the horny layer is seen (haematoxylin-eosin stain)

Several immunohistochemical studies have been performed in CPH, with inconsistent and often conflicting results, even between lesions of the same patient [28]. The expression of the hyperproliferative keratin (K) 16 has often been found increased [18, 28, 46, 56] but has also been reported normal [21, 34]. The expression of the hyperproliferative K6 has been reported increased [29, 56]; however, the expression of the cell cycle-associated antigen MIB-1/Ki-67 has been found normal [21, 29, 34, 52], increased [18, 19, 42, 56] or even decreased [22, 51]. K2e, expressed in the granular epidermal layer, is often reported decreased [18, 34, 66]. The expression of K9, found in the suprabasal palmoplantar epidermal layers, has also been often found decreased [21, 28, 34, 46, 51] but may be normal [18, 42, 66]. K10 has been found, according to the studies, normal [28, 56], decreased [42, 56] or increased [21, 51]. p53 expression in diseased epidermis has been found normal [21] or increased [19]. K7 and K20 were not expressed in diseased epidermis (as in the non-diseased one) [18]. Nuclear phospho-STAT3 expression was found diminished [56]. In one study, connexin 26 was found normal in one case and decreased in another, and on the basis of this finding, it was postulated that CPH may encompass two subtypes [21]; however, the wide variability of immunohistochemical profiles makes distinction of CPH into different subtypes questionable, at least on the basis of the antigenic profiles studied so far. Among other epidermal differentiation-associated antigens that have been studied, filaggrin was found decreased [18, 29, 42], loricrin decreased [42] and involucrin decreased [18, 42] or normal [29]. K5/14 [56], calprotectin, p63 and CD138/syndecan [29] were reportedly normally expressed in diseased epidermis. The expression of LEKTI and corneodesmosin was found decreased in three cases and slightly increased in two cases, whereas kallikrein 5 was found increased [29].

Electron-microscopic examination, performed in a few cases of CPH, has identified intracytoplasmic separation/breakage [66] and vacuolation of corneocytes [18], decreased maturation of keratinocytes [20], reduction of keratin bundles and keratohyalin granules [73], shorter keratin filaments in the spinous layer [66] and increased lipids in the horny layer [73]. Regarding attachment structures, two studies found them normal [18, 66], whereas another study noted early degradation of desmosomes in the upper granular layer and corneodesmosomes in the lower horny layer [26].

Differential Diagnosis

The clinical diagnosis of CPH has been very seldom suggested [1, 50]; however, the lesions have characteristic clinical features, so that CPH can be suspected on clinical grounds by physicians aware of this condition. CPH has usually been (mis) diagnosed clinically as porokeratosis [1, 3, 9, 12, 17, 41, 42] or Bowen disease [1, 6, 8, 29, 41, 42, 50], more rarely as psoriasis [8, 9], eczema/dermatitis [9, 10], actinic keratosis [29, 41], tinea [17, 50], squamous- [10, 41] or basal-cell carcinoma [6], keratosis *sulcatum* [22], irritated seborrheic keratosis [10], ulcerated fibroma [10] or *granuloma annulare* [29]. Dermatoscopic examination can aid in the diagnosis by showing the characteristic keratotic edge surrounding the hypokeratotic centre of the lesion. The definite diagnosis requires microscopic examination which shows the characteristic and specific finding, i.e. a sharp decrease of the horny layer. Of note, a microscopic aspect of CPH has been reported as an incidental finding in some clinically unrelated conditions occurring on the extremities (mainly palms and soles), such as neoplasms (SCC, poroma, dermatofibroma), verrucae, inflammatory processes (*lichen amyloidosus*, granulomatous inflammation associated to a ruptured epidermoid cyst), scars and fibrosing granulation tissue. This condition, reported under the term of 'pseudo-circumscribed palmar or plantar hypokeratosis' [73], has been tentatively attributed to a reaction pattern to trauma. Although it is microscopically indistinguishable from 'primary' CPH, it does not share the characteristic clinical appearance of CPH. A case of a lesion showing clinicopathologic features of CPH has been reported, which contained a cornoid lamella and was therefore diagnosed as solitary porokeratosis mimicking CPH [75]. Hypokeratosis has also been observed in a patient with multiple lesions of Bowen disease of the palms [76]. Microscopically, CPH should be distinguished from pitted keratolysis, which also shows defects in the horny layer; however, this disease – which also affects plantar skin – is due to Gram-positive bacteria that can be seen with special stains (Gram, PAS, Giemsa or methenamine silver), as coccoid or filamentous forms, within the horny layer; besides, the clinical setting is different.

Etiopathogenesis

Although CPH presents stereotypical clinicopathologic features, its aetiopathogenesis remains so far unclear. The disease was initially considered as a benign clonal epidermal malformation [1]; this hypothesis is consistent with the exceptional congenital cases reported [35, 44, 64], but is not supported by the late onset of the disease noted in the vast majority of cases. Repetitive (minor) trauma has been considered as a possible aetiologic factor as CPH mostly affects the dominant hand, so that CPH has been thought of as a 'forme fruste' of epidermolysis bullosa [10]. In fact, prior trauma (incision wound, cut, bird bite) or burn has been recalled by 12 patients [4, 6, 17, 36, 37, 45, 47, 57], and gardening, rubbing and the practice of embroidery have been considered as possible triggering factors [10, 29, 72]. Furthermore, features of CPH (in the so-called pseudo-CPH) have been considered as a possible reaction pattern to previous trauma [74]. However, correlation with dominant handedness is not invariable, and in half of the published cases, no triggering event preceding the onset of CPH was recalled by the patients; besides, even in cases with prior traumatisms, these occurred several years or decades before the diagnosis of CPH, so that their role in the provocation of CPH does not seem obvious. The role of HPV has been discussed as HPV-4 and HPV-6 have been detected in two cases [11, 17]; however, 18 other cases that were tested for HPV by various methods (immunohistochemistry, *in situ* hybridization, liquid-phase PCR, electron microscopy) proved HPV negative [1, 13, 14, 17, 18, 20, 22, 27, 31, 37, 42, 43, 45, 63, 65] so that the role of HPV in CPH seems, at least in the majority of cases, unlikely. The presence of corynebacteria has been occasionally reported on histological examination [22]; however, cultures, both bacterial [21] and mycological [30, 39], have remained sterile, and no lesion-specific bacteria were detected by 16 s microbial rRNA analysis [18] so that the role of any microorganism remains unproven. CPH has been regarded as a disorder of epidermal differentiation/keratinization involving the granular and horny layers [18, 20, 30, 42, 51]; however, the alterations in the expression of keratins and other epidermal differentiation antigens are inconsistent or even contradictory, even among lesions developing in the same patient [28] so that no universal theory based on the role of alterations in epidermal differentiation can be formulated. It has been hypothesized that CPH could be due to a clonal expansion of keratinocytes [56], which would lose their capacity to differentiate into hyperkeratotic palmoplantar corneocytes [28]. We have hypothesized that CPH may be due to an accelerated process of corneocyte desquamation, as suggested by the altered expression of molecules involved in this process, such as LEKTI, corneodesmosin and kallikrein 5 [29]. This hypothesis is supported by electron-microscopic findings of early production of Odland bodies and early degradation of (corneo)desmosomes in the uppermost epidermal layers, causing impairment of intercellular cohesion [26]. In fact, the pathogenesis of CPH is probably multifactorial. The disease could be due to the clonal expansion of abnormally differentiated keratinocytes, which would be unable to maintain their cohesion in the upper epidermal layers. Repeated micro-traumatisms could trigger the lesions, on a background of locally increased desquamation.

Therapy

No consistently efficient treatment for CPH exists. Various local physical and medical treatments have been tried with variable success. Excision has been performed in several patients [8, 13, 14, 50, 29, 41, 42, 45, 51, 56, 63] and no recurrences were reported in some of them [8, 50, 56, 63]. Cryotherapy (occasionally extended) proved successful in five patients [16, 32, 46, 58, 60] but was not efficient in two other cases [40, 48]. Successful treatment was reported in one patient after three sessions with the 10600-nm CO_2 fractional laser [54]. In one 17-year-old patient, a 2-month treatment with calcipotriol ointment led to practically complete regression of the lesion [38]. Another patient was improved with extended, 4.5-year application of calcipotriol ointment under occlusion [68]; however, vitamin D derivatives (calcipotriol, calcitriol, maxacalcitol) proved inefficient in the majority of patients in whom they were tried [10, 17, 18, 25, 26, 29, 44, 45, 47, 50, 54, 58]. One patient reportedly achieved slight improvement with a combination of calcipotriol and local betamethasone, but the treatment was discontinued because of irritation [60]. Partial remission was obtained with photodynamic therapy in one patient [19]. 5-Fluorouracil (5-FU) led to clearance of one of the lesions in one patient, but the lesion recurred 3 months after treatment discontinuation [31]. 5-FU and imiquimod produced slight improvement in one patient [22]; however, 5-FU proved unsuccessful in three other patients [17, 48, 67] and in the remaining lesions of the patient in whom one lesion responded [31]. Calcineurin inhibitors (tacrolimus/pimecrolimus) were mostly ineffective [18, 48, 56]; they achieved little improvement in one case [60]. Heparinoid-containing products failed in one case [56] and proved effective in another one [62]. The following treatments were invariably inefficient: local corticosteroids [1, 2, 8–10, 12, 15–18, 34, 36, 40, 47–49, 52, 54, 56, 58, 59, 61], vitamin A and retinoids (retinoic acid, tazarotene) [1, 2, 18, 40, 45, 54], emollients and hydrocolloid dressings [16, 29, 40, 52], antifungals (ketoconazole, clotrimazole) [36, 59], keratolytics (urea) [1, 18], zinc sulphate [18] and antibiotics [40]. It seems therefore that physical treatments (namely excision and cryotherapy) achieve better results than medical ones; however, excision may be uncomfortable on the palms, especially in the case of large lesions. Considering the asymptomatic and usually benign nature of the lesions, on the one hand, and the moderate efficacy of existing treatments, on the other, refraining from treatment appears as a reasonable, not infrequently adopted, option [5, 17, 22, 27, 50, 60].

Prognosis and Course

The course of CPH is chronic and benign. The lesions usually enlarge slowly over some months or years and then remain stable [2, 9, 15, 17–19, 21, 30, 32, 34, 40, 48, 57]. Remarkably, in one patient, bilateral lesions on the fingers resolved completely without treatment within 2 years after the biopsy [10]. The prognosis is in the vast majority of cases benign. However, the lesions of CPH may exceptionally harbour changes of *in situ* carcinoma (actinic keratosis or Bowen disease); therefore, follow-up of the patients for the possible development of keratinocytic neoplasms within the lesions seems advisable.

Conclusions

CPH is a rare, poorly known and probably underrecognized palmoplantar dermatosis, despite the fact that it has characteristic macroscopic and microscopic features, which enable physicians aware of the disease to suggest the diagnosis clinically.

The diagnosis can be confirmed by histopathological examination of a skin biopsy taken from the border of the lesion. The pathogenesis of CPH remains elusive, even though several theories have been proposed. The disease responds poorly to local medical treatments, but considering its usually benign nature, it does not necessarily warrant aggressive treatment. The study of more cases will hopefully shed more light on the pathogenesis of this enigmatic condition and help in discovering a satisfactory treatment.

References

1. Pérez A, Rütten A, Gold R, Urbina F, Misad C, Izquierdo MJ, Requena C, Aliaga A, Kutzner H, Requena L. Circumscribed palmar or plantar hypokeratosis: a distinctive epidermal malformation of the palms or soles. J Am Acad Dermatol. 2002;47:21–7.
2. Obermoser G, Zelger B. "Multifocal" circumscribed palmar hypokeratosis: malformation or not? J Am Acad Dermatol. 2003;49:1197–8.
3. Vives R, Valcayo AM, Hernandez R, Larringaga B. Hipoqueratosis palmar circunscrita. Actas Dermosifiliogr. 2003;94:491–2.
4. De Bloom JR 2nd, Ting W, Stone MS, Arpey CJ. Circumscribed palmar hypokeratosis. J Am Acad Dermatol. 2004;51:319–21.
5. Burnett JW, Harvey VM. Circumscribed palmar or plantar hypokeratosis: report of two additional cases. J Am Acad Dermatol. 2004;51:843.
6. Rütten A, Wecker-Brosi H, Gruhlke G, Kutzner H, de Castro LC, Requena L. Zirkumscripte akrale Hypokeratose. Hautarzt. 2004;55:1060–3.
7. Jeong YI, Chang SE, Lee MW, Choi JH, Moon KC, Koh JK. A case of circumscribed palmar hypokeratosis. Korean J Dermatol. 2004;42:111–3.
8. Mensing CH, Schleusner VH, Sander CA, Mensing H. Circumscribed palmar or plantar hypokeratosis: two cases of a recently described entity of unknown origin. Am J Dermatopathol. 2005;27:247–9.
9. García J, Catacora J, Montesinos P. Circumscribed palmar hypokeratosis: report of a clinical case. Folia Dermatol (Peru). 2005;16:137–9.
10. Resnik KS, DiLeonardo M. Circumscribed palmar hypokeratosis: new observations. Am J Dermatopathol. 2006;28:112–6.
11. Böer A, Falk TM. Circumscribed palmar hypokeratosis induced by papilloma virus type 4. J Am Acad Dermatol. 2006;54:908–9.
12. Lee SE, Kim YC, Kim SC. Circumscribed palmar or plantar hypokeratosis: report of a Korean case and published work review. J Dermatol. 2006;33:403–5.
13. Murata M, Saito Y, Mitsuto I. A case of circumscribed palmar hypokeratosis (in Japanese). Japan J Clin Dermatol. 2006;60:27–9.
14. Oshima M, Murao K, Takahashi O, Arase S. Circumscribed palmar or plantar hypokeratosis. Rinsho Derma (Tokyo). 2006;48:1679–81.
15. Jarrett P, Sutton T. Circumscribed palmar hypokeratosis. Australas J Dermatol. 2007;48:57–9.
16. Boffa MJ, Degaetano JS. Circumscribed palmar hypokeratosis: successful treatment with cryotherapy. J Eur Acad Dermatol Venereol. 2007;21:420–1.
17. Berk DR, Böer A, Bauschard FD, Hurt MA, Santa-Cruz DJ, Eisen AZ. Circumscribed acral hypokeratosis. J Am Acad Dermatol. 2007;57:292–6.
18. Ishiko A, Dekio I, Fujimoto A, Kameyama K, Sakamoto M, Benno Y, Amagai M, Nishikawa T. Abnormal keratin expression in circumscribed palmar hypokeratosis. J Am Acad Dermatol. 2007;57:285–91.
19. Benoit S, Seitz CS, Hamm H, Vetter-Kauczok CS, Bröcker EB. Circumscribed palmar hypokeratosis: partial remission by photodynamic therapy. Br J Dermatol. 2007;157:804–6.

20. Barry CI, Glusac EJ, Kashgarian M, Gwin K, McNiff JM. Circumscribed palmar hypokeratosis: two cases and a review of the literature. J Cutan Pathol. 2008;35:484–7.
21. Tanioka M, Miyagawa-Hayashino A, Manabe T, Toichi E, Miyachi Y, Takahashi K. Circumscribed palmo-plantar hypokeratosis: a disease with two subtypes. J Invest Dermatol. 2009;129:1045–7.
22. Cribier B, Fabre F, Merlio C, Antoni-Bach N. Hypokératose acrale circonscrite: forme plantaire et forme du dos du doigt (deux cas). Ann Dermatol Venereol. 2009;136:32–6.
23. Shen A, Markus R, Tschen J. Circumscribed palmar or plantar hypokeratosis (abstr). J Cutan Pathol. 2009;36:132.
24. Tutrone W, Niedt G, Salob S. A case of erythematous hand depressions. Arch Dermatol. 2009;145:195–200.
25. Fueyo-Casado A, Mallo-Garcia S, Martinez-Gonzalez C, Santos-Juanes J. Circumscribed palmar hypokeratosis. J Am Acad Dermatol. 2009;61:1090–1.
26. Yamamoto O, Yoshida Y, Adachi K, Yamada N. Abnormal cell attachment in circumscribed palmar hypokeratosis: ultrastructural observations. Br J Dermatol. 2011;164:1395–6.
27. Blanco-Barrios S, Cañueto J, Santos-Briz A, Unamuno P. Circumscribed palmar hypokeratosis associated with disseminated superficial actinic porokeratosis. Am J Dermatopathol. 2011;33:e21–3.
28. Yasuda M, Abe M, Suto M, Okada E, Nagai Y, Tamura A, Ishikawa O, Takahashi K. Circumscribed palmar hypokeratosis on both hands: distinct keratin expression in multiple depressed lesions. Br J Dermatol. 2011;164:211–3.
29. Kanitakis J, Lora V, Chouvet B, Zambruno G, Haftek M, Faure M. Circumscribed palmoplantar hypokeratosis: a disease of desquamation? Immunohistological study of five cases and literature review. J Eur Acad Dermatol Venereol. 2011;25:296–301.
30. Tosi D, Sala F, Crosti C. Circumscribed palmar or plantar hypokeratosis: report of an Italian case. Indian J Dermatol. 2011;56:211–3.
31. Wilk M, Zelger BG, Zelger B. Circumscribed palmar hypokeratosis: Successful treatment with fluorouracil cream. Dermatol Ther (Heidelb). 2011;1:11–4.
32. Butler LK, Kiracofe EA, Marks VJ. Circumscribed acral hypokeratosis: successful treatment of a potentially premalignant condition. Arch Dermatol. 2012;148:1427–8.
33. Nishimura M, Nishie W, Nakazato S, Nemoto-Hasebe I, Fujita Y, Shimizu H. Circumscribed palmar hypokeratosis: correlation between histopathological patterns and dermoscopic findings. Br J Dermatol. 2012;167:221–2.
34. Akasaka K, Maesawa C, Takahashi K, Masuda T, Akasaka T. Circumscribed palmar or plantar hypokeratosis: two cases and a review of published work. J Dermatol. 2012;39:314–5.
35. Arbesman J, Loss LC, Helm KF, Rothman IL. A congenital case of circumscribed acral hypokeratosis. Pediatr Dermatol. 2012;29:485–7.
36. DeBoyes T, Sherrod Q, El-Masry M, Williams EA, Chiu MW. Circumscribed palmar hypokeratosis. Int J Dermatol. 2012;51:486–8.
37. Riveiro-Falkenbach E, Rodríguez-Peralto JL. Circumscribed palmar hypokeratosis associated to a burn scar. Am J Dermatopathol. 2013;35:246–7.
38. Batalla A, de la Torre C. Circumscribed plantar hypokeratosis responding to topical calcipotriol. J Dermatol Case Rep. 2013;4:129–31.
39. Rocha LK, Nico MM. Circumscribed palmoplantar hypokeratosis: report of two Brazilian cases. An Bras Dermatol. 2013;88:623–6.
40. Lekić B, Janković B, Nikolić M. Circumscribed palmar hypokeratosis – the first case from south-east Europe. Acta Dermatovenerol Croat. 2013;21:39–42.
41. Groysman T, Rothfleisch J, Baldassano MF. Circumscribed palmar or plantar hypokeratosis: first report on a nonacral site with unique histologic features. Am J Dermatopathol. 2013;35:491–3.
42. Kawashima H, Kawachi Y, Fujisawa Y, Furuta J, Nakamura Y, Ishii Y, Ichikawa E, Otsuka F. Circumscribed palmar hypokeratosis: implication of suppression of early epidermal differentiation. Eur J Dermatol. 2013;23:261–2.

43. Houk L, Kauh Y, Lee J. Circumscribed palmar hypokeratosis: a new acral anomaly (abstr). J Am Acad Dermatol. 2007;56(Suppl. 2):AB83.
44. Santamarina-Albertos A, Noguera-Morel L, Feito-Rodríguez M, Beato-Merino MJ, de Lucas-Laguna R. Congenital circumscribed acral hypokeratosis. Pediatr Dermatol. 2013;30:e102–3.
45. Erkek E, Çetin ED, Sezer E, Sahin S. Circumscribed acral hypokeratosis: a report of 2 cases and a brief review of the literature. Cutis. 2014;93:97–101.
46. Kanayama Y, Fukai K, Sugawara K, Tsuruta D. Circumscribed palmoplantar hypokeratosis in a barber: Successful treatment using cryotherapy. J Dermatol. 2015;42:818–9.
47. Amakata M, Teraki Y. Case of circumscribed hypokeratosis on the dorsum of the index finger. J Dermatol. 2015;42:754–6.
48. Mitkov M, Balagula Y, Lockshin B. Circumscribed plantar hypokeratosis. Int J Dermatol. 2015;54:e203–5.
49. Polańska A, Bowszyc-Dmochowska M, Żaba R, Adamski Z, Pazdrowski J, Dańczak-Pazdrowska A. High-frequency ultrasonography (20 MHz) in circumscribed palmar hypokeratosis – new observations. Arch Med Sci. 2016;12:1389–91.
50. Ramos-Garibay A, Navarrete-Franco G, Venadero-Albarrán F, Domínguez-Gómez A, Trejo-Acuña JR, Salazar-DelValle JJ, Domínguez-Ugalde G, Rivera-Ramírez MO, Martínez-Ortega J, Gutiérrez-Bravo R, Martínez-Burillo G, Jurado S-CF. Circumscribed hypokeratosis: report on a series of 7 Mexican cases and review of the literature. Am J Dermatopathol. 2016;38:399–408.
51. Iwasaki A, Harada K, Maeda T, Nogita A, Matsumoto Y, Tsuboi R. Case of circumscribed palmar hypokeratosis in a patient with palmoplantar keratoderma. J Dermatol. 2016;43:1441–3.
52. Topin-Ruiz S, Debarre JM, Blanchard E, Kettani S, Valmier PJ, Martin L, Le Corre Y. Hypokératose acrale circonscrite (HAS): utilité diagnostique de la dermoscopie. Ann Dermatol Venereol. 2017;144:197–202.
53. Peña-Romero AG, Toussaint-Caire S, Domínguez-Cherit J. Periodic acid-schiff stain in circumscribed hypokeratosis. Am J Dermatopathol. 2017;39:709–11.
54. Lee JW, Kim DS, Park CO. Circumscribed palmoplantar hypokeratosis: successful treatment with the 10 600-nm carbon dioxide fractional laser. J Eur Acad Dermatol Venereol. 2017;31:e473–4.
55. Vilas Boas da Silva PT, Rodríguez-Lomba E, Avilés-Izquierdo JA, Ciudad-Blanco C, Suárez-Fernández R. Dermoscopic features of circumscribed palmar hypokeratosis. JAMA Dermatol. 2017;153:609–11.
56. Toyoshima A, Osada SI, Umebayashi Y, Manabe M. Mutually exclusive expression pattern of keratin markers for differentiation and proliferation in circumscribed palmar hypokeratosis. Br J Dermatol. 2017;177:e122–4.
57. Nazzaro G, Ponziani A, Brena M, Cavicchini S. Dermoscopy confirms diagnosis of circumscribed plantar hypokeratosis. J Am Acad Dermatol. 2017;76(2S1):S43–5.
58. Abignano G, Kapadia A, Lettieri G, Goodfield M, Emery P, McGonagle D, Del Galdo F, Mikeljevic J. Use of optical coherence tomography for the diagnosis of preclinical lesions of circumscribed palmar hypokeratosis. Clin Exp Dermatol. 2017;42:192–5.
59. D'Silva NC, Behrens E, Sturgeon A, Stetson C. Circumscribed palmar hypokeratosis. Dermatol Online J. 2018;24(3)
60. Aranguren-López I, Vildósola-Esturo S, Arias-Camisón I, López-Pestaña A. Circumscribed plantar hypokeratosis. Actas Dermosifiliogr. 2019;110:619–21.
61. Boix-Vilanova J, Montis-Palos MC, Giacaman A, Antón-Valentí E. Circumscribed palmar hypokeratosis: treatment with cryotherapy. Actas Dermosifiliogr. 2019;110:174–6.
62. Yamazaki Y, Munetsugu T, Satoh T. Circumscribed palmar hypokeratosis with sweating disturbance: successful treatment with a heparinoid-containing moisturizer. Eur J Dermatol. 2019;29:559–61.
63. Giacaman-von der Weth MM, Partarrieu-Mejías F, Ferrer-Guillén B, Hernández-Bel P. Circumscribed palmar hypokeratosis. J Cutan Pathol. 2019;46:713–6.

64. Bassi A, Oranges T, Massi D, Piccolo V, Mazzatenta C, Neri I. Congenital circumscribed plantar hypokeratosis. Int J Dermatol. 2020;59:e367–9.
65. Wechter T, Kantor R, Siamas K, Alapati U. Circumscribed palmoplantar hypokeratosis: a case report and review of the literature. Dermatol Online J. 2020;26:13030.
66. Kawai T, Kabata Y, Shinkuma S, Oginezawa M, Hayashi R, Hayatsu M, Abe RJ. Intracytoplasmic abnormality of corneocytes in circumscribed palmar or plantar hypokeratosis: ultrastructural observations. J Eur Acad Dermatol Venereol. 2020;34:e709–11.
67. Bibb LA, Rash JP, King R. Malignant circumscribed acral hypokeratosis. JAAD Case Rep. 2020;6:214–6.
68. Tognetti L, Fiorani D, Suppa M, Cinotti E, Fontaine M, Marmol VD, Rubegni P, Perrot JL. Examination of circumscribed palmar hypokeratosis with line-field confocal optical coherence tomography: dermoscopic, ultrasonographic and histopathologic correlates. Indian J Dermatol Venereol Leprol. 2020;86:206–8.
69. Rizo-Potau D, Marti-Marti I, Martin-Ortega E. Circumscribed acral hypokeratosis: a benign localized lesion in the palm. Indian J Dermatol Venereol Leprol. 2020; https://doi.org/10.4103/ijdvl.IJDVL_1095_19. Online ahead of print.
70. Nguyen J, Rutnin S, Rubin A. Circumscribed acral hypokeratosis. Cutis. 2013;91:18–20.
71. Urbina F, Pérez A, Requena L, Rütten A. Circumscribed palmar or plantar hypokeratosis 10 years after the first description: what is known and the issues under discussion. Actas Dermosifiliogr. 2014;105:574–82.
72. Kanitakis J, Lora V, Balme B, Roby J. Premalignant circumscribed palmar hypokeratosis: a new form of circumscribed palmar hypokeratosis? Dermatology. 2010;220:143–6.
73. Urbina F, Misad C, González S. Circumscribed palmar hypokeratosis: clinical evolution and ultrastructural study after prolonged treatment with topical calcipotriol. J Eur Acad Dermatol Venereol. 2005;19:491–4.
74. Groysman T, Baldassano MF. "Pseudo-circumscribed palmar or plantar hypokeratosis (Pseudo-CPH)": a histologic pattern secondary to trauma; further characterization of a known entity. Am J Dermatopathol. 2016;38:359–62.
75. Kim JH, Shim J, Park SW, Shin HT, Park JH, Lee DY. A case of solitary porokeratosis mimicking circumscribed palmar hypokeratosis. Ann Dermatol. 2015;27:233–4.
76. Nakai K, Yoneda K, Moriue J, Moriue T, Kubota Y. Hypokeratosis of multiple Bowen's disease of the palms. Dermatol Sin. 2017;35:100–1.

Necrotizing Infundibular Crystalline Folliculitis and Necrotizing Eosinophilic Folliculitis

Steven Kossard

Introduction

Although both necrotizing infundibular crystalline folliculitis (NICF) [1] and necrotizing eosinophilic folliculitis (NEF) [2] share necrosis as a feature, they are totally distinct in both their clinical and histopathological features. NICF was initially described as a perforating transepidermal process with urate-like crystals [3]. Subsequently, the folliculosebaceous nature has become recognized, although the necrotizing process is not clinically apparent, but on histopathology only the superficial infundibular ostial epithelium remains with total loss of follicular remnants [4]. In contrast necrotizing eosinophilic folliculitis (NEC) was initially defined as a disorder linked to atopy and presenting with gross nodular, inflammatory, ulcerative and necrotic lesions and not purely as an eosinophilic folliculitis [2]. NEF has also appeared as a florid variant of facial eosinophilic folliculitis accompanied by follicular mucinosis [5, 6]. NEF remains to be defined as an entity and ultimately may represent a complex presentation triggered by a highly activated innate immune response to follicular microbial super antigens in the setting of eosinophilic folliculitis. In contrast NICF is increasingly recognized as a distinctive entity that is folliculocentric. The development of NICF as a consequence of antitumour therapy with EGFR, VEGF [7] and PD-I inhibitors [8] offers an opportunity to explore the pathogenic process that underpins this enigmatic disorder. Relatively few cases of both forms of necrotizing folliculitis have been reported and many aspects remain unchartered.

S. Kossard (✉)
Kossard Dermatopathologists, Laverty Pathology, Macquarie Park, NSW, Australia

F. Rongioletti, B. R. Smoller (eds.), *New and Emerging Entities in Dermatology and Dermatopathology*, https://doi.org/10.1007/978-3-030-80027-7_5

Necrotizing Infundibular Crystalline Folliculitis

Clinical Features

NICF has distinct clinical features that can be recognized. The process is often eruptive with multiple folliculocentric pale fibrillar and waxy plugs that are localized particularly to the folliculosebaceous skin sites over the forehead (Fig. 1a) and back [1, 4, 9–12]. The follicular nature of the process has been recognized and shares

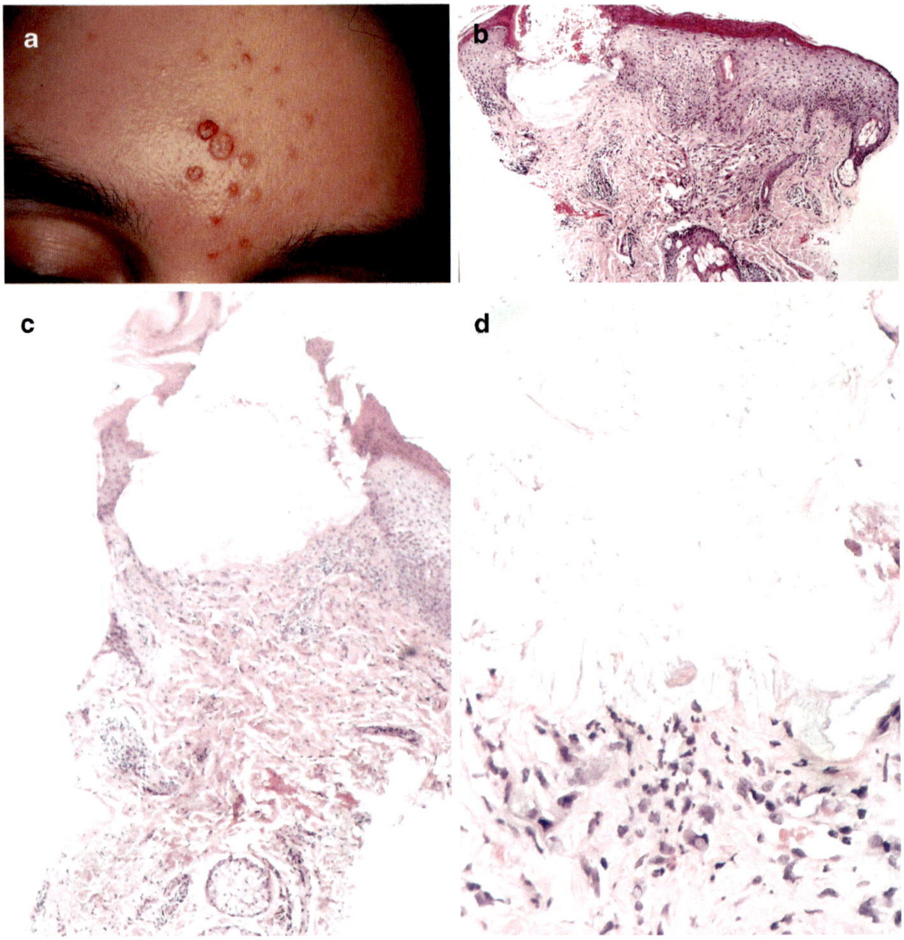

Fig. 1 (**a**) Clinical presentation with matted waxy fibrillar follicular plugs on the forehead. (**b**)Epidermal parakeratosis, dilated follicular cavity, superficial infundibular ostial remnant and bare interface of crystalline contents with dermis (H&E, ×40). (**c**) Base and sides of bare cavity lacking a lining as a result of infundibular necrosis (H&E, ×100). (**d**) Detail of cavity with minimal dermal inflammation at the base and no granulomatous response to vertically orientated crystalline filaments (H&E, ×250)

features with keratotic perforating disorders. The process is relatively uncommon, and in a tabulation of 21 published cases, the patients were 16–85 years old and most were elderly [8]. Acneiform lesions predominated on the forehead. The eruption usually was synchronous and nonrecurrent. The process can spontaneously remit and usually settles with topical treatments. NICF has developed in patients receiving antitumour targeted therapies with EGFR and VEGF [7], both of which are known to trigger follicular eruptions. A patient receiving PD-1 inhibitor developed dermatomal NICF in the area of previous herpes zoster [8]. This induction of NICF by these biological-based therapies offers potential fresh insights into the activation of elusive pathogenic pathway for NICF.

Histopathology

NICF has a distinctive histopathology with distended infundibular cavities filled by a pale sebaceous plug containing urate-like crystalline filaments (Fig. 1b). The base of the cavities lacks an epithelial lining and is bounded by a bare dermis (Fig. 1c). The interface with the dermis shows only scant inflammation without a granulomatous component (Fig. 1d). Although the crystalline material was initially viewed as a transepidermal elimination of dermally located crystalline material [3], this has not been demonstrated on histopathology. The orifice of the cavity is often lipped by parakeratosis [2] and the orifice expanded [6]. The crystalline contents polarize and at least partially consist of tonofilaments demonstrated on ultrastructure [4] but are likely to be more complex. A physical and chemical reaction to the mix sebum, cholesterol yeast and bacteria may play a role in crystal formation. Mucin has also been demonstrated as a component of the amorphous sebaceous mix [11]. The infundibular nature of the process can be difficult to recognize due to the consumption of the infundibular epithelial wall leaving only the orifice [1].

Work-Up

No work-up is necessary for NICF except for a biopsy to confirm diagnosis and a review of the medical history in reference to previous destructive folliculitis such as acne, bacterial or viral scarring folliculitis and whether the patient is receiving antitumour biological inhibitor agents.

Differential Diagnosis

Both the clinical and histopathological aspects of NICF are distinctive, but the condition is rare and is not a widely recognized entity. The clinical presentation may appear as a folliculitis, an acneiform process or an unusual perforating disorder. The crystalline infundibular pathology admixed with yeast and bacteria may be observed incidentally in skin biopsies without the clinical features of NICF [1]. Although initially viewed as a transepidermal elimination of urate-like crystals, the follicular nature of NICF has been recognized and the crystals linked to sebum production admixed with organisms and not as dermally sourced crystals. Significantly, in the setting of antitumour therapy with EFGR and VEGF that are known to induce inflammatory folliculitis as a common side effect [13], NICF has developed as a distinct recognizable presentation.

Etiopathogenesis

The aetiopathogenesis of NICF remains undetermined. Crystalline pattern of folliculitis may be seen within expanded infundibular canals without the full clinical or histopathological features of NICF. Clinically NICF is usually eruptive and diffuse with distinctive waxy fibrillar plugged follicular ostia. Nonetheless, this indicates the likely infundibular localization of the process and the capacity of the mix of sebum admixed with yeast and bacteria to undergo crystallization shared with NICF. However, in NICF only the orifical infundibular component remains and the rest of the follicle is no longer retained. The reason for this paradoxical feature remains to be determined. The development of NICF after antitumour therapy with EFGR and VEGF raises the issue whether there is a basic folliculogenic stem cell pathway that is activated and disrupted leading to this enigmatic histopathology.

Therapy

Most reported cases of NICF have been treated by topical corticosteroids, topical keratolytics agents, antimycotic agents or emollients [1, 8]. Spontaneous resolution may also occur. In the cases of NICF induced by antitumoural therapies, one patient who received a VEGF inhibitor (bevacizumab) and then subsequently an EGFR inhibitor (panitumumab), cyclical recurrences developed after each administration [7]. A second patient had continuous lesions until the EGFR inhibitor (erlotinib) was stopped. The true drug-related association of NICF with this class of agents is documented in these cases.

Prognosis and Course

NICF usually is a self-limited process that can be either spontaneous or following topical treatments such as topical corticosteroids or keratolytics often without a relapse. In the case of antitumour biologic therapy-related NICF, the occurrence appears uncommon and manageable.

Necrotizing Eosinophilic Folliculitis

Clinical Features

Disorders classified as eosinophilic folliculitis are by definition characterized by follicular pustules that are pruritic and dominated by eosinophils on histopathology rather than neutrophils. Pruritus is often a feature and three main subtypes have been classified as Ofuji's disease, eosinophilic folliculitis of infancy and HIV-related eosinophilic folliculitis [14–17]. The arciform pustular eruption of Ofuji's disease usually localized to the face serves as a clinical indicator, but there are no distinctive features for this group of disorders that often require histopathology for diagnosis. However, eosinophilic folliculitis can occur in diverse settings such as follicular tinea, parasitic infestation and follicular mucinosis [18] or as an independent process.

NEF has rarely been reported as an acute form of eosinophilic folliculitis, but the basis for the necrosis remains uncertain as does the pathogenic forces resulting in ulcerative, erosive pustular lesions which can be nodular or emerge as crusted plaques with a dark eschar. NEF was originally used to define a series of ten atopic individuals with diverse clinical features including three cases presenting as Ofuji's disease anchored by distinctive histopathology including vasculitis. A subsequent case report documented a woman who developed extensive ulcerative and crusted lesions with an explosive onset on her face (Fig. 2a). A specific diagnosis could not be reached with the clinical presentation and required histopathology.

Histopathology

The histopathology of NEF is not distinctive and by definition requires the presence of prominent follicular eosinophilic spongiosis and variable eosinophilic follicular micro abscesses (Fig. 2b–d). This feature is not limited to conditions currently defined clinically as eosinophilic folliculitis. Eosinophils are not solely present and are accompanied by lymphocytes and to a variable degree neutrophil and histiocytes that may play a key pathogenic role particularly in the necrotizing subset. The histopathological basis for the clinical necrosis and ulceration in NEF at this time remains uncertain. Vasculitis and the presence of extensive toxic eosinophil degranulation are expressed as collagen necrosis and dermal flame figures in atopy-related NEF. Follicular mucinosis may also be apparent in follicles containing eosinophils [18], and there is overlap with follicular mucinosis that is eosinophil rich.

Work-Up

NEF at present is not a well-defined entity either clinically or by histopathology. Due to the acute nature of NEF and the potentially destructive and scarring nature of the process, work-up needs to be broad including FBC, metabolic screen and

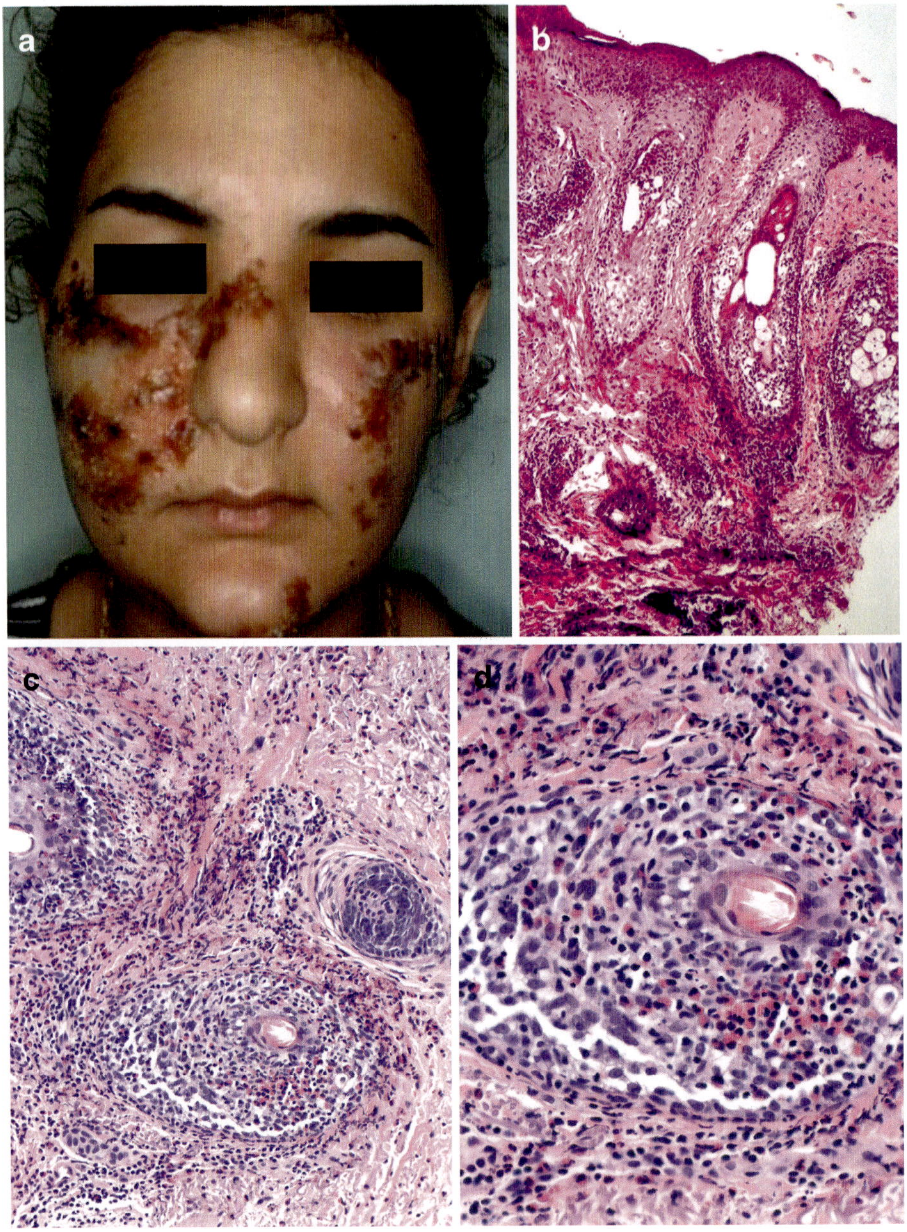

Fig. 2 (**a**) Erosive, necrotizing and crusted facial lesions in patient with pustular and dark eschars. (**b**) Histopathology with folliculocentric inflammation and follicular spongiosis that showed mucinosis (H&E, ×40). (**c**) Follicular and perifollicular inflammation dominated by eosinophils and lymphocytes (H&E, ×100). (**d**) Detail of follicle with eosinophilic spongiosis, lymphocytes and scattered neutrophils (H&E, ×250)

possibly elevated IgE as a reflection of atopy. Other investigations that may be needed are dependent on the medical history and presentation and further potential associations. By definition skin biopsy must reveal eosinophilic folliculitis to consider this as a diagnosis. Bacterial cultures may be required to address the potential inciting cofactor of bacteria in the pathogenesis of NEF and for therapy at presentation due to the clinical features with a potentially destructive outcome.

Differential Diagnosis

The nosology of eosinophilic folliculitis itself remains uncertain, and it is doubtful that all the current forms are necessarily unified pathogenically. The basis for the acute necrotizing aspect seen in the setting of atopy as well as an acute necrotizing facial eruption remains unknown. Clinically the facial presentation had an initial differential diagnosis that included pyoderma faciale, halogenoderma and impetigo, and the diagnosis emerged subsequently on histopathology and bacterial cultures which were negative. Although the presentation could be viewed as an acute flare of Ofuji's disease, the pustular aspect was such that cephalexin was combined with indomethacin as initial treatment, but the antibiotic was ceased. Currently NEF is not fully characterized to form a distinct entity for the purpose of differential diagnosis.

Etiopathogenesis

Aetiopathogenesis of NEF is difficult to determine due to its rarity and its indefinite status in respect to eosinophilic folliculitis per se as a crucial pathogenic factor. Eosinophil granules are toxic to tissue producing flame figures and tissue necrosis. Well's syndrome with eosinophilic cellulitis is the prototype for eosinophilic flame figures, and at times the syndrome can present with bullous lesions [19], but a necrotizing form has not been documented. In the group of atopic patients with NEF, eosinophilic vasculitis was noted as a basis for the necrosis [2]. The latter is seen particularly with allergic granulomatous polyangiitis that may also have eosinophilic flame figs [20]. and may share features with NEF. Activation of the Th2 pathway linked to atopy has been suggested as a pathogenic factor [2]. Both lymphocytes and neutrophils contribute to inflammatory cascade and may be driving forces. NEF related to atopy often responded to dapsone that targets neutrophils [2] raising the issue whether the marked reaction is connected to the sudden activation of innate immunity.

Therapy

There are too few cases of NEF to assess the most appropriate therapy. Indomethacin has been chosen as it is the most effective treatment for non-necrotizing forms of eosinophilic folliculitis, particularly Ofuji's disease [21]. Due to the erosive and pustular nature of NEF, indomethacin has been combined with cephalexin as bacterial culture may reveal *Staphylococcus aureus* and in one case of NEF recurred when the antibiotic was ceased [2]. In the case of atopy-related NEF, a wide variety of agents were used, particularly dapsone. In one patient cephalexin resulted in clearing the NEF, but microbial cultures in this series of patients only revealed *Staphylococcus epidermidis* in two patients despite their atopic background [2]. Both NEF and other variants of eosinophilic folliculitis may be difficult to control and subject to flares.

Prognosis and Course

The prognosis and course of NEF is difficult to determine given the uncertainty of a defined entity. The process is often a challenge to control, and therapy was varied but usually included indomethacin or dapsone before responding but subject to flares.

Conclusions Regarding NICF and NES

NICF is increasingly recognized as an entity with distinctive clinical and histopathological features, despite having an enigmatic pathogenesis. In contrast, the nosology of NEF remains undefined. NEF is likely to represent a heterogeneous process due to the varied clinical presentations and the uncertain role of eosinophilic folliculitis that is the defining criterion, and this also applies to the subset of patients presenting with necrotizing clinical features.

References

1. Denisjuk N, Hilty N, Pfaltz M, Kempf W. Necrotizing infundibular crystalline folliculitis: a clinicopathological study. J Am Acad Dermatol. 2012;66:823–6.
2. Magro CM, Crowson AN. Necrotising eosinophilic folliculitis as a manifestation of the atopic diathesis. Int J Dermatol. 2000;39:672–7.
3. Lucke TW, Fallowfield MF, Evans A, et al. Transepidermal elimination of urate-like crystals: a new perforating disorder? Brit J Dermatol. 1999;141:310–4.
4. Kossard S, Scurry J, Killingsworth M. Necrotizing infundibular crystalline folliculitis. Brit J Dermatol. 2001;145:165–8.
5. Kossard S. Necrotizing eosinophilic folliculitis with mucinosis. Australas J Dermatol. 2003;44:298–301.
6. Fallah F, Dunlop K, Kossard S. Successful treatment of recalcitrant necrotizing eosinophilic folliculitis using indomethacin and cephalexin. Australas J Dermatol. 2006;47:281–5.

7. Fattouh K, Collet-Benzaquen D, Provensal AM, et al. Necrotizing infundibular crystalline folliculitis (NICF) induced by anti-tumoral therapies: report of 2 cases. Am J Dermatopathol. 2017;39:764–6.
8. Fischer AS, Pei S, Shields BE, et al. Dermatomal necrotizing infundibular crystalline folliculitis following herpes zoster in a patient on PD-1 inhibitor therapy. J Cutan Pathol. 2020;47:502–5.
9. Cadoso JC, Leonard J, Carton J, Calonje E. Multiple follicular papules on bac of an elderly man. Necrotizing infundibular crystalline folliculitis (NICF). JAMA Dermatol. 2013;149:1233–4.
10. Saxer-Sekulic N, Vion-Gauthery B, Gurken K. Necrotizing infundibular crystalline folliculitis: a case report of an exceptional lesion of unknown etiology. Dermatopathology. 2014;1:3–6.
11. Fraga GR, Gadzia JE, Abraham JL, Machan M. Necrotizing infundibular crystalline folliculitis manifesting as a perforating mucinosis: a case report. Am J Dermatopathol. 2013;35:757–60.
12. Yim S, Yang J, Nam JH, Chae SW. A case of necrotizing infundibular crystalline folliculitis. Int J Dermatol. 2019;58:846–8.
13. Liza A, Agero C, Dusza W, et al. Dermatologic side effects associated with the epidermal growth factor receptor inhibitors. J Am Acad Dermatol. 2006;55:657–70.
14. Ofugi S, Ogino A, Horio T, et al. Eosinophilic pustular folliculitis. Acta Dermatol Venereol. 1970;50:195–203.
15. Nervi SJ, Schwartz RA, Dmochowski M. Eosinophilic pustular folliculitis: a 40-year retrospective. J Am Acad Dermatol. 2006;55:285–9.
16. Katoh M, Nomura T, Miyachi Y, Kabashima K. Eosinophilic pustular folliculitis: a review of the Japanese published works. J Dermatol. 2013;40:15–20.
17. Tang MB, Tan E, Chua SH. Eosinophilic pustular folliculitis (Ofugi's disease) : a review of 23 adult cases. Australas J Dermatol. 2003;44:44–7.
18. Munoz-Aceituno E, Vega-Gonzalez R, Martinez-Palazuelos S, et al. Association between eosinophilic folliculitis and follicular mucinosis. A case series. Int J Dermatol. 2020; https://doi.org/10.1111/ijd.14980.
19. Fugimoto N, Wakabayashi M, Kato T, et al. Wells' syndrome associated with Churg-Strauss syndrome. Clin Exp Dermatol. 2011;36:46–8.
20. Gillian AE, Bruckner AL, Howard RM, et al. Bullous "cellulitis" with eosinophilia : a case report and review of Wells' syndrome in childhood. Pediatrics. 2005;116:e149–55.
21. Ota T, Hata Y, Tanikawa A, et al. Eosinophilic pustular folliculitis (Ofugi's disease) indomethacin as a first choice of treatment. Clin Exp Dermatol. 2001;26:179–81.

Annular Erythema: New and Revisited Variants

Chiara Colato, Martina Maurelli, and Giampiero Girolomoni

Introduction

Several skin diseases present with cutaneous annular lesions. Some of these disorders are variants of common diseases including psoriasis, lichen planus, lupus erythematosus, tinea, urticaria, sarcoidosis, and drug eruptions [1]. Other disorders are less frequent but typically feature annular lesions including erythema annulare centrifugum, granuloma annulare, erythema gyratum repens, erythema chronicum migrans, and erythema marginatum. In addition, there are rare variants of annular erythema whose distinction and diagnosis may be challenging. These variants are discussed here. In general, they are all benign disorders, but their nosographic positioning, etiopathogenesis, and treatment are still debated or unknown.

Annually Recurring Erythema Annulare Centrifugum

Introduction Annually recurring erythema annulare centrifugum (AR-EAC) is a rare EAC variant characterized by the appearance of annular plaques usually localized to the extremities and recurring strikingly in the same period of the year. The lesions regress spontaneously after a variable period of days to few weeks [2–4].

C. Colato (✉)
Section of Pathology, Department of Diagnostics and Public Health, University of Verona, Verona, Italy
e-mail: chiara.colato@aovr.veneto.it

M. Maurelli · G. Girolomoni
Section of Dermatology and Venereology, Department of Medicine, University of Verona, Verona, Italy

F. Rongioletti, B. R. Smoller (eds.), *New and Emerging Entities in Dermatology and Dermatopathology*, https://doi.org/10.1007/978-3-030-80027-7_6

Clinical Features Only 14 cases have been described. Patient age ranged from 16 to 83 years, with a mean age of 47 years. In most cases AR-EAC has been observed in women with a M:F = 1:2.4. The disorder is characterized by annular erythematous plaques that enlarge centrifugally with central clearing (Fig. 1a). A fine scale may be present inside the advancing edge. In most cases, lesions involve the extremities, in particular thighs and legs, and less frequently the trunk with moderate pruritus. Annual recurrences are more commonly in summer or spring.

Histopathological Features The epidermis presents with mild acanthosis, patchy spongiosis, slight parakeratosis, and mild exocytosis. An inflammatory perivascular lympho-histiocytic infiltrate of variable intensity is present in the papillary and mid-dermis, with occasional eosinophils (Fig. 1b).

Etiopathogenesis The majority of cases are idiopathic. It has been hypothesized that AR-EAC is the result of a hypersensitivity reaction to some external or internal causative factors (insect bite, infectious diseases, hormonal disturbances, drugs, and neoplasms) [3, 4]. An association with hereditary lactate dehydrogenase M-subunit deficiency has been described in three cases.

Differential Diagnosis EAC, erythema papulatum centrifugum, and other annular erythematous skin diseases, such as erythema chronicum migrans, erythema marginatum, and urticaria.

Prognosis Benign disorder, but it may recur for years. The lesions resolve spontaneously without leaving skin marks.

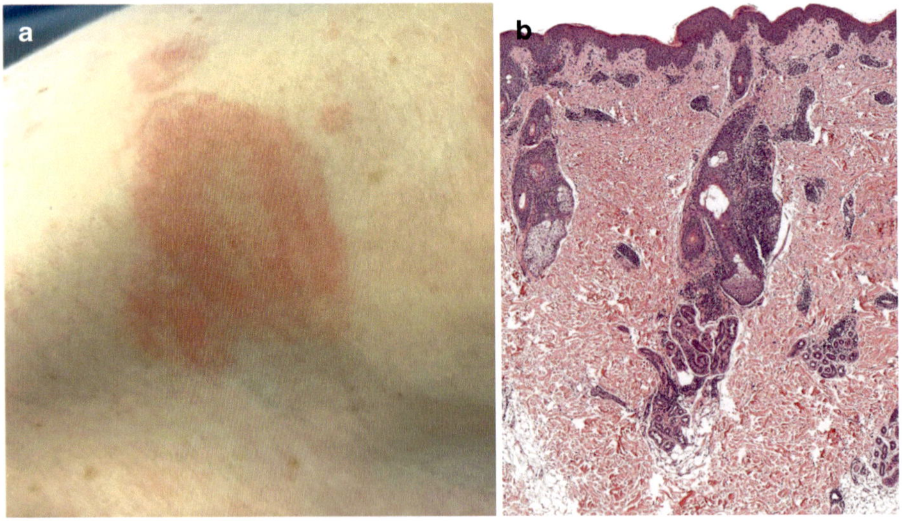

Fig. 1 Annual recurring erythema annulare centrifugum. (**a**) Female, 34 years old. Erythematous self-healing annular plaques, presenting for 3 years always in spring. (**b**) An inflammatory perivascular lympho-histiocytic infiltrate of variable intensity in the dermis, with occasional eosinophils (hematoxylin & eosin, ×100)

Therapy Topical medium-high potency corticosteroids and a brief course of systemic corticosteroids lead to a faster disappearance of the lesions.

Neutrophilic Figurate Erythema

Introduction Neutrophilic figurate erythema (NFE) originally described to occur in infancy is a rare benign inflammatory dermatosis characterized by annular or polycyclic indurated erythematous plaques and histologically by an inflammatory infiltrate with numerous neutrophils and nuclear debris without signs of vasculitis [5–7].

Clinical Features Only five cases in pediatric patients have been reported with a male to female prevalence, M:F = 1:4. The age range is from 9 months to 2 years [6]. About 20 cases have been described in adults, with a female prevalence M:F = 1:2.5 [5]. Lesions are annular or polycyclic plaques with raised, firm erythematous border and trailing scales (Fig. 2a). Blisters and purpuric lesions have also been reported [7]. They are asymptomatic or mildly pruritic [5–7]. In adults, NFE manifests as a single lesion, whereas in all infants' lesions are multiple. Lesions are mainly localized on the trunk and limbs [5].

Histopathological Features Lesions show normal epidermis without or very limited spongiosis or parakeratosis. The dermis is dominated by a superficial and deep perivascular and interstitial infiltrate with numerous neutrophils and nuclear dust. Lymphocytes, histiocytes, and rare plasma cells and eosinophils may be present

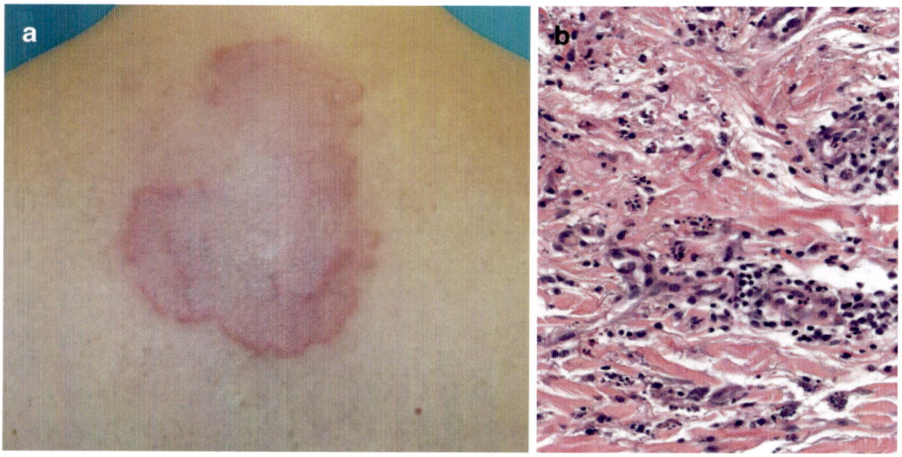

Fig. 2 Neutrophilic figurate erythema. Age and sex. (**a**) Annular plaque of 9 × 7 cm with central clearing on the back (permission). (**b**) Normal appearing epidermis. In the upper and mid-dermis, there is a moderate inflammatory infiltrate composed of numerous neutrophils, nuclear debris, lymphocytes and histiocytes, rare plasma cells, and eosinophils (hematoxylin & eosin, ×100)

(Fig. 2b). Focal extravasated erythrocytes have been described, but no signs of vasculitis are evident [5–7].

Etiopathogenesis The majority are idiopathic and have been hypothesized to be a hypersensitivity reaction to an unidentified antigen.

Differential Diagnosis Erythema gyratum repens, erythema marginatum, tinea corporis, Sweet syndrome, paraneoplastic neutrophilic figurate erythema, granuloma annulare, erythema annulare centrifugum, erythema chronicum migrans, erythema gyratum atrophicans transiens neonatale, annular erythematous lesions, eosinophilic annular erythema and annular erythema of infancy, urticaria, and small vessel vasculitis.

Prognosis Benign, with lesions persisting for weeks or months.

Therapy Topical and systemic steroids, dapsone, colchicine.

Palpable Migratory Arciform Erythema

Introduction Palpable migratory arciform erythema (PMAE) is a very rare cutaneous disease first described by Clark et al. in 1974 as a unique entity in the set of lymphocytic infiltrations of the skin [8]. Since then, only 15 cases of PMAE have been reported. Its nosological classification is still controversial: over time, it has been considered as a distinct skin disease, a subtype of T-cell pseudolymphoma, a rare variant of Jessner-Kanof disease, or a variant of erythema annulare centrifugum [8–11]. An alternative term used to identify this entity is erythema migrans arciforme et palpable [10].

Clinical Features PMAE preferentially affects adult individuals with slight gender predisposition (male to female ratio of 1.5:1) and mean age of onset 49 years. Most cases (67%) have been reported from Europe. The predilection site of PMAE is the upper trunk with back, neck, arms, and thighs being additional sites [9, 10, 12]. The lesions are usually asymptomatic, but itchy or a burning sensation has been reported in some patients. The clinical picture is characterized by multiple annular erythematous lesions with sharply elevated borders that rapidly enlarge with centrifugal arciform progression and central clearing, sometimes growing to a diameter of 20 cm or more (Fig. 3a). The lesions are strictly dynamic and change within days or week, with occurrence of new lesions and/or spontaneous regression of existing ones. This distinctive clinical evolution justifies the term "migratory" [8, 9]. Serological screening for *Borrelia*, *Treponema pallidum*, and viral infections and testing for antinuclear antibodies are always negative [12].

Histopathologic Features The histological findings show a moderate to abundant perivascular and periadnexal lymphocytic infiltrate throughout the reticular dermis, with no epidermal involvement and a lack of plasma cells (Fig. 3b). No interstitial infiltrates or mucin deposition is found. Lymphocytes are predominantly T cells

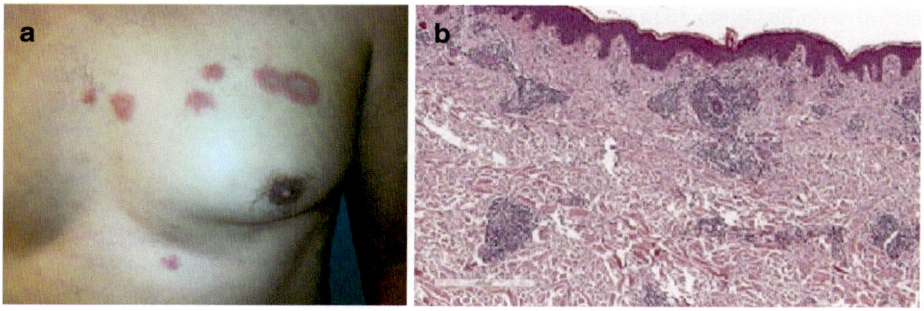

Fig. 3 Palpable migratory annular erythema. Age and sex. (**a**) Multiple annular erythematous plaques on the trunk. (**b**). Epidermis is uninvolved and a perivascular and periadnexal lymphocytic infiltrate is seen throughout the reticular dermis

(CD4 > CD8+) with a small B-cell and histiocytic component. CD1a+ cells are absent and CD30+ cells are below 1% [9, 10]. Direct immunofluorescence analysis is always negative [9, 12]. TCR-ϒ gene rearrangement study usually demonstrates polyclonality. Only one case revealed a clonal TCR-ϒ gene rearrangement [12] (Fig. 4).

Etiopathogenesis The etiology is unknown. Although a good response to antibiotic treatment was observed in most of the reported cases, evidence of infection was never found. An iatrogenic etiology was suggested for two patients taking diclofenac for fibromyalgia, but the lesions recurred a few weeks after drug withdrawal. Based on current knowledge, an auto-inflammatory/reactive process triggered by a variety of stimuli seems to be the most likely cause [12].

Differential Diagnosis The clinical differential diagnosis includes Jessner-Kanof, lupus erythematosus tumidus, deep erythema annulare centrifugum, erythema chronicum migrans, polymorphous light eruption, granuloma annulare, and annular plaque of mycosis fungoides [12].

Prognosis PMAE typically runs a chronic course and often tends to recur after weeks despite treatment attempts. Complete spontaneous regression of the lesions has only been described in isolated cases after years of persistence [9, 12].

Therapy Topical steroid, penicillins, cephalosporins, and PUVA or UVA-1 phototherapy have been used with variable results. Recently, low-dose hydroxychloroquine has been indicated as a possible treatment for steroid-refractory or relapsing PMAE [12].

Eosinophilic Annular Erythema

Introduction Eosinophilic annular erythema (EAE) is a rare, benign skin disorder that was first described by Kahofer et al. in 2000 as a recurrent annular erythema with marked tissue eosinophilia and absence of "flame figures" [13]. It is still a matter of debate whether EAE represents an annular variant of Wells syndrome or a separate entity [14, 15]. The condition was originally believed to be closely related to annular erythema of infancy, but currently is regarded as distinct [14, 16].

Clinical Features About 40 cases of EAE in adults and fewer than 10 cases in children have been reported. Among adult patients, there is a slight female preponderance (female:male ratio 1.14:1), and age at onset varies from 20 to 85 years [16]. Lesions generally occur on the trunk and extremities with rare involvement of the face, axilla, groin, or palms and soles [15]. They are usually asymptomatic, sometimes itchy or tender [15, 16].

EAE presents in one of two patterns: as a figurate/centrifugum-type pattern resembling deep erythema annulare centrifugum or as an urticarial/annular-type pattern reminiscent of granuloma annulare [14]. It begins as solitary or multiple recurring erythematous nodules or papules that evolve into annular, polycyclic, or gyrate plaques with central clearing and elevated erythematous border. The plaques may vary in size from 1 to 30 cm, correlating to their duration and heal without sequelae or rarely with hyperpigmentation [15, 16]. A single case of bullous eosinophilic annular erythema has been reported [17]. Laboratory tests usually are noncontributory although in some cases may show peripheral eosinophilia. It has been associated with various systemic diseases including underlying neoplasms, autoimmune disease, and infections [15, 16].

Histological Features Histologically, EAE is characterized by a dense superficial and deep perivascular and interstitial lympho-histiocytic infiltrate with abundant eosinophils. Basal vacuolar degeneration and dermal mucin deposition have been described in a few cases. Classically, "flame figures" or granulomatous reactions are absent, but their presence has been reported in long-lasting lesions in some patients [14, 15]. Direct immunofluorescence is negative [17].

Etiopathogenesis The etiology is not still understood. Currently the entity is considered as a hypersensitive reaction to various unidentified triggers that cause release of IL-5 and increase in eosinophil chemotaxis. IL-4 and IL-13 released by activated eosinophils can be important in pathogenesis [16, 18].

Differential Diagnosis The main differential diagnosis of EAE is Wells syndrome; other differential diagnoses include annular erythema of infancy, figurate erythemas, urticaria, urticarial bullous pemphigoid, subacute lupus erythematosus, and insect-bite and drug reactions.

Prognosis EAE typically runs a chronic relapsing and remitting course. Rarely, the disease can be self-limited and could resolve with no treatments [19].

Therapy Generally, EAE is resistant to multiple treatments and there is currently no gold-standard treatment. Systemic steroids and antimalarials are the usual first-line option. Other therapeutic options include dapsone, indomethacin, cyclosporine, nicotinamide, and ultraviolet B phototherapy [16]. Recently, dupilumab and mepolizumab have been suggested as new safe and effective therapeutic options for this rare disease [16, 18]. The proper management of coexisting diseases has proven to be helpful in increasing the efficacy of EAE treatment, prolonging the remission period, and decreasing the relapse rate.

Annular Lichenoid Dermatitis of Youth

Introduction Annular lichenoid dermatitis of youth (ALDY) is a rare dermatosis first described by Annessi et al. in 2003 in 23 Italian children and adolescents [20]. Since then, about 60 cases have been described [21]. It is still a debated entity, given its similarity with mycosis fungoides, but increasing evidence supports the hypothesis that ALDY is a reactive lichenoid dermatosis, closely related to lichen planus [22].

Clinical Features ALDY mainly occurs in children and young people at a mean age of 11 years and with slight male preponderance [20], but adults may also be affected [23–26]. Therefore, it has been recommended "annular lichenoid dermatitis" as a more suitable name for this entity [23]. Most patients are from Italy and West Europe, especially from the Mediterranean area [20, 21, 23, 24] with anecdotal reports from America, Japan, and Iran [21, 25]. The clinical picture is characterized by solitary or multiple annular brownish-red patches with raised borders and hypopigmented centers without scaling or skin atrophy. Lesions typically occur on the flanks and groin and less commonly on the axillae or the neck. Lesions may or may not be distributed in a bilateral and symmetrical fashion [20, 24]. The condition is mostly asymptomatic with occasional mild pruritus.

Histopathological Features The histological hallmark of ALDY is an interface dermatitis affecting specifically the tips of the rete ridges with massive apoptosis of keratinocytes limited to this area and thus configuring a squared base [20]. The

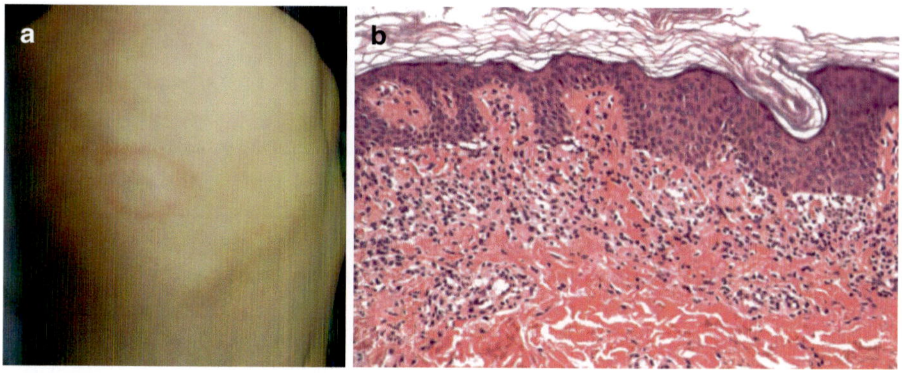

Fig. 4 Annular lichenoid dermatitis of youth. (**a**) Annular thin plaque on the flank with an erythematous edge and hypopigmented center. (**b**) Patchy lichenoid lymphocytic infiltrate in the superficial dermis restricted to the tips of elongated and squared rete ridges with basal layer vacuolization and same necrosis of keratinocytes; dermal fibroplasia beneath the rete tips was also present (hematoxylin & eosin, ×100)

infiltrate consists of small lymphocytes, few histiocytes, and scattered melanophages. The T cells are mostly of CD4+ T cells in the dermis and mainly CD8+ T-cells in the epidermis, as in other lichenoid dermatoses. No epidermotropism is observed and molecular studies are negative for monoclonal T-cell receptor rearrangement [24].

Etiopathogenesis The precise etiopathogenesis of this condition is unknown although immunohistochemical findings suggest a T-cell-mediated cytotoxic reaction against keratinocytes, analogous to other lichenoid dermatoses [23, 24]. Hepatitis B vaccination has been suggested as a possible trigger in one case [26], and an association with *Borrelia* infection has been reported in another case series from Austria [27]. Testing for autoimmunity, viral infections, or allergies failed to find any relevant etiologic factor.

Differential Diagnosis The clinical appearance of ALDY can simulate inflammatory morphea, vitiligo, annular erythemas, patch-type granuloma annulare, or mycosis fungoides, whereas histopathological differential diagnosis includes primarily inflammatory vitiligo and particularly mycosis fungoides [20, 22, 24, 28].

Prognosis ALDY may resolve spontaneously [20, 21, 24], but in most cases runs a chronic course with high relapse frequency.

Therapy Therapeutic options include topical and systemic corticosteroids, calcineurin inhibitors (tacrolimus or pimecrolimus), and phototherapy. Most patients respond well to corticosteroids, but recurrence after discontinuation is frequent. Other treatments used with variable response are photochemotherapy (psoralen-UV-A), systemic and topical antibiotics, and eosin 2% [20, 24]. Recently, cyclosporine has been successfully used in a resistant case [29].

Conclusions

Dermatology encompasses a huge number of skin diseases. Classification and nosographic attribution change according to availability of new information and details, which modify disease interpretation. Over time, there are periods of lumping alternating with time splitting skin diseases. In the case of annular skin diseases, we witnessed in the last few decades the description of new rare entities differing only slightly (splitting), in part because describing a new entity may be rewarding. We propose now to lump some of these diseases differing only marginally based on the clinical and histological features.

EAC and AR-EAC may easily represent different aspects of the same disease, as EAC also is reported to frequently recur, even if not with striking timing of AR-EAC [2]. Some authors consider EAC a clinical reaction pattern that does not represent a specific clinico-pathological entity [30]. PMAE is hardly distinguishable from the deep type of EAC and Jessner-Kanof disease, as well as lupus tumidus. EAE and NFE are very similar clinically, differing only in the relative proportion of eosinophils and neutrophils, which, however, are both present in each of these disorders. As long as the etiopathogenesis remains unknown, it will be difficult to establish whether the annular erythemas are variant reaction patterns or separate clinico-pathological entities.

References

1. Trayes KP, Savage K, Studdiford JS. Annular lesions: diagnosis and treatment. Am Fam Physician. 2018;98:283–91.
2. García Muret MP, Pujol RM, Gimenez-Arnau AM, Barranco C, Gallardo F, Alomar A. Annually recurring erythema annulare centrifugum: a distinct entity? J Am Acad Dermatol. 2006;54:1091–5.
3. Mandel VD, Ferrari B, Manfredini M, Giusti F, Pellacani G. Annually recurring erythema annulare centrifugum: a case report. J Med Case Rep. 2015;9:236.
4. Anedda J, Atzori L, Agosta D, Ferreli C, Atzori MG, Pilloni L, Rongioletti F. Annually recurring acro-erythema. G Ital Dermatol Venereol 2020. Online ahead of print.
5. Maurelli M, Colato C, Tessari G, Girolomoni G. Neutrophilic figurate erythema: report of a new case in an adult and comparison between adult and paediatric cases. Eur J Dermatol. 2016;26:634–5.
6. Hamidi S, Prose NS, Selim MA. Neutrophilic figurate erythema of infancy: a diagnostic challenge. J Cutan Pathol. 2019;46:216–20.
7. Wu YH, Hsiao PF. Neutrophilic figurate erythema. Am J Dermatopathol. 2017;39:344–50.
8. Clark WH, Mihm MC, Reed FJ, Ainworth AM. The lymphocytic infiltrates of the skin. Hum Pathol. 1974;5:25–43.
9. Abeck D, Ollert MW, Eckert F, Szeimies RM, Tiemann M, Braun-Falco O, et al. Palpable migratory arciform erythema. Clinical morphology, histopathology, immunohistochemistry, and response to treatment. Arch Dermatol. 1997;133:763–6.
10. Lohrisch I, Alexandrakis E, Maywurm H, Petres J. Erythema migrans arciforme et palpabile (T-Zell-Pseudolymphom). Hautarzt. 1990;41:78–82.
11. Patterson JW. Weedon's skin pathology. 5th ed. Oxford: Churchill Livingstone Elsevier; 2020. p. 281.
12. Tognetti L, Cinotti E, Fimiani M, Rubegni P. Palpable migratory arciform erythema: hydroxychloroquine as a possible therapeutic option. G Ital Dermatol Venereol. 2019;154:357–60.
13. Kahofer P, Grabmaier E, Aberer E. Treatment of eosinophilic annular erythema with chloroquine. Acta Derm Venereol. 2000;80:70–1.
14. Rongioletti F, Fausti V, Kempf W, Rebora A, Parodi A. Eosinophilic annular erythema: an expression of the clinical and pathological polymorphism of Wells syndrome. J Am Acad Dermatol. 2011;65:e135–7.
15. El-Khalawany M, Al-Mutairi N, Sultan M, Shaaban D. Eosinophilic annular erythema is a peculiar subtype in the spectrum of Wells syndrome: a multicentre long-term follow-up study. J Eur Acad Dermatol Venereol. 2013;27:973–9.
16. Zychowska M, Tutka K, Reich A. Mepolizumab therapy for recalcitrant eosinophilic annular erythema in an adult: a case report and review of treatment options. Dermatol Ther. 2020;10:893–9.
17. Kato K, Namiki T, Tokoro S, Takayama K, Yokozeki H. Bullous eosinophilic annular erythema. J Dermatol. 2017;44:e42–3.
18. Maione V, Caravello S, Cozzi C, et al. Refractory eosinophilic annular erythema treated successfully with dupilumab. J Dtsch Dermatol Ges. 2020;18:1031–2.
19. Prajapati V, Cheung-Lee M, Schloss E, et al. Spontaneously resolving eosinophilic annular erythema. J Am Acad Dermatol. 2012;67:e75–7.

20. Annessi G, Paradisi M, Angelo C, et al. Annular lichenoid dermatitis of youth. J Am Acad Dermatol. 2003;49:1029–36.
21. Debois D, Dargent JL, Ngendahayo P, Roquet-Gravy PP. Annular lichenoid dermatitis of youth: a case report and literature review. Ann Dermatol Venereol. 2018;145:365–75.
22. Cesinaro AM. Annular lichenoid dermatitis (of youth); report of a case with lichen planus-like features. Am J Dermatol. 2017;39:914–5.
23. Cesinaro AM, Sighinolfi P, Greco A, et al. Annular lichenoid dermatitis of youth … and beyond: a series of 6 cases. Am J Dermatopathol. 2009;31:263–7.
24. Di Mercurio M, Gisondi P, Colato C, et al. Annular lichenoid dermatitis of youth: report of six new cases with review of the literature. Dermatology. 2015;231:195–200.
25. Mahmoudi H, Ghanadan A, Fahim S, Moghanlou S, Etesami I, Daneshpazhooh M. Annular lichenoid dermatitis of youth: report on two adult cases and one child. J Dtsch Dermatol Ges. 2019;17:1173–6.
26. Sans V, Leaute-Labreze C, Vergier B, Taieb A. A further case of annular lichenoid dermatitis of youth: role of the anti-hepatitis immunization. Pediatr Dermatol. 2008;25:577–9.
27. Wilk M, Zelger BG, Emberger M, Zelger B. Annular lichenoid dermatitis (of youth) immunohistochemical and serological evidence for another clinical presentation of borrelia infection in patients of Western Austria. Am J Dermatopathol. 2017;39:177–80.
28. Kazlouskaya V, Trager JD, Junkins-Hopkins JM. Lichenoid dermatitis of youth: a separate entity or on the spectrum of mycosis fungoides? Case report and review of the literature. J Cutan Pathol. 2015;42:420–6.
29. Stojkovic-Filipovic J, Lekic B, Brasanac D, Lalosevic J, Gajic-Veljic M, Nikolic M. Annular lichenoid dermatitis of youth - recurrent case of rare skin disease treated with cyclosporine. Dermatol Ther. 2020;33:e13285.
30. Ziemer M, Eisendle K, Zelger B. New concepts on erythema annulare centrifugum: a clinical reaction pattern that does not represent a specific clinicopathological entity. Br J Dermatol. 2009;160:119–26.

Frontal Fibrosing Alopecia

Camila Jaramillo, Paolo Romanelli, and Mariya Miteva

Introduction

Frontal fibrosing alopecia (FFA) is characterized by irreversible scarring alopecia of the temporo-frontal, periauricular, and occipital hairline and irreversible non-scarring alopecia of the eyebrows and body hair. The etiology is still vaguely understood and there is no cure [1]. Described by Kossard in 1994 as a variant of lichen planopilaris (LPP) affecting the frontal hairline primarily seen in postmenopausal women, FFA is a lymphocytic cicatricial alopecia in a pattern distribution. Unlike LPP, FFA usually lacks associated mucus membrane and skin lesions [2].

Epidemiology and Genetics

Prevalence of FFA has increased over the past years including among premenopausal women and men [3, 4]. In men it may be under recognized since early/only involvement of the facial hair could be mistaken for alopecia areata. A recent multicenter retrospective study on the frequency of the different types of alopecia at 22 hair clinics among Europe, America, Africa, and Australia showed that FFA was the most frequent cause of cicatricial alopecia in all studied geographical areas [5].

Age of onset ranges from mid teenage years to the eighth decade of life with median and mean ages of onset commonly being in the sixth decade [6]. The most

C. Jaramillo (✉)
Nova Southeastern University, Dr. Kiran C. Patel College of Medicine,
Ft. Lauderdale, FL, USA
e-mail: cj1091@mynsu.nova.edu

P. Romanelli · M. Miteva
Miller School of Medicine, Dr. Phillip Frost Department of Dermatology and Cutaneous Surgery University of Miami, Miami, FL, USA

F. Rongioletti, B. R. Smoller (eds.), *New and Emerging Entities in Dermatology and Dermatopathology*, https://doi.org/10.1007/978-3-030-80027-7_7

common comorbidity is thyroid disease, with arterial hypertension and dyslipidemia, respectively, following [6]. Four genetic variants have been significantly associated with FFA in genome-wide studies, and it has been estimated that the genome-wide single nucleotide polymorphism heritability for FFA is 46.66%. The strongest effect on FFA susceptibility is observed at 6p21.1 which is located within the MHC region [7]. Fine mapping in genomic studies has suggested that the class I allele HLA-B*07:02 has indicated to confer a fivefold increase in risk of FFA. Further, a potential causal missense variant in CYP1B1 has been implicated, encoding a homonymous xenobiotic- and hormone-processing enzyme [7].

Clinical Features

Moreno-Arrones et al. have described the three most common types of FFA presentations [8]. *Pattern type I or the "linear pattern"* is the most common and has an intermediate prognosis (Fig. 1). Only a third of such patients treated have shown not to progress after 1 year of treatment with oral dutasteride and a topical corticosteroid [8], while the rest have progressed with a mean frontal and temporal increment of 0.63 and 0.24 cm, respectively. *Pattern type II or "the irregular pattern"* is the second most common and has the worst prognosis [8]. It has more significant hairline recession (at least 50% decrease of normal hair density behind the frontal hairline), perifollicular erythema, and hyperkeratosis (Fig. 2). In addition, the majority of the patients (86.1%) have shown to progress despite the same treatment [8]. Both patterns I and II have shown complete eyebrow loss after 1 year of treatment [8]. *Pattern III or the "pseudo-fringe/double-line pattern"* is the least common and has the best prognosis (Fig. 3). There is decreased temporo-frontal hairline recession, eyebrow involvement, perifollicular erythema and hyperkeratosis, facial papules, glabellar red dots, and depression of frontal veins than the other two patterns [8]. Treatment has shown to confer stability of the disease at 1-year follow-up, and eyebrow involvement is significantly less and slower than the other two patterns [8].

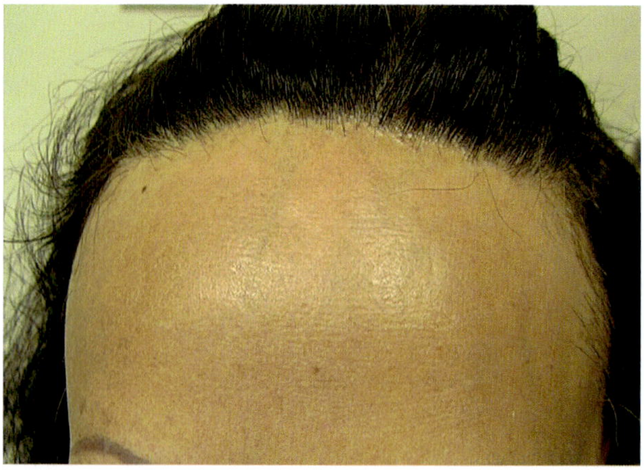

Fig. 1 Type I linear pattern FFA: a band of uniform hairline recession, note the lonely hairs marking the preexisting hairline

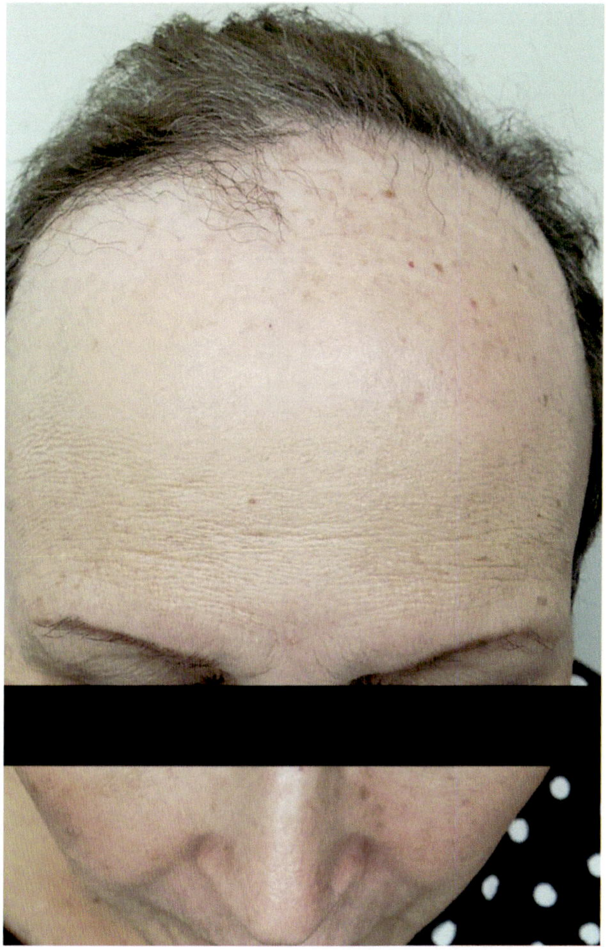

Fig. 2 Type II irregular pattern FFA is associated with the worst prognosis: by definition there is at least 50% decrease of normal hair density behind the frontal hairline which can be appreciated on the image

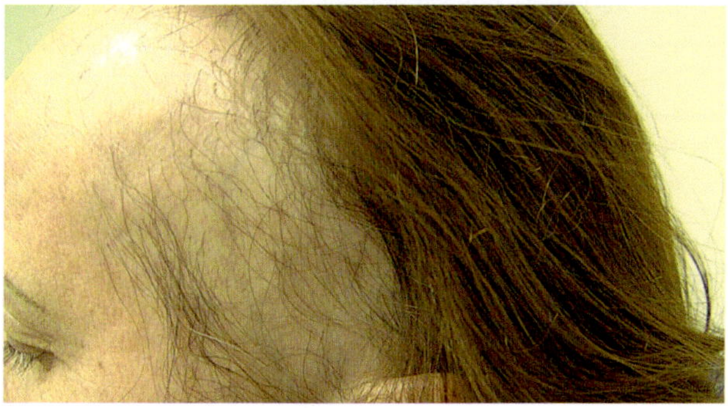

Fig. 3 Type III pseudo-fringe/double-line pattern FFA: note the temporal unaffected primitive hairline

Atypical Patterns

Atypical clinical presentations of FFA include the androgenetic-like alopecia (AGA-like) pattern, which spares the paramedian frontal hairline as well as the cockade pattern, which includes bilateral oval patches of alopecia temporally, with sparing of a band of temporal hairlines, in addition to typical recession of the frontal hairline [9]. The ophiasis-like pattern consists of continuous involvement of the hairline from frontal to occipital regions [9]. We have described a case of FFA involving a band of alopecia along the frontotemporal scalp extending into two symmetrical triangles along the parietal scalp reminiscent of the Greek letter upsilon (υ) [10]. There is also a patchy (focal) FFA atypical presentation that requires histology for the diagnosis [11].

Eyebrows

Over 80% of patients with FFA have also concurrent eyebrow loss [3, 4] with 40% presenting with eyebrow loss as initial manifestation. A clue to distinguish FFA from alopecia areata (AA) limited to the eyebrows is the symmetrical involvement and pattern of regrowth in distinct directions in FFA [12] (Fig. 4). In difficult cases, a biopsy can help establish the diagnosis.

Lonely Hairs, Facial Papules, Glabellar Red Dots, Prominent Veins

Lonely hairs (3 to 7 cm long, which may or may not be accompanied by peripilar casts and peripilar erythema) [13], glabellar red dots [14], and prominently visible frontal veins [4] have been described in FFA. Yellow facial papules or just facial papules [4] around the temporal area show significant associations with Hispanic/

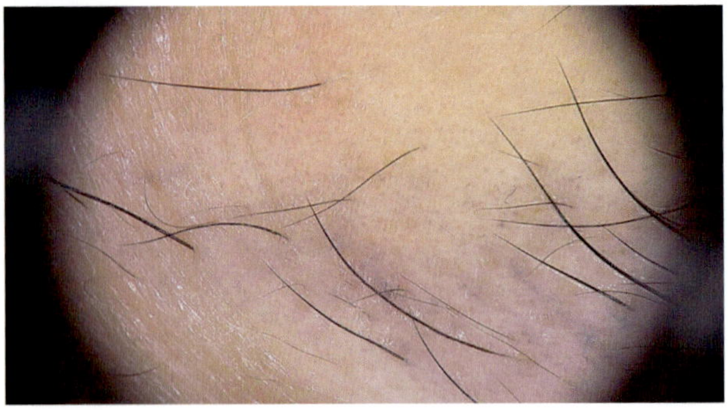

Fig. 4 Trichoscopy image of eyebrow involvement in FFA – note the yellow dots, multiple pinpoint blue-gray dots, short thin hairs, and hairs regrowing in different directions (FotoFinder, ×40)

Latino ethnicity, premenopausal age, and more severe disease [15]. In fact, eyelash loss, facial papules, and body hair involvement are associated with increasing severity of FFA [4]. There are two main hypotheses behind the pathophysiology of the papules, one being lichenoid inflammation of the vellus follicles [16] and the second being sebaceous hyperplasia without vellus involvement, in which there is a loss of perifollicular elastic tissue which makes sebaceous glands more visible superficially [17]. Pirmez et al. showed improvement of the papules secondary to isotretinoin 20 mg daily for 3 months [17].

Follicular erythematous dots and reticulate erythema have been associated with FFA on the face, chest, and hip [14, 18–20]. Termed glabellar red dots, these is a clinical sign of vellus follicle involvement. Because perifollicular erythema occasionally continues to manifest despite advancement of hairline recession, follicular red dots might not be representative of inflammation but instead could also indicate perifollicular changes such as atrophy or vascular changes [14].

Lichen Planus Pigmentosus (LPPigm)

LPPigm is a separate disease that presents as diffuse or reticulated macules on sun-exposed areas and in flexures [21]. Dermoscopy of LPPigm has identified vascular pseudo-network patterns, blue-gray dots arranged in circles, speckled blue-gray dots, dotted patterns, rhomboid, and asymmetric pigmented follicular openings. Focal and diffuse erythema along with telangiectatic vessels and loss of facial vellus hairs have also been reported [22]. The diagnosis of LPPigm can precede the diagnosis of FFA up to 3 years and is twice as common among premenopausal than postmenopausal women [21]. LPPigm should be distinguished from pigmented contact dermatitis (Riehl's melanosis) and hydroxychloroquine-induced hyperpigmentation [22]. Histologically, LPPigm shows vacuolar/interface dermatitis, melanophages, orthokeratosis, and epidermal atrophy [23]. We recently showed that LPPigm in FFA can also show follicular involvement of the vellus follicles (lichenoid folliculitis) [24].

Preauricular Lines

Female patients with FFA have increased preauricular lines compared to age-matched controls regardless of age, with no correlation to disease severity [25].

Updated Criteria for the Diagnosis

Vaño-Galvan et al. proposed updated criteria for the diagnosis of FFA. Diagnosis requires two major criteria or one major criterion and two minor criteria [26]. These criteria intend to take into account atypical cases and allow the differential diagnosis of FFA with other entities (Table 1).

Table 1 Diagnostic criteria for FFA

Major criteria:
1. Cicatricial alopecia of the frontal, temporal, or temporo-frontal scalp on examination in the absence of follicular keratotic papules on the body
2. Diffuse bilateral eyebrow alopecia
Minor criteria:
1. Typical trichoscopic features: perifollicular erythema, follicular hyperkeratosis, or both 2. Histopathologic features of cicatricial alopecia in the pattern of FFA and lichen planus pigmentosus (LPPigm) on biopsy 3. Involvement (hair loss or perifollicular erythema) of additional FFA sites: occipital area, facial hair, sideburns, or body hair 4. Noninflammatory facial papules

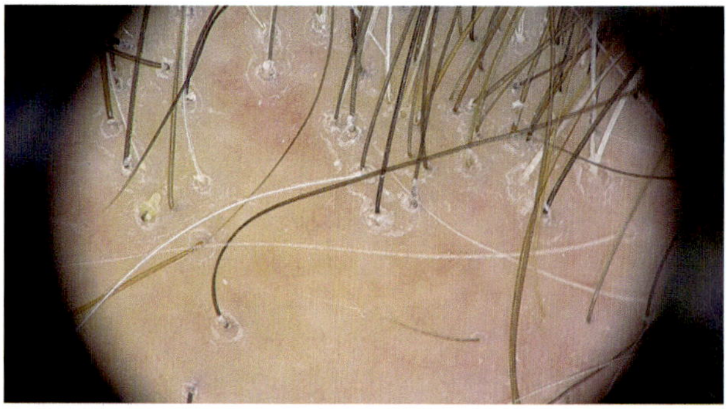

Fig. 5 Trichoscopy of the affected hairline in FFA shows loss of vellus hairs, prominent peripilar casts, and focal erythema (FotoFinder, ×40)

Trichoscopy

Scalp trichoscopic features of FFA include loss of follicular openings, absence of vellus hairs at the hairline, peripilar casts (layered scales that concentrically encircle the emerging hair shafts), perifollicular erythema [27], and blue-gray and classic white dots [28] (Fig. 5). Some authors have described that perifollicular erythema may persist without progression in hairline recession and therefore are not an indicator of inflammation [27]; however, Pedrosa et al. demonstrated that perifollicular erythema and scaling were independently associated with severe FFA in a multivariate analysis [3].

The most common trichoscopic findings on the eyebrows include yellow dots, multiple pinpoint dots, vellus hairs, black dots, dystrophic hairs, and tapering hairs in decreasing order of frequency (see Fig. 4). Although most of these correspond to viable follicles unseen in non-cicatricial alopecia, these are usually unrelated to such a diagnosis [29]. Hairs regrowing in different directions is also a common feature [12]. Fibrotic tracts are also seen in the eyebrows, which signify permanent hair follicle loss [30].

Sideburns in FFA usually lack peripilar casts but are affected with transparent proximal hair emergence surrounded by patches of smooth skin with increased pallor. FFA presenting with sideburn involvement should not be missed due to a lack of peripilar casts and erythema [31].

Body hair has shown to be decreased on the extremities, axilla, and pubic area [4, 32]. Limb and truncal body hair loss affects approximately 24% of patients, whereas axillary and pubic hair affects 21% and 18% of patients, respectively [4]. Trichoscopy of the limbs ranges from alopecic patches to complete alopecia [30, 33]. In the forearms, very fine peripilar casts and transparent proximal hair emergencies have been identified [34].

Histopathologic Features

FFA is a lymphocytic cicatricial alopecia characterized by follicular dropout, absence or atrophy of the sebaceous glands, lichenoid inflammatory infiltrate, and concentric perifollicular fibrosis around the affected follicles (Fig. 6) [35, 36].

Inflammation involving the lower follicular levels [37], increased apoptotic activity in the outer root sheaths [38], and simultaneous involvement of vellus, terminal anagen and telogen follicles by lichenoid inflammation, and perifollicular fibrosis [39] are considered clues to distinguish from LPP. However, distinction is not possible without the clinical information. Although pathology is not necessary for the diagnosis of established FFA cases, biopsying early/subtle cases is crucial in halting the progression, especially because there may be preservation of vellus hairs in early FFA that delays the correct diagnosis [40]. The inflammatory pattern in early FFA is composed of lymphohistiocytic inflammation of the vellus follicles, atrophy of the sebaceous glands, and absence of perifollicular lamellar fibrosis, which is similar to the pattern seen in biopsies from affected limbs [34, 40] (Fig. 7). Later stages of FFA have manifested with concentric perifollicular fibrosis and a

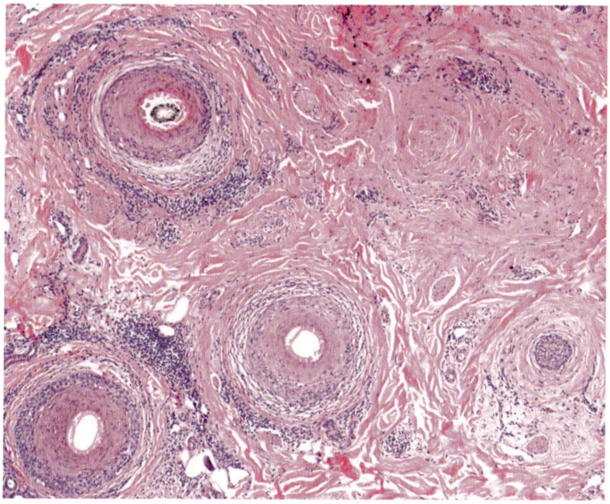

Fig. 6 Pathology of FFA shows altered follicular architecture with areas of follicular dropout and affected hair follicles by perifollicular fibrosis and lichenoid inflammatory infiltrate. There are apoptotic cells in the outer root sheath (horizontal sections, H&E, × 10)

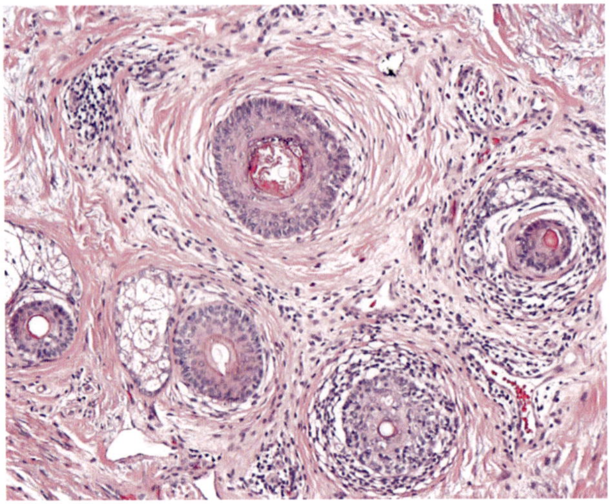

Fig. 7 Pathology of an early case of FFA with only focal patchy presentation – note the lack of perifollicular fibrosis but the inflammatory lichenoid infiltrate involving the vellus follicles (horizontal sections, H&E, × 10)

perifollicular lichenoid lymphocytic infiltrate around the infundibuloisthmic portion of the hair follicle [41]. Novel observations in pathology include fat tissue infiltration at the isthmus level, in the arrector pili muscle, and sweat coils positioned in the reticular dermis [1]. We also determined histological evidence for epidermal and dermal atrophy in biopsies from the alopecic band in treatment-naïve FFA patients compared to unaffected scalp [42].

Workup

The classic presentation of a cicatricial hairless band involving the frontotemporal hairline rarely poses diagnostic difficulty. Trichoscopy can help detect fine peripilar casts in early or atypical cases such as patchy FFA and guide the side for the biopsy (dermoscopy-guided biopsy) [43]. In our experience, with the dermoscopy-guided approach, a single biopsy of 3 mm could be sufficient for the diagnosis in cosmetically sensitive areas such as the frontal scalp.

Differential Diagnosis

Differential diagnosis includes traction alopecia, alopecia areata (ophiasis), LPP, Graham Little-Piccardi-Lassueur syndrome, or even androgenetic alopecia [26]. Peripilar casts are also seen in lupus erythematosus, and the presentation may be similar to FFA in cases involving the frontal hairline, especially because DLE and FFA can be associated [44]. There is also fibrosing alopecia in a pattern distribution (FAPD) which is clinically distinctive and also characterized by pattern hair loss with evidence of follicular inflammation and fibrosis [45, 46]. Considerable overlap exists among FFA, LPP, and FAPD [47, 48], and some authors consider these entities part of the same spectrum especially based on their similar histological features.

Etiopathogenesis

Epithelial-to-mesenchymal transition (EMT) is imperative for wound healing, and embryonic development, and is seen in fibrotic disease. EMT occurs within the epithelial stem cell niche of human scalp hair follicles in LPP and other primary cicatricial alopecias such as FFA [49]. During the transition, epithelial cells undertake a fibroblast-like role secondary to nuclear suppression of factors such as Snail1 and upregulation of proteins such as fibronectin. Abnormal expression of Snail has been acknowledged in the fibrotic dermis of FFA, which may suggest that EMT may be involved in the disease's etiology [49]. EMT is preceded by a CD8+ cell-mediated attack and subsequently fibrosis develops.

It is proposed that what differentiates FFA and LPP is that FFA is EMT predominant, whereas LPP is cytotoxic T-cell attack predominant. FFA also has hormonal and epigenetic influences that are not seen in LPP [50]. Androgenetic changes and age-related decline in dehydroepiandrosterone activity or estrogen decline is associated with FFA [51, 52]; however, normal or low [35, 53, 54] sex steroid levels and the involvement of non-androgen-dependent hair follicles may argue against this association being causative [53].

Possible associations of FFA with skin care products have been discussed [32]. The pathogenesis behind how sunscreen might lead to FFA has been postulated but not identified. A commonly discussed theory is that the sunscreen enters the follicular infundibulum and produces a lichenoid reaction that leads to the development of autoimmune disease [32, 55, 56]. This implies that decreased clearance of exogenous substances from follicles secondary to age-dependent decline in sebum synthesis could explain why postmenopausal women are mainly affected [57].

Although authors [32, 55, 58] have collected data confirming that titanium dioxide nanoparticles may be present along hair shafts, their suggestion that these nanoparticles also elicit a T-cell-mediated response remains hypothetical. The identification of the titanium species on the hair shafts was also present on the hair shafts of nearly all healthy controls [59] making the supposition unreliable. The photocatalytic properties of titanium dioxide have been established [60, 61]; however, the particles are usually coated with a nonreactive chemical to prevent the release of reactive oxygen species to the tissue [57]. There is also the hypothesis that systemic absorption of chemical UV filters may lead to endocrine-disrupting effects secondary to estrogen-like activity previously reported [62]. Besides genetic factors, environmental variables, such as contact allergens, could be causative in FFA and may be influencing its increased incidence; however, the precise etiology of the pathology is yet to be demonstrated [63]. For this reason, clinicians should consider that there is insufficient data supporting that sunscreen contributes to the development of

FFA before recommending its avoidance. In our practice, mineral sunscreens containing pure zinc applied away from the hairline and eyebrows are recommended over chemical sunscreens.

Therapy

Currently, 5-α-reductase inhibitors (finasteride and dutasteride), intralesional steroids, and hydroxychloroquine have the highest level of evidence for treating FFA, while the remaining therapies have varying results [64, 65]. Most recently, in a retrospective observational study on 224 patients with FFA, stabilization showed a statistically significant association with an increasing dose of dutasteride (88%, 91%, and 84% with a weekly treatment of 5 or 7 doses of 0.5 mg ($n = 32$), $P < 0.005$). Donovan et al. showed that intralesional triamcinolone 10 mg/ml with 0.125 mL per eyebrow can lead to successful regrowth of eyebrow hair with a low chance of atrophy [66]. Of note, Rakoska et al. assessed the efficacy of systemic retinoids in treating FFA. No further progression of hairline recession after 12 months of treatment was achieved by 76% (23/29) of patients treated with oral isotretinoin (20 mg daily), 73% (8/11) of patients treated with oral acitretin (20 mg daily), and 43% (6/14) of patients treated with oral finasteride (5 mg daily) [67]. Thus, the use of systemic retinoids may be beneficial for the stabilization of frontal hairline in patients with FFA.

Strazzulla et al. demonstrated that patients treated with 0.3% tacrolimus were significantly more likely to prevent further hairline regression, eyebrow loss, and decreased active inflammation after 3 months compared with patients treated with clobetasol/betamethasone. Overall, median times to stabilization were 11.9 months for tacrolimus and 13.2 months for clobetasol/betamethasone [68]. It was also found that patients treated with doxycycline, tetracycline, or minocycline were more likely to experience medication side effects compared with other treatments [68]. FFA progression can also be halted with PPAR-γ agonists [4, 17, 67, 69–71].

Prognosis and Course

Disease stabilization is commonly defined as no further hairline recession, eyebrow loss, or evidence of active inflammation such as follicular erythema or follicular hyperkeratosis. A majority of patients have shown to be able to reach stabilization with treatment after an average of 10.4 months, but the average may be sooner, as this data had a lack of follow-ups before those 10 months [68]. It has been found that a younger age of onset is associated with decreased disease intensity and that a family history of hair disorders does not affect prognosis [68].

Conclusions

FFA is a chronic lymphocytic cicatricial alopecia of unknown etiology. It shares characteristics with traction alopecia, systemic lupus erythematosus, lichen planus pigmentosus, androgenetic alopecia, fibrosing alopecia in a pattern distribution, and others. FFA is not limited to the hairline; it also presents on the forehead, face, trunk, and limbs. Further, its presentation comes in typical and atypical patterns. Fortunately, histopathologic and trichoscopic findings used in conjunction with the updated diagnostic criteria by Vaño-Galvan et al. should assist clinicians in obtaining an accurate diagnosis. The Frontal Fibrosing Alopecia Severity Index may then be used to describe severity and monitor progression. Treatment and prognosis vary depending on severity at presentation; however, reduced progression with treatment has been demonstrated in most patients.

References

1. Miteva M, Castillo D, Sabiq S. Adipose infiltration of the dermis, involving the arrector pili muscle, and dermal displacement of eccrine sweat coils. Am J Dermatopathol. 2019;41(7):492–7.
2. Kossard S. Postmenopausal frontal fibrosing alopecia: scarring alopecia in a pattern distribution. Arch Dermatol. 1994;130:770–4.
3. Pedrosa AF, Duarte AF, Ventura F, Haneke E, Correia O. Frontal fibrosing alopecia: a cross-sectional study of 108 patients followed at a single center. J Dermatol Case Rep. 2017;11:35–42. https://doi.org/10.3315/jdcr.2017.1247.
4. Vano-Galvan S, Molina-Ruiz AM, Serrano-Falcon C, et al. Frontal fibrosing alopecia: a multicenter review of 355 patients. J Am Acad Dermatol. 2014;70:670–8.
5. Vañó-Galván S, Saceda-Corralo D, Blume-Peytavi U, Cucchía J, Dlova NC, Gavazzoni Dias MFR, et al. Frequency of the types of alopecia at twenty-two specialist hair clinics: a multicenter study. Skin Appendage Disord. 2019;5(5):309–15. https://doi.org/10.1159/000496708.
6. Kanti V, Constantinou A, Reygagne P, Vogt A, Kottner J, Blume-Peytavi U. Frontal fibrosing alopecia: demographic and clinical characteristics of 490 cases. J Eur Acad Dermatol Venereol. 2019;33(10):1976–83. https://doi.org/10.1111/jdv.15735.
7. Tziotzios C, Petridis C, Dand N, et al. Genome-wide association study in frontal fibrosing alopecia identifies four susceptibility loci including HLA-B*07:02. Nat Commun. 2019;10(1):1150. https://doi.org/10.1038/s41467-019-09117-w.
8. Moreno-Arrones O, Saceda-Corralo D, Fonda-Pascual P, Rodrigues-Barata A, Buendía-Castaño D, Alegre-Sánchez A, et al. Frontal fibrosing alopecia: clinical and prognostic classification. J Eur Acad Dermatol Venereol. 2017;31:1739–45. https://doi.org/10.1111/jdv.14287.
9. Rossi A, Grassi S, Fortuna MC, Garelli V, Pranteda G, Caro G, et al. Unusual patterns of presentation of frontal fibrosing alopecia: a clinical and trichoscopic analysis of 98 patients. J Am Acad Dermatol. 2017;77(1):172–4. https://doi.org/10.1016/j.jaad.2017.02.012.
10. Goldman C, Diaz A, Miteva M. A novel atypical presentation of frontal fibrosing alopecia involving the frontoparietal scalp. Skin Appendage Disord. 2020;6(4):250–3. https://doi.org/10.1159/000508388.
11. Contin LA, de Almeida Ledá YL, Caldeira Nassif K, Suárez Restrepo MV. Patchy frontal fibrosing alopecia: description of an incomplete clinical presentation. Skin Appendage Disord. 2017;3(4):190–2. https://doi.org/10.1159/000475821.

12. Waśkiel-Burnat A, Rakowska A, Kurzeja M, et al. The value of dermoscopy in diagnosing eyebrow loss in patients with alopecia areata and frontal fibrosing alopecia. J Eur Acad Dermatol Venereol. 2019;33(1):213–9. https://doi.org/10.1111/jdv.15279.
13. Tosti A, Miteva M, Torres F. Lonely hair: a clue to the diagnosis of frontal fibrosing alopecia. Arch Dermatol. 2011;147:1240.
14. Pirmez R, Donati A, Valente NS, Sodré CT, Tosti A. Glabellar red dots in frontal fibrosing alopecia: a further clinical sign of vellus follicle involvement. Br J Dermatol. 2014;170(3):745–6.11.
15. Mervis JS, Borda LJ, Miteva M. Facial and extrafacial lesions in an ethnically diverse series of 91 patients with frontal fibrosing alopecia followed at a single center. Dermatology. 2019;235(2):112–9. https://doi.org/10.1159/000494603.
16. Donati A, Molina L, Doche I, Valente NS, Romiti R. Facial papules in frontal fibrosing alopecia: evidence of vellus follicle involvement. Arch Dermatol. 2011;147(12):1424–7.
17. Pirmez R, Duque-Estrada B, Barreto T, Quintella DC, Cuzzi T. Successful treatment of facial papules in frontal fibrosing alopecia with oral isotretinoin. Skin Appendage Disord. 2017;3:111–3.
18. López-Pestaña A, Tuneu A, Lobo C, Ormaechea N, Zubizarreta J, Vildosola S, et al. Facial lesions in frontal fibrosing alopecia (FFA): clinicopathological features in a series of 12 cases. J Am Acad Dermatol. 2015;73(6):987.e1–6.
19. Billero V, Oberlin KE, Miteva M. Red dots in a net-like pattern on the upper chest: a novel clinical observation in frontal fibrosing alopecia and fibrosing alopecia in pattern distribution. Skin Appendage Disord. 2018;4(1):47–9.
20. Meyer V, Sachse M, Rose C, Wagner G. Follicular red dots of the hip in frontal fibrosing alopecia – do we have to look twice? J Dtsch Dermatol Ges. 2017;15(3):327–8.
21. Dlova NC. Frontal fibrosing alopecia and lichen planus pigmentosus: is there a link? Br J Dermatol. 2013;168(2):439–42. https://doi.org/10.1111/j.1365-2133.2012.11146.x.
22. Pirmez R, Duque-Estrada B, Donati A, Campos-do-Carmo G, Valente NS, Romiti R, Sodré CT, Tosti A. Clinical and dermoscopic features of lichen planus pigmentosus in 37 patients with frontal fibrosing alopecia. Br J Dermatol. 2016;175(6):1387–90. https://doi.org/10.1111/bjd.14722.
23. Vega ME, Waxtein L, Arenas R, Hojyo T, Dominguez-Soto L. Ashy dermatosis and lichen planus pigmentosus: a clinicopathologic study of 31 cases. Int J Dermatol. 1992;31(2):90–4.
24. Miteva M, Goldberg LJ. Lichenoid folliculitis in facial lichen planus pigmentosus-A clue to frontal fibrosing alopecia? J Cutan Pathol. 2020;47(10):983–5. https://doi.org/10.1111/cup.13715.
25. Nanda S, De Bedout V, Hirt PA, Castillo DE, Mesquita T, Scott L, et al. Increased preauricular wrinkles in frontal fibrosing alopecia compared to age-matched controls: a prospective study of 64 patients. Ski Appendage Disord. 2020;6(1):11–3.
26. Vañó-Galván S, Saceda-Corralo D, Moreno-Arrones ÓM, Camacho-Martinez FM. Updated diagnostic criteria for frontal fibrosing alopecia. J Am Acad Dermatol. 2018;78(1):e21–2. https://doi.org/10.1016/j.jaad.2017.08.062.
27. Fernández-Crehuet P, Rodrigues-Barata AR, Vañó-Galván S, et al. Trichoscopic features of frontal fibrosing alopecia: results in 249 patients. J Am Acad Dermatol. 2015;72:357–9.
28. Waśkiel A, Rakowska A, Sikora M, et al. Trichoscopy in lichen planopilaris: an update. Dermatol Rev. 2018;105(1):63–75.
29. Anzai A, Pirmez R, Vincenzi C, Fabbrocini G, Romiti R, Tosti A. Trichoscopy findings of frontal fibrosing alopecia on the eyebrows: a study of 151 cases. J Am Acad Dermatol. 2019;17:S0190–9622(19)33298-0. https://doi.org/10.1016/j.jaad.2019.12.023.
30. Chew AL, Bashir SJ, Wain EM, et al. Expanding the spectrum of frontal fibrosing alopecia: a unifying concept. J Am Acad Dermatol. 2010;63:653–60.
31. Cervantes J, Miteva M. Distinct trichoscopic features of the sideburns in frontal fibrosing alopecia compared to the frontotemporal scalp. Skin Appendage Disord. 2017;4(1):50–4. https://doi.org/10.1159/000479116.

32. Aldoori N, Dobson K, Holden CR, McDonagh AJ, Harries M, Messenger AG. Frontal fibrosing alopecia: possible association with leave-on facial skin care products and sunscreens; a questionnaire study. Br J Dermatol. 2016;175(4):762–7. https://doi.org/10.1111/bjd.14535.
33. Miteva M, Camacho I, Romanelli P, et al. Acute hair loss on the limbs in frontal fibrosing alopecia: a clinicopathological study of two cases. Br J Dermatol. 2010;163:426–8.
34. Miteva M. Frontal fibrosing alopecia involving the limbs shows inflammatory pattern on histology. Am J Dermatopathol. 2020;42(3):226–9. https://doi.org/10.1097/dad.0000000000001500.
35. Kossard S, May-Sen L, Barbara W. Postmenopausal frontal fibrosing alopecia: a frontal variant of lichen planopilaris. J Am Acad Dermatol. 1997;36(1):59–66. https://doi.org/10.1016/s0190-9622(97)70326-8.
36. Sperling LC. Scarring alopecia and the dermatopathologist. J Cutan Pathol. 2001;28:333–42.
37. Wong D, Goldberg LJ. The depth of inflammation in frontal fibrosing alopecia and lichen planopilaris: a potential distinguishing feature. J Am Acad Dermatol. 2017;76:1183–4.
38. Poblet E, Jimenez F, Pascual A, et al. Frontal fibrosing alopecia versus lichen planopilaris: a clinicopathological study. Int J Dermatol. 2006;45:375–80.
39. Miteva M, Tosti A. The follicular triad: a pathological clue to the diagnosis of early frontal fibrosing alopecia. Br J Dermatol. 2012;166:440–2.
40. Miteva M, Sabiq S. A new histologic pattern in 6 biopsies from early frontal fibrosing alopecia. Am J Dermatopathol. 2019;41(2):118–21. https://doi.org/10.1097/dad.0000000000001247.
41. Ma SA, Imadojemu S, Beer K, Seykora JT. Inflammatory features of frontal fibrosing alopecia. J Cutan Pathol. 2017;44(8):672–6. https://doi.org/10.1111/cup.12955.
42. Saceda-Corralo D, Desai K, Pindado-Ortega C, Moreno-Arrones OM, Vañó-Galván S, Miteva M. Histological evidence for epidermal and dermal atrophy of the alopecic band in treatment-naïve patients with frontal fibrosing alopecia. J Eur Acad Dermatol Venereol. 2020. doi: https://doi.org/10.1111/jdv.16792.
43. Miteva M, Tosti A. Dermoscopy guided scalp biopsy in cicatricial alopecia. J Eur Acad Dermatol Venereol. 2013;27(10):1299–303. https://doi.org/10.1111/j.1468-3083.2012.04530.x.
44. Gaffney DC, Sinclair RD, Yong-Gee S. Discoid lupus alopecia complicated by frontal fibrosing alopecia on a background of androgenetic alopecia. Br J Dermatol. 2013;169(1):217–8. https://doi.org/10.1111/bjd.12287.
45. Zinkernagel MS, Med C, Trüeb RM. Fibrosing alopecia in a pattern distribution: patterned lichen planopilaris or androgenetic alopecia with a lichenoid tissue reaction pattern? Arch Dermatol. 2000;136(2):205–11. https://doi.org/10.1001/archderm.136.2.205.
46. Ramanauskaite A, Trüeb RM. Facial papules in fibrosing alopecia in a pattern distribution (cicatricial pattern hair loss). Int J Trichol. 2015;7:119–22.
47. Trüeb RM, Torricelli R. Lichen planopilaris simulating postmenopausal frontal fibrosing alopecia. Kossard. 1998;49(5):388–91. Germanica. https://doi.org/10.1007/s001050050760.
48. Macpherson M, Hohendorf-Ansari P, Trüeb RM. Nail involvement in frontal fibrosing alopecia. Int J Trichol. 2015;7(2):64–6. https://doi.org/10.4103/0974-7753.160107.
49. Imanishi H, Ansell DM, Chéret J, et al. Epithelial-to-MESENCHYMAL stem cell transition in a human organ: lessons from lichen planopilaris. J Investig Dermatol. 2018;138(3):511–9. https://doi.org/10.1016/j.jid.2017.09.047.
50. Harries MJ, Jimenez F, Izeta A, et al. Lichen planopilaris and frontal fibrosing alopecia as model epithelial stem cell diseases. Trends Mol Med. 2018;24(5):435–48. https://doi.org/10.1016/j.molmed.2018.03.007.
51. Tziotzios C, Stefanato CM, Fenton DA, Simpson MA, McGrath JA. Frontal fibrosing alopecia: reflections and hypotheses on aetiology and pathogenesis. Exp Dermatol. 2016;25(11):847–52. https://doi.org/10.1111/exd.13071.
52. Gaspar NK. DHEA and frontal fibrosing alopecia: molecular and physiopathological mechanisms. An Bras Dermatol. 2016;91(6):776–80. https://doi.org/10.1590/abd1806-4841.20165029.

53. Macdonald A, Clark C, Holmes S. Frontal fibrosing alopecia: a review of 60 cases. J Am Acad Dermatol. 2012;67:955–61.
54. Ranasinghe GC, Piliang MP, Bergfeld WF. Prevalence of hormonal and endocrine dysfunction in patients with lichen planopilaris (LPP): a retrospective data analysis of 168 patients. J Am Acad Dermatol. 2017;76(2):314–20. https://doi.org/10.1016/j.jaad.2016.05.038.
55. Debroy Kidambi A, Dobson K, Holmes S, et al. Frontal fibrosing alopecia in men: an association with facial moisturizers and sunscreens. Br J Der matol. 2017;177:260–1.
56. Cranwell WC, Sinclair R. Sunscreen and facial skincare products in frontal fibrosing alopecia: a case-control study. Br J Dermatol. 2019;180(4):943–4.
57. Robinson G, McMichael A, Wang SQ, Lim HW. Sunscreen and frontal fibrosing alopecia: a review. J Am Acad Dermatol. 2020;82:723–8.
58. Kumaran MS, Razmi TM, Vinay K, Parsad D. Clinical, dermoscopic, and trichoscopic analysis of frontal fibrosing alopecia associated with acquired dermal macular hyperpigmentation: a cross sectional observational case-control study. J Am Acad Dermatol. 2018;79(3):588–91. https://doi.org/10.1016/j.jaad.2018.03.001.
59. Thompson CT, Chen ZQ, Kolivras A, Tosti A. Identification of titanium dioxide on the hair shaft of patients with and without frontal fibrosing alopecia: a pilot study of 20 patients. Br J Dermatol. 2019;181(1):216–7.
60. Fujishima A, Rao TN, Tryk DA. Titanium dioxide photocatalysis. J Photochem Photobiol C: Photochem Rev. 2000;1(1):1–21.
61. Skocaj M, Filipic M, Petkovic J, Novak S. Titanium dioxide in our everyday life; is it safe? Radiol Oncol. 2011;45(4):227–47.
62. Wang J, Pan L, Wu S, et al. Recent advances on endocrine disrupting effects of UV filters. Int J Environ Res Public Health. 2016;13(8):782.
63. Aerts O, Bracke A, Goossens A, Meuleman V, Lambert J. Titanium dioxide nanoparticles and frontal fibrosing alopecia: cause or consequence? J Eur Acad Dermatol Venereol. 2018;33(1):e45–6. https://doi.org/10.1111/jdv.15161.
64. Gamret AC, Potluri VS, Krishnamurthy K, Fertig RM. Frontal fibrosing alopecia: efficacy of treatment modalities. Int J Women's Health. 2019;11:273–85. https://doi.org/10.2147/ijwh.s177308.
65. Lajevardi V, Ghodsi SZ, Goodarzi A, Hejazi P, Azizpour A, Beygi S. Comparison of systemic mycophenolate mofetil with topical clobetasol in lichen planopilaris: a parallel-group, assessor- and analyst-blinded, randomized controlled trial. Am J Clin Dermatol. 2015;16:303–11.
66. Donovan JC, Samrao A, Ruben BS, Price VH. Eyebrow regrowth in patients with frontal fibrosing alopecia treated with intralesional triamcinolone acetonide. Br J Dermatol. 2010;163(5):1142–4. https://doi.org/10.1111/j.1365-2133.2010.09994.x.
67. Rakowska A, Gradzińska A, Olszewska M, Rudnicka L. Efficacy of isotretinoin and acitretin in treatment of frontal fibrosing alopecia: retrospective analysis of 54 cases. J Drugs Dermatol. 2017;16(10):988–92.
68. Strazzulla LC, Avila L, Li X, Lo Sicco K, Shapiro J. Prognosis, treatment, and disease outcomes in frontal fibrosing alopecia: a retrospective review of 92 cases. J Am Acad Dermatol. 2018;78(1):203–5. https://doi.org/10.1016/j.jaad.2017.07.035.
69. Chiang C, Sah D, Cho BK, Ochoa BE, Price VH. Hydroxychloroquine and lichen planopilaris: efficacy and introduction of lichen planopilaris activity index scoring system. J Am Acad Dermatol. 2010;62:387–92.
70. Pedrosa AF, Duarte AF, Haneke E, Correia O. Yellow facial papules associated with frontal fibrosing alopecia: a distinct histologic pattern and response to isotretinoin. J Am Acad Dermatol. 2017;77:764–6.
71. Samrao A, Chew AL, Price V. Frontal fibrosing alopecia: a clinical review of 36 patients. Br J Dermatol. 2010;163:1296–300.

Terra Firma-Forme Dermatosis and Dermatosis Neglecta

Claudio Guarneri, Fabrizio Guarneri, and Serafinella Patrizia Cannavò

Terra Firma-Forme Dermatosis

This benign condition of unknown origin characterized by a dirty skin appearance, terra firma-forme dermatosis, was originally described in 1987 by Duncan, Tschen, and Knox (hence the eponymic name "Duncan's dirty dermatosis") [1]. The reason for the choice of this Latin name, which literally means "solid ground," was not explained by the authors in the article, but is probably due to the earthy aspect of lesions.

Epidemiology The frequency of terra firma-forme dermatosis is unknown. As of December 2020, the literature includes approximately 260 cases, mostly published as case reports and only a few case series, with a maximum study population of 79 patients [2]. Based on these data, the disease seems to be rather infrequent. However, many cases are not recognized, usually for lack of knowledge about the condition rather than for diagnostic difficulties, or not reported because of the benign course and rapid and complete resolution, so the picture resulting from literature is probably an underestimate. Younger people are affected more frequently, but cases were observed in all periods of life: the mean age of patients is ~18 years, and the age range is 3 months–94 years. Females are slightly more represented than males, while there is no difference between ethnicities [3].

C. Guarneri (✉)
Department of Biomedical and Dental Sciences and Morpho Functional Imaging, University of Messina, Messina, Italy
e-mail: cguarneri@unime.it

F. Guarneri · S. P. Cannavò
Department of Clinical and Experimental Medicine, University of Messina, Messina, Italy
e-mail: fguarneri@unime.it; cannavop@unime.it

F. Rongioletti, B. R. Smoller (eds.), *New and Emerging Entities in Dermatology and Dermatopathology*, https://doi.org/10.1007/978-3-030-80027-7_8

Etiopathogenesis Cause(s) and pathogenetic mechanism(s) of terra firma-forme dermatosis have not been defined yet. Some authors hypothesized an alteration of keratinocyte maturation, with retention of melanin, as well as inadequate cleansing, at least in an initial phase, with subsequent buildup and compaction of dirt and scales [1, 4, 5]. Atopic dermatitis is frequently associated, and some authors suggested that it could play a role in the etiopathogenesis, because of the epidermal barrier defects and the probably less frequent bathing and use of skin sponges [6].

Clinical Aspects Physical examination of the skin shows localized or extensive, clear-cut, brownish-gray-black patches, sometimes palpable papillomatous or pseudoverrucous plaques, with a dirt-like appearance; light scaling may also be present. The lesions may have a reticulated pattern, with interspersed areas of normal skin. Usually no symptoms are reported. The neck and trunk are the most common localizations, but all body areas may be involved (Figs. 1, 2, 3, and 4) [7–11].

Histopathology Since cutaneous biopsy and its microscopic examination are ordinarily not necessary for the diagnosis of terra firma-forme dermatosis, literature data on the histopathological aspects of this condition are limited to 20 cases [3]. Hematoxylin-eosin stain typically reveals lamellar hyperkeratosis, whorled hyperkeratosis in focal areas, keratin whorls and globules, acanthosis, papillomatosis, and hypermelanosis in the basal epidermal layer and hyperkeratotic areas. No inflammatory infiltrate is usually seen (Fig. 5) [3, 11]. These histopathological features may be indistinguishable from other benign papillomatous conditions, such as acanthosis nigricans, confluent and reticulated papillomatosis, and epidermal nevi.

Some authors also described superficial dermal infiltration of lymphocytes. Periodic acid-Schiff (PAS) staining may inconstantly reveal fungi in the stratum corneum [12]. Electron microscopy, used in this condition only for research purposes, shows disorganized and delayed keratinization, persistence of desmosomes, and abundance of melanin in basal keratinocytes [13].

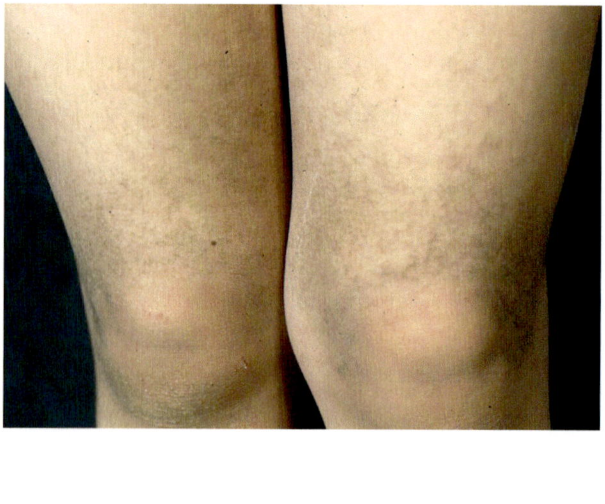

Fig. 1 Diffuse hyperkeratosis and hyperpigmentation of the lower limbs in a 16-year-old boy

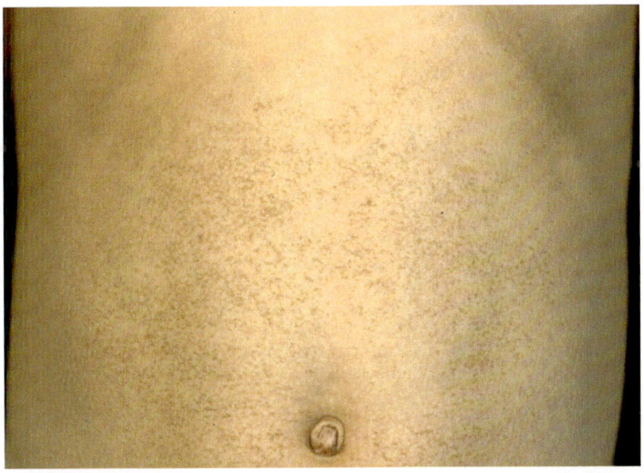

Fig. 2 Asymptomatic hyperpigmentation in a dirty-appearing typical skin pattern on the trunk of a 10-year-old boy

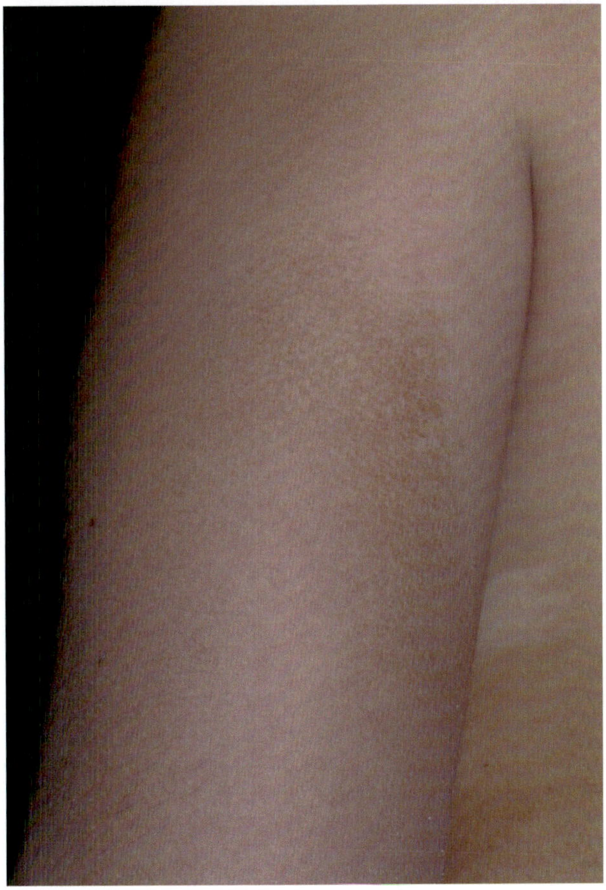

Fig. 3 Subtle brown-blackish pigmentation of the lateral aspect of the trunk and of the dorsal surface of the arm in 9-year-old boy. Alcohol swabbing revealed a pink linear area of normal skin

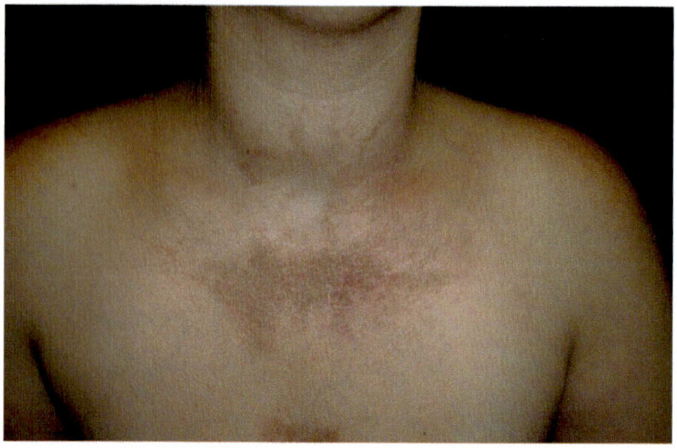

Fig. 4 Dirt-like hyperpigmented patch lesions on the anterior neck, sternum, and intermammary cleft in a 15-year-old girl. Note the frictional erythema, from vigorous scrubbing by the patient, at the periphery of the sternal lesion

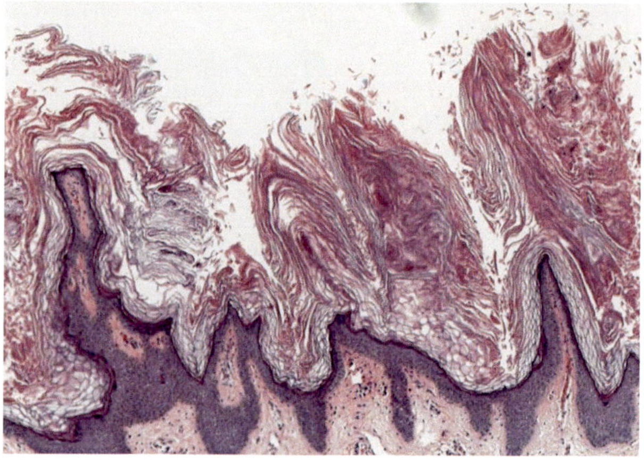

Fig. 5 Histopathology of terra firma-forme dermatosis: acanthosis nigricans-like features showing hyperkeratosis, keratin whorls, papillomatosis, hypermelanosis of the basal epidermal layer. (Courtesy of Franco Rongioletti, Milan)

Workup The recognition of the typical clinical characteristics of the disease in lesions described by patients as similar to patches of dirt, but appeared despite normal hygiene and resistant to all cleaners, is the main element for the diagnosis of terra firma-forme dermatosis. Removal of the dark pigment through rubbing with gauze pads soaked in 70% isopropyl alcohol easily and immediately confirms the clinical suspicion. Recently, this procedure was named by some authors with the acronym SMART (skin modified by alcohol rubbing test) [7–12, 14, 15]. Dermoscopy, commonly used in dermatological clinical practice, reveals a mosaic pattern, with polygonal yellowish-brown clods/scales and a pigmented pseudonetwork (Fig. 6) [16, 17]. Cytology and skin swabs, sometimes performed in the suspicion of bacterial or fungal infections, do not appear relevant for diagnosis [7, 8]. Wood's light examination reveals chalk-white fluorescence of the lesions [18]. Experimental observations with reflectance confocal microscopy confirmed in a noninvasive manner the thickening and ultrastructural modifications of the stratum

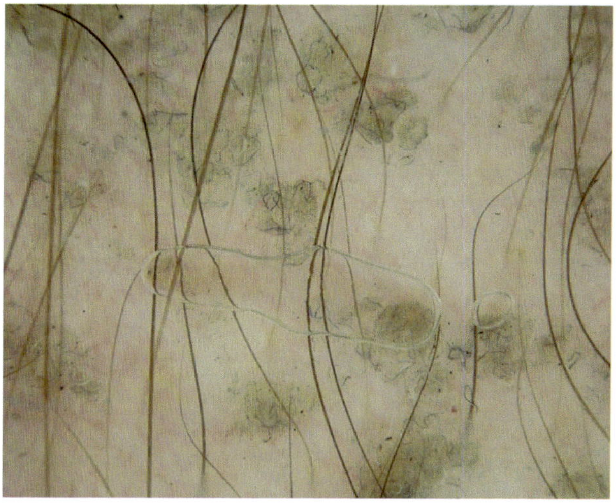

Fig. 6 Dermoscopy of terra firma-forme dermatosis showing a mosaic pattern, with polygonal yellowish-brown clods/scales. (Courtesy of Franco Rongioletti, Milan)

corneum observed in optic and electron microscopy and also allowed to visualize the intracorneal keratin whorls, which appear as hyper-refractile areas [19].

Etiopathogenesis Terra firma-forme dermatosis is considered to be a disorder of keratinization caused by abnormal development and delayed release of keratinocytes. Adhesion between keratinocytes is increased with retention of sebum, melanin, and microorganisms, leading to the formation of brown patches and thickened plaques.

Differential Diagnosis Although the clinical diagnosis of terra firma-forme dermatosis is usually not difficult, in particular cases many differential diagnoses should be considered, which include dermatosis neglecta, acanthosis nigricans, confluent and reticulated papillomatosis, dirty neck syndrome, post-inflammatory hyperpigmentation, ichthyosis, tinea versicolor, intertriginous granular parakeratosis, verrucous epidermal nevi, frictional melanosis, macular amyloidosis, hyperkeratotic head and neck *Malassezia* dermatosis, melasma, livedo racemosa, ashy dermatosis, Dowling-Degos syndrome, acroangiodermatitis of Mali, epidermolytic hyperkeratosis of the nipple and areola, and scalp discoloration from selenium sulfide shampoo [3].

Treatment As mentioned above, rubbing with 70% isopropyl alcohol is sufficient to clear the hyperpigmented lesions. Peculiar patients described in the literature have been successfully treated with topical urea-based keratolytics (associated with topical anti-inflammatory drugs), ammonium lactate or other alpha hydroxy acid salts, retinoids, salicylic acid, or even acetone or CO_2 laser in extreme cases [3, 10].

Prognosis and Course Once diagnosed, the condition usually responds completely to therapy and rarely relapses. Patients should be reassured about the benignity of dermatosis.

Dermatosis Neglecta

Introduction

Dermatosis neglecta was described for the first time in 1995 by Poskitt, Wayte, Wojnarowska, and Wilkinson, who coined this term to underline the etiological role of self-neglect behavior in its genesis [20]. Indeed, this condition is caused by inadequate washing/cleaning of a body area (hence the alternative name "unwashed dermatosis"), with consequent accumulation of sebum, sweat, corneocytes, and bacteria, which ultimately results in the formation of one or more hyperpigmented plaques, hyperkeratotic or verrucous, with cornflake-like scales, and usually asymptomatic [21, 22]. The lack of inflammation led in 1999 Ruiz-Maldonado et al. [23] to suggest a change of the denomination of the disease, from the original "dermatitis" to the more appropriate "dermatosis." Dermatosis neglecta equally affects both genders and all age groups.

Clinical Features

The dermatosis is characterized by localized hyperpigmented patches or verrucous plaques with adherent, flaking scale involving the trunk, limbs, face, genitalia, and surgical sites. Lesions are generally asymptomatic. Multiple reasons are reported in literature for self-neglect behaviors: the most common are physical disability, neurological problems, psychiatric illness, localized pain/hyperesthesia, and personal or socially induced beliefs [22, 24]. Diagnosis is based, other than on the characteristics of the lesions, on a complete and careful clinical history, which should reveal if and why the patient washed inadequately. Diagnostic suspicion may be easily confirmed when disappearance of hyperpigmented lesions is observed with adequate washing [24, 25]. Dermoscopy has been used in a few cases [17, 26, 27] and shows irregularly distributed cornflake-like dark-brown scales.

Histopathological Features

Skin biopsy and histopathology are rarely performed; in the rare cases reported in literature, the picture was nonspecific, with orthokeratotic hyperkeratosis, mild acanthosis, papillomatosis, and absence of inflammatory infiltrate [28, 29].

Differential Diagnosis Various conditions must be considered as possible differential diagnoses: terra firma-forme dermatosis, acanthosis nigricans, verrucous nevi, confluent reticulated papillomatosis of Gougerot and Carteaud, hyperkeratotic pityriasis versicolor, post-inflammatory hyperpigmentation, vagabond's disease, Darier's disease, and X-linked ichthyosis [28, 30, 31].

Treatment Adequate washing is sufficient to achieve rapid and complete *restitutio ad integrum*; in particularly severe cases, keratolytic agents may be required [24, 31]. Associated disorders (e.g., psychiatric illness) should be assessed and managed.

References

1. Duncan WC, Tschen JA, Knox JM. Terra firma-forme dermatosis. Arch Dermatol. 1987;123:567–9.
2. Aslan NÇ, Güler Ş, Demirci K, Isiyel E. Features of terra firma-forme dermatosis. Ann Fam Med. 2018;16:52–4.
3. Sechi A, Patrizi A, Savoia F, Leuzzi M, Guglielmo A, Neri I. Terra firma-forme dermatosis: a systematic review. Int J Dermatol. 2021;60:933–43.
4. O'Brien TJ, Hall AP. Terra firma-forme dermatosis. Australas J Dermatol. 1997;38:163–4.
5. Raveh T, Gilead LT, Wexler MR. Terra firma-forme dermatosis. Ann Plast Surg. 1997;39:542–5.
6. Neri I, Savoia F, Tengattini V, Sechi A, Rucci P, Patrizi A. Terra firma-forme dermatosis is underestimated in children and is associated with atopic dermatitis. J Eur Acad Dermatol Venereol. 2018;32:e421–2.
7. Guarneri C, Guarneri F, Cannavò SP. Terra firma-forme dermatosis. Int J Dermatol. 2008;47:482–4.
8. Borgia F, Cannavò SP. Terra firma-forme dermatosis. Clin Case Rep. 2014;2:19.
9. Santarpia M, Guarneri C. Terra firma-forme dermatosis. Eur J Intern Med. 2016;34:e1–2.
10. Unal E, Guarneri C, Chokoeva AA, Wollina U, Tchernev G. Terra firma-forme dermatosis. Wien Med Wochenschr. 2017;167:66–9.
11. Unal E, Lotti J, Fioranelli M, Roccia MG, Lotti T, Guarneri C, et al. Duncan's dermatosis: from the "terra firma-forme" to a possible syndromic condition. The story of a dirty disease. J Biol Regul Homeost Agents. 2017;31(2 Suppl. 2):39–44.
12. Panchal K, Bhalla N, Salunke P, Jerajani H. Extensive terra firma forme dermatosis [TFFD]: A rare presentation. Indian Dermatol Online J. 2015;6:458–9.
13. Chen HS, Li FG, Zhu Y, Wang T, Fan YM. Penile terra firma-forme dermatosis in a child: ultrastructural observation and topical ethacridine lactate and tacrolimus treatment. Eur J Dermatol. 2019;29:222–4.
14. Greywal T, Cohen PR. Non-invasive methods to establish the diagnosis of terra firma-forme dermatosis: the SMART (skin modified by alcohol rubbing test) evaluation and dermoscopy. Dermatol Online J. 2016; 22.
15. Cohen PR. Terra firma-forme dermatosis: rubbing with alcohol establishes the diagnosis. Skinmed. 2020;18:51–2.
16. Abdel-Razek MM, Fathy H. Terra firma-forme dermatosis: case series and dermoscopic features. Dermatol Online J 2015; 21.
17. Errichetti E, Stinco G. Dermoscopy in terra firma-forme dermatosis and dermatosis neglecta. Int J Dermatol. 2017;56:1481–3.
18. Ozturk DE. Chalk-white fluorescence under wood light in a case of terra firma-forme dermatosis. Clin Exp Dermatol. 2021;46:165–6.
19. Lora V, Ardigò M, Catricalà C, Cota C. Terra firma-forme dermatosis. J Cutan Pathol. 2014;41:141–3.
20. Poskitt L, Wayte J, Wojnarowska F, Wilkinson JD. 'Dermatitis neglecta': unwashed dermatosis. Br J Dermatol. 1995;132:827–9.
21. Pérez-Rodríguez IM, Muñoz-Garza FZ, Ocampo-Candiani J. An unusually severe case of dermatosis neglecta: a diagnostic challenge. Case Rep Dermatol. 2014;6:194–9.
22. Saha A, Seth J, Bindal A, Samanta AB, Gorai S, Sharma A. Dermatosis neglecta: an increasingly recognized entity with review of literature. Indian J Dermatol. 2016;61:450–2.

23. Ruiz-Maldonado R, Durán-McKinster C, Tamayo-Sánchez L, Orozco-Covarrubias ML. Dermatosis neglecta: dirt crusts simulating verrucous nevi. Arch Dermatol. 1999;135:728–9.
24. Qadir SN, Ejaz A, Raza N. Dermatosis neglecta in a case of multiple fractures, shoulder dislocation and radial nerve palsy in a 35-year-old man: a case report. J Med Case Rep. 2008;2:347.
25. Gómez-Fernández C, Casado Verrier B, Sanz Canalejas L, Moreno Alonso de Celada R, Herranz Pinto P. Cornflake-like scales on the ankles and feet. Cleve Clin J Med. 2010;77:8489.
26. Moon J, Park HS, Yoon HS, Cho S. A case of dermatosis neglecta caused by an inappropriate habit of applying a moisturizer. Ann Dermatol. 2017;29:657–9.
27. Piccolo V, Russo T, Delorenze LM, Argenziano G. Perinevic dermatosis neglecta: clinical and dermoscopic description. An Bras Dermatol. 2019;94:361–2.
28. Erker E, Sezer E. Dermatosis neglecta presenting as a brown verrucous plaster. Acta Dermatovenerol Croat. 2012;20:123–5.
29. Richter LL, Miller RM, Hillman JD, Chiu MW. Bilateral thick crusts on the legs. Int J Dermatol. 2013;52:133–5.
30. Saha A, Seth J, Sharma A, Biswas D. Dermatitis neglecta – a dirty dermatosis: report of three cases. Indian J Dermatol. 2015;60:185–7.
31. Lucas JL, Brodell RT, Feldman SR. Dermatosis neglecta: a series of case reports and review of other dirty-appearing dermatoses. Dermatol Online J. 2006;12:5.

Papular Epidermal Nevus with "Skyline" Basal Cell Layer (PENS)

James Anderson-Vildósola, Isabel Colmenero, and Antonio Torrelo

Introduction

The term "papular epidermal nevus with 'skyline' basal cell layer" (PENS) was first used in 2011 to describe a previously unreported type of keratinocyte nevus with distinctive clinical and histopathologic features in five infants [1]. After the initial description of PENS, numerous cases have been reported, including familial cases and cases with associated extracutaneous features, the so-called PENS syndrome.

Clinical Features

Individual PENS lesions are congenital or appear soon after birth. They consist of hyperkeratotic papules with a rough, flat surface (Fig. 1), with size ranging from 1 to 30 mm. They can be located anywhere on the skin surface. Their shape can vary, presenting as round, comma-shaped, rectangular, or polygonal discrete papules. Rarely, the lesions are arranged following the lines of Blaschko [2]. Color ranges from white to brown, and some can show a fine overlying scale. Lesions can be solitary or multiple. PENS predominantly occurs as a sporadic condition; however, there have been several reports of familial cases [3–8].

The association PENS with extracutaneous features is called the PENS syndrome [3–7]. Mild neurological abnormalities have been documented, such as epilepsy, psychomotor delay, and mental retardation [3–7]. Other features include bilateral Achilles tendon shortening, peculiar facies, a curved penis, and hypospadias [9, 10]. Table 1 summarizes published extracutaneous features concomitant with PENS.

J. Anderson-Vildósola · I. Colmenero · A. Torrelo (✉)
Departments of Dermatology and Pathology, Hospital Infantil Universitario Niño Jesús, Madrid, Spain
e-mail: atorrelo@aedv.es

F. Rongioletti, B. R. Smoller (eds.), *New and Emerging Entities in Dermatology and Dermatopathology*, https://doi.org/10.1007/978-3-030-80027-7_9

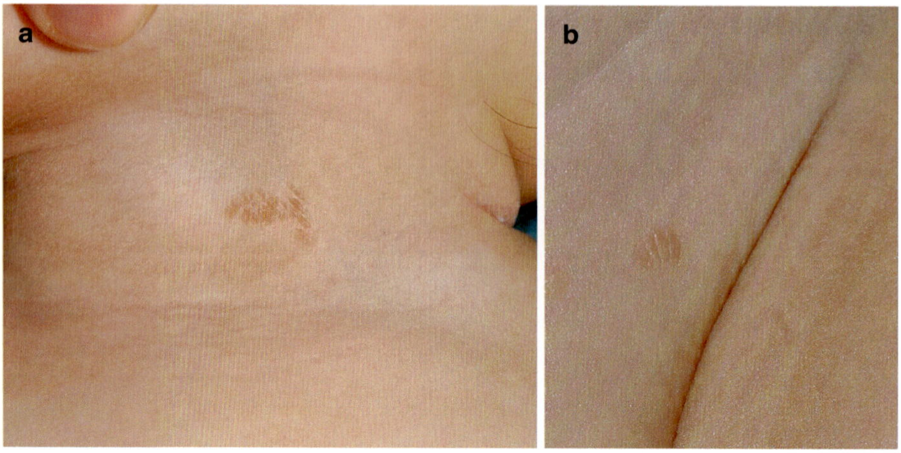

Fig. 1 (**a**), A hyperkeratotic papule on the neck of an infant. (**b**), A round, hyperkeratotic papule with pebbled surface on the groin of an infant

Table 1 Summary of published extracutaneous features of PENS

Reference	Sex	Reported extracutaneous manifestation	Familial
Tadini et al. [3]	F	Speech impairment, disturbance in language structure, and dyslexia	No
	M	Defective dentition, nystagmus, diplopia, mild dizziness, left eye divergent strabismus, and epilepsy	No
	M	Partial epilepsy, psychomotor delay, difficulties in learning, and behavior	No
	M	Motor clumsiness, psychomotor retardation, and attention deficit with hyperactivity	Yes
	F	Dyslexia and psychomotor delay	No
Rodríguez-Díaz et al. [9]	M	Bilateral shortening of Achilles tendon, functional systolic murmur, mild neurosensorial hypoacusia of left ear, mild psychomotor delay, and peculiar facies	No
Pernet et al. [12]	M	Autism spectrum disorder	No
Luna et al. [10]	M	Mild developmental delay, curved penis, and hypospadias	No
Balestri et al. [13]	F	Epileptic seizures	No
Zahn et al. [5]	M	Mild mental retardation, motor clumsiness	Yes
Rizzoli et al. [6]	F	Multiple pilomatricomas and febrile seizures	Yes
	F	Multiple pilomatricomas and febrile seizures	Yes
Beteta-Gorriti et al. [7]	F	Right hydronephrosis	Yes
Pardo et al. [14]	M	Left stiff neck (thinning of the hydromyelia cavity at C5-T1), motor, cognitive, and language neurodevelopmental retardation	No
	F	Right renal aplasia	No

Histopathologic Features

Histopathology shows diffusely compact orthokeratotic hyperkeratosis. Acanthosis is seen, with a peculiar pattern of broad rectangular rete ridges. The basal cell layer shows a striking palisaded arrangement of basal cell nuclei (Fig. 2) [1]. The basal cell layer thus resembles the "skyline" or "eyeliner" pattern of Bowen disease [11]. The dermis has no remarkable changes and adnexal structures appear normal. The epidermis surrounding PENS looks normal, and the demarcation between normal-appearing and lesional skin is abrupt.

Workup

The diagnosis of PENS is made by a correlation of clinical and histologic features. Presently there are no guidelines for the management of PENS, but neurological assessment for any underlying neurodevelopmental abnormality seems reasonable, especially in patients with multiple PENS lesions, as well as inquiring about similar lesions in family members.

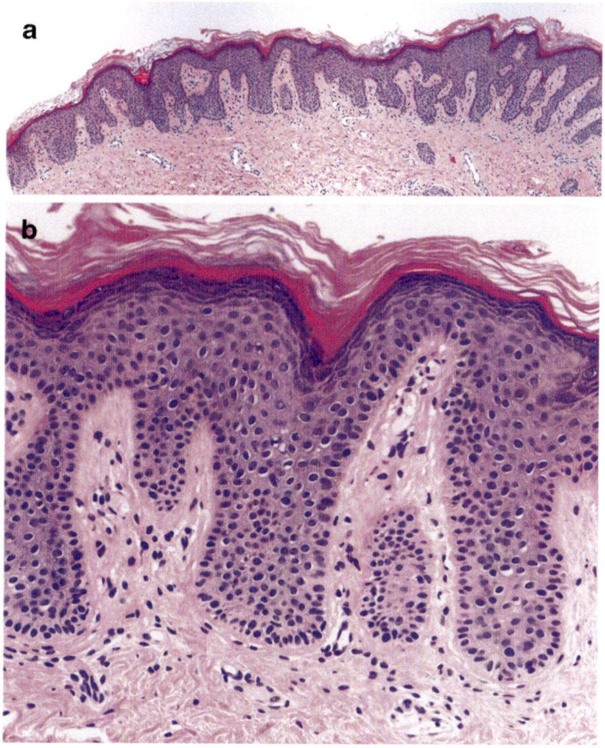

Fig. 2 (**a**), Acanthosis with broad rectangular rete ridges; the basal cell layer shows a striking palisading of basal cell nuclei (H&E stain, original magnification 4x). (**b**), A detail showing the skyline pattern of the basal cell layer (H&E stain, original magnification 40x)

Differential Diagnosis

Keratinocyte epidermal nevi (KEN) are present at birth but are distributed in a linear or whorled pattern following Blaschko lines. From a genetic standpoint, a significant proportion of KEN lesions demonstrate activating mutations in FGFR3 and PIK3CA, which have not been found in PENS [1]. Waxy keratoses of childhood (kerino-keratosis papulosa) is another entity to be considered, although the lesions are different in shape, distribution, and number. By far the most defining hallmark of PENS, which differentiates this entity from other keratinocyte-derived conditions, is the histological finding of the characteristic "skyline" basal cell layer.

Etiopathogenesis

Gene testing for common mutations in FGFR3 and PIK3CA causing keratinocyte nevi failed to reveal a pathogenetic change. No other causal genetic mutations have been found to date. Inheritance and presence of PENS in different members of a family may suggest gonadal mosaicism or a dominant nonlethal condition requiring second-hit mutations to develop the skin lesions [3, 4].

Therapy

There is no specific literature on how to treat PENS. Most lesions are small and do not require treatment. For cosmetic reasons, local destruction or removal can be considered.

Prognosis and Course

The lesions tend to remain stable in morphology although they can grow in accordance with the growth of the patient. Neurological prognosis seems to be favorable as the observed deficiencies subside during infancy or adolescence [5]. There have been no reports of malignancy developing in these types of lesions.

References

1. Torrelo A, Colmenero I, Kristal L, Navarro L, Hafner C, Hernández-Martín A, Requena L, Happle R. Papular epidermal nevus with "skyline" basal cell layer (PENS). J Am Acad Dermatol. 2011;64:888–92.

2. Faure E, Tadini G, Brena M, Cassulini LR. Papular epidermal nevus with "skyline" basal cell layer (PENS) following a Blaschko linear pattern. Pediatr Dermatol. 2013;30:e270–1.
3. Tadini G, Restano L, Happle R, Itin P. PENS syndrome: a new Neurocutaneous phenotype. Dermatology. 2012;224:24–30.
4. Brena M, Besagni F, Boneschi V, Tadini G. Familial Papular epidermal nevus with "skyline" basal cell layer. Pediatr Dermatol. 2014;31:e33–5.
5. Zahn CA, Itin P. Papular epidermal nevus with "skyline" basal cell layer syndrome – natural course: case report and literature review. Case Rep Dermatol. 2017;9:1–5.
6. Rizzoli L, Balestri R, Rech G, Zorzi MG, Speziali L, Pedrolli A, Girardelli CR. Familial papular epidermal nevus with "skyline" basal cell layer and multiple pilomatricomas: a new association? Pediatr Dermatol. 2018;35:e147–50.
7. Beteta-Gorriti V, de Dios-Velázquez Á, Yuste M, Santos-Briz Á, Román-Curto C, Cañueto J. Familial papular epidermal nevus with "skyline" basal cell layer. Pediatr Dermatol. 2018;35:e191–2.
8. Santos Silva LF, Miroux-Catarino A, Pimentel BV, Amaro CS, Viana IF. Familial cases of PENS: a review of the literature. Am J Dermatopathol. 2020;42:593–6.
9. Rodríguez-Díaz E, Gonzalvo P, Colmenero I, Requena L, Hernández-Martín A, Torrelo A. Papular epidermal nevus with "skyline" basal cell layer (PENS) with Extracutaneous findings: brief report. Pediatr Dermatol. 2013;30:e54–6.
10. Luna PC, Pannizardi AA, Martin CI, Vigovich F, Casas JG, Larralde M. Papular epidermal nevus with skyline basal cell layer (PENS): three new cases and review of the literature. Pediatr Dermatol. 2016;33:296–300.
11. Saglam O, Salama M, Meier F, Chaffins M, Ma C, Ormsby A, Lee M. Immunohistochemical staining of palisading basal cells in Bowen's disease and basal involvement in actinic keratosis: contrasting staining patterns suggest different cells of origin. Am J Dermatopathol. 2008;30:4.
12. Pernet C, Munoz J, Bessis D. Syndrome PENS (papular epidermal nevus with "skyline" basal cell layer). Ann Dermatol Vénéréologie. 2015;142:41–5.
13. Balestri R, Rizzoli L, Rech G, Girardelli CR. Dermoscopy of Papular epidermal nevus with skyline basal cell layer. Pediatr Dermatol. 2017;34:e99–e101.
14. Pardo Domínguez C, del Boz GJ, Fúnez Liébana R. Papular epidermal nevus with «skyline»: 3 nuevos casos. Actas Dermosifiliogr. 2020;111:185–7.

Grover Disease with Focus on New Histopathological Patterns

Maria-Teresa Fernández-Figueras and Lluís Puig

Introduction

The entity we are dealing with in this chapter is one of the most curious and mysterious cutaneous disorders. While most dermatological entities have been known for long periods of time, it was not until 1970 that Ralph Weir Grover described six patients with a process that he denominated "transient acantholytic dermatosis" [1]. Shortly after its discovery, a persistent variant of this condition was described, and the denomination of Grover disease (GD) was definitely coined to encompass the spectrum of clinical and histological presentations [2]. The rather nonspecific clinical appearance of this process, which resembles other banal dermatoses, explains why it had been overlooked until recent times. However, it does not justify the little progress made over subsequent years on its knowledge. GD seems to be resisting most attempts to elucidate its pathogenesis and behavior patterns.

The habit of RW Grover of performing Tzanck tests in patients with peculiar transient eruptions was crucial to identify a group of patients with lesions characterized by acantholysis with dyskeratosis [3]. When these cases were analyzed histologically, he realized that despite the resemblance of three of them to Darier disease, and the other three to Hailey-Hailey disease, they had a common clinical presentation that precluded these diagnoses. Grover's seminal paper [1] provides a complete clinicopathological description of the disease, and thereafter, the histopathological characterization of the process was precisely established with the support of AB Ackerman [4] and has been reappraised in recent years [5, 6].

M.-T. Fernández-Figueras (✉)
Anatomic Pathology, Hospital Universitari General de Catalunya. Grupo Quironsalud and Universitat Internacional de Catalunya, Sant Cugat del Vallés (Barcelona), Spain

L. Puig
Dermatology, Hospital de la Santa Creu i Sant Pau, Barcelona, Spain
e-mail: lpuig@santpau.cat

F. Rongioletti, B. R. Smoller (eds.), *New and Emerging Entities in Dermatology and Dermatopathology*, https://doi.org/10.1007/978-3-030-80027-7_10

GD most commonly affects middle-aged males; it has been described in different ethnic groups [7], but most reported cases correspond to Caucasian individuals. Peaks of incidence typically occur in spring and winter [8]. The relevance of GD has been growing as life expectancy increases, cases associated with transplantation, neoplasms and their treatments have become more common, and the ability of making this diagnosis clinically and histopathologically has improved.

Clinical Features

The most frequent form of presentation is an eruption of papules and or papulovesicles in individuals in their 60s that tend to disappear spontaneously, lasting from a few days to several months [5, 9]. Yet, some cases may relapse or persist over years [2, 10]. The male to female ratio ranges from 2:1 [5, 11] to 7:1 [10], according to different series. The lesions are most frequently located on the trunk (Fig. 1 a, b), followed by proximal portions of the limbs. Nonetheless, atypical cases, often related to comorbidities, can be extensive or widespread, involving any topographic location [12]. Exceptionally, GD lesions can adopt unilateral [13] or bilateral [14] Blaschkoid distribution.

Typical lesions are small papules or papulovesicles with frequent formation of crusts and erosions, but some patients present with a predominantly vesicular or bullous eruption that can acquire a pseudo-herpetic appearance. Keratotic or pustulous lesions are frequently described, whereas erythematous plaques [15], nodules [16], and mucosal involvement [10] are exceptional. Patients with dark skin can develop hypopigmented macules [17]. Secondary infection by bacteria or herpes simplex can exhibit a conspicuous pustular presentation [18] and may lead to Kaposi varicelliform eruptions [19]. Most patients complain of pruritus, which may be severe. Sometimes the itch is disproportionate to the small number of lesions [20], although up to one quarter of patients are asymptomatic [9]. In general, chronic and persistent cases tend to be less itchy [20].

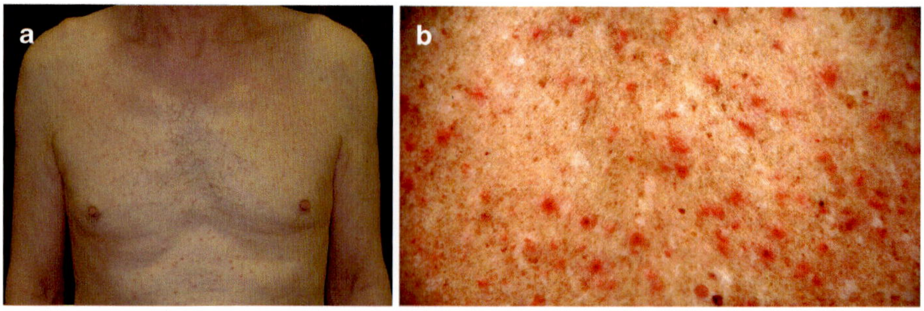

Fig. 1 Grover's disease (**a**). Widespread papular eruption on the trunk and arms. (**b**). Erythematous papules with some crusts on the trunk in a patient with prostate carcinoma

Development of GD is often associated with other dermatological conditions as a Koebner phenomenon [20]. Conversely, Wolf's isotopic response in relation to a previous herpes zoster infection might explain the zosteriform distribution in some patients [21].

Histological Features

The most constant finding of GD is the presence of acantholysis secondary to desmosomal dissolution [22], which can be located basally or in the upper layers of the epidermis resembling pemphigus vulgaris or pemphigus foliaceus (Fig. 2). In addition, keratinocytes often undergo different degrees of individual keratinization. The acantholytic dyskeratotic cells with a nuclear halo denominated "corps ronds" migrate to the epidermal surface where they evolve to form dyskeratotic elements with nuclear remnants known as "grains" (Fig. 3). This abrupt keratinization differs from the usual apoptosis found in lichenoid eruptions and is typical of the group of dermatoses with acantholytic dyskeratosis. In GD these changes can perfectly

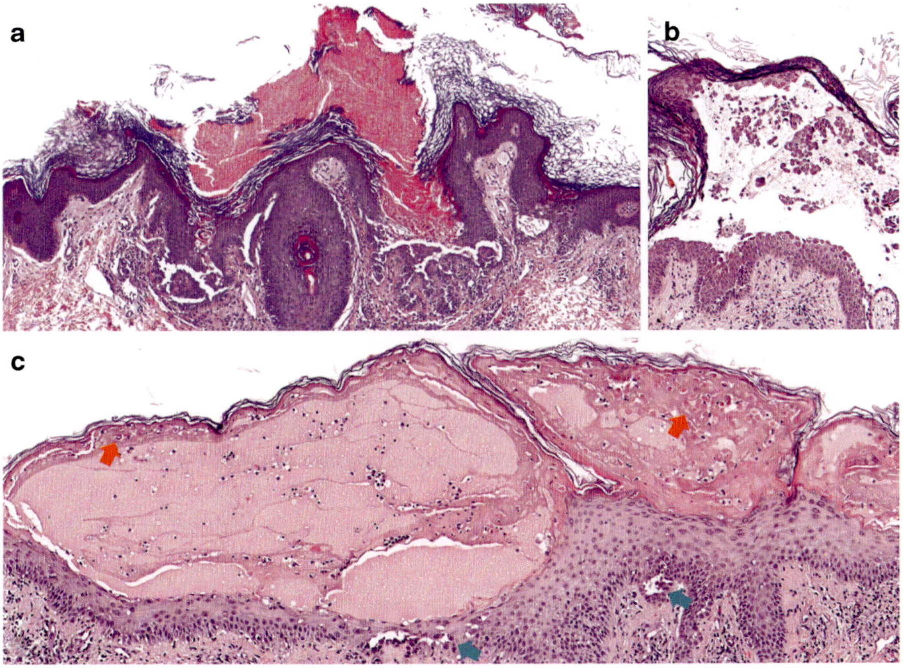

Fig. 2 (**a**) Darier-like pattern in a young patient with Grover disease associated with BRAF inhibitors. (**b**) Epidermis with a dilapidated brick wall appearance typical of Hailey-Hailey disease. (**c**) Vesiculobullous lesion with pemphigus-like suprabasal acantholysis (blue arrows) and superficial acantholytic dyskeratosis (orange arrow). The plasma that accumulated within the blister suggests the existence of previous spongiotic changes

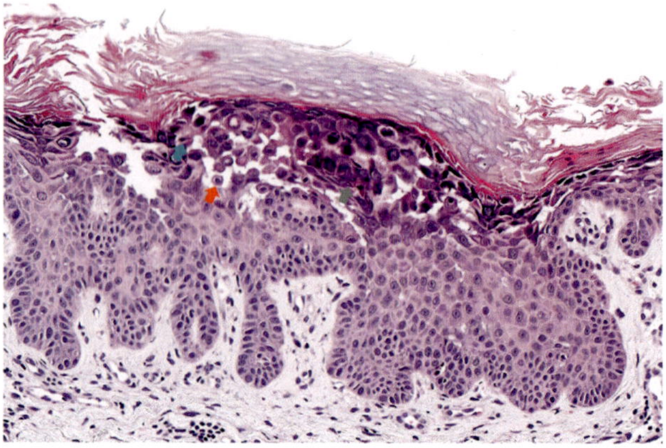

Fig. 3 Epidermis with lentiginous silhouette showing acantholytic dyskeratosis with "corps ronds" (orange arrow) and "grains" (blue arrow), as well as an incipient area of epidermolytic hyperkeratosis (gray arrow)

simulate Darier disease or Hailey-Hailey disease when acantholysis predominates throughout the epidermis (Fig. 2). Spongiosis is also common, although usually mild and nonspecific for diagnostic purposes. In recent years, new histological patterns have been described widening the histopathologic spectrum of GD and allowing recognition of cases that could have been missed or misinterpreted. Among the newly recognized histological variants, vesicular, bullous, and pseudo-herpetic GD are those more often mentioned in the literature [5, 23, 24]. These three names basically describe the same phenomenon, the formation of a large area of dermoepidermal separation, which corresponds to a vesicle (less than 5 mm in diameter) or bulla (5 mm or more). The existence of acantholysis with dyskeratosis justifies the "pseudo-herpetic" denomination [23]. A lentiginous epidermal silhouette (Figs. 3 and 4b) [5, 25, 26] sometimes with keratinocytic atypia, (Fig. 1b) [5, 27] and dysmaturation, is one of the more misleading appearances. Other patterns described in GD are lichenoid (Fig. 1c and d), porokeratosis-like (Fig. 4a) [5, 28], and with epidermolytic hyperkeratosis (Fig. 3) [6, 29]. Difficult cases may require the study of serial sections; nonetheless, areas of epidermal involvement larger than 2 mm are not rare. Underlying these epidermal changes, there is often a dermal infiltrate containing mainly lymphocytes intermixed with scattered macrophages and some eosinophils and neutrophils, which can be abundant in some cases [5, 30]. Capillary vessels within these areas display endothelial tumefaction and mild erythrocyte extravasation [5].

Workup

Dermoscopy with the use of polarized light can contribute to the diagnosis of GD. The most characteristic pattern is a star-like yellow to brown structure corresponding to the central plug that can overlie a pinkish structureless area [31] and present a thin whitish halo [32] or a white radiating pattern containing linear and hairpin vessels [33]. Using reflectance confocal microscopy, acantholytic

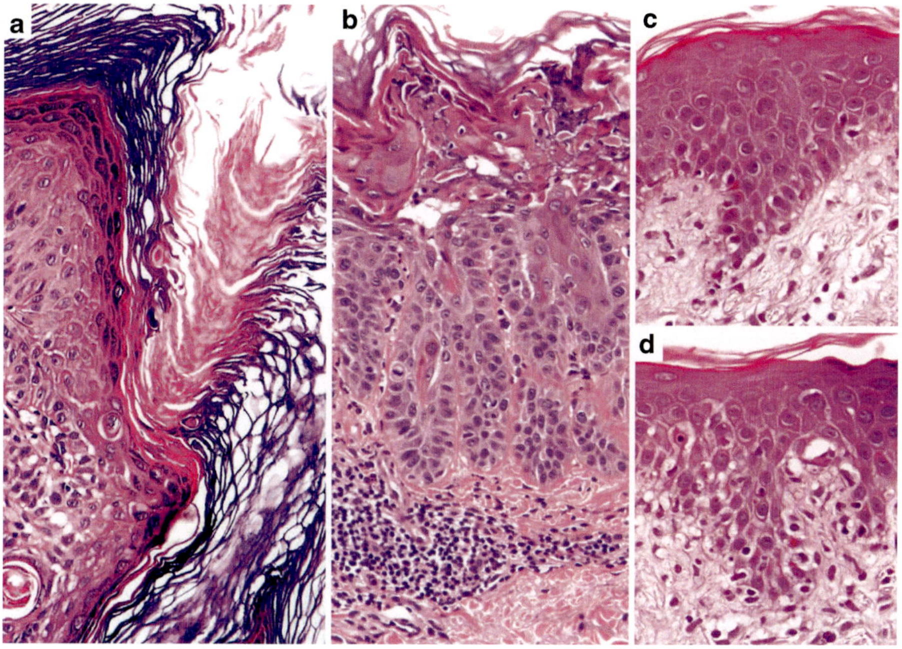

Fig. 4 (**a**) Porokeratosis-like pattern at the edge of a hair follicle (**b**) lentiginous and dysmaturative pattern simulating an inflamed actinic keratosis (**c** and **d**) lichenoid pattern with serrated silhouette (**c**) and lymphocytic infiltrate with apoptosis (**d**)

keratinocytes look as round, bright cells, dyskeratotic cells show a target-like appearance with dark center and peripheral reflecting halo, and intraepidermal clefts give the impression of dark spaces [32]. Since GD is not a systemic disorder, blood tests are only advisable to preclude the association with underlying diseases or the development of superinfections [18, 34, 35], which require microbiological confirmation. Immunofluorescence studies have failed to reveal a consistent pattern of abnormalities, with occasional mild deposition of Ig and/or C3 within the epidermis, either at the basal layer or with intercellular distribution [36].

Differential Diagnosis

Clinically, the main differential diagnoses of GD are folliculitis, arthropod bites, miliaria rubra, prurigo simplex, and papular drug eruptions. A drug eruption can also be considered histologically in cases with neutrophilic or eosinophilic rich infiltrates and when lichenoid features predominate. Darier and Hailey-Hailey disease, as well as pemphigus vulgaris or pemphigus foliaceus, can be microscopically indistinguishable from Grover disease in some sections. The absence of immune deposits is especially significant in the differential diagnosis with pemphigus [24,

37]. The combination of several microscopic patterns in the same specimen, the absence of a family history, and the anatomical distribution of lesions allow differentiation from them. Nevertheless, coexistence of GD with blistering diseases can be occasionally observed [37, 38].

Some biopsies can resemble porokeratosis, but the epidermis lacks its typical appearance [5, 28]. Warty dyskeratomas [39] and acantholytic dyskeratotic acanthomas [40] can be included in the differential diagnosis of GD when patients develop a small number of lesions, but in acanthomas the size of lesions tends to be larger.

As regards papular acantholytic dyskeratosis of the anogenital and genitocrural area [41], familial dyskeratotic comedones [42], and comedonal Darier disease [43], their distinctive location and comedonal silhouette allow differentiation from GD. Nonetheless, localized GD with Blaschkoid distribution can be impossible to differentiate from eruptive linear Darier disease [13] or congenital acantholytic dyskeratotic epidermal nevus following Blaschko lines [44]. The same occurs with relapsing linear acantholytic dermatosis [42, 43], considering a localized form of Hailey-Hailey disease caused by a postzygotic ATP2C1 mutation.

Galli-Galli disease is a rare genodermatosis that is considered a variant of Dowling-Degos disease. Both diseases share the same keratin 5 gene (KRT5) mutation and histologically a lentiginous epidermal silhouette that is always associated with acantholysis in the former, whereas it is sporadic and discrete in the latter [45]. Cases with atypical disseminated distribution involving the extremities and torso that fail to present the usual flexural involvement do not show the same mutation [46, 47].

GD with dysmaturative changes simulates actinic keratosis. Furthermore, this appearance can be accompanied by a lentiginous silhouette that resembles solar lentigo. However, since most biopsies are taken from the back, the absence of actinic elastosis contributes to rule out these diagnoses [5, 25, 27].

Finally, it is important to keep in mind that both acantholysis and dyskeratosis can appear incidentally in many biopsies, individually or combined, and are not rarely seen at the edges of epidermal neoplasms [48].

Etiopathogenesis

The etiopathogenesis of GD remains unknown. In spite of the similarity to Darier and Hailey-Hailey disease, GD has not been associated with abnormalities in the ATP2A2, ATP2C1, or keratin 5 genes [14, 49]. GD has been related to many triggers and conditions that do not seem to have a direct role in its development. The best-known exacerbating factors are heat and sweating, which were considered responsible for the occlusion of the acrosyringial portion of eccrine glands. However, acantholytic involvement of the acrosyringia is currently not deemed important, despite former conjectures [5, 50, 51]. Ultraviolet or ionizing irradiations are common triggers, but their direct contribution is unclear [9], especially considering that phototherapy has been used as a treatment [52]. Many dermatological conditions as well as xerosis or a dry ambience have likewise been implicated in the development of GD, but their main contribution might well be impairment of the epidermal integrity [16]. Finally, renal failure and dialysis have been commonly implicated in the development of GD, and in one csase complete resolution followed renal transplantation [53].

The most frequent comorbidities in patients with GD are malignant hematological and non-hematological neoplasms [9]. Bone marrow and solid organ transplantation, targeted therapies, and immune checkpoint inhibitors have also been associated with development of GD, often giving raise to atypical forms that some authors denominate “Grover-like” (Fig. 2a). Atypical extensive forms tend to involve at least one region besides the trunk and are associated with malignancy (61%), recent chemotherapy (38%), and recent transplantation (20%) [12].

Autoimmunity does not seem to be involved in the pathogenesis of GD. However, the damage of desmosomal structures caused by the disease may expose sequestered antigens to the immune system, stimulating the development of autoantibodies. This process can explain the development of bullous disorders such as pemphigus or pemphigoid in some GD patients [38, 54, 55].

Therapy

There are few studies with a high level of evidence because all articles are case reports or case series, and frequent spontaneous resolution of the disease and publication bias impair the interpretation of results. Topical mid-high potency corticosteroids are the mainstay of symptomatic treatment, alone or in combination with antibiotics, calcipotriol or calcineurin inhibitors. Second-line treatment includes low-dose (10–20 mg/day) retinoids (isotretinoin or acitretin) and/or low-dose systemic corticosteroids (approximately 20 mg prednisone equivalent daily). Phototherapy (nbUVB, UVA1) and photochemotherapy (PUVA) have been repeatedly reported as successful therapeutic options [9].

Prognosis and Course

GD resolves spontaneously within weeks to months in 40% of patients [9], but it can be persistent and recur repeatedly for years.

Conclusions: GD is generally transient and often asymptomatic but can cause severe itching. In recent years new histopathological patterns have been described widening the microscopic spectrum of GD.

References

1. Grover RW. Transient acantholytic dermatosis. Arch Dermatol. 1970;101:426–34.
2. Simon RS, Bloom D, Ackerman AB. Persistent acantholytic dermatosis. A variant of transient acantholytic dermatosis (Grover disease). Arch Dermatol. 1976;112:1429–31.
3. Krivo JM, Ackerman AB, Lepaw MI. In memoriam: Dr Ralph Wier Grover: friend, teacher, and dermatologist. J Am Acad Dermatol. 2010;62:e3.
4. Chalet M, Grover R, Ackerman AB. Transient acantholytic dermatosis: a reevaluation. Arch Dermatol. 1977;113:431–5.
5. Fernández-Figueras M-T, Puig L, Cannata P, Cuatrecases M, Quer A, Ferrándiz C, Ariza A. Grover disease: a reappraisal of histopathological diagnostic criteria in 120 cases. Am J Dermatopathol. 2010;32:541–9.
6. Bearden JN, Essary LR, Cockerell CJ. Grover disease with features of epidermolytic hyperkeratosis. Am J Dermatopathol. 2014;36:358–9.
7. Parsons JM. Transient acantholytic dermatosis (Grover's disease): a global perspective. J Am Acad Dermatol. 1996;35:653–66.
8. Harvell JD, Selig DJ. Seasonal variations in dermatologic and dermatopathologic diagnoses: a retrospective 15-year analysis of dermatopathologic data. Int J Dermatol. 2016;55:1115–8.
9. Bellinato F, Maurelli M, Gisondi P, Girolomoni G. Clinical features and treatments of transient acantholytic dermatosis (Grover's disease): a systematic review. J Dtsch Dermatol Ges. 2020; https://doi.org/10.1111/ddg.14202.
10. Davis MDP, Dinneen AM, Landa N, Gibson LE. Grover's disease: Clinicopathologic review of 72 cases. Mayo Clin Proc. 1999;74:229–34.
11. Scheinfeld N, Mones J. Seasonal variation of transient acantholytic dyskeratosis (Grover's disease). J Am Acad Dermatol. 2006;55:263–8.
12. Gantz M, Butler D, Goldberg M, Ryu J, McCalmont T, Shinkai K (2017) Atypical features and systemic associations in extensive cases of Grover disease: a systematic review. J am Acad Dermatol.77:952–7.e1.
13. di Meo N, Ulessi B, Trevisini S, Noal C, Nan K, Vichi S, Trevisan G. Monolateral Grover's disease with Blaschkoid distribution. Acta Dermatovenerol Croat. 2017;25:31–311.
14. Asahina A, Ishiko A, Saito I, Hasegawa K, Sawamura D, Nakano H. Grover's disease following multiple bilateral Blaschko lines: a rare clinical presentation with genetic and electron microscopic analyses. Dermatology (Basel). 2012;225:183–7.
15. Erythematous plaque variant of transient acantholytic dermatosis. - Abstract - Europe PMC. https://europepmc.org/article/med/3731869. Accessed 15 Nov 2020.
16. Aldana PC, Khachemoune A. Grover disease: review of subtypes with a focus on management options. Int J Dermatol. 2020;59:543–50.
17. Rowley MJ, Nesbitt LT, Carrington PR, Espinoza CG. Hypopigmented macules in acantholytic disorders. Int J Dermatol. 1995;34:390–2.
18. Bunce PA, Stanford DG. Grover's disease secondarily infected with herpes simplex virus and Staphylococcus aureus: case report and review. Australas J Dermatol. 2013;54:e88–91.
19. Karray M, Kwan E, Souissi A (2020) Kaposi Varicelliform Eruption. StatPearls.
20. Quirk CJ, Heenan PJ. Grover's disease: 34 years on. Australas J Dermatol. 2004;45:83–6; quiz 87–88.
21. Lee HJ, Jung KE, Kim HS, Lee JY, Kim HO, Park YM. Zosteriform transient acantholytic dermatosis. J Dermatol. 2014;41:104–5.
22. Hashimoto K, Fujiwara K, Tada J, Harada M, Setoyama M, Eto H. Desmosomal dissolution in Grover's disease, Hailey-Hailey's disease and Darier's disease. J Cutan Pathol. 1995;22:488–501.
23. Capusan TM, Herrero-Moyano M, Fraga J, Llamas-Velasco M. Clinico-pathological study of 4 cases of Pseudoherpetic Grover disease: the same as vesicular Grover disease. Am J Dermatopathol. 2018;40:445–8.

24. Li YM, Milikowski C, Galimberti F. Case of bullous Grover disease. Am J Dermatopathol. 2020; https://doi.org/10.1097/DAD.0000000000001756.
25. Cooper SM, Dhittavat J, Millard P, Burge S. Extensive Grover's-like eruption with lentiginous "freckling": report of two cases. Br J Dermatol. 2004;150:350–2.
26. Melwani PM, Parsons AC, Sangueza OP. Early histopathologic changes in Grover disease. Am J Dermatopathol. 2010;32:565–7.
27. Aljarbou OZ, Asgari M, Al-Saidi N, Silloca-Cabana EO, Alathamneh M, Sangueza OP. Grover disease with epidermal Dysmaturation pattern: a common histopathologic finding. Am J Dermatopathol. 2018;40:642–6.
28. Montoya C, Arias LM, Salazar M, Flórez HA. Porokeratosis-like Grover disease: more than an Acantholytic pattern. Actas Dermosifiliogr. 2019;110:332–4.
29. Bardazzi F, Pepe F, Malosso M, Loi C, Baraldi C, Misciali C, Patrizi A. Epidermolytic hyperkeratosis: one more pattern of Grover disease. Int J Dermatol. 2020; https://doi.org/10.1111/ijd.15055.
30. Togo S, Ozawa K, Fujii A, Tanii T, Tsuruta D, Ishii N, Hashimoto T, Tadokoro T, Isei T. Neutrophil-rich variant of persistent bullous Grover's disease. Acta Derm Venereol. 2019;99:1282–3.
31. Specchio F, Argenziano G, Tiodorovic-Zivkovic D, Moscarella E, Lallas A, Zalaudek I, Longo C. Dermoscopic clues to diagnose acantholytic dyskeratosis. Dermatol Pract Concept. 2015;5:59–60.
32. Lacarrubba F, Boscaglia S, Nasca MR, Caltabiano R, Micali G. Grover's disease: dermoscopy, reflectance confocal microscopy and histopathological correlation. Dermatol Pract Concept. 2017;7:51–4.
33. de Abreu L, Guimarães Cordeiro NG, Buçard AM, Quintella DC, Argenziano G. Dermoscopy of Grover disease. J Am Acad Dermatol. 2017;76:S60–3.
34. Aldabagh B, Patel RR, Honda K. Leukemia cutis in association with Grover's disease. Am J Dermatopathol. 2011;33:e41–3.
35. García-Río I, Delgado-Jimenez Y, Aragüés M, Fernández-Herrera J, Fraga J, García-Díez A. A case of Grover's disease with syringoma-like features and leukemia cutis. J Cutan Pathol. 2006;33:443–6.
36. Bystryn JC. Immunofluorescence studies in transient acantholytic dermatosis (Grover's disease). Am J Dermatopathol. 1979;1:325–7.
37. Magdaleno-Tapial J, Valenzuela-Oñate C, Martínez-Doménech Á, García-Legaz-Martínez M, Carballeira-Braña A, Sánchez-Carazo JL, Pérez-Ferriols A, Alegre-de Miquel V. Coexistence of pemphigus Foliaceus and Grover disease after a radical surgery for basal cell carcinoma. Am J Dermatopathol. 2019;41:744–6.
38. Matsudate Y, Urano Y, Hashimoto T. Grover's disease in a patient with pemphigus vulgaris. Int J Dermatol. 2017;56:1052–4.
39. Kaddu S, Dong H, Mayer G, Kerl H, Cerroni L. Warty dyskeratoma - "follicular dyskeratoma": analysis of clinicopathologic features of a distinctive follicular adnexal neoplasm. J Am Acad Dermatol. 2002;47:423–8.
40. Goldenberg A, Lee RA, Cohen PR. Acantholytic dyskeratotic acanthoma: case report and review of the literature. Dermatol Pract Concept. 2014;4:25–30.
41. Al-Muriesh M, Abdul-Fattah B, Wang X, Zhao M, Chen S, Huang C. Papular acantholytic dyskeratosis of the anogenital and genitocrural area: case series and review of the literature. J Cutan Pathol. 2016;43:749–58.
42. Van Geel NA, Kockaert M, Neumann HA. Familial dyskeratotic comedones. Br J Dermatol. 1999;140:956–9.
43. Llamas-Velasco M, Kempf W, Cavelier-Balloy B, Camarero-Mulas C, Gomez-Vazquez MM, Rütten A, Fraga J, Fernández-Figueras MT. Comedonal Darier's disease: six additional cases and a review of this entity. J Dtsch Dermatol Ges. 2020; https://doi.org/10.1111/ddg.14179.

44. Huh WK, Fujiwara K, Takahashi H, Kanitakis J. Congenital acantholytic dyskeratotic epidermal naevus following Blaschko's lines versus segmental Darier's disease. Eur J Dermatol. 2007;17:130–2.
45. Hanneken S, Rütten A, Pasternack SM, et al. Systematic mutation screening of KRT5 supports the hypothesis that Galli-Galli disease is a variant of Dowling-Degos disease. Br J Dermatol. 2010;163:197–200.
46. Yang A, Cheung K, Kossard S, Murrell DF. Atypical disseminated variant of Galli-Galli disease: a review of the literature. Am J Dermatopathol. 2020;42:484–90.
47. Rongioletti F, Fausti V, Christana K, Montinari M, Parodi A, Fiocca R. Atypical variant of galli-galli disease (Grover-like eruption with lentiginous freckling) in a liver transplant patient. Am J Dermatopathol. 2011;33:504–7.
48. Gaertner EM. Incidental cutaneous reaction patterns: Epidermolytic hyperkeratosis, Acantholytic Dyskeratosis, and Hailey-Hailey-like Acantholysis: a potential marker of premalignant skin change. J Skin Cancer. 2011; https://doi.org/10.1155/2011/645743.
49. Powell J, Sakuntabhai A, James M, Burge S, Hovnanian A. Grover's disease, despite histological similarity to Darier's disease, does not share an abnormality in the ATP2A2 gene. Br J Dermatol. 2000;143:658.
50. Antley CM, Carrington PR, Mrak RE, Smoller BR. Grover's disease (transient acantholytic dermatosis): relationship of acantholysis to acrosyringia. J Cutan Pathol. 1998;25:545–9.
51. Hashimoto K, Moiin A, Chang MW, Tada J. Sudoriferous acrosyringeal acantholytic disease. A subset of Grover's disease J Cutan Pathol. 1996;23:151–64.
52. Powell JB, Gach JE. Phototherapy in the elderly. Clin Exp Dermatol. 2015;40:605–10.
53. González-Sixto B, Rosón E, De La Torre C, Garcia-Doval I, Cruces M. Grover's disease in a patient undergoing peritoneal dialysis with resolution after renal transplant. Acta Derm Venereol. 2007;87:561–2.
54. Ellenbogen E, Geller S, Azrielant S, et al. Grover disease and bullous pemphigoid: a clinicopathological study of six cases. Clin Exp Dermatol. 2019;44:524–7.
55. Phillips C, Kalantari-Dehaghi M, Marchenko S, Chernyavsky AI, Galitovskiy V, Gindi V, Chun S, Paslin D, Grando SA. Is Grover's disease an autoimmune dermatosis? Exp Dermatol. 2013;22:781–4.

The Spectrum of Acquired Elastolytic Disorders

T. Gambichler

Introduction

Fibrillar elastin and collagen are two of the basic extracellular matrix (ECM) components significantly contributing to the maintenance of skin structure, elasticity, and, hence, resilience. They each form an architecturally distinct meshwork that confers elastic recoil properties to the skin. The formation of elastic fibers is complex and not yet fully understood. Tropoelastin – the crucial building component of elastin – is expressed by the *ELN* gene, and the mature form of the protein is secreted into the ECM [1, 2]. Tropoelastin accumulates on the cell surface, first as small particles and then as larger spherules which are associated coacervates of tropoelastin. Tropoelastin is subjected to oxidase (LOX) and LOX-like (LOXL) enzymes at a subset of lysines which subsequently participate in aldol condensation and Schiff base reactions to form cross-links [1, 2]. The forming elastin is introduced to microfibrils (fibrillin-1) in the ECM by members of the fibulin protein family where the elastin fibers are assembled. The resulting protein elastin is a highly stable and robust structure with an impressive ability to confer recoil to human tissues such as the skin. A dense mass of elastic fibers characterizes the reticular dermis and is crucial for the overall elasticity of the skin. In general, the most mature, thicker elastin fibers are found deep in the dermis, where they function as an interpenetrating elastin network [1–4].

As mentioned above, the fundamental building component of elastin is tropoelastin encoded by the *ELN* gene, whose expression is highest before birth and during the first years of life. Thereafter, tropoelastin gene expression, and, thus, elastin formation, decreases significantly. In middle-aged subjects, only a small fraction of elastin is still produced [1–4]. Hence, adults have to rely mostly on the elastin that was deposited in the first few years of life. As a consequence, damage to elastin in

T. Gambichler (✉)
Department of Dermatology, Ruhr-University Bochum, Bochum, Germany
e-mail: t.gambichler@klinikum-bochum.de

F. Rongioletti, B. R. Smoller (eds.), *New and Emerging Entities in Dermatology and Dermatopathology*, https://doi.org/10.1007/978-3-030-80027-7_11

the skin of adults following injuries (e.g., burns), loss during the aging process or through elastolytic disorders, and the lack of robust endogenous elastin synthesis will not be repaired efficiently, thereby leading to loss of skin elasticity [1–5].

At least in part, cutis laxa (CL), acrokeratoelastoidosis, and anetoderma (AD) may belong to the inherited cutaneous elastolytic disorders [6, 7]. In CL, for example, various gene defects have been identified resulting in complex cutaneous as well as non-cutaneous clinical manifestations, e.g., Williams-Beuren syndrome and Menkes disease [8]. However, the pathomechanisms of acquired elastolytic skin diseases are poorly understood given the paucity of reported patients and limited research in this field. Several acquired disorders in which loss of dermal elastic tissue results in prominent clinical and histopathological features have been observed, including acquired CL (ACL), AD, annular elastolytic giant cell granuloma (AEGCG), mid-dermal elastolysis (MDE), papular elastorrhexis (PE), perifollicular elastolysis (PFE), fibroelastolytic papulosis (FEP), and sporadic acrokeratoelastoidosis (SAKE) [7, 9–14]. In the following brief review, we will focus on acquired elastolytic skin disorders.

Anetoderma

Clinical Features

AD is a benign asymptomatic elastolytic skin disease characterized by well-circumscribed, focal areas of flaccid skin usually manifesting on the trunk and proximal extremities. AD presents as round to oval atrophic depressions, wrinkled patches, or herniated sac-like protrusions. Once present, AD tends to be active over decades. It usually affects middle-aged women. Different subtypes of AD have previously been distinguished, including primary (idiopathic) AD, secondary AD from a preceding skin disease, drug-induced AD, familial AD, and AD associated with prematurity. Today, terms such as the Jadassohn-Pellizzari, Schweninger-Buzzi, and Alexander types are antiquated [6, 15]. Secondary AD usually develops in areas of pathologic skin, including acne vulgaris, varicella, sarcoidosis, tuberculosis, mastocytosis, nodular amyloidosis, lupus erythematosus, etc. Drug-induced AD can be induced by penicillamine. Familial (autosomal-dominant) AD is very rare. Premature AD is observed in premature neonates (24 to 29 weeks of gestational age).

Histopathological Features

On hematoxylin-eosin stain, the skin looks relatively normal, perhaps with some signs of inflammation. With special elastic tissue stain, there is almost complete loss of elastic fibers from the papillary to the reticular dermis sometimes accompanied by perivascular infiltrates with histiocytes and plasma cells. On electron microscopy, elastophagocytosis and small fragmented elastic fibrils may be observed in lesional skin.

Etiopathogenesis

The underlying pathomechanisms of AD are uncertain. Loss of elastic tissue may be due to a decrease in elastin synthesis, increase in elastin degradation, decrease in elastolytic enzyme inhibitors, and/or increased elastin phagocytosis [16–18].

Workup

In order to differentiate AD from other acquired elastolytic disorders (e.g., MDE), diagnosis should be confirmed by histopathology. Since primary AD may be associated with antiphospholipid syndrome, antibody status should be evaluated [15, 18].

Cutis Laxa

Clinical Features

ACL can be either localized or generalized. Generalized ACL may occur after an inflammatory skin disorder. Most frequently adults are affected. Generalized elastolysis also manifesting in the bronchioloalveolar tract appears to have a poor prognosis. Some cases have been described after drug intake or infectious diseases. A rare subtype of ACL represents Marshall's syndrome or postinflammatory elastolysis and cutis laxa that is characterized by acute inflammatory skin lesions (urticarial, papulous) resulting in destruction of elastic tissue, skin wrinkling, and severe physical disfigurement in young children [9]. Nevertheless, ACL is relatively often observed in patients with monoclonal gammopathy and related disorders. Localized ACL usually affects the extremities. It may be associated with underlying diseases such as rheumatoid polyarthritis, syphilis, sarcoidosis, amyloidosis, and, again, monoclonal gammopathy. Patients with only cutaneous involvement have a good prognosis, and life expectancy is usually normal [19–32].

Histopathological Features

Histopathology reveals a decrease in elastic tissue in the entire dermis. Giant cells may also be seen phagocyting elastic fibers. ACL is also associated with dermal inflammatory infiltrates. On electron microscopy, the elastic fiber structure is often irregularly fragmented [8, 22–24].

Etiopathogenesis

Heritable types of CL have variable transmissions and clinical expressions including autosomal dominant, autosomal recessive, and X-linked recessive [20, 21]. ACL is more frequent and characterized by a later onset. All types of CL have progressive loose and sagging skin with reduced elasticity usually manifesting with large skin folds. ACL can follow the beginning of an inflammatory condition, which increases the degradation of elastic fibers.

Annular Elastolytic Giant Cell Granuloma

Clinical Features

AEGCG is characterized by annular, polycyclic erythematous lesions with raised borders predominantly affecting ultraviolet (UV)-exposed skin, including the face, neck, arms, and the upper back (Fig. 1). Diabetes mellitus is the systemic disease most frequently associated with this condition. AEGCG usually manifests in the

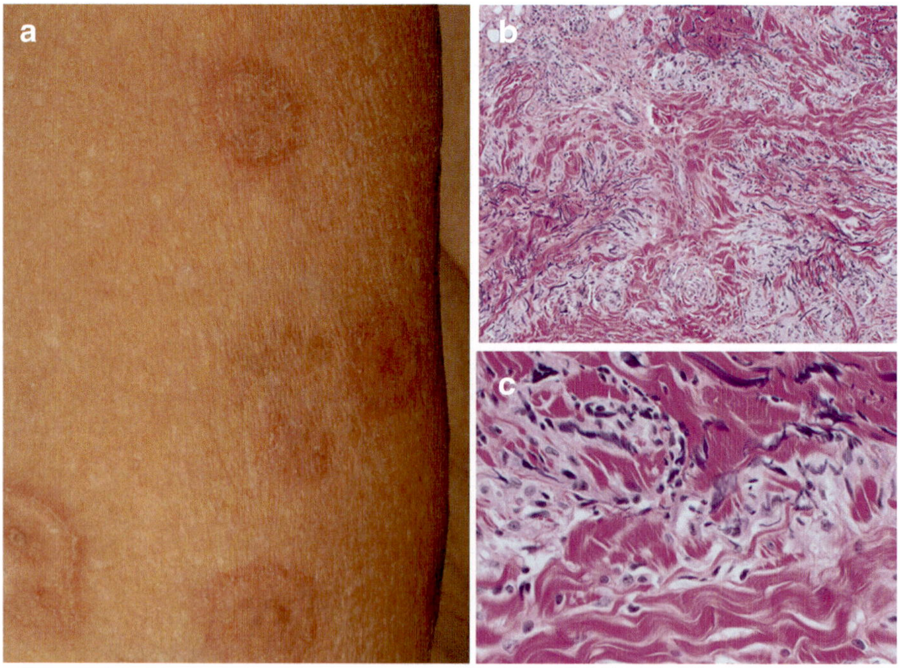

Fig. 1 Showing annular skin lesions on the left arm of a 59-year-old diabetic patient (**a**). Histopathology revealed a granulomatous reaction (**b**) and elastophagocytosis by multinucleate giant cells (**c**) including the absence of collagen necrobiosis. A diagnosis of annular elastolytic giant cell granuloma was made

fourth to the seventh decade with a male preponderance to equal gender occurrence [33–37].

Histopathological Features

AEGCG represents as granulomatous reaction with elastolysis, phagocytosis of the elastic fibers by multinucleate giant cells (Fig. 1), and absence or reduction of elastin fibers.

Differential Diagnosis

Histopathological hallmarks also include absence of collagen necrobiosis, or mucin deposition, as observed in necrobiosis lipoidica and granuloma annulare, respectively.

Etiopathogenesis

Pathogenesis of AEGCG is barely understood. Initially described as actinic granuloma, atypical necrobiosis lipoidica, and Miescher's granuloma of the face, it is proposed an UV-induced cellular immunological reaction wherein the elastin immunopathogenicity of elastin fibers may play a crucial role resulting in AEGCG [33–37].

Mid-Dermal Elastolysis

MDE is a rare acquired skin disease characterized by selective loss of elastic fibers confined to the mid-dermis (Fig. 2). MDE usually affects younger Caucasian females. Most commonly found skin lesions include well-circumscribed patches of fine wrinkles (type I), perifollicular papular protrusions (type II), and persistent reticular erythema and wrinkles (type III). Skin lesions are predominantly observed on the trunk and proximal extremities [5, 38–41].

Histopathological Features

Hematoxylin-eosin staining does not reveal significant changes that could aid in diagnosing MDE. Disease-defining histopathological findings identified by elastica stains (e.g., Orcein stain, Verhoeff-van Gieson stain) include a band-like or focal

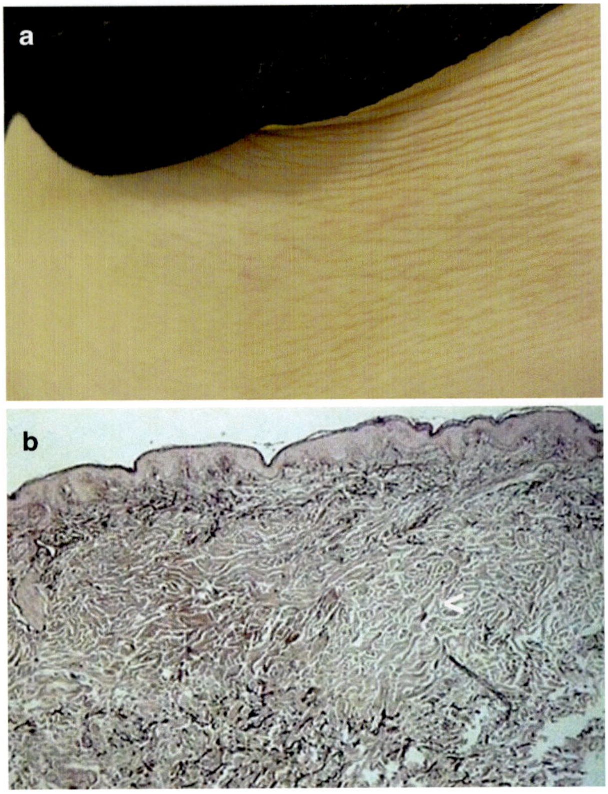

Fig. 2 A 32-year-old woman presented with fine wrinkling under her breasts without evidence of inflammation (**a**). On histopathology, almost complete loss (<) of elastic fibers was observed in the mid-dermis (**b**). The clinical and histopathological findings were consistent with the diagnosis of mid-dermal elastolysis

loss of elastic fibers in the mid-dermis. In contrast, no histological alterations are found in the papillary and deeper reticular dermis.

Etiopathogenesis

The pathogenesis of MDE remains unclear. However, some insights into MDE pathomechanisms have been gained during the last decades [5, 19]. Current data on MDE patients suggest that cooperation of different cell populations resident in the mid-dermis (e.g., macrophages, fibroblasts) may result in enhanced elastolytic activity due to matrix metalloproteinases overexpression as well as a concomitant decreased expression of tissue inhibitor of matrix metalloproteinases. Such enhanced elastolytic activity might then produce the zonal degradation and loss of elastic tissue in the mid-dermis. However, the causes leading to enhanced elastolytic activity in MDE remain elusive but are very likely multifactorial, including genetic predisposition, preceding inflammation, and (auto)immune processes.

Moreover, the capacity of elastic fiber remodeling and renewal through LOXL and fibulins appears to be diminished in lesional skin of MDE patients [38–41]. In previous studies and case reports, MDE was frequently reported to be associated with granuloma annulare, atopic dermatitis, Sweet's syndrome, and different (auto) immune processes such as rheumatoid arthritis, Hashimoto thyroiditis, Grave's disease, systemic lupus erythematosus, type I diabetes, dermatitis herpetiformis, and the presence of antiphospholipid antibodies [5]. Other pathogenetic factors previously discussed in MDE include the influence of sex hormones and UV radiation.

Papular Elastorrhexis

Clinical Features

PE usually affects females in the second decade of life. It is clinically characterized by asymptomatic non-follicular small firm white papules on the trunk. There exists no history for preceding trauma and inflammatory processes or other associated systemic conditions [7, 11].

Histopathological Features

Marked fragmentation or even complete loss of elastic fibers can be observed in the reticular dermis. Sparse inflammatory infiltrates may also be observed. Collagen bundles can be thickened and homogenized.

Differential Diagnosis

Other acquired elastolytic disorders may be considered as differential diagnoses, including nevus anelasticus (NA) and eruptive collagenoma (EC). Ryder et al. [13], however, recently suggested that it is not possible to definitely differentiate whether these three conditions represent the same disease state, multiple distinct diagnoses, or different points of the same disease spectrum. Ryder et al. [13] argued that the considerable similarities in the clinical and histopathological features, combined with similar times of disease onset, similar localization of lesions, and lack of history of trauma, inflammation, family history, or systemic manifestations, indicate that NA, PE, and EC are the same entity, whereby the term PE likely describes the clinical and histopathologic picture at best [7, 12, 42].

Perifollicular Elastolysis

Clinical Features

PFE is a relatively common acquired elastolytic disease characterized by tiny grayish/whitish, discretely wrinkled lesions associated with loss of elastic fibers surrounding hair follicles and balloon-like protrusions over the face and upper back. However, other affected sites (intertriginous) and associated conditions (atopic dermatitis) have been described [43].

Histopathological Features

Histopathologic investigation predominantly reveals almost complete loss of elastic fibers around hair follicles in the absence of inflammatory infiltrates, vessel involvement, or collagen anomalies. An increased amount of mucin may be also observed around involved hair follicles [7, 43, 44].

Etiopathogenesis

PE is usually associated with acne vulgaris due to an elastase-producing strain of *S. epidermidis.*

Fibroelastolytic Papulosis

FEP is a rare, relatively new acquired fibroelastolytic disorder that presents clinically as whitish/yellowish papules and plaques most commonly occurring on the neck of elderly patients (Fig. 3a). To date, the term FEP encompasses two elastolytic conditions, i.e. pseudoxanthoma elasticum-like papillary dermal elastolysis (PXE-PDE) and white fibrous papulosis of the neck (WFPN). and papillary dermal elastosis (PDE) [10, 45–50].

Clinical Features

In PXE-PDE, firstly described by Rongioletti and Rebora [10], small yellowish coalescing papules are observed tending to develop into cobblestone plaques on the neck (Fig. 4), thus simulating inherited pseudoxanthoma elasticum [10, 45].

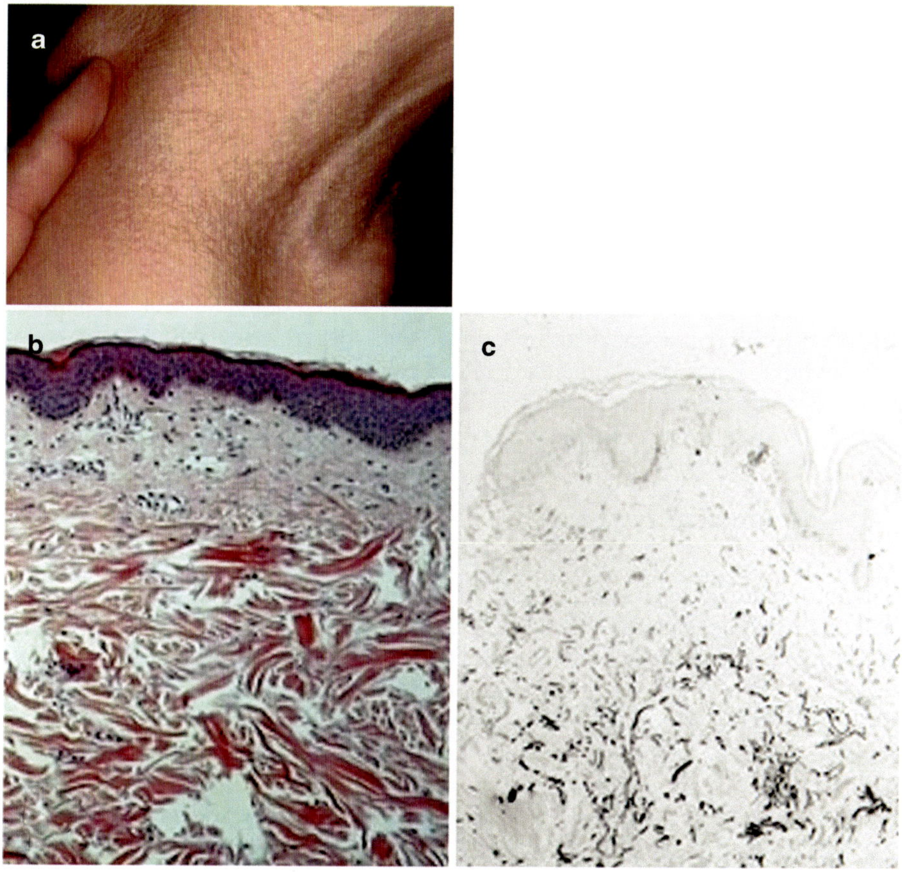

Fig. 3 Showing tiny yellowish papules on the neck of an elderly woman (**a**). Routine histopathology revealed increased density of the collagen network including thickening of collagen bundles (**b**). Elastica stain showed loss of the elastic fibers in the papillary and upper reticular dermis (**c**). A diagnosis of fibroelastolytic papulosis was made (courtesy of Franco Rongioletti, Milan, Italy)

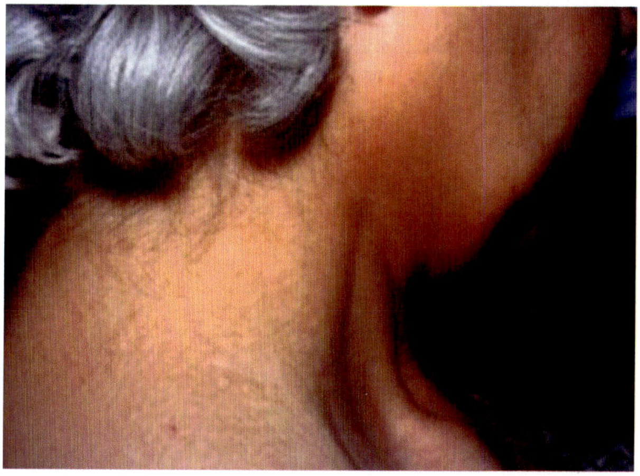

Fig. 4 An elderly woman presented with multiple yellowish papules around her neck clinically consistent with a diagnosis of pseudoxanthoma elasticum-like papillary dermal elastolysis (courtesy of Franco Rongioletti, Milan, Italy)

Predilection sites include the neck, supraclavicular fossae, and flexural areas. In contrast to pseudoxanthoma elasticum, systemic involvement has never been reported in PXE-PDE. Although the epidemiology of PXE-PDE is predominately in females after the fifth decade of life, recent case reports have documented PXE-PDE in young females as well [51]. To date, more than 50 cases have been reported under the term PXE-PDE [49].

Similar to PXE-PDE, WFPN presents with multiple whitish, round, small papules on the neck. It is a rare condition, first described in elderly Japanese. As mentioned before, it is believed to belong to the broader category of FEP [12, 46, 48]. The lesions of WFPN present on the posterior, occipital, or lateral neck, sometimes extending to the supraclavicular area, upper back, or rarely the axilla as numerous 2–3 mm (up to 6 mm) non-follicular white or pale firm discrete papules that tend not to coalesce into plaques, in contrast to PXE-PDE.

Histopathological Features

FEP may comprise a spectrum of very similar acquired elastolytic disorders among PXE-PDE that appears to be the most reported and best investigated condition so far (52). As proposed by Rongioletti et al. [45], marked reduction or loss of oxytalan and elaunin fibers in the papillary elastic plexus is the histologic hallmark of PXE-PDE (Fig.3b,c). The main histopathological feature of WFPN on routine hematoxylin-eosin stains is a distinct area of thickened collagen bundles arranged haphazardly in the papillary and upper to mid-reticular dermis. Mild hyperorthokeratosis and a sparse perivascular lymphocytic infiltrate can be seen in the superficial dermis.

Sporadic Acrokeratoelastoidosis

Clinical Features

SAKE manifests with multiple, usually bilateral, asymptomatic, yellowish/whitish, aggregated, small papules on the thenar and hypothenar eminences of the palms and more rarely on the soles. This very infrequent form of focal acral keratoderma of unknown cause typically manifests during childhood. As per the limited published literature on this disease, there appears to be no sex or racial predilection [53].

Histopathological Features

On routine histology focal hyperkeratosis, acanthosis, and thickened granular layer are observed in the epidermis. Elastica stains usually reveal elastorrhexis – the histopathological hallmark of SAKE – and loss of elastic fibers in the deep dermis [7]. The presence of abnormal dense granules in lesional dermal fibroblasts indicates the possibility of SAKE representing the outcome of abnormal secretion of elastic fibers rather than that of fiber degradation as its name suggests [54]. Given the histopathological similarities, one may speculate that SAKE is also a clinical variant of PE.

Treatment Approaches for Acquired Elastolytic Disorders

The management of acquired elastolytic disorders remains extremely challenging. Once elastolytic activity and consecutive loss of elastic tissue has spread, the likelihood of successful management of already lost elastic tissue is very poor. A variety of interventions have been tried in many of the aforementioned conditions, including vitamin E, clofazimine, tretinoin, colchicine, mycophenolate mofetil, corticosteroids, hydroxychloroquine, dapsone, and carbon dioxide laser. However, no convincing benefit was reported using these regimens. The best responses to treatment may be achieved by reduction of inflammatory processes and thus stop of disease progression. Given the importance of elastin for the elasticity of the skin and its loss in the aging process and acquired elastolytic disorders, it is not surprising that various attempts have been made to elevate elastin levels. Therapies aiming to regenerate elastin in elastic tissues should consider all the molecules implicated in elastin fiber formation, for example, including fibrillins, fibulins, and LOX/LOXL enzymes. Since elastic fibers predominantly consist of elastin, the integration of sufficient tropoelastin into elastin fibers seems to be the major target. Currently, however, effective therapy regimens are limited due to the obvious physical challenge of transferring materials (e.g., proteins) and/or treatments across the epidermis and into the dermis [1–5].

References

1. Vindin H, Mithieux SM, Weiss AS. Elastin architecture. Matrix Biol. 2019;84:4–16.
2. Wise SG, Weiss AS. Tropoelastin. Int J Biochem Cell Biol. 2009;41(3):494–7.
3. Baldwin AK, Simpson A, Steer R, Cain SA, Kielty CM. Elastic fibres in health and disease. Expert Rev Mol Med. 2013 Aug 20;15:e8.
4. Kielty CM, Sherratt MJ, Shuttleworth CA. Elastic fibres. J Cell Sci. 2002:15;115(Pt 14):2817–28.
5. Gambichler T, Mamali K, Scheel CH. A brief literature update on mid-dermal elastolysis with an emphasis on pathogenetic and therapeutic aspects. J Clin Aesthet Dermatol. 2020;13(9):18.

6. Fukayama M, Miyagaki T, Akamata K, Suzuki S, Tanaka M, Sato S. Japanese familial anetoderma: a report of two cases and review of the published work. J Dermatol. 2018;45(12):1459–62.
7. Andrés-Ramos I, Alegría-Landa V, Gimeno I, et al. Cutaneous elastic tissue anomalies. Am J Dermatopathol. 2019;41(2):85–117.
8. Gara S, Litaiem N. Cutis Laxa (Elastolysis). In: StatPearls. Treasure Island (FL): StatPearls Publishing; 2020.
9. Fontenelle E, Almeida AP, Souza GM. Marshall's syndrome. An Bras Dermatol. 2013;88(2):279–82.
10. Rongioletti F, Rebora A. Pseudoxanthoma elasticum—like papillary dermal elastolysis. J Am Acad Dermatol. 1992;26:648–50.
11. Lewis KG, Bercovitch L, Dill SW, Robinson-Bostom L. Acquired disorders of elastic tissue: part II. Decreased elastic tissue. J Am Acad Dermatol. 2004;51(2):165–85.
12. Dokic Y, Tschen J. White fibrous papulosis of the axillae and neck. Cureus. 2020;12(4):e7635.
13. Ryder HF, Antaya RJ. Nevus anelasticus, papular elastorrhexis, and eruptive collagenoma: clinically similar entities with focal absence of elastic fibers in childhood. Pediatr Dermatol. 2005;22(2):153–7.
14. Tronnier M. Cutaneous disorders characterized by elastolysis or loss of elastic tissue. J Dtsch Dermatol Ges. 2018;16(2):183–91.
15. Cook JC, Puckett Y. Anetoderma. In: StatPearls. Treasure Island (FL): StatPearls Publishing; 2020.
16. Venencie PY, Bonnefoy A, Gogly B, Groult N, Kut C, Pellat B, Hornebeck, et al. Increased expression of gelatinases a and B by skin explants from patients with anetoderma. Br J Dermatol. 1997;137:517–25.
17. Ghomrasseni S, Dridi M, Gogly B. Anetoderma: an altered balance between metalloproteinases and tissue inhibitors of metalloproteinases. Am J Dermatopathol. 2002;24:118–29.
18. Kim JE, Sohn KM, Woo YJ, Jeong KH, Kim M, Lee JD, Lee JY, Park HJ, Kim GM, Park CJ, Yu DS, Kang H. A Clinicoimmunohistopathologic Study of Anetoderma: Is Protruding Type More Advanced in Stage Than Indented Type? J Immunol Res. 2016;2016:4325463.
19. Gambichler T. Mid-dermal elastolysis revisited. Arch Dermatol Res. 2010;302:85–93.
20. Letard P, Schepers D, Albuisson J, et al. Severe phenotype of cutis laxa type 1B with antenatal signs due to a novel homozygous nonsense mutation in EFEMP2. Mol Syndromol. 2018;9(4):190–6.
21. Mohamed M, Kouwenberg D, Gardeitchik T, Kornak U, Wevers RA, Morava E. Metabolic cutis laxa syndromes. J Inherit Metab Dis. 2011;34(4):907–16.
22. Gkogkolou P, Hildebrandt K, Broekaert S, Metze D, Sengle G, Böhm M. Cutis laxa acquisita: novel insights into impaired elastic fibre regeneration [published correction appears in Br J Dermatol. 2018;178(1):307]. Br J Dermatol. 2017;176(3):832–5.
23. Dantas SG, Trope BM, de Magalhães TC, Azulay DR, Quintella DC, Ramos-E-Silva M. Blepharochalasis: A rare presentation of cutis laxa. Blefarocalasia: una presentación rara de cutis laxo. Actas Dermosifiliogr. 2019;110(4):327–9.
24. Berk DR, Bentley DD, Bayliss SJ, Lind A, Urban Z. Cutis laxa: a review. J Am Acad Dermatol. 2012;66(5).
25. Yürekli A, Açıkgöz G, Can İ, Çalışkan E, Yavan İ. A case of Marshall's syndrome (postinflammatory elastolysis). Indian J Dermatol Venereol Leprol. 2017;83(2):218–20.
26. Jain A. Acquired cutis Laxa. Turk J Haematol. 2020;37(3):212–3. https://doi.org/10.4274/tjh.galenos.2020.2020.0121.
27. Shalhout SZ, Nahas MR, Drews RE, Miller DM. Generalized acquired cutis laxa associated with monoclonal gammopathy of dermatological significance. Case Rep Dermatol Med. 2020;2020:7480607.
28. Koskelainen S, Zhao F, Kalimo H, Baumann M, Kiuru-Enari S. Severe elastolysis in hereditary gelsolin (AGel) amyloidosis. Amyloid. 2020;27(2):81–8.

29. Jachiet M, Harel S, Saussine A, et al. Cutis laxa associated with monoclonal gammopathy: 14 new cases and review of the literature. J Am Acad Dermatol. 2018;79(5):945–7.
30. Shalhout SZ, Nahas MR, Drews RE, Miller DM. Generalized acquired cutis laxa associated with monoclonal gammopathy of dermatological significance. Case Rep Dermatol Med. 2020;2020:7480607.
31. Gonzalez Santiago TM, Lehman JS, Buonaccorsi JN, Kalaaji AN, Wieland CN. Frequency of cutis laxa-like clinical features and elastolysis in scleromyxedema: a retrospective clinicopathologic study of 19 patients with scleromyxedema. J Cutan Pathol. 2016;43(3):246–51.
32. Chavarot N, Battistella M, Vignon M, et al. Cutis laxa for diagnosis of γ1-heavy-chain deposition disease: report of four cases. J Dermatol. 2018;45(10):1211–5.
33. Hanke CW, Bailin PL, Roenigk HH Jr. Annular elastolytic giant cell granuloma. A clinicopathologic study of five cases and a review of similar entities. J Am Acad Dermatol. 1979;1(5):413–21.
34. Hassan R, Arunprasath P, Padmavathy L, Srivenkateswaran K. Annular elastolytic giant cell granuloma in association with Hashimoto's thyroiditis. Indian Dermatol Online J. 2016;7(2):107–10.
35. Müller FB, Groth W. Annular elastolytic giant cell granuloma: a prodromal stage of mid-dermal elastolysis? Br J Dermatol. 2007;156(6):1377–9.
36. Arora S, Malik A, Patil C, Balki A. Annular elastolytic giant cell granuloma: a report of 10 cases. Indian Dermatol Online J. 2015;6(Suppl 1):S17–20.
37. Mittal R, Meena M, Saha D. Actinic granuloma of the conjunctiva in young women. Ophthalmology. 2013;120(9):1786–9.
38. Patroi I, Annessi G, Girolomoni G. Mid-dermal elastolysis: a clinical, histologic, and immunohistochemical study of 11 patients. J Am Acad Dermatol. 2003;48(6):846–51.
39. Gambichler T, Mahjurian-Namari M, Reininghaus L, Schmitz L, Skrygan M, Schulze HJ, Schaller J, Girolomoni G. Lysyl oxidase-like-2 mutations and reduced mRNA and protein expression in mid-dermal elastolysis. Clin Exp Dermatol. 2019;44(1):47–51.
40. Gambichler T, Reininghaus L, Skrygan M, Schulze HJ, Schaller J, Colato C, Girolomoni G. Fibulin protein expression in mid-dermal elastolysis and anetoderma: a study of 23 cases. Acta Derm Venereol. 2016;96(5):708–10.a.
41. Gambichler T, Skrygan M, Reininghaus L, Schulze HJ, Schaller J, Hessam S, Colato C, Girolomoni G, Heitzer E. Lysyl oxidase-like 2 promoter hypermethylation in mid-dermal elastolysis. Br J Dermatol. 2016;175(6):1354–6.b.
42. Wang AR, Kent K, Jagdeo J, Robinson-Bostom L, Bercovitch L. Nevus anelasticus: how should such lesions be classified? J Cutan Pathol. 2014;41(6):519–23.
43. Ramachandran V, Hinds B, Marsch AF. Intertriginous perifollicular elastolysis: a report of 2 cases. JAAD Case Rep. 2020;6(7):612–5. Published 2020.
44. Amano H, Kishi C, Motegi S, Aoyama K, Shimizu A, Ishikawa O. Perifollicular elastolysis with atopic dermatitis. J Dermatol. 2014;41(3):231–2.
45. Rongioletti F, Izakovic J, Romanelli P, Lanuti E, Miteva M. Pseudoxanthoma elasticum-like papillary dermal elastolysis: a large case series with clinicopathological correlation. J Am Acad Dermatol. 2012;67(1):128–35.
46. Wang X, Sun J. Fibroelastolytic papulosis with vacuolar interface dermatitis: a new observation. Australas J Dermatol. 2020;61(1):e101–2.
47. Setó-Torrent N, Iglesias-Sancho M, Arandes-Marcocci J, Fernández-Figueras MT. Pseudoxanthoma elasticum-like papillary dermal elastolysis in non-exposed skin. An Bras Dermatol. 2020;95(2):247–9.
48. Balus L, Amantea A, Donati P, Fazio M, Giuliano MC, Bellocci M. Fibroelastolytic papulosis of the neck: a report of 20 cases. Br J Dermatol. 1997;137(3):461–6.
49. Panagou E, Ratynska M, Heelan K. Pseudoxanthoma elasticum-like papillary dermal elastolysis: a case report and review of literature. Int J Dermatol. 2019;58(1):93–7.
50. Patterson AT, Beasley KJ, Kobayashi TT. Fibroelastolytic papulosis: histopathologic confirmation of disease spectrum variants in a single case. J Cutan Pathol. 2016;43(2):142–7.

51. Gambichler T, Reininghhaus L, Schaller J. Early-onset pseudoxanthoma elasticum-like papillary dermal elastolysis. J Eur Acad Dermatol Venereol. 2016;30:446–7.
52. Rongioletti F, Rebora A. Fibroelastolytic patterns of intrinsic skin aging: pseudoxanthoma-elasticum-like papillary dermal elastolysis and white fibrous papulosis of the neck. Dermatology. 1995;191(1):19–24.
53. Sonthalia S, Aboobacker S. Acrokeratoelastoidosis. 2020. In: StatPearls [Internet]. Treasure Island (FL): StatPearls Publishing; 2020 Jan. PMID: 30725752.

Post-Irradiation Pseudo-Sclerodermatous Panniculitis

Sarah M. Al-Naqshabandi, Luis Requena Caballero, and Omar P. Sangueza

Introduction

In 1993, Winkelmann and associates [1] described a peculiar type of panniculitis secondary to radiotherapy. These authors reported four cases of women with breast cancer that were treated by radical mastectomy and megavoltage X-ray radiotherapy. The patients developed indurated erythematous plaques on the irradiated skin after 1–6 months following radiotherapy.

Histopathologically, the lesions demonstrated lymphoplasmocytic infiltrates in the dermis and subcutaneous septa with areas of sclerosis and thickening of collagen bundles. In some cases, lipophagic granulomas were seen at the periphery of the fat lobules. Radiation-induced changes including dilated sclerotic blood vessels, endothelial cell hyperplasia, fibrosis associated with involution of epidermal appendages, and fibroblasts were also present. The authors named this condition post-irradiation pseudo-sclerodermatous panniculitis.

No additional cases of this entity were reported until 2001 when Carrasco et al. [2] reported another four additional cases of this entity. All patients received post-operative radiotherapy on the anterior chest, and one of them also received radiotherapy on the abdominal skin because of painful bone metastases from breast carcinoma.

Another study was conducted in 2013 by Pielasinski and Requena [3]. These authors reported three more cases with additional histopathological findings besides the panniculitis. These findings included dermal vessels with sclerotic walls and atypical bizarre fibroblasts with large pleomorphic and hyperchromatic nuclei

S. M. Al-Naqshabandi · O. P. Sangueza (✉)
Departments of Pathology and Dermatology, Wake Forest University School of Medicine, Winston-Salem, NC, USA
e-mail: osanguez@wakehealth.edu

L. R. Caballero
Department of Dermatology, Fundacion Jimenez Diaz, Madrid, Spain

F. Rongioletti, B. R. Smoller (eds.), *New and Emerging Entities in Dermatology and Dermatopathology*, https://doi.org/10.1007/978-3-030-80027-7_12

between collagen bundles of the dermis. These additional histopathological findings provided further evidence to the pathogenic role of radiotherapy in the development of this rare variant of panniculitis.

Clinical Features

Cutaneous effects of X-ray irradiation include acute and chronic radiodermatitis [4]. Early or acute changes consist of variable erythema, accompanied by edema in the more severe cases. This is usually followed by loss of hair and post-inflammatory hyperpigmentation. Currently, the severe changes seen in cases of radiodermatitis of some years ago, such as vesiculation, erosion, or ulceration, are not usually seen anymore, because the dosage is more precisely controlled. Pseudo-sclerodermatous panniculitis presents with indurated, erythematous, and edematous plaques in sites treated with megavoltage photons with or without electron beam therapy, usually after breast carcinoma (Fig.1). Lesions can develop anywhere from 1 month up to 17 years after irradiation therapy.

Histopathologic Features

Microscopically, at scanning magnification, the biopsies show normal epidermis and nearly normal dermis, with a few dilated lymphatic vessels throughout the dermis as the only dermal abnormality (Fig. 2a). Classic histopathologic features of chronic radiodermatitis, such as atrophy of epidermal appendages, thrombosed or sclerotic blood vessels in the superficial dermis, endothelial cell hyperplasia, fibrosis, and atypical fibroblasts, are not seen in most cases, although it might be present

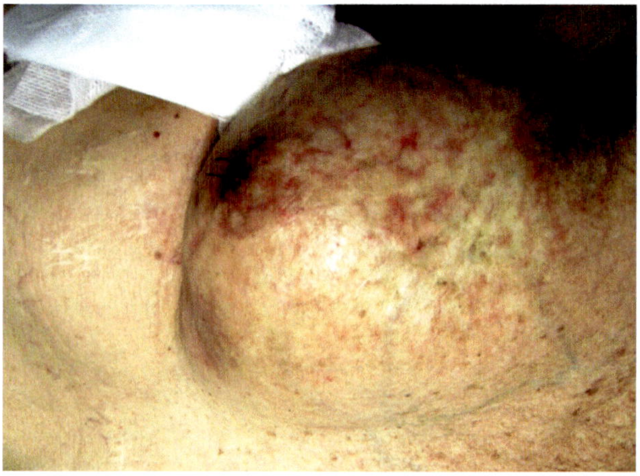

Fig. 1 Pseudo-sclerodermatous panniculitis. Indurated, erythematous, and edematous plaque on the irradiated skin after five months following radiotherapy for breast carcinoma (Courtesy of F. Rongioletti, Milan, Italy)

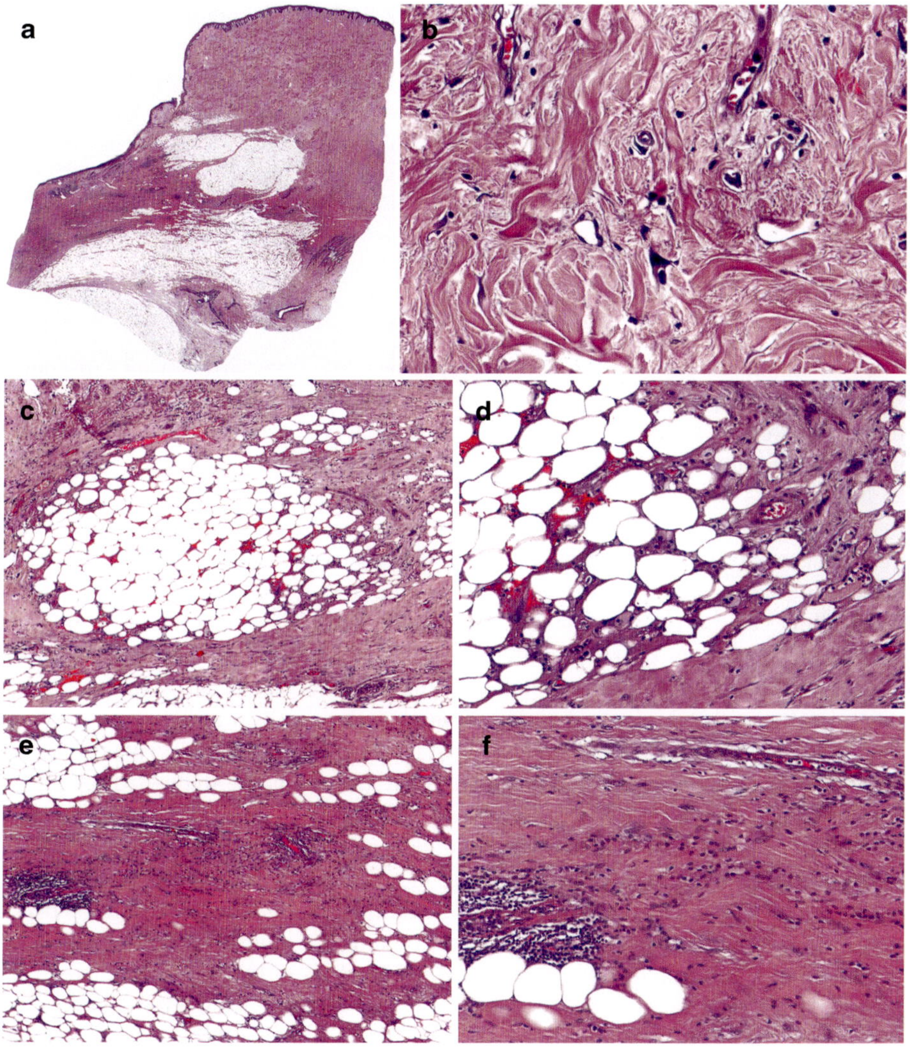

Fig. 2 (**a**): Low power demonstrating diffuse sclerosis of the entire dermis extending into the subcutaneous tissue. (**b**): Higher magnification to highlight the sclerosis, dilated blood vessels, and the presence of fibroblasts with bizarre nuclei. (**c**): Subcutaneous fat with lobules of irregular size and shape. (**d**): Higher magnification showing prominent fibroblasts and foamy histiocytes. (**e**): Collections of lymphoplasmacytic infiltrates and areas of sclerosis. (**f**): Higher magnification to show a detail of the inflammatory infiltrate and sclerosis

(Fig. 2b). The main changes are present in the subcutaneous tissue and consist of predominantly lobular panniculitis, with subcutaneous fat lobules showing necrotic adipocytes and dense inflammatory infiltrates composed mainly of foamy histiocytes (Fig. 2c–f). Lipophagic granulomas, in the form of small aggregations of foamy histiocytes around necrotic adipocytes, are seen in some lobules (Fig. 2c–d).

Sparse lymphocytes and plasma cells are also scattered throughout the fat lobules (Fig. 2e–f). The septa of the subcutaneous tissue appear thickened with an eosinophilic appearance, and they are composed of thick collagen bundles separated by thin ones. No inflammatory infiltrate is present within the septa. In all reported cases, serial sections failed to demonstrate metastatic breast carcinoma in the subcutaneous tissue [2].

Differential Diagnosis

The histopathologic differential diagnosis of post-irradiation pseudo-sclerodermatous panniculitis includes other septal and lobular panniculitides with thickening of the septa of subcutaneous fat, namely, necrobiosis lipoidica, deep morphea, and lupus panniculitis.

Necrobiosis lipoidica is characterized by palisading granulomas which extend from the deep dermis into the upper part of the connective tissue of the subcutaneous septa resulting in a septal panniculitis. The involvement of the subcutis in necrobiosis lipoidica is a result of a deep extension of the dermal process. There are no descriptions of necrobiosis lipoidica affecting the subcutaneous tissue alone. Necrobiosis lipoidica presents with palisading granulomas with histiocytes surrounding areas of collagen degeneration within widened septa [5–7]. In the dermis there are alternating horizontal bands of inflammatory cells and fibrosis involving the full thickness of the dermis. In late-stage lesions, lymphocytes and plasma cells, sometimes with lymphoid follicle formation, are present in the thickened septa [7]. The dramatic thickening of the septa results in decreased size of the fat lobules, but in contrast with the lesions of post-irradiation pseudo-sclerodermatous panniculitis, there are no inflammatory infiltrates within the fat lobule.

Scleroderma may also extend into the septa of subcutaneous fat from the deep dermis, but sometimes the process is entirely subcutaneous with no involvement of the epidermis, cutaneous adnexa, or dermis [8–12]. The most characteristic histopathologic finding in deep morphea is the presence of a marked thickening of the septa of the subcutaneous fat. As a consequence of the thickening, collagen also replaces the fat normally present around the eccrine coils and below them, giving the false impression that sweat glands have ascended into the dermis. When the sclerotic process involves both dermis and subcutis, the full thickness of the specimen appears homogeneously eosinophilic. The spaces between collagen bundles disappear, with atrophy of the adnexal structures, blood vessels, and nerves, remaining only the muscle fibers of arrector pili. Inflammatory infiltrate is present only in active lesions; it consists of aggregations of lymphocytes surrounded by plasma cells at the junction of the thickened septa and the fat lobules. Plasma cells may also be present arranged interstitially between the sclerotic collagen bundles. In contrast with post-irradiation pseudo-sclerodermatous panniculitis, lesions of deep morphea show little or no inflammatory infiltrate within the fat lobule.

Morphea has also been described after radiotherapy for breast cancer with lesions located entirely within the treatment field [13–15]. In contrast with post-irradiation pseudo-sclerodermatous panniculitis, the histopathologic changes in these cases of post-irradiation morphea were confined to the dermis.

Most authors consider eosinophilic fasciitis, also named Shulman's syndrome, as a variant of scleroderma [16–22]. Clinically the process is characterized by its sudden onset, sometimes after intense physical activity. The lesions consist of a symmetrical induration of the skin and subcutaneous tissues of the limbs. Usually, there is a gradual improvement of the lesions, even without any treatment, and the majority of affected patients experience complete recovery after some years [19]. Histopathologically, lesions of eosinophilic fasciitis are quite similar to those of subcutaneous scleroderma. They show edema and thickening of the interlobular fibrous septa of the subcutaneous fat and the deep fascia. Both the septa and the fascia show inflammatory infiltrate of lymphocytes, histiocytes, plasma cells, and abundant numbers of eosinophils [20–22]. In contrast with eosinophilic fasciitis, cases of post-irradiation pseudo-sclerodermatous panniculitis showed no inflammatory infiltrate in the septa, and eosinophils were not seen in the inflammatory infiltrate of the fat lobules.

Lichen sclerosus et atrophicus has also been described on the trunk after radiation therapy for breast cancer [23, 24]. However, in these cases the histopathologic features were confined to the epidermis and superficial dermis. They consisted of thinning of the epidermis, vacuolar alteration of the basal layer, subepidermal edema with homogenization of the collagen or sclerotic collagen in later lesions, and a moderate diffuse or perivascular inflammatory infiltrate mostly composed of lymphocytes in the mid-dermis. In contrast with post-irradiation pseudo-sclerodermatous panniculitis, the lesions of lichen sclerosus et atrophicus after radiation therapy showed no anomalies in the subcutaneous fat.

Lupus erythematosus profundus, also named lupus panniculitis, is a chronic recurrent panniculitis that is present in approximately 1 to 3% of patients with cutaneous lupus erythematosus. Occasionally, lesions of lupus panniculitis may show epidermal and dermal changes of discoid lupus erythematosus, namely, atrophy of the epidermis, vacuolar alteration of the dermo-epidermal junction, thickened basement membrane, interstitial mucin between collagen bundles of the dermis, and superficial and deep perivascular inflammatory infiltrates of lymphocytes involving the dermis [11, 25]. However, more often, the changes are confined to the subcutaneous fat, with no anomalies in the dermis or epidermis. Lupus panniculitis is mostly a lobular panniculitis with inflammatory infiltrate predominantly composed of lymphocytes and sclerosis of the fat lobules. A characteristic feature, found in over half of the patients, is the presence of lymphoid follicles in the subcutaneous septa [26, 27]. These lymphoid follicles may show germinal centers and numerous plasma cells at the periphery, which in some cases extend interstitially between collagen bundles of the septa of the subcutis. Sometimes, necrosis of adipocytes is sparse or absent in lupus panniculitis. Another important finding is the presence of nuclear dust, an infrequent finding in other variants of lobular panniculitis, so peculiar, that it has been proposed as a clue to the diagnosis of lupus panniculitis [28].

Collagen bundles of subcutaneous septa appear to be thick and sclerotic, and they also contain an interstitial inflammatory infiltrate of lymphocytes and plasma cells. Lipophagic granulomas within the fat lobules are not usually seen in lesions of lupus panniculitis but characterize post-irradiation pseudo-sclerodermatous panniculitis.

Etiopathogenesis

The pathogenesis of PIPP is unknown. Pathogenetic theories include hormonal or immune-mediated factors and genetic predisposition, causing vascular injury following external beam radiotherapy. It is interesting that all cases of PIPP reported to date have occurred in women. It is possible that hormonal or immune-mediated factors may play a role in the pathogenesis of this lesion. A delayed immune-mediated reaction to neoantigens induced by radiation has been suggested as a potential mechanism of disease for PIPP [29]. External beam radiotherapy results in greater penetration and concentration of radiation in deep tissues. This mode of radiotherapy causes less radiation dermatitis but increased damage to subcutaneous tissue in the form of fibrosis [3, 30, 31]. More acutely, radiation-induced endothelial cell damage activates inflammatory mediators, including cytokines such as transforming growth factor-β1 (TGF-β1), which increases vascular endothelial permeability, inflammation, and fibrosis [31, 32]. Late effects of radiation on normal tissues have been shown to be associated with genetic factors. Molecular studies have identified single nucleotide polymorphisms in candidate genes, associated with TGF-β1 and retinoic acid, mediators linked to the development of fibrosis following radiotherapy [30, 33, 34, 35]. It is possible, by extension, that genetic polymorphisms may also be associated with an increased risk of radiation vasculopathy and PIPP. Thus, there may be multiple confounding factors influencing the development of PIPP in certain individuals.

Therapy

There is no effective treatment for post-irradiation pseudo-sclerodermatous panniculitis [2].

Prognosis and Course

Progressive improvement of the subcutaneous induration was observed without any treatment in all patients during the months after radiotherapy withdrawal [2].

Conclusions

In conclusion, post-irradiation pseudo-sclerodermatous panniculitis is a rare complication that may appear in the subcutaneous tissue of patients receiving megavoltage radiotherapy. Clinically the lesions consist of indurated plaques that raise a diagnosis of subcutaneous metastatic disease, but histopathologic changes are characteristic and distinctive.

References

1. Winkelmann RK, Grado GL, Quimby S, et al. Pseudo-sclerodermatous panniculitis after irradiation: an unusual complication of megavoltage treatment of breast carcinoma. Mayo Clin Proc. 1993;68:122–7.
2. Carrasco L, Moreno C, Pastor MA, et al. Postirradiation pseudosclerodermatous panniculitis. Am J Dermatopathol. 2001;23:283.
3. Pielasinski U, Machan S, Camacho D, et al. Postirradiation pseudosclerodermatous panniculitis: three new cases with additional histopathologic features sup- porting the radiotherapy etiology. Am J Dermatopathol. 2013;35:129.
4. Fajardo LF, Berthrong M. Radiation injury in surgical pathology. Part I Am J Surg Pathol. 1978;2:159–99.
5. Muller SA, Winkelmann RK. Necrobiosis lipoidica diabeticorum. A clinical and pathological investigation of 171 cases. Arch Der- Matol. 1966;93:272–81.
6. Ackerman AB. Hisologic diagnosis of inflammatory skin Diseases. Philadelphia: Lea & Febiger; 1978. p. 424.
7. Alegre VA, Winkelmann RK. A new histopathologic feature of necrobiosis lipoidica diabeticorum: lymphoid nodules. J Cutan Pathol. 1988;15:75–7.
8. Doyle JA, Connolly SM, Winkelmann RK. Cutaneous and subcutaneous inflammatory sclerosis syndromes. Arch Dermatol. 1982;118:886–90.
9. Whittaker SJ, Smith NP, Russel JR. Solitary morphoea profunda. Br J Dermatol. 1989;120:431–40.
10. Su WPD, Person JR. Morphea profunda. A new concept and a histopathologic study of 23 cases. Am J Dermatopathol. 1981;3:251–60.
11. Winkelmann RK. Panniculitis in connective tissue disease. Arch Dermatol. 1983;119:336–44.
12. Person JR, Su WPD. Subcutaneous morphoea: a clinical study of sixteen cases. Br J Dermatol. 1979;100:371–80.
13. Fischer M, Bormann G, Wohlrab J, et al. Radiogene Morphaea. Hautarzt. 1999;50:507–10.
14. Blesel NR, Stapleton KM, Commens C, Ahern VA. Radiation- induced localized scleroderma in breast cancer patients. Australas J Dermatol. 1999;40:99–102.
15. Schaffer JV, Carroll C, Dvoretsky I, et al. Postirradiation morphea of the breast presentation of two cases and review of the literature. Dermatology. 2000;200:67–71.
16. Jarrat M, Bybee JD, Ramsdell W. Eosinophilic fasciitis: an early variant of scleroderma. J Am Acad Dermatol. 1979;1:221–6.
17. Cramer SF, Kent L, Abramowsky C, et al. Eosinophilic fasciitis. Arch Pathol Lab Med. 1982;106:85–91.
18. Lee P. Eosinophilic fasciitis—new associations and current perspectives (editorial). J Rheumatol. 1981;8:6–8.
19. Micher CJ Jr, Doyle JA, Ginsburg WW. Eosinophilic fasciitis. Report of 15 cases. Mayo Clin Proc. 1981;56:27–34.

20. Barnes L, Rodnan GP, Medsger TA Jr, et al. Eosinophilic fasciitis. A pathologic study of twenty cases. Am J Pathol. 1979;96:493–518.
21. Tamura T, Saito Y, Ishikawa H. Diffuse fasciitis with eosinophilia. Histological and electron microscopic study. Acta Derm Venereol (Stockh). 1979;59:325–31.
22. Naschitz JE, Boss JH, Misselvich I, Yeshurum D, Rosner I. The fasciitis-panniculitis syndromes. Clinical and pathological features. Medicine. 1996;75:6–16.
23. Yates VM, King CM, Dave VK. Lichen sclerosus et atrophicus following radiation therapy. Arch Dermatol. 1985;121:1044–7.
24. Tournillac I, Dandurand M, Guillot B. Lichen sclereux bulleux apres radiotherapie. Ann Dermatol Venereol. 1998;125:121–3.
25. Izumi AK, Takiguchi P. Lupus erythematosus panniculitis. Arch Dermatol. 1983;119:61–4.
26. Sanchez NP, Peters MS, Winkelmann RK. The histopathology of lupus erythematosus panniculitis. J Am Acad Dermatol. 1981;5:673–80.
27. Harris RB, Duncan SC, Ecker RI, et al. Lymphoid follicles in subcutaneous inflammatory disease. Arch Dermatol. 1979;115:442–3.
28. Ackerman AB, Jacobson M, Vitale P. Clues to diagnosis in dermatopathology, Vol. I. Chicago: ASCP Press; 1991. p. 397–400. 89;16:379–82.
29. Dalle S, Skowron F, Ronger-Savlè S, Balme B, Thomas L. Pseudosclerodermatous panniculitis after irradiation and bronchiolitis obliterans organizing pneumonia: simultaneous onset suggesting a common origin. Dermatology. 2004;209:138.
30. Giotopoulos G, Symonds RP, Foweraker K, et al. The late radiotherapy normal tissue injury phenotypes of telangiectasia, fibro- sis and atrophy in breast cancer patients have distinct genotype-dependent causes. Br J Cancer. 2007;96:1001.
31. Rodemann HP, Bamberg M. Cellular basis of radiation-induced fibrosis. Radiother Oncol. 1995;35:83.
32. Collette S, Collette L, Budiharto T, et al. Predictors of the risk of fibrosis at 10 years after breast conserving therapy for early breast cancer – a study based on the EORTC trial 22881–10882 'boost versus no boost'. Eur J Cancer. 2008;44:2587.
33. Terrazzino S, La Mattina P, Gambaro G, et al. Common variants of GSTP1, GSTA1, and TGFβ are associated with the risk of radiation-induced fibrosis in breast cancer patients. Int J Radiat Oncol Biol Phys. 2012;83:504.
34. Forrester HB, Li J, Leong T, McKay MJ, Sprung CN. Identification of a radiation sensitivity gene expression profile in primary fibroblasts derived from patients who developed radiotherapy-induced fibrosis. Radiother Oncol. 2014;111:186.
35. Shirsat HS, Walsh NM, McDonald LJ, Rutledge R, Porter G, Barnes PJ. Postirradiation pseudo-sclerodermatous panniculitis with involvement of breast parenchyma: a dramatic example of a rare entity and a pitfall in diagnosis. J Cutan Pathol. 2016;43(5):444–50.

Linear Focal Elastosis and PXE-Like Fibroelastolytic-Elastotic Papulosis Disorders

Jacqueline M. Junkins-Hopkins and Leslie Robinson-Bostom

Introduction

Elastic tissue disorders include a variety of conditions defined by the pattern and location of elastic tissue alteration and, at times, collagen changes, together with the defining clinical presentation. The elastic tissue may be increased, decreased, fragmented, or clumped or may undertake unique morphologic histopathologic appearances. Disorders characterized by histopathologic loss of elastic tissue (elastolysis) include conditions such as cutis laxa (hereditary and post-inflammatory causes), mid-dermal and perifollicular elastolysis, pseudoxanthoma elasticum-like papillary dermal elastolysis, white fibrous papulosis of the neck, papular elastorrhexis, and anetoderma. Increased elastic tissue is seen in entities such as nevus elasticus (elastoma), dermatofibrosis lenticularis disseminata (Buschke-Ollendorff syndrome), pseudoxanthoma elasticum (PXE) (acquired and hereditary), linear focal elastosis, late-onset focal dermal elastosis, elastosis perforans serpiginosa, elastoderma, and elastofibroma dorsi [1].

This chapter is devoted to primarily discussing linear focal elastosis and disorders with altered dermal connective tissue and unique elastic tissue abnormalities that clinically mimic PXE. The fibroelastolytic papulosis (FEP) disorders, including PXE-like papillary dermal elastolysis (PXE-PDE), white fibrous papulosis of the neck (WFPN), and papillary dermal elastosis (PDE), are included in the chapter on elastolysis. Given the variable presence of elastosis as well as elastolysis in FEP, these conditions are also discussed in this chapter. "Late-onset" focal dermal elastosis (LOFDE) has similar clinical features; thus, a more encompassing term

J. M. Junkins-Hopkins (✉)
Dermatologist, Dermatopathologist, Consultant, Cutaneous Lymphoma, Geisinger Medical Center, Danville, PA, USA

L. Robinson-Bostom
Division of Dermatopathology, Department of Dermatology, The Warren Alpert Medical School of Brown University, Providence, RI, USA

F. Rongioletti, B. R. Smoller (eds.), *New and Emerging Entities in Dermatology and Dermatopathology*, https://doi.org/10.1007/978-3-030-80027-7_13

fibroelastolytic and elastotic papulosis (FEEP) is proposed to include LOFDE with the other FEP disorders. All of these conditions have nearly identical clinical presentations; thus, a biopsy stained for elastic tissue, in addition to hematoxylin and eosin (H and E) stains, is required to confirm the diagnosis. Commonly used stains include Verhoeff elastic stain, often with van Gieson counterstain (VVG), but elastic fibers can also be identified with orcein, Weigert resorcin-fuchsin, Gomori aldehyde-fuchsin [1, 2], and Luna stains [3]. The ultimate diagnosis requires correlation of the characteristic elastic tissue features with the clinical presentation (Table 1).

Elastic fibers are complex extracellular molecules created by a multistep hierarchical assembly process involving several key proteins, the discussion of which is beyond the scope of this chapter and is discussed elsewhere [1, 4–6]. Elastic fibers are composed primarily of an elastin core surrounded by a microfibril scaffolding. Elastin is initially secreted as the precursor tropoelastin by elastogenic cells, such as fibroblasts. This self-aggregates (coacervation) and is further cross-linked with desmosine by lysyl oxidase, creating stable elastin aggregates that become deposited onto a mantle of microfibrils, rich in fibrillin-1 (FBN-1). Further cross-linking of microfibrils and elastin creates the stable elastic fiber. In addition to elastin and FBN-1, other key proteins that contribute to elastogenesis include members of the fibulin family of extracellular matrix molecules (especially FBLN 4 and FBLN 5), found at the elastin-microfibril interface and/or in the elastin core, and latent TGFβ-binding protein-4 (LTBP4), which aids in elastic fiber assembly through interactions with FBLN 5. The resultant thick elastic fibers are found in the reticular dermis. This differs from the papillary dermal elastic tissue, which is composed of thin elaunin fibers, composed predominantly of microfibrils, and a smaller component of elastin that merges with thin oxytalan fibers composed only of microfibrils, which radiate perpendicular to the base of the epidermis as brush-like bundles. These thinner papillary dermal oxytalan and elaunin fibers connect to the thicker reticular dermal elastic fibers [7].

Elastogenesis starts during gestation and is complete before adolescence with essentially no new elastic fibers formed in adult tissue skin under normal circumstance [5, 6]. Chronologically aged skin undergoes clinical changes, resulting in "temporary wrinkles" (fade with stretching of the skin), associated with ultrastructural features characterized by disintegrating and immature-appearing elastic fibers. These changes, theorized to represent an attempt at elastic tissue repair, can also be seen in conditions such as fibroelastolytic papulosis [8]. Degradation of elastic tissue also occurs in association with elastases found in inflammatory cells such as neutrophils and macrophages and fibroblasts. Further metabolism of elastin by elastase activity can occur with other enzymes such as the metalloproteases, while inhibition of elastase and other factors helps to balance the elastic fiber destruction [1]. The exact pathogenesis of elastic tissue disorders is not well established, but alterations of the process of assembly and metabolism, as well as mechanical stress and aging, likely contribute to these increases and decreases in elastic fibers.

Table 1 Differentiating features of PXE and PXE-like disorders

Disorder	Age/sex	Morphology	Distribution	Histology	Association or others
PXE/PDE	Elderly F Rare younger	2–4 mm yellow non-follicular papules coalescing to cobblestone plaques	Symmetric; lateral neck, supraclavicular, nape, axillae> abdomen, forearms, chest	H&E: Sparse papillary dermal melanophages; −/+ mild epidermal atrophy +/− mild perivascular lymphocytes +/− mild papillary dermal fibrosis Elastic stain: Papillary dermis: Band-like loss/ significantly decreased elastic fibers Occasional fragmentation and clumping of elastic fibers Mild subepidermal increase in normal elastic fibers	No systemic associations Rare familial In spectrum of FEP
PXE	F > M Second or third decade	1–5 mm yellow papules coalescing into cobblestone yellow plaques with slack skin	Neck, axillae, groin, other flexural sites	H and E and von Kossa stains: Calcified fragmented, curled, thickened elastic fibers in reticular dermis	Mutation ABCC6 gene Angioid streaks, cardiovascular disease
White fibrous papulosis of the neck	Mean age 60 years; rare younger F = M	White, 2–3 mm non-coalescing papules	Posterior> lateral neck; less common axilla, upper trunk	Variable loss of elastic fibers in papillary dermis Thick collagen bundles in papillary and upper/mid reticular dermis. May be morphea-like	In spectrum of FEP

(continued)

Table 1 (continued)

Disorder	Age/sex	Morphology	Distribution	Histology	Association or others
Papillary dermal elastosis	Two reports: Women in their 30s	Similar to PXE-PDE	Similar to PXE-PDE	Focal clumps of elastic fibers alternating with absent or diminished elastic fibers in papillary dermis	Only two case reports In spectrum of FEP
Type II mid-dermal elastolysis/perifollicular elastolysis	Adolescent and older	1–3 mm gray/white perifollicular wrinkled patches or papular protrusions	Face, upper back: Acne distribution	Perifollicular loss of elastic tissue +/− mucin	Associated with acne vulgaris associated bacterial elastolysis
Late-onset focal dermal elastosis	Elderly; rarely 30–40 yrs. F> > M	1–5 mm white to yellow non-follicular papules	Neck, popliteal and axillary fossae, volar arms, groin, rare chest, acral	Increased aggregates of normal-appearing or thickened branching elastic fibers in the upper, mid, and deep reticular dermis	Clinical overlap with PXE-PDE Rare familial Probable relationship with FEP spectrum
Dermatofibrosis lenticularis disseminata (Buschke-Ollendorff)	Children and adolescents	Skin-colored or yellow papules, nodules, plaques	Trunk, extremities	Elastoma: Increased antler-like thickened elastic fibers reticular dermis; may have collagenoma	Autosomal dominant; LEMD3 mutations Subset with X-ray (+) osteopoikilosis hands/feet, hips, long bones
Papular elastorrhexis	Children/adolescents F > M	Skin-colored 3–5 mm non-follicular non-fusing papules	Trunk, limbs	Reduced, fragmented, and/or loss of elastic fibers upper and mid dermis Collagen may be thickened/homogenized	May be abortive B-O syndrome

PDE pseudoxanthoma elasticum-like papillary dermal elastolysis, *F* female, *M* male, *PXE* pseudoxanthoma elasticum

Linear Focal Elastosis

Clinical Features

Linear focal elastosis (LFE) was first reported by Burket, Zelickson, and Padilla in 1989 [9] as a distinct clinical presentation of "layered, symmetric, palpable yellow lines extending on both sides of the vertebral column" of the lower back. These asymptomatic linear yellow-orange lesions have a horizontally layered arrangement along skin cleavage (Langer lines) [10, 11] often crossing the spine of the mid to lower back (Fig. 1a). The authors designated this as "linear focal elastosis (elastotic striae)," acknowledging the clinical similarity to striae, although patients with LFE rarely present with concomitant striae distensae [12–15]. Since their initial report, there have been slightly over 50 cases reported confirming and expanding on this clinical-pathologic entity [9–39]. LFE is typically seen in men ages 60 years and older, but the condition is often present for years to decades [12, 17]; thus, the age of onset is often younger, and LFE is reported in adolescents [15, 21, 25, 32–34] and rarely in children as young as 7 years [22]. Most cases arise in men, but there are a few reports of LFE in women [18, 20, 21, 25]. LFE has been reported in White, Asian, Turkish [32], and Black [10, 14] patients, with a skew toward Asian patients reported in the literature [38, 15, 22, 24]. A family history is rarely reported [10, 31, 33].

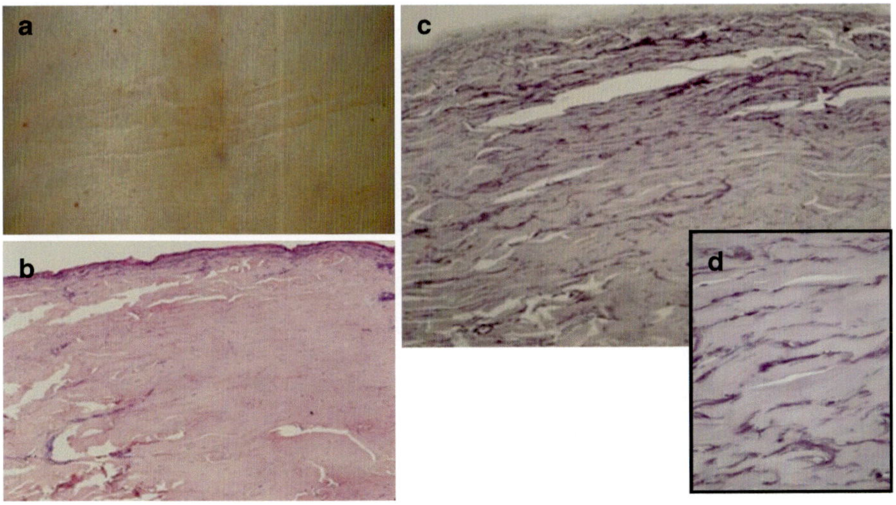

Fig. 1 Linear focal elastosis (courtesy of Franco Rongioletti, MD). (**a**): Horizontally arranged linear yellow depressed plaques on the lower back. (**b**): Layered arrangement of thickened intradermal collagen bundles with interspersed faintly basophilic material. H and E stain x100. (**c**): Elastic stain demonstrates thickened wavy elongated elastic fibers in the reticular dermis with normal papillary dermal elastic fibers. Orcein stain x200. (**d**): The fibers are thickened and elongated, with split ends imparting a "paintbrush" morphology. Orcein stain x400

Rarely, involvement of the upper back [24], shoulders, lower extremities [21, 25, 39], and in one report, the face [28] has been described. Early lesions may have an erythematous hue [21, 22, 24, 38]. Pruritus has been reported [38], but the lesions are usually asymptomatic. Aside from frequent reports of a preceding growth spurt [34, 38], events reported prior to the development of LFE are sporadic. Rarely other events are noted, such as prominent weight loss [14], blunt trauma [22], pregnancy [38], and strenuous exercise [11, 39], but cause and effect has not been established. Some patients have classic striae distensae in other areas of the body [13–15, 20, 31, 34]. There are no specific systemic or other cutaneous associations with this disorder.

Histopathologic Features

The histopathologic features of elastic tissue alteration will vary, depending on the age and morphology of the clinical lesion. An elastic stain is necessary to confirm the diagnosis, although on biopsies from the static established palpable yellowish lesions (around two years duration) [33], the abnormality can be identified on routine H and E-stained sections as abundant light pink-staining delicate fibrillar-appearing material splaying the adjacent more eosinophilic collagen bundles. Basophilic fibers have also been described [12], and the collagen bundles may appear thickened (Fig. 1b) [15]. On an elastic tissue stain, the abnormal elastic fibers appear as wavy, fragmented, and/or aggregated and agglutinated fibers (Fig. 1c) [9, 19]. The fibers may be elongated, with split ends imparting a "paint-brush" morphology (Fig. 1d) [15, 21, 36]. The increased elastic tissue is present in the mid reticular dermis, with preservation of normal elastic tissue architecture of the upper reticular and papillary dermis. If a recent onset erythematous atrophic lesion is biopsied (around two months) [33], there may be evidence of elastolysis, with the elastic fibers appearing thin, fragmented, and/or diminished, suggesting elastic tissue degeneration [24, 33].

Ultrastructurally, numerous fragmented elastic fibers have been described [9, 12, 19] with variable amounts of fine reticular or granular material in the matrix, consistent with microfibrils [12]. Microfibrils have been identified adjacent to fragmented elastic fibers, suggesting regenerative activity [24]. Elastic microfibrils connected with intracytoplasmic filaments of fibroblasts also suggest active elastogenesis [12]. Specimens taken from 1 cm beyond the lesion shows normal elastic tissue.

Differential Diagnosis

The histopathologic features on routine H and E-stained sections may be minimal, resulting in a misdiagnosis of normal skin if one is not aware of the subtle splaying of collagen by the elastic tissue on H and E [29]. The prominent dermal connective tissue alteration may simulate a collagenoma or morphea (Fig. 1).

The most frequently encountered clinical differential of linear focal elastosis is striae distensae, which presents as broad linear bands that vary in morphology, based on the evolutionary stage [40]. Early lesions are erythematous to violaceous or hyperpigmented, while older lesions are white or hypopigmented, flat, wrinkled, or atrophic. The locations are dependent in part on the trigger, but tend to be on the arms, thighs, hips, lower flank, abdomen, and breast, in contrast to LFE, which is limited to the back. Triggers of striae distensae such as corticosteroid use or hormonal changes are typically absent in patients with linear focal elastosis. Growth spurts may precede both conditions. Biopsies of mature striae distensae will show a flattened epidermis, with horizontal arrangement of compact straight, thin eosinophilic elastic fibers parallel to the epidermis. Early lesions show dermal edema and a perivascular lymphocytic infiltrate [40]. Elastic stains demonstrate diminished elastic fibers in contrast to increased elastic tissue seen in LFE.

A single report of linear lumbar localized lysis of elastic fibers that is morphologically identical to linear focal elastosis has been reported in a 20-year-old Filipino woman [35]. The biopsy showed a localized area of elastolysis in the mid dermis with a paucity of fragmented elastic fibers in the upper reticular dermis. Citing similar presentations in the literature [22, 24, 32], the authors proposed these represent a distinct condition they termed linear focal elastolysis. However, this likely represents an evolutionary early degenerative stage of LFE.

From a purely histopathologic point of view, the differential of localized increased elastic tissue will include "late onset" focal dermal elastosis (LOFDE), dermatofibrosis lenticularis disseminata (Buschke-Ollendorff syndrome), and elastoma, all of which show histopathologic features of increased dermal elastic tissue, but with clinical papules, nodules, and/or plaques that are distinct from the linear bands present on the lower back in LFE. Additionally, in contrast to fragmented or paint brush-like elastic fibers of LFE, the elastic fibers are often normal or thickened and have been described as "antler-like" on elastic stains in Buschke-Ollendorff [1]. LOFDE presents with numerous small papules, coalescing into cobblestone plaques on flexural sites, with increased normal-appearing elastic tissue in the dermis [41].

Etiopathogenesis

With specific regard to linear focal elastosis, the pathogenesis has not been confirmed. Electron microscopy demonstrating microfibrils adjacent to fragmented elastic fibers [12, 24] and maturing elastic fibers in sequential development have been observed, supporting a theory of active elastogenesis [12]. It may be a process of both degeneration and regeneration [24, 33]. Choi et al. [24] demonstrated fine fragmented and diminished elastic fibers, with electron microscopic evidence of degeneration of elastin in a patient with new-onset (6 months) erythematous linear bands, while a patient with stable (2 years duration) lesions showed massive elastic fibers with microfibrils adjacent to these fragmented fibers, consistent with elastogenesis. Other authors report similar biopsy findings of clinically erythematous early lesions demonstrating diminished elastic fibers, while increased elastic fibers were noted in older white lesions [33]. Some feel LFE is a subtype of striae distensae, or LFE and striae distensae represent the same process at different evolutionary stages, possibly representing a degenerative and/or regenerative process of striae distensae [11, 13–15, 18, 34]. LFE rarely may arise contiguous with striae [20, 15] leading some to propose a keloidal-like repair of striae [15], challenging the possibility of de novo synthesis of abnormal elastic tissue. In one series, 45% reported a growth spurt, including two patients with growth of >9 cm/year, prior to the LFE [38]; thus, a relation to striae distensae is plausible [34, 38].

There have been no other potential triggers established. Some have attributed the process of combined degenerative and regenerative elastic fiber alteration to be a hamartomatous or nevoid proliferation of elastic tissue [19]. This notion of elastolysis playing a role in LFE etiopathogenesis has been disputed, favoring instead a separate entity of linear lumbar elastolysis [35].

Treatment

There are no effective treatments for LFE. Retinoid therapy has been attempted without success [33].

Prognosis

LFE is a benign chronic but stable condition that has no associated systemic conditions.

Conclusion

LFE is a benign chronic cutaneous elastic tissue disorder characterized by horizontal linear yellowish plaques that cross the spine in the mid and lower back and histologically show increased wavy, fragmented, agglutinated, or aggregated elastic fibers layered between thickened collagen bundles. These are morphologically different from striae distensae, but may coexist with striae. Thus, LFE has been theorized to represent an evolutionary form of striae distensae, representing a later stage in which reparative elastogenesis has taken place.

PXE-Like Fibroelastolytic and Elastotic Papulosis Disorders (PXE-FEEP)

Introduction

PXE-like fibroelastolytic and elastotic papulosis disorders (PXE-FEEP) include pseudoxanthoma elasticum-like papillary dermal elastolysis (PXE-PDE), white fibrous papulosis of the neck (WFPN), papillary dermal elastosis (PDE), and "late-onset" focal dermal elastosis (LOFDE). These are acquired cutaneous elastic tissue disorders that present with similar appearing yellow or white superficial dermal papules on the neck and non-sun-exposed flexural sites. These entities clinically may simulate PXE [42, 44, 45], but they lack the systemic associations and dermal calcified fragmented elastic fibers that define PXE. All have elastic tissue abnormalities that distinguish them, but due to the overlapping clinical and histopathologic features, the term fibroelastolytic papulosis (FEP) was proposed to include PXE-PDE,WFPN [8, 43, 46–49], and PDE [50, 51]. Elastolysis is present on biopsy; thus, they are also discussed in "The Spectrum of Acquired Elastolytic Disorders". LOFDE is a clinically similar entity, but differs by the presence of increased elastic fibers instead of elastolysis [52]. The more inclusive term FEEP reflects the clinical overlap with FEP and LOFDE. The discussion below incorporates features initially ascribed to the individual entities.

Clinical Features

Pseudoxanthoma Elasticum-like Papillary Dermal Elastolysis (PXE-PDE)

PXE-PDE was first reported by Rongioletti and Rebora in 1992 [42], and the features were further detailed in 2012 [43]. There have been at least 50 cases reported in the literature [42–44, 46, 48–50, 53–77], some of which are described in the (FEP) spectrum [46–49, 73, 75], but the condition may be under reported [43]. Nearly all patients with PXE-PDE are women, with a mean age around 60, but there are reports of cases in the fourth decade and younger [58, 65]. The lesions invariably arise symmetrically on the lateral neck and at times on the nape as 2–4 mm (range 1–6 mm) yellowish, non-follicular soft papules coalescing into plaques with a cobblestone appearance resembling PXE . Other sites of involvement include supraclavicular and outer axillary regions (Fig. 2a,b), flexor forearms/antecubital fossa, chest, abdomen, and inguinal region. On dermoscopic evaluation, these appear as flesh-colored or normochromic non-follicular papules forming plaques, with linear or arboriform vessels [63, 70, 77]. These areas of hypopigmented or whitish-yellowish discoloration coalesce into cobblestone plaques, which may be surrounded by a peripheral skin-colored or erythematous background [72, 76] corresponding to vascular ectasia noted on histology [76]. This is distinct from the purplish-red background previously noted in PXE [74]. PXE-PDE is typically asymptomatic but may be mildly pruritic. The lesions are indolent and may be found incidentally. Frontal fibrosing alopecia of the occiput occurred coincidentally with PXE-PDE of the nape [72], but in general, there are no consistently reported associated disorders. Specifically, these patients do not have ophthalmologic or cardiac conditions, in contrast to patients with PXE. Rare reports of familial occurrence include two sisters in their 70s with PXE-PDE [55].

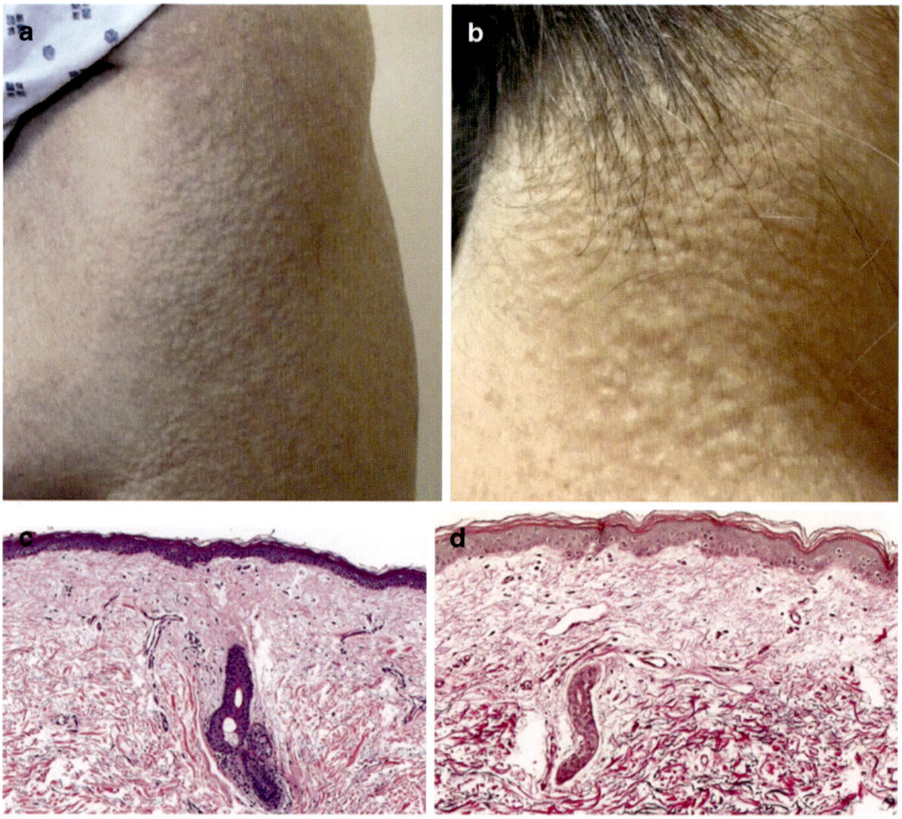

Fig. 2 Pseudoxanthoma elasticum-like papillary dermal elastolysis. (**a**): Multiple 2–5 mm skin-colored papules on the lateral flank and along the edge of the axillary vault. These show coalescence into cobblestone plaques. (**b**): Multiple 2–4 mm yellowish papules on the lateral neck. These are non-follicular and focally coalesce into cobblestone plaques. (**c**): Mild epidermal atrophy with expansion of the papillary dermis, noted as a band of more delicate collagen (H and E stain 100X). (**d**): Elastic tissue stain demonstrates near-complete loss of papillary dermal elastic fibers. There is a normal to slightly increased amount of morphologically elastic tissue in the underlying reticular dermis (VVG stain 100X)

White Fibrous Papulosis of the Neck (WPN)

WFPN was first reported by Shimizu in 1985 and was further characterized by the authors and designated a distinct entity in 1989 [78]. Several cases have since been reviewed [79], and some are described under the broader category of FEP, highlighting overlapping features of PXE-PDE and WFPN [46–48, 73]. Classic WFPN typically presents in middle age and older age groups, usually after age 40, with a mean age slightly younger than classic PXE-PDE. It has been reported as young as 26 years [80]. Both men and women are affected, with a reported predominance in men [78]. The lesions of WFPN present on the posterior, occipital, or lateral neck, sometimes extending to the supraclavicular area, upper back, or rarely the axilla [79] as numerous 2–3 mm (up to 6 mm) non-follicular white or pale firm discrete papules that tend not to coalesce into plaques, in contrast to PXE-PDE [43, 78, 79]. On dermoscopy, these appear as well-circumscribed homogeneous white areas with short thin vessels, not associated with a hair follicle [80]. There are no systemic associations.

Papillary Dermal Elastosis (PDE)

PDE was first reported in 2009 by Wang et al. as multiple pruritic 1–2 mm non-follicular papules on the lower neck and back [81], similar to other FEP (Fig. 3a). A second case of similar white to red pruritic papules involving the back, scapula, and lumbosacral region was reported [51]. The cases thus far reported have been in women in their 30s. There are no systemic associations. PDE is included in the spectrum of FEP, along with WFPN and PXE-PDE [48, 51, 75], but the literature is too sparse to draw conclusions regarding the pathogenesis.

Late-Onset Focal Dermal Elastosis (LOFDE)

LOFDE was first reported by Tajima et al. in 1995 as a PXE-like disorder similar to PXE-PDE but with elastosis instead of elastolysis on biopsy [52]. Only a handful of cases have been reported [41, 45, 52, 82–90]. Most reported patients are over age 65 years, with the average age of onset in the mid-50s. Patients present with indolent 1–5 mm firm yellow dermal papules that coalesce into cobblestone plaques, most often involving the neck and flexural sites, especially the antecubital and popliteal fossae, volar forearms, thighs, and groin (Fig. 4a). Other reported sites of involvement include the shoulders, upper back, axillae, anterior chest, and abdomen. A single case of dorsal hand/wrist involvement has been reported [82]. The lesions are usually asymptomatic but may be pruritic. Unlike PXE, systemic and ocular associations are absent. Rare familial occurrence has been reported [82].

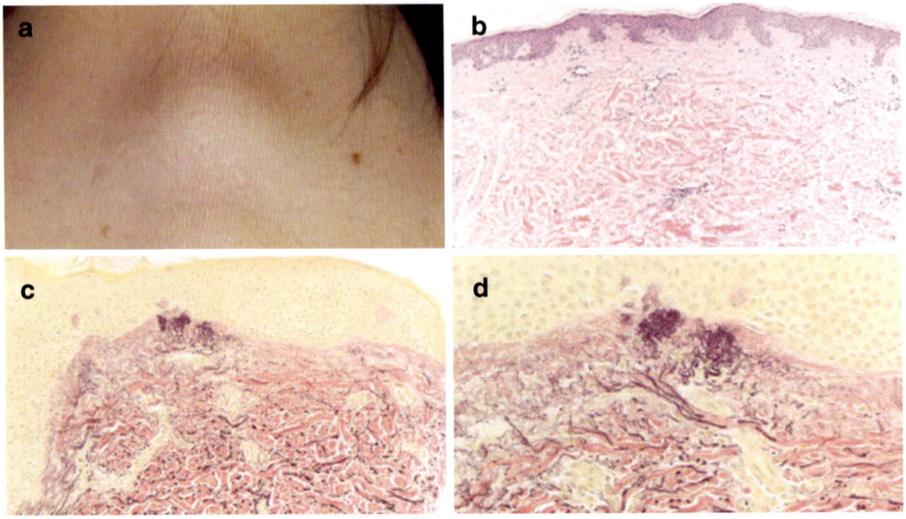

Fig. 3 Papillary dermal elastosis. (**a**): Multiple 1–2 mm skin-colored papules on the nape of the neck. (**b**): Routine H and E shows an unremarkable epidermis and dermis (H and E stain, 100x). (**c**): Elastic stain demonstrating clumped and curled papillary dermal elastic fibers arising in a band of decreased papillary dermal elastic fibers (VVG stain 200x). (**d**): Higher-power view of the clumped and curled papillary dermal elastic fibers (VVG stain 400x)

This disorder was originally termed late-onset focal dermal elastosis, acknowledging the late onset of lesions in comparison to PXE, and acknowledging the prevalence in elderly patients similar to PXE-PDE, suggesting a process related to intrinsic aging [89]. However, some patients noted onset of lesions in their 30s [45, 82]; thus, an alternative term, focal dermal elastosis, has been proposed [41].

Histopathologic Features

The histopathologic features of the FEEP disorders overlap [46, 48, 51, 75], as these disorders may represent a continuum of elastolysis and elastogenesis, with variable prominence or fibrosis of dermal collagen. On H and E stains, the biopsy will usually appear as "normal skin," and all of the disorders require elastic tissue stains, such as Verhoeff-van Gieson, orcein, or Weigert to confirm the diagnosis. One must review levels of the specimen if initial sections show no abnormalities on elastic stains, especially if a punch biopsy centered around the lesion is not bisected. Rarely, there will be no discernable findings, despite a strong clinical suspicion, requiring repeat biopsy [48].

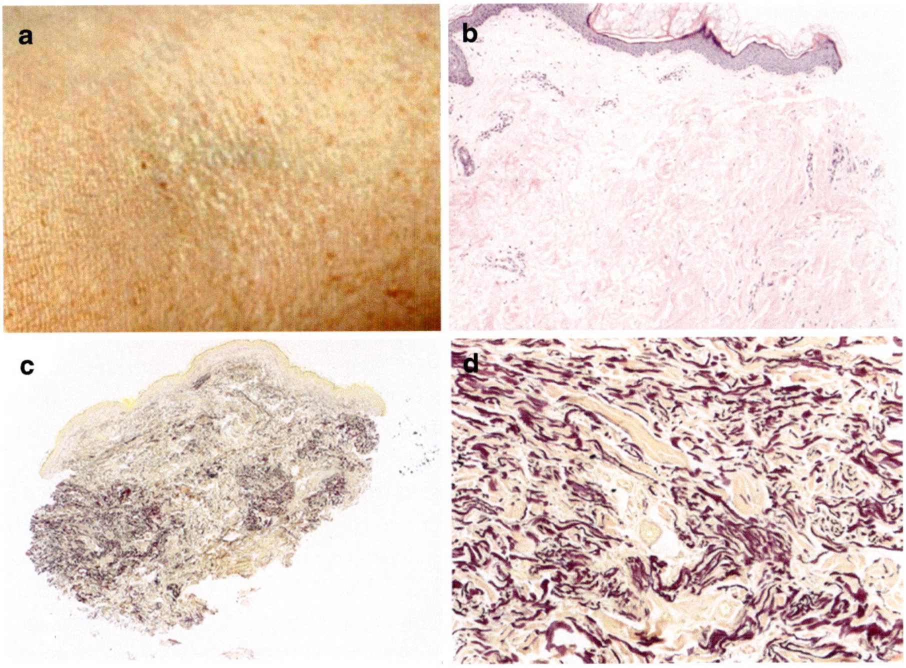

Fig. 4 Late-onset focal dermal elastosis. (**a**): Multiple 2–3 mm yellow papules in the antecubital fossa. (**b**): Normal-appearing biopsy except for mild epidermal atrophy, sparse superficial perivascular lymphocytic infiltrate, subtle nodular connective tissue prominence, and foci of thickened collagen bundles in the reticular dermis (H and E stain 100x). (**c**): Elastic stain demonstrating nodular zones of increase elastic tissue with foci of thickened and aggregated elastic fibers in the reticular dermis (VVG stain 40x). (**d**): Higher magnification of the thickened, clumped, and branched elastic fibers (VVG 400x)

Immunohistochemical stains for elastic fibers are not routinely used in diagnosis but have contributed to our knowledge of the elastic tissue abnormalities in these entities. These include anti-elastin and anti-fibrillin-1 [56, 84]. Antibodies to serum amyloid P (SAP) component shows differential staining of the papillary dermal elastic fibers, due to the target of the microfibril mantle surrounding the elastic fiber. Thus, oxytalan fibers in the papillary dermis show homogenous staining due to a predominantly microfibril composition, while the elastin core that characterizes elaunin fibers and elastic fibers in the reticular dermis results in a tubular staining pattern of the mantle of microfibrils [61]. This stain has been shown to be more sensitive than conventional stains, such as orcein, in highlighting tiny residual elastic fibers seen in cases of papillary dermal elastolysis [61], but it is not routinely used. Assessment by direct immunofluorescence using antibodies to fibrillins 1 and 2 (anti-Fib1, 2), anti-microfibril-associated glycoprotein 1 (MAGP-1) and MAGP-4 [27], and anti-elastin has been reported.

The histopathologic features of the specific subtypes are outlined below.

Pseudoxanthoma Elasticum-like Papillary Dermal Elastolysis (PXE-PDE)

On routine H and E stains, there are minimal changes that include an unremarkable or mildly atrophic epidermis (Fig. 2c) and sparse melanophages in the papillary dermis, the latter of which is a clue to the diagnosis [43]. Aside from pigment incontinence, the papillary and reticular dermis are usually unremarkable, but might show a mild nonspecific perivascular lymphocytic infiltrate and rarely papillary dermal fibrosis [43]. Dilated vessels may be present [63, 77]. Oxytalan and elaunin elastic fibers usually seen as perpendicular and parallel candelabra-like plexi in the papillary dermis are absent or reduced [43, 50]. This subepidermal band of elastolysis is documented with elastic stains. Additionally, expansion of the papillary dermis may be evident (Fig. 2d). This is all that is required to confirm the diagnosis; however, similar changes can be seen in aged skin. Fragmented, thickened, and clumped fibers have been described in the reticular dermis [43] or at the junction of the papillary and reticular dermis [53], but in general, morphologic aberrations in elastic fibers are not a feature of PXE-PDE [42]. Calcium deposition is absent on H and E and von Kossa stains.

Immunohistochemical stains with anti-SAP [61], anti-elastin, and anti-Fib1 [56] document loss of elastic fibers in the papillary dermis. On direct immunofluorescence, antibodies directed against elastin, Fib-1, Fib-2, MAGP-1, and MAGP-4 show complete absence of immunoreactivity in the papillary dermis [27]. Beneath this zone, elastic fibers have been reported to be normal [43], but subpapillary elastotic changes have been described as an accumulation of structurally normal elastic fibers [27, 48, 57, 59]. Accordingly, DIF shows staining with the abovementioned microfibril-associated antibodies within the subpapillary and mid-reticular dermal elastotic areas, indicating an accumulation of normal elastic fibers [27]. This elastosis may be under reported, as images of reported cases of PDE-PXE appear to show increased elastic tissue staining in the upper reticular dermis, just beneath the elastolytic zone [1, 43, 44, 48, 56–61, 65].

Ultrastructural features include absence of oxytalan and elaunin fibers in papillary dermis with granular and finely fibrillar degeneration of elastic fibers at the periphery and a widened microfibril-dense zone with less compaction of the skeleton of elastic fibers [8]. Accumulations of short and coarse elastic fibers and globules with peripheral granulations in the peripheral portion have also been described [55]. Immature elastic fibers with minimal elastin formation are seen in the upper reticular dermis [8, 42]. Fibroblasts with prominent rough endoplasmic reticulum, cisterna-like dilations, and abundant elongated dendritic processes have been identified in the affected area, but not in the adjacent normal skin, suggesting abnormal elastogenesis and cell activation [55].

White Fibrous Papulosis of the Neck

The main histopathologic feature noted on routine H and E stains is a distinct area of thickened collagen bundles arranged haphazardly in the papillary and upper to mid reticular dermis [46, 78, 79]. The epidermis may show slight decrease in melanin on a Fontana-Masson stain [78]. Mild hyperorthokeratosis and a sparse perivascular lymphocytic infiltrate can be seen in the superficial dermis. Papillary dermal elastolysis with morphologically normal or rarely slightly fragmented elastic fibers may be seen on elastic stains in up to 50% of patients [78]. Electron microscopy documents increased diameter of collagen bundles, as compared to non-lesional skin [78].

Papillary Dermal Elastosis

Routine H and E stained sections of PDE do not show significant changes (Fig. 3b), with the exception of slight superficial perivascular inflammation, although on close inspection of the images in the case of Val-Bernal et al., increased elastic fibers can be identified in dermal papillae as subtle granular or fibrillar basophilic material [51]. The diagnosis requires an elastic stain, which will show foci of clumped, granular, and curled elastic fibers within dermal papillae (Fig. 3c) [81], replacing the usual pattern of papillary dermal oxytalan and elaunin fiber architecture. These elastotic clumps are seen along the base of the epidermis within dermal papillae [51] or may appear to arise within a subepidermal band of diminished normal-appearing elastic fibers, resulting in alternating areas of clumped elastic fibers and areas of elastolysis (Fig. 3d) [81]. Some cases may show overlapping features of PDE and other subtypes of FEP. In such instances, the subepidermal band of fibroelastolysis may be more prominent, with only foci of elastic clumping [48]. Elastotic globules and melanophages are not seen. The reticular dermal elastic fibers appear normal.

Late-Onset Focal Dermal Elastosis

LOFDE lesions are unremarkable on H and E stains, although thickened collagen bundles with a fascicular appearance have been described on H and E (Fig. 4b) [45]. Elastic stains reveal a focal increase in elastic tissue in the upper, mid, and at times deep reticular dermis. The elastic fibers are normal appearing but closely packed and may present as focal aggregates in the reticular dermis or as large amounts of thickened and branching or interlacing elastic fibers (Fig. 4c,d) [45, 82]. The elastic fibers in the papillary dermis are not increased. Images of several reported cases suggest that there may be an element of elastic tissue loss, but this has not been previously reported as a feature of LOFDE [41, 45, 52, 82, 85–88]. Fragmentation or calcification of elastic fibers and inflammatory changes are absent. Solar elastosis has been noted [87] but is not a characteristic feature.

Differential Diagnosis

The main histopathologic differential of the FEEP disorders is that of normal skin if one reviews a biopsy without appropriate clinical information. Sparse melanophages in the papillary dermis may suggest post-inflammatory pigment incontinence or a late lichenoid tissue reaction, but interface alteration is absent in FEEP. The differential diagnosis generated by the clinical lesions includes PXE, along with the spectrum of PXE-like FEEP: PXE-PDE, WFPN, PDE, and LOFDE. Other conditions with connective tissue aberrations and similar discrete dermal papules include perifollicular elastolysis, papular elastorrhexis, dermatofibrosis lenticularis disseminata, eruptive collagenomas, and acne scars. An elastic tissue stain and correlation with the clinical distribution and lesion morphology will be sufficient to differentiate these papular conditions. Less likely, other miscellaneous disorders, such as eruptive xanthoma, milia, and steatocystoma/vellus hair cysts, may present with similar small dermal papules, but a routine biopsy will easily exclude these.

Differentiating between the spectrum of FEEP disorders may be difficult, as the clinical presentation may be identical, and additionally, there is histopathologic overlap. Discriminating features can be found in Table 1. However, adopting the more unifying term of FEEP avoids a need to distinguish these disorders on a practical level. In general, PXE-PDE papules are yellow and often fuse into confluent plaques, while WFPN and PDE are more white and non-confluent. Nearly all patients with PXE-PDE have been in elderly women, while WFPN is seen more often in men, with a slightly younger mean age of onset. The presentation of the two reported cases of PDE in women in their 30s is distinct, as are the discrete foci of clumped and curled elastic fibers in the dermal papillae. LOFDE clinically mimics FEEP disorders, but increased aggregates of elastic fibers in the reticular dermis distinguish LOFDE from other FEEP. While elastolysis of the papillary dermis has not been formally reported in LOFDE, many of the images in prior reports appear to show a thin band of diminished elastic tissue staining [41, 45, 52, 82, 85–88]; thus, if only the surface is sampled, this may be difficult to distinguish from the other FEEP disorders.

PXE is the most critical diagnosis to exclude, as the clinical lesions are similar to PXE-PDE, with yellow papules coalescing to form cobblestone plaques that eventually become lax due to the elastic tissue abnormalities. Clinically it is differentiated by a hereditary history, presentation at a younger age, presence of a mutation on the ABCC6 gene [1], and absence of cardiovascular and retinal abnormalities. A biopsy will show granular, fragmented, curled, frayed, and thick calcified elastic fibers in the reticular dermis, which are notable as basophilic material in the reticular dermis on H and E and highlighted by a von Kossa stain [1].

PXE-like primary systemic light chain amyloidosis and amyloid elastosis are rare cutaneous manifestations of amyloidosis in which deposition of amyloid is present around pilosebaceous structures and present with yellow papules that coalesce into cobblestone plaques [91]. In the case reported by Wat et al., a woman in her 50s presented with PXE-like lesions on the neck and bilateral antecubital fossa. Other signs of systemic amyloidosis, including macroglossia and carpel tunnel syndrome, were present. Biopsy showed the amyloid deposition around a pilosebaceous unit, as well as papillary dermal and reticular dermal amyloid. The absence of elastic fiber amyloid deposition differentiates this from amyloid elastosis, which has also been reported to present with PXE-like plaques. The elastic fibers are normal, with no thickening, fragmentation, or truncation, differentiating this from the spectrum of FEEP.

Juxtaclavicular beaded lines are yellowish 2 mm papules on the neck, which have a similar appearance as PXE-PDE, but are arranged in a linear fashion, often in a V-distribution. This is not an uncommon finding and has been reported in white and dark-skinned individuals, often in older age groups or after corticosteroid usage. Biopsies show prominent sebaceous glands. These papules are felt to likely represent normal pilosebaceous structures that are naturally arranged along linear Langer lines of tension and become more prominent if the overlying and surrounding skin atrophies [92].

There are other entities that present with similar small dermal papules that usually occur off the neck and flexural sites but may occasionally enter the differential diagnosis. Mid-dermal elastolysis is characterized by elastolysis, but this occurs in the mid-reticular dermis and not the papillary dermis [1, 43, 93]. The *type I* variant clinically has no overlap with the FEEP disorders and, instead, presents as patches of circumscribed finely wrinkled skin. Type II (perifollicular) mid-dermal elastolysis may present with dermal papules or protrusions, but these are follicular based and are frequently seen on the trunk and proximal extremities. It arises in all ages, but more common in younger white female patients. The elastolysis occurs in the mid reticular dermis, around hair follicles, while the papillary dermis is spared. *Acne scars* may show similar appearing small yellowish papules, but these are follicular and are more frequent on the face and trunk. Histologically there is perifollicular elastolysis due to scar-like fibrosis. PXE-PDE may enter the clinical and histopathologic diagnosis if only the perifollicular dermis without the follicle is present in the initial sections of the biopsy. Papular elastorrhexis occurs in children and adolescence with 3–5 non-follicular skin-colored discrete papules on the trunk and extremities, with histology showing absent or diminished elastic fibers throughout the reticular dermis [94]. This entity is considered by some to represent the same entity as eruptive collagenoma and or an abortive form of Buschke-Ollendorff syndrome (dermatofibrosis lenticularis disseminata), which is an autosomal dominantly inherited disorder associated with a mutation in the LEMD3 gene [45], characterized by widespread elastomas and collagenomas. These patients usually present by adolescence and often have osteopoikilosis, which are densities that occur in the epiphyses and metaphyses of long bones and are detected on X-rays of the hands, feet, and hips [45]. The elastic tissue abnormality noted on biopsies of the yellow papules is characterized by thick antler-like elastic fibers. Birt-Hogg Dubé syndrome is a hereditary condition due to a defect in the folliculin codifying gene (FLCN), characterized by numerous white dome-shaped dermal papules involving the face/head, neck, and upper back/arms, in association with renal tumors and pulmonary pseudocysts. Biopsies show hamartomas of the hair follicle and associated mesenchyme, including fibrofolliculomas, trichodiscomas, and perifollicular fibromas [95, 96]. Fox Fordyce disease typically presents in young and premenopausal women on the axillary vault (in contrast to the axillary folds) and other apocrine-rich sites, such as the groin and anogenital region as 1–2 mm yellowish or skin-colored papules, characterized histologically by perifollicular foamy xanthomatous histiocytes [97].

Etiopathogenesis

Pseudoxanthoma Elasticum-like Papillary Dermal Elastolysis (PXE-PDE)

The exact cause of PXE-PDE is not known. Initially, it was considered a form of intrinsic aging, based on the older age of onset and absence of oxytalan fibers, which also characterizes intrinsic aging [42, 43]. Arguments against this theory include the rare occurrence in patients in their 40s and younger [58], absence of the condition in men, and immunohistochemical studies showing different findings in PXE-PDE versus normal aged skin [56]. Ohnishi Y et al. documented loss of papillary dermal elastin and fibrillin-1 in lesions of PXE-PDE and only fibrillin-1 loss in normal aged skin, while in young skin, immunohistochemical staining with both antibodies was intact. The findings suggest a multifactorial cause not solely due to aging [56]. The rare reports of familial cases suggest a small role for genetic factors [55]. The occurrence of PXE-PDE in four patients undergoing glucocorticoid therapy led the authors to postulate a role of glucocorticosteroids through downregulation of elastin gene expression and elastin mRNA, in vitro [64]. Despite the frequent occurrence on the lateral neck, ultraviolet light exposure is not felt to play a significant role, as solar elastosis is not a histopathologic feature, and non-sun-exposed sites are often affected. The occurrence of PXE-PDE in two sisters who wore a religious nun habit since adolescence [54], in two additional nuns [64], and in several women who chronically wear a hijab [44] lends further evidence against a role for chronic UV radiation. Although elastolysis is the primary diagnostic feature, several cases additionally have reported elastotic changes in the subpapillary dermis on elastic stains [57, 59]. Moreover, increased elastic tissue is observed beneath the band of elastolysis in photos of prior reported cases suggesting this may be an under-recognized feature [1, 43, 44, 48, 56, 59, 61, 65]. Ultrastructural findings of absent, degenerating, and immature elastic fibers with adjacent fibroblasts showing signs of activation are features promoted to represent ongoing elastolysis and repair by elastogenesis. This theory would explain this concomitant elastosis. Some have implied that the clinical lesion may, in part, be related to increased dermal elastic tissue, rather than the elastolysis [48, 57]. Herniation of the fibroelastolytic or elastotic alteration through compromised papillary dermis may accentuate the lesion.

WFPN

There has not been much speculation as to the cause of WFPN, aside from the contribution of intrinsic aging, similar to PXE-PDE. Accumulation of fibrous tissue has been attributed to abnormal elastogenesis and fibroblast activation seen ultrastructurally, representing the consequence of fibroblasts compensating for the loss of elastic tissue [55]. Similarly, WFPN, fibroblasts with abundant rough endoplasmic reticulum, and mitochondria support a theory of increased fibroblast activity and overproduction of collagen as a consequence of elastolysis [78]. Under this concept, the rare cases of PDE could also represent an evolutionary stage of PXE-PDE, given that the main histopathologic difference between the two disorders is the presence of clumped elastic fibers in PDE.

Late-Onset Focal Dermal Elastosis

LOFDE, as with other FEEP disorders, does not have a definitive etiopathogenesis. There may be a component of intrinsic aging, but this does not accommodate the younger presentations. Other theories offered include a genetically determined characteristic of elastic tissue properties that contribute to a response to repetitive mechanical stress in flexural elastic tissue [85]. An age-related local increase in elastic tissue production, analogous to acquisition of skin tags and other common acquired skin lesions, possibly due to loss of homeostatic growth regulating gene control mechanisms has also been proposed [86].

Treatment

There is no effective topical treatment for the FEEP disorders. Topical retinoids, antioxidants, and topical steroids have been tried without success. Physical modalities provide some hope for cosmetic improvement, especially considering their success in improving the appearance of photo-aged skin and dermal scarring. Non-ablative fractional resurfacing was helpful in a case of PXE-PDE. At least a 50% improvement of the texture and appearance was appreciated after three treatments [69]. In a case of a 26-year-old with numerous clinical lesions, felt to be WFPN, but with equivocal supportive images, eight sessions of non-ablative fractional photothermolysis laser treatments using a fractionated 1550 nm erbium glass laser resulted in 60–70% improvement by the opinion of the patient and 50–70% by blinded dermatologists [80].

Prognosis

FEEP disorders are benign and indolent. Once established, there is no widespread progression. There are no systemic associations. The lesions are usually asymptomatic, apart from mild pruritus in a subset, so treatment is not necessary. The main concern is usually that of cosmesis. In the case of LOFDE, it will be important to exclude Buschke-Ollendorff syndrome with genetic testing and/or plain films of the hands/feet, long bones, and/or hips, although not all cases will present with osteopoikilosis [1].

Conclusion

A subset of elastic tissue disorders present with non-follicular yellow or white papules on the neck and axillae that may coalesce into cobblestone plaques, simulating PXE, but instead showing increased or decreased elastic tissue without the calcifications that typify PXE. These include PXE-PDE, WFPN, and PDE, which show papillary dermal elastolysis and variably increased reticular dermal collagen and rarely with clumped elastic fibers in the papillary dermis. These are included in the spectrum of FEEP. LOFDE has similar clinical lesions but with increased masses of reticular dermal elastic tissue. The spectrum of FEEP has clinical and histopathologic overlap. Ultrastructural evidence of elastogenesis and elastic tissue degeneration in these disorders suggests that these may be variants of the same condition at different evolutionary stages. These conditions are benign, indolent, and chronic. There are no systemic associations and they pose only a cosmetic concern. Therapy is limited to physical modalities, such as laser therapy.

References

1. Andrés-Ramos I, Alegría-Landa V, Gimeno I, Pérez-Plaza A, Rütten A, Kutzner H, Requena L. Cutaneous Elastic Tissue Anomalies. Am J Dermatopathol. 2019. Feb;41(2):85–117.
2. Kazlouskaya V, Malhotra S, Lambe J, Idriss MH, Elston D, Andres C. The utility of elastic Verhoeff-Van Gieson staining in dermatopathology. J Cutan Pathol. 2013;40(2):211–25.
3. Kligman LH. Luna's technique. A beautiful stain for elastin. Am J Dermatopathol. 1981 Summer;3(2):199–201.
4. Kielty CM, Sherratt MJ, Shuttleworth CA. Elastic fibres. J Cell Sci. 2002;115(Pt 14):2817–28.
5. Shin SJ, Yanagisawa H. Recent updates on the molecular network of elastic fiber formation. Essays Biochem. 2019;63(3):365–76.
6. Schmelzer CEH, Hedtke T, Heinz A. Unique molecular networks: formation and role of elastin cross-links. IUBMB Life. 2020;72(5):842–54.
7. Cotta-Pereira G, Guerra Rodrigo F, Bittencourt-Sampaio S. Oxytalan, elaunin, and elastic fibers in the human skin. J Invest Dermatol. 1976;66(3):143–8.
8. Rongioletti F, Rebora A. Fibroelastolytic patterns of intrinsic skin aging: pseudoxanthoma-elasticum-like papillary dermal elastolysis and white fibrouspapulosis of the neck. Dermatology. 1995;191(1):19–24.
9. Burket JM, Zelickson AS, Padilla RS. Linear focal elastosis (elastotic striae). J Am Acad Dermatol. 1989;20(4):633–6.
10. Moiin A, Hashimoto K. Linear focal elastosis in a young black man: a new presentation. J Am Acad Dermatol. 1994;30(5 Pt 2):874–7.
11. Florell AJ, Wada DA, Hawkes JE. Linear focal elastosis associated with exercise. JAAD Case Rep. 2017;3(1):39–41.
12. Hagari Y, Mihara M, Morimura T, Shimao S. Linear focal elastosis. An ultrastructural study. Arch Dermatol. 1991;127(9):1365–8.
13. White GM. Linear focal elastosis: a degenerative or regenerative process of striae distenae? J Am Acad Dermatol. 1992;27(3):468.
14. Hashimoto K. Linear focal elastosis: Keloidal repair of striae distensae. J Am Acad Dermatol. 1998;39(2 Pt 2):309–13.

15. Jeong JS, Lee JY, Kim MK, Yoon TY. Linear focal elastosis following striae distensae: further evidence of keloidal repair process in the pathogenesis of linear focal elastosis. Ann Dermatol. 2011;23(Suppl 2):S141–3.
16. Vogel PS, Cardenas A, Ross EV, Cobb MW, Sau P, James WD. Linear focal elastosis. Arch Dermatol. 1995;131(7):855–6.
17. Palmer J, Madison KC, Stone MS. Asymptomatic linear bands across the back. Linear focal elastosis. Arch Dermatol. 1995;131(9):1070–1, 1073–4.
18. Trüeb RM, Fellas AS. [Linear focal elastosis (elastotic striae)]. Hautarzt. 1995;46(5):346–8.
19. Tamada Y, Yokochi K, Ikeya T, Nakagomi Y, Miyake T, Hara K. Linear focal elastosis: a review of three cases in young Japanese men. J Am Acad Dermatol. 1997;36(2 Pt 2):301–3.
20. Hagari Y, Norimoto M, Mihara M. Linear focal elastosis associated with striae distensae in an elderly woman. Cutis. 1997;60(5):246–8. quiz 250.
21. Breier F, Trautinger F, Jurecka W, Hönigsmann H. Linear focal elastosis (elastotic striae): increased number of elastic fibres determined by a video measuring system. Br J Dermatol. 1997;137(6):955–7.
22. Chang SE, Park IJ, Moon KC, Koh JK. Two cases of linear focal elastosis (elastotic striae). J Dermatol. 1998;25(6):395–9.
23. Parsad D. Linear focal elastosis. Indian J Dermatol Venereol Leprol. 1998;64(6):299–300.
24. Choi SW, Lee JH, Woo HJ, Park CJ, Yi JY, Song KY, Kim HO. Two cases of linear focal elastosis: different histopathologic findings. Int J Dermatol. 2000;39(3):207–9.
25. Ramlogan D, Tan BB, Garrido M. Linear focal elastosis. Br J Dermatol. 2001;145(1):188–90.
26. Arroyo MP, Soter NA. Linear focal elastosis. Dermatol Online J. 2001;7(2):18. No abstract available.
27. Akagi A, Tajima S, Kawada A, Ishibashi A. Coexistence of pseudoxanthoma elasticum-like papillary dermal elastolysis and linear focal dermal elastosis. J Am Acad Dermatol. 2002;47(2 Suppl):S189–92.
28. Inaloz HS, Kirtak N, Karakok M, Ozgoztasi O. Facial linear focal elastosis: a case report. Int J Dermatol. 2003;42(7):558–60.
29. Pui JC, Arroyo M, Heintz P. Linear focal elastosis: histopathologic diagnosis of an uncommon dermal elastosis. J Drugs Dermatol. 2003;2(1):79–83.
30. Péc J, Chromej I. Linear focal elastosis: what's new? J Eur Acad Dermatol Venereol. 2004;18(3):247–9.
31. Whalen JG, English JC 3rd. Case study on linear focal elastosis. Dermatol Nurs. 2006;18(5):469–71.
32. Adişen E, Ilter N, Erdem O, Gürer MA. Early onset linear focal elastosis in a Turkish boy. Turk J Pediatr. 2007;49(4):441–3.
33. Seo JK, Chun JS, Jung SY, Hwang SW, Sung HS, Lee D. A case of linear focal elastosis with a family history. Ann Dermatol. 2010;22(2):209–11.
34. Jang WS, Lee JW, Yoo KH, Park KY, Han TY, Li K, Seo SJ, Hong CK. Could a growth spurt cause linear focal elastosis like striae distensae? Ann Dermatol. 2012;24(1):81–3.
35. Cohen PR, Tschen JA. Linear lumbar localized lysis of elastic fibers: a distinctive clinical presentation of mid-dermal elastolysis. J Clin Aesthet Dermatol. 2013;6(7):32–9.
36. Clement BC, Forster C, Logemann N. Focal linear elastosis in a patient with joint hypermobility syndrome. Dermatol Online J. 2018;15:24(1).
37. Zink AGS, Steimle-Grauer A, Hein R, Biedermann T. Image gallery: Linear focal elastosis mimicking striae distensae. Br J Dermatol. 2018;178(4):e278.
38. Seol JE, Kim DH, Cho GJ, Park SH, Jung SY, Kim H. Linear focal elastosis: a case report and institutional case series of 22 patients. Australas J Dermatol. 2019;60(3):e261–3.
39. Kaur I, Jakhar D, Bhattacharya SN, Sharma S. Linear focal elastosis localized to bilateral knee of a marathon runner. J Postgrad Med. 2019;65(1):60–1.
40. Singh G, Kumar LP. Striae distensae. Indian J Dermatol Venereol Leprol. 2005;71:370–2.
41. Knapp M, Carpenter CE, Shea K, Stowman A, Pierson JC. Focal dermal elastosis: a proposed update to the nomenclature. Am J Dermatopathol. 2020;42(10):774–5.

42. Rongioletti F, Rebora A. Pseudoxanthoma elasticum-like papillary dermal elastolysis. J Am Acad Dermatol. 1992;26(4):648–50.
43. Rongioletti F, Izakovic J, Romanelli P, Lanuti E, Miteva M. Pseudoxanthoma elasticum-like papillary dermal elastolysis: a large case series with clinicopathological correlation. J Am Acad Dermatol. 2012;67(1):128–35.
44. Aljoudi SB, Abduljabbar MH, Hariri JO. A case series of pseudoxanthoma Elasticum-like disorders. Indian J Dermatol. 2019;64(6):482–5.
45. Wang AR, Fonder MA, Telang GH, Bercovitch L, Robinson-Bostom L. Late-onset focal dermal elastosis: an uncommon mimicker of pseudoxanthoma elasticum. J Cutan Pathol. 2012;39(10):957–61.
46. Balus L, Amantea A, Donati P, Fazio M, Giuliano MC, Bellocci M. Fibroelastolytic papulosis of the neck: a report of 20 cases. Br J Dermatol. 1997;137(3):461–6.
47. Jagdeo J, Ng C, Ronchetti IP, Wilkel C, Bercovitch L, Robinson-Bostom L. Fibroelastolytic papulosis. J Am Acad Dermatol. 2004;51(6):958–64.
48. Patterson AT, Beasley KJ, Kobayashi TT. Fibroelastolytic papulosis: histopathologic confirmation of disease spectrum variants in a single case. J Cutan Pathol. 2016 Feb;43(2):142–7.
49. Oiso N, Kato M, Kawada A. Fibroelastolytic papulosis in an elderly woman with a 30-year history: overlapping between pseudoxanthoma elasticum-like papillary dermal elastolysis and white fibrous papulosis of the neck. Eur J Dermatol. 2014;24(6):688–9.
50. Alves R, Ferreira L, Vale E, Bordalo O. Pseudoxanthoma elasticum papillary dermal elastolysis: a case report. Dermatol Res Pract. 2010;2010
51. Val-Bernal JF, González-Vela MC, León-Castillo A, Armesto S. Papillary Dermal Elastosis. Am J Dermatopathol. 2017;39(2):150–2.
52. Tajima S, Shimizu K, Izumi T, Kurihara S, Harada T. Late-onset focal dermal elastosis: clinical and histological features. Br J Dermatol. 1995;133(2):303–5.
53. el-Charif MA, Mousawi AM, Rubeiz NG, Kibbi AG. Pseudoxanthoma elasticum-like papillary dermal elastolysis: a report of two cases. J Cutan Pathol 1994;21(3):252–255.
54. Vargas-Díez E, Peñas PF, Fraga J, Aragües M, García-Díez A. Pseudoxanthoma elasticum-like papillary dermal elastolysis. A report of two cases and review of the literature. Acta Derm Venereol. 1997;77(1):43–5.
55. Orlandi A, Bianchi L, Nini G, Spagnoli LG. Familial occurrence of pseudoxanthoma-elasticum-like papillary dermal elastolysis. J Eur Acad Dermatol Venereol. 1998 Mar;10(2): 175-8. P
56. Ohnishi Y, Tajima S, Ishibashi A, Inazumi T, Sasaki T, Sakamoto H. Pseudoxanthoma elasticum-like papillary dermal elastolysis: report of four Japanese cases and an immunohistochemical study of elastin and fibrillin-1. Br J Dermatol. 1998;139(1):141–4.
57. Tajima S, Ohnishi Y, Akagi A, Sasaki T. Elastotic change in the subpapillary and mid-dermal layers in pseudoxanthoma elasticum-like papillary dermal elastolysis. Br J Dermatol. 2000;142(3):586–8.
58. Byun JY, DO MO, Kim SH, Choi HY, Myung KB, Choi YW. Pseudoxanthoma elasticum-like papillary dermal elastolysis developed in early middle age. J Dermatol. 2007;34(10):709–11.
59. Lee HS, Song HJ, Hong WK, Shin JH, Choi GS. Pseudoxanthoma elasticum-like papillary dermal elastolysis with solar elastosis. J Eur Acad Dermatol Venereol. 2008;22(3):368–9.
60. López V, Revert A, Santonja N, Jordá E. Pseudoxantoma elasticum-like dermal elastolysis: a case report. Dermatol Online J. 2011;17(4):13.
61. Revelles JM, Machan S, Pielasinski U, Camacho D, Vallés L, Santonja C, Kutzner H, Requena L. Pseudoxanthoma elasticum-like papillary dermal elastolysis: immunohistochemical study using elastic fiber cross-reactivity with an antibody against amyloid P component. Am J Dermatopathol. 2012;34(6):637–43.
62. Abdullah L, Abbas O. Dermacase: Can you identify this condition? Pseudoxanthoma elasticum–like papillary dermal elastolysis. Can Fam Physician. 2012;58(7):765, 768.
63. Ito T, Fujita Y, Nomura T, Abe R, Shimizu H. Dermoscopy of pseudoxanthoma elasticum-like papillary dermal elastolysis. J Am Acad Dermatol. 2013 Oct;69(4):e202–3.

64. Pranteda G, Muscianese M, Marmo G, Fidanza L, Pranteda G, Tamburi F, Bottoni U, Nisticò S. Role of steroid therapy in pseudoxanthoma elasticum-like papillary dermal elastolysis. Int J Immunopathol Pharmacol. 2013;26(4):1013–8.
65. Gambichler T, Reininghhaus L, Schaller J. Early-onset pseudoxanthoma elasticum-like papillary dermal elastolysis. J Eur Acad Dermatol Venereol. 2016;30(3):448–9.
66. Vázquez-Osorio I, Rosón E, Suárez-Peñaranda JM, Vázquez-Veiga H. Pseudoxanthoma elasticum-like papillary dermal elastolysis. Actas Dermosifiliogr. 2015;106(4):333–6.
67. Fukuda H, Mukai H, Otani A, Oharaseki T, Takahashi M. Dermoscopic findings of pseudoxanthoma elasticum-like papillary dermal elastolysis. Eur J Dermatol. 2017;27(1):99–100. https://doi.org/10.1684/ejd.2016.2911.
68. Valbuena V, Assaad D, Yeung J. Pseudoxanthoma elasticum-like papillary dermal elastolysis: a single case report. J Cutan Med Surg. 2017;21(4):345–347.
69. Foering K, Torbeck RL, Frank MP, Saedi N. Treatment of pseudoxanthoma elasticum-like papillary dermal elastolysis with nonablative fractional resurfacing laser resulting in clinical and histologic improvement in elastin and collagen. J Cosmet Laser Ther. 2018;20(7–8):382–384.
70. Ribeiro CP, Abuawad YG, Swiczar BCC, Valente NYS. Pseudoxanthoma elasticum-like papillary dermal elastolysis. An bras Dermatol. 2017 Nov-Dec;92(6):897-898.
71. Panagou E, Ratynska M, Heelan K. Pseudoxanthoma elasticum-like papillary dermal elastolysis: a case report and review of literature. Int J Dermatol. 2019;58(1):93–7.
72. Tengattini V, Alessandrini A, Misciali C, Patrizi A, Piraccini BM. Pseudoxanthoma elasticum-like papillary dermal elastolysis in frontal fibrosing alopecia. J Dtsch Dermatol Ges. 2018 Sep;16(9):1136–1138.
73. Ho D, Jagdeo J. Fractionated carbon dioxide laser treatment of Fibroelastolytic papulosis with excellent cosmetic result and resolution of pruritus. J Drugs Dermatol. 2015;14(11):1354–7.
74. Kawashima S, Togawa Y, Miyachi H, Matsue H. Dermoscopic features of pseudoxanthoma elasticum. Clin Exp Dermatol. 2018;43(2):175–9.
75. Wang X, Sun J. Fibroelastolytic papulosis with vacuolar interface dermatitis: a new observation. Australas J Dermatol. 2020;61(1):e101–2.
76. Mercuri SR, Cestone E, Bearzi P, Rizzo N, Paolino G. Dermoscopical and pathological findings in pseudoxanthoma elasticum-like papillary dermal elastolysis. G Ital Dermatol Venereol. 2020;155(5):692–3.
77. Setó-Torrent N, Iglesias-Sancho M, Arandes-Marcocci J, Fernández-Figueras MT. Pseudoxanthoma elasticum-like papillary dermal elastolysis in non-exposed skin. An Bras Dermatol. 2020;95(2):247–249.
78. Shimizu H, Kimura S, Harada T, Nishikawa T. White fibrous papulosis of the neck: a new clinicopathologic entity? J Am Acad Dermatol. 1989;20(6):1073–7.
79. Dokic Y, Tschen J. White fibrous papulosis of the axillae and neck. Cureus. 2020;12(4):e7635.
80. Lueangarun S, Panchaprateep R. White fibrous papulosis of the neck treated with fractionated 1550-nm erbium glass laser: a case report. J Lasers Med Sci. 2016;7:256–8.
81. Wang AR, Lewis K, Lewis M, Robinson-Bostom L. Papillary dermal elastosis: a unique elastic tissue disorder or an unusual manifestation of pseudoxanthoma elasticum-like papillary dermal elastolysis? J Cutan Pathol. 2009;36(9):1010–3.
82. Camacho D, Machan S, Pielasinski U, Revelles JM, del Carmen FM, Santonja C, Requena L. Familial acral localized late-onset focal dermal elastosis. Am J Dermatopathol. 2012;34(3):310–4.
83. Tajima S, Inazumi T, Kobayashi T. A case of acrogeria associated with late-onset focal dermal elastosis. Dermatology. 1996;192(3):264–8.
84. Tajima S, Tanaka N, Ohnishi Y, Ishibashi A, Kajiya H, Osakabe T, Seyama Y, Sakamoto H. Analysis of elastin metabolism in patients with late-onset focal dermal elastosis. Acta Derm Venereol. 1999;79(4):285–7.
85. Limas C. Late onset focal dermal elastosis: a distinct clinicopathologic entity? Am J Dermatopathol. 1999;21(4):381–3.

86. Kossard S. Pseudoxanthoma-like late-onset focal dermal elastosis. Australas J Dermatol. 2005;46(1):47–50.
87. Higgins HJ, Whitworth MW. Late-onset focal dermal elastosis: a case report and review of the literature. Cutis. 2010;85(4):195–7.
88. Tian S, Chen Z. Late-onset focal dermal elastosis. Eur J Dermatol. 2012;22(3):399–400. https://doi.org/10.1684/ejd.2012.1664.
89. Chappell J, Kozel J, Hurley MY, Vidal CI. A yellow Papular eruption on the arms, legs, and neck: a rare masquerader. Skinmed. 2016;14(6):465–6.
90. Hanami Y, Nakamura T, Yamamoto T. Case of late-onset focal dermal elastosis. J Dermatol. 2018;45(12):e339–40.
91. Wat H, Wu DC, Mahmood MN. Brassard a primary systemic (amyloid light-chain) amyloidosis masquerading as pseudoxanthoma elasticum: recognizing a novel clinicopathological pattern. JAMA Dermatol. 2014;150(10):1091–4.
92. Woldow AB, Houk LD, Samie FH. Juxtaclavicular beaded lines: a presentation of sebaceous gland hyperplasia. Dermatol Online J. 2009;
93. Gambichler T, Mamali K, Scheel C. A brief literature update on mid-dermal Elastolysis with an emphasis on Pathogenetic and therapeutic aspects. J Clin Aesthet Dermatol. 2020;13(9):E53–8.
94. Jiang M, Bu W, Chen X, Gu H. A case of papular elastorrhexis. Postepy Dermatol Alergol. 2019;36(1):117–8.
95. Lencastre A, Ponte P. ApetatoM, Nunes L, Lestre S. Birt-Hogg-Dubé syndrome An Bras Dermatol. 2013;88(6 Suppl 1):203–5.
96. Shvartsbeyn M, Mason AR, Bosenberg MW, Ko CJ. Perifollicular fibroma in Birt-Hogg-Dubé syndrome: an association revisited. J Cutan Pathol. 2012;39(7):675–9.
97. Vega-Memije ME, Pérez-Rojas DO, Boeta-Ángeles L, Valdés-Landrum P. Fox-Fordyce disease: report of two cases with perifollicular xanthomatosis on histological image. An Bras Dermatol. 2018;93(4):562–5.

Rare Variants of Keratosis Pilaris

Hatice B. Zengin, Tatsiana Pukhalskaya, and Bruce R. Smoller

Introduction

Keratosis pilaris (KP), commonly referred to as "chicken skin," is a hereditary skin disorder with altered follicular keratinization [1]. It is among the most common skin conditions and is frequent in otherwise asymptomatic patients visiting a dermatologist for other reasons [2].

In addition to commonly observed forms of KP, including KP rubra, there are also rare variants, i.e., KP atrophicans (KPA), erythromelanosis follicularis faciei et colli (EFFC), as well as papular, profuse, precocious KP (see Fig. 1). Although these rare variants demonstrate a wide spectrum of clinical presentations, they all feature a prominent plug of keratin within the follicular opening.

KPA encompasses a group of conditions in which the abnormality in follicular keratinization is accompanied by atrophy and scarring alopecia [3]. It is phenotypically related to keratosis pilaris and there is significant overlap between the subtypes [3]. In fact, it has been suggested that rather than one heterogeneous disease, KPA might be a feature shared by various clinical entities [4]. The above conditions include keratosis pilaris atrophicans faciei (KPAF) as well as atrophoderma vermiculatum (AV) and keratosis follicularis spinulosa decalvans (KFSD) (Fig. 1).

KPAF is also known as ulerythema ophryogenes that literally means "scarring of the eyebrows." This condition was first described by Wilson in 1878 as folliculitis rubra [3].

H. B. Zengin (✉) · T. Pukhalskaya · B. R. Smoller
Department of Pathology and Laboratory Medicine, University of Rochester Medical Center (URMC), Rochester, NY, USA
e-mail: Hatice_zengin@urmc.rochester.edu

F. Rongioletti, B. R. Smoller (eds.), *New and Emerging Entities in Dermatology and Dermatopathology*, https://doi.org/10.1007/978-3-030-80027-7_14

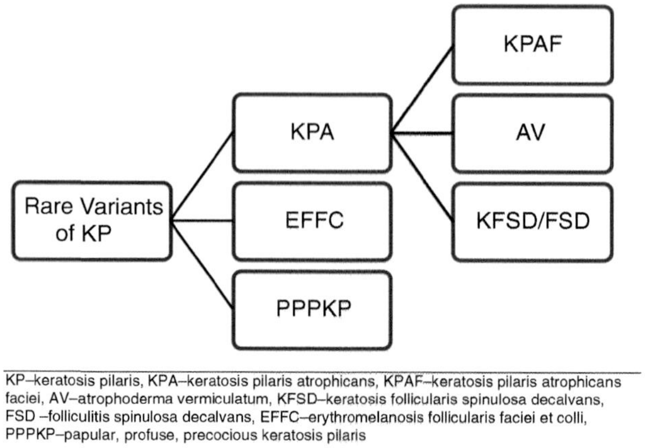

Fig. 1 Rare variants of keratosis pilaris. KP keratosis pilaris, KPA keratosis pilaris atrophicans, KPAF keratosis pilaris atrophicans faciei, AV atrophoderma vermiculatum, KFSD keratosis follicularis spinulosa decalvans, FSD folliculitis spinulosa decalvans, EFFC erythromelanosis follicularis faciei et colli, PPPKP papular, profuse, precocious keratosis pilaris

Another subtype of KPA, atrophoderma vermiculatum, is topographically limited to cheeks [5]. This condition was first described by Unna in 1894 under the name "ulerythema acneiforme" [6]. It is also known as honeycomb atrophy [7]. In fact, there are multiple different names of this condition in the literature with "atrophoderma vermiculatum" used most commonly through the years [7].

Compared to the above entities, KFSD was described later in 1926 by Siemens [3]. It is generally viewed as a more severe form of KPAF [3, 8].

Next rare variant of KP, erythromelanosis follicularis faciei et colli (EFFC), has significant clinical overlap with KP rubra and may represent a disease spectrum with individual differences in pigmentation [9, 10]. It was first described in 1960 by Kitamura et al. in six Japanese males [11]. In some cases it presents concomitantly with classic keratosis pilaris on other body parts [12, 13].

Papular, profuse, precocious KP (PPPKP), recently described by Emeline Castela et al., is characterized by an early onset (<18 months old) and significant involvement of the cheeks and extremities [14].

Clinical Presentation

In addition to the typical findings of KP, KPA shows variable degrees of inflammation with secondary atrophy and scarring [1, 15, 16]. The clinical presentation usually begins on the patient's face and may further involve their scalp, resulting in fibrosing alopecia [15, 16].

KPAF initially presents with small follicular keratotic papules and associated erythematous halo on the lateral third of the eyebrows [3, 15, 16]. With further

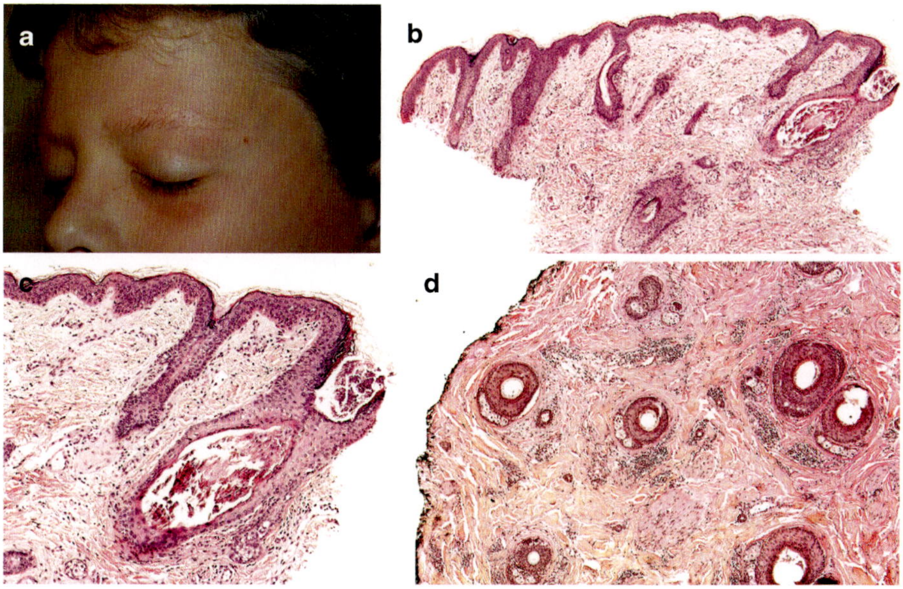

Fig. 2 KPAF and KFSD. (**a**) Keratosis pilaris atrophicans faciei (KPAF). Erythema with scar like follicular depressions and loss of hair in the eyebrows resulting in atrophy and permanent loss of hairs. (**b**) KPAF - H&E, X2. Histopathology showing a decrease in number of follicular structures, a widened follicular infundibulum with plugging, and a superficial perivascular infiltrate with slight dermal fibrosis. (**c**) KPAF – H&E, X4. Close-up of a widened follicular infundibulum with plugging and a slight infiltrate including plasma cells. (**d**) Keratosis follicularis spinulosa decalvans (KFSD). Scalp biopsy (horizontal section) – H&E, X4. Decrease of follicular structures with dilation of the follicular infundibulum and perifollicular fibrosis with a moderately dense inflammatory cell infiltrate. (Courtesy of Annalisa Patrizi, Iria Neri and Cosimo Misciali, Bologna, Italy)

progression, papules may extend to the entire eyebrow, cheeks, and forehead leading to permanent atrophy and alopecia (Fig. 2a). Although the disease usually subsides after puberty, irreversible hair loss may have already occurred by that time [3, 15, 16].

Similar to KPAF, atrophoderma vermiculatum classically manifests on the face (mainly cheeks) presenting with keratotic papules, erythema, and milia [3, 15, 16]. It usually spares the eyebrows and scalp, but may involve the upper lip, ears, neck, and extremities [3, 15, 16]. The lesions slowly progress into small atrophic pitting resulting in a reticular, honeycomb, or worm-eaten appearance of the patient's cheeks (Fig. 3a). Perifollicular inflammation generally ceases after puberty, but progressive disease is also described [3, 15, 16]. Spontaneous improvement of the erythema and reticulated atrophy may also be seen [17]. Important to add that both KPAF and AV usually present in a symmetrical fashion; however, unilateral cases have also been reported [15, 18].

KFSD usually begins during infancy with keratotic follicular and sometimes erythematous papules on the malar area and nose [3, 15, 16]. It may spread

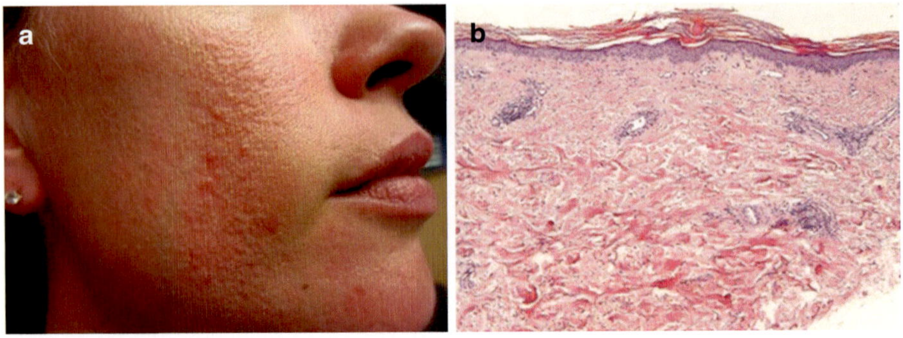

Fig. 3 (**a**) Atrophoderma vermiculatum(AV). This figure shows multiple follicular papules, surrounding erythema, and early worm-eaten appearance of the lesion on the cheek. (**b**) AV – H&E, X4. This figure shows hyperkeratosis in the follicular orifice, atrophic epidermis, dilated capillaries, and perivascular lymphocytic inflammation

during childhood to the scalp, neck, and trunk [3, 15, 16]. Papules tend to develop into patchy cicatricial alopecia involving the patient's eyebrows, eyelashes, and scalp [3, 15, 16]. Thinning of axillary and pubic hair may also occur [16]. The autosomal dominant variant of the disease is characterized by more pronounced erythema, persistent pustular inflammation, crusting, and desquamation on the scalp [16, 19]. In addition, common accompanied findings of KFSD include widespread KP, thickened cuticles, and hyperkeratosis of calcaneal region [4, 15]. Extracutaneous features may include photophobia, keratitis, blepharitis, and enamel hypoplasia [15, 20]. The X-linked variant of the disease usually remits at puberty, while in contrast, the autosomal dominant variant exacerbates [16, 19].

Erythromelanosis follicularis faciei et colli commonly demonstrates the triad of sharply demarcated erythema, hyperpigmentation, and follicular papules located on cheeks and preauricular region [21]. The lesions are uniformly located on both sides of the body, although a unilateral presentation of EFFC is also possible [15]. They can further spread to the pinna, neck, and eyebrows [22]. The accompanied erythema might be associated with focal telangiectasia [21]. Prominent KP with perifollicular erythema on the arms and thighs is a common finding [22]. The patients are overall asymptomatic, but pruritus and photosensitivity can occur [22]. In fact, pigmentation in EFFC can occur as a result of exposure to sunlight in the predisposed skin [23]. The affected skin has granular appearance with diminished vellus hair and a rough sensation upon palpation [21]. It is important to add that absence of scarring and atrophy differentiates this subtype from KPA [24].

Another rare variant papular, profuse, precocious KP displays extensive red to pink follicular papules on the cheeks and extremities [14]. Buttock involvement can be seen while the trunk and flexures are usually spared [14]. Compared to KP and KPR, the size of the individual lesions is larger (2–3 mm) [14, 15]. The patients with PPPKP can improve spontaneously [14].

Histopathology

All forms of KPA typically show follicular hyperkeratosis in the follicular orifice and hypergranulosis of the infundibulum and isthmus [15]. It is hard to differentiate variants based on histology, which varies depending on the stages of the disease [4]. Earlier stages display an acute neutrophilic inflammation and associated edema in the epidermis and dermis [25]. In contrast, advanced disease shows a decrease in number of follicular structures, widened follicular infundibulum with plugging, atrophic hair follicles, and a superficial perivascular infiltrate with dermal fibrosis leading to alopecia (Fig. 2b,c) [3, 25]. Atrophic sebaceous glands, comedones, and milia are among the other findings in this entity [7, 26]. In KFSP there is a decrease of follicular structures with dilation of the follicular infundibulum and perifollicular fibrosis with an inflammatory cell infiltrate leading to cicatricial alopecia (Fig. 2d). Variable acanthosis, papillomatosis, and trapped hair shafts have also been described in KFSD [27]. AV can additionally show epidermal atrophy, dilated capillaries, and decreased elastic fibers in the dermis (Fig. 3b) [28]. EFFC commonly demonstrates increased basilar pigmentation in addition to hyperkeratosis and follicular plugging [21, 29]. Perivascular and peri-adnexal inflammation, follicular dilatation, dilated blood vessels in the upper dermis, as well as decreased diameter of hair shafts are frequently identified [21, 29]. Furthermore, there are no unique features in the histological presentation of PPPKP compared to other forms of keratosis pilaris.

Differential Diagnosis

Since all rare variants of KP have follicular plugging as a common denominator, these entities might be easily mistaken for each other, as well as for KP itself, especially in the initial stages of the disease. The late-stage scarring and atrophy, particularly in the KPA spectrum, might be helpful in distinguishing this variant from EFFC [21]. In addition, other conditions with similar clinical pictures should be acknowledged in this section. These include, but are not limited to, lichen spinulosus, phrynoderma, juvenile pityriasis rubra pilaris, lichen planopilaris, acne vulgaris, trichostasis spinulosa, and eruptive vellus hair cysts [30].

Lichen spinulosus (LS) is characterized by follicular keratotic papules on the extensor surfaces of the extremities, back, face, and neck [31]. Histology of the papule reveals a keratotic plug in the dilated infundibulum and less often perifollicular fibrosis and atrophy of sebaceous glands. There is an abundant perifollicular inflammation in comparison to KP [31]. Interestingly, LS has previously been suggested to be a variant of KP [31].

Phrynoderma is a skin manifestation of vitamin A deficiency manifesting with skin xerosis as well as formation of follicular keratotic papules [32].

Clinically similar to KP, juvenile pityriasis rubra pilaris presents with small follicular papules with a central keratin plug and perifollicular erythema [33]. In addition to perivascular and perifollicular inflammation, a characteristic "checkerboard" pattern of parakeratosis (alternating vertical and horizontal ortho- and parakeratosis) can be seen upon histology [33].

Lichen planopilaris (LP) is characterized by keratotic follicular lesions and associated erythema at the margins of the scarring alopecia [34]. Lichenoid inflammation involving the perifollicular epithelium and variable perifollicular fibrosis are the major histologic findings [34].

Another similar entity, eruptive vellus hair cysts (EVHC), might occur as multiple, asymptomatic papules on the chest or axilla in children or young adults [35]. Histology reveals small epidermoid cysts containing multiple vellus hair [35]. Trichostasis spinulosa (TS) might be in the differential for EVHC and KP, as well [36]. Clinical features of this entity include comedo-like lesions or horny, spinous plugs on the face, while histology depicts hyperkeratosis of dilated hair follicles with retention of multiple vellus hairs [36].

Poikiloderma of Civatte (PC) could be similar to EFFC as it presents with red to brownish, reticular, and symmetrically distributed patches on the neck, upper chest, and face [21, 37]. Microscopy of the lesion reveals variable telangiectasia, melanin incontinence, mild epidermal atrophy, and sparse perivascular inflammation [38].

Etiopathogenesis

KP atrophicans faciei has an autosomal dominant inheritance with incomplete penetrance (genetic locus 18p11.2). It is viewed as a marker for certain syndromes such as Noonan, Rubinstein-Taybi, Cornelia de Lange, and cardio-facio-cutaneous syndrome [26, 39, 40]. There is an association of KPAF and woolly hair [41]. KPAF may also be linked to low levels of vitamin A and iron [42]. Similar to KPAF, AV is presumed to have an autosomal dominant inheritance with a well-documented familial incidence [43]. Men and women tend to be equally affected [7]. It is documented to be in association with leukokeratosis oris, ipsilateral congenital cataracts, and Loeys-Dietz, Rombo, and Down syndromes [44–48]. On the other hand, KFSD has both X-linked recessive and autosomal dominant (folliculitis spinulosa decalvans) modes of inheritance [49, 50]. The X-linked variant is characterized by the mutation in the MBTPS2 gene located on Xp22.11 [49, 50]. Both sporadic and familial cases have been reported in the literature [8, 51, 52]. This condition is rarely associated with Noonan syndrome and mental retardation [3, 49]. The cause appears to be hyperkeratosis at the follicular orifice of the infundibulum [25].

EFFC mainly affects adolescents [9]. Nevertheless, it has also been reported in children and adults [9]. Familial cases have also been described with suggestions of an autosomal recessive mode of inheritance [13, 23, 53–55]. The possibility of a spontaneous mutation has also been proposed [56]. It has been also viewed as a polyetiological disorder (i.e., familial and environmental) with the possibility of chromosomal instability [53].

In contrast to the conditions above, PPPKP is not inherited or yet known to be associated with other conditions or syndromes [14].

Therapy, Prognosis, and Course

Treatment of KPA is challenging and there is no satisfactory option. Symptomatic treatment includes use of keratolytics and topical retinoids [57]. Gerbig reported a good response to external application of tazarotene, although some authors have shown retinoids to be ineffective [57]. Additionally, pulsed dye laser or intense pulsed light showed marked reduction in erythema with a low incidence of side effects [58]. Topical and systemic antibiotics are not helpful against KPA [25]. For severe forms, especially in the inflammatory stages, systemic retinoids might be effective [59]. It is important to add that due to the chronic nature of the disease, treatment effects must be weighed against the possibility of severe side effects [3].

Analogous to KPA, there is no adequate treatment option yet existing for EFFC. Most of the lesions usually recur shortly after the treatment is discontinued [60]. Emollients, keratolytic, tacalcitol ointment, metronidazole, hydroquinone 4%, chemical peel, and laser systems have been used with variable results [55, 61–64].

Regarding the treatment options for PPPKP, the best clinical response was observed with a combination of propylene glycol, lactic acid, oleic acid, and glycerin [14]. These authors emphasize that treatment with this agent must be restricted to small areas to avoid toxicity [14].

Conclusions

We believe that the rare variants of keratosis pilaris represent a challenging group of clinically and histologically similar conditions that require careful investigation and proper classification. Due to the limited knowledge of their existence, these entities might be underdiagnosed. However, the chronic and sometimes disfiguring nature, association with genetic syndromes, as well as cosmetic impact emphasize the importance of establishing an early diagnosis, treatment, and the overall acknowledgment of their individual differences.

References

1. Hwang S, Schwartz RA. Keratosis pilaris: a common follicular hyperkeratosis. Cutis. 2008;82(3):177–80.
2. Pennycook, K.B, McCready T.A. Keratosis pilaris, in StatPearls; 2021. Treasure Island (FL).

3. Arnold AW, Buechner SA. Keratosis pilaris and keratosis pilaris atrophicans faciei. J Dtsch Dermatol Ges. 2006;4(4):319–23.
4. Oranje AP, van Osch LD, Oosterwijk JC. Keratosis pilaris atrophicans. One heterogeneous disease or a symptom in different clinical entities? Arch Dermatol. 1994;130(4):500–2.
5. Das A, Podder I. Atrophoderma vermiculatum. Indian Pediatr. 2014;51(8):679.
6. PG U. DieHistopathologiederHautkrankheiten. Berlin: Hirschwald; 1894. p. 1102.
7. Frosch PJ, et al. Atrophoderma vermiculatum. Case reports and review. J Am Acad Dermatol. 1988;18(3):538–42.
8. Verma R, et al. Keratosis follicularis spinulosa decalvans. Indian J Dermatol Venereol Leprol. 2016;82(2):214–6.
9. Al Hawsawi K, et al. Erythromelanosis follicularis faciei: a case report and review of the literature. Case Rep Dermatol. 2015;7(3):335–9.
10. Watt TL, Kaiser JS. Erythromelanosis follicularis faciei et colli. A case report. J Am Acad Dermatol. 1981;5(5):533–4.
11. Kitamura K, et al. Erythromelanosis follicularis faciei. Hautarzt. 1960;11:391–3.
12. Volks N, Folster-Holst R. Erythromelanosis follicularis faciei–a variant of keratosis pilaris? J Dtsch Dermatol Ges. 2015;13(1):51–4.
13. Lalit G, et al. Familial erythromelanosis follicularis faciei et colli with extensive keratosis pilaris. Int J Dermatol. 2011;50(11):1400–1.
14. Castela E, et al. Papular, profuse, and precocious keratosis pilaris. Pediatr Dermatol. 2012;29(3):285–8.
15. Wang JF, Orlow SJ. Keratosis pilaris and its subtypes: associations, new molecular and pharmacologic etiologies, and therapeutic options. Am J Clin Dermatol. 2018;19(5):733–57.
16. Callaway SR, Lesher JL Jr. Keratosis pilaris atrophicans: case series and review. Pediatr Dermatol. 2004;21(1):14–7.
17. Barron DR, et al. Folliculitis ulerythematosus reticulata: a report of four cases and brief review of the literature. Pediatr Dermatol. 1987;4(2):85–9.
18. Dajani ZA, Kerns MJ, Mutasim DF. Unilateral keratosis pilaris atrophicans faciei mimicking follicular mucinosis. J Am Acad Dermatol. 2011;64(5):e71–2.
19. Di Lernia V, Ricci C. Folliculitis spinulosa decalvans: an uncommon entity within the keratosis pilaris atrophicans spectrum. Pediatr Dermatol. 2006;23(3):255–8.
20. Fong K, et al. MBTPS2 mutation in a British pedigree with keratosis follicularis spinulosa decalvans. Clin Exp Dermatol. 2012;37(6):631–4.
21. Rather S, Yaseen A, Mukhija M. Erythromelanosis follicularis faciei et colli - a cross-sectional, descriptive study. Indian J Dermatol. 2016;61(3):308–13.
22. Arif T, et al. Erythromelanosis follicularis faciei et colli: a clinicoepidemiologic study. Pediatr Dermatol. 2018;35(1):e70–1.
23. Augustine M, Jayaseelan E. Erythromelanosis follicularis faciei et colli: relationship with keratosis pilaris. Indian J Dermatol Venereol Leprol. 2008;74(1):47–9.
24. Sardana K, et al. An observational analysis of erythromelanosis follicularis faciei et colli. Clin Exp Dermatol. 2008;33(3):333–6.
25. Baden HP, Byers HR. Clinical findings, cutaneous pathology, and response to therapy in 21 patients with keratosis pilaris atrophicans. Arch Dermatol. 1994;130(4):469–75.
26. Pierini DO, Pierini AM. Keratosis pilaris atrophicans faciei (ulerythema ophryogenes): a cutaneous marker in the Noonan syndrome. Br J Dermatol. 1979;100(4):409–16.
27. Romine KA, Rothschild JG, Hansen RC. Cicatricial alopecia and keratosis pilaris. Keratosis follicularis spinulosa decalvans. Arch Dermatol. 1997;133(3):381–4.
28. Jansen T, Sander CA, Altmeyer P. Atrophodermia vermiculata: case report and review of the literature. J Eur Acad Dermatol Venereol. 2003;17(1):70–2.
29. Kim MG, et al. Quantitative histopathologic findings of erythromelanosis follicularis faciei et colli. J Cutan Pathol. 2001;28(3):160–4.
30. Thomas M, Khopkar US. Keratosis pilaris revisited: is it more than just a follicular keratosis? Int J Trichol. 2012;4(4):255–8.

31. Friedman SJ. Lichen spinulosus. Clinicopathologic review of thirty-five cases. J Am Acad Dermatol. 1990;22(2 Pt 1):261–4.
32. Logan WS. Vitamin A and keratinization. Arch Dermatol. 1972;105(5):748–53.
33. Albert MR, Mackool BT. Pityriasis rubra pilaris. Int J Dermatol. 1999;38(1):1–11.
34. Mehregan DA, Van Hale HM, Muller SA. Lichen planopilaris: clinical and pathologic study of forty-five patients. J Am Acad Dermatol. 1992;27(6 Pt 1):935–42.
35. Esterly NB, Fretzin DF, Pinkus H. Eruptive vellus hair cysts. Arch Dermatol. 1977;113(4):500–3.
36. Panchaprateep R, Tanus A, Tosti A. Clinical, dermoscopic, and histopathologic features of body hair disorders. J Am Acad Dermatol. 2015;72(5):890–900.
37. Katoulis AC, et al. Poikiloderma of Civatte: a clinical and epidemiological study. J Eur Acad Dermatol Venereol. 2005;19(4):444–8.
38. Scattone L, et al. Histopathologic changes induced by intense pulsed light in the treatment of poikiloderma of Civatte. Dermatol Surg. 2012;38(7 Pt 1):1010–6.
39. Gomez Centeno P, et al. Rubinstein–Taybi syndrome and ulerythema ophryogenes in a 9-year-old boy. Pediatr Dermatol. 1999;16(2):134–6.
40. Borradori L, Blanchet-Bardon C. Skin manifestations of cardio-facio-cutaneous syndrome. J Am Acad Dermatol. 1993;28(5 Pt 2):815–9.
41. McHenry PM, Nevin NC, Bingham EA. The association of keratosis pilaris atrophicans with hereditary woolly hair. Pediatr Dermatol. 1990;7(3):202–4.
42. Hecht H. Keratosis pilaris rubra atrophicans ficiei. Arch Dermatol Syphilol. 1948;58(1):41–6.
43. KA A. Follicular syndromes with inflammation and atrophy. In: Fitzpatrick TB, Wolff K, Freed-berg IM, Austen KF, editors. Fitzpatrick's dermatology in general medicine. New York: McGraw-Hill; 1979.
44. Seville RH. Chlorpromazine dermatitis in nurses. Br J Dermatol. 1956;68(10):332–5.
45. Bhoyrul B, Jones H, Blackford S. Extensive unilateral atrophoderma vermiculatum associated with ipsilateral congenital cataract. Clin Exp Dermatol. 2016;41(2):159–61.
46. van Dijk FS, et al. Atrophoderma Vermiculatum: a cutaneous feature of Loeys-Dietz syndrome. JAMA Dermatol. 2015;151(6):675–7.
47. van Steensel MA, Jaspers NG, Steijlen PM. A case of Rombo syndrome. Br J Dermatol. 2001;144(6):1215–8.
48. Costa M. Atrophoderma reticulata (two cases). Nederl tijdschr v geneesk (pt (2)). 1926;70:1587.
49. Sanke S, et al. Keratosis follicularis spinulosa decalvans with associated mental retardation: response to isotretinoin. Int J Trichol. 2017;9(3):138–9.
50. Aten E, et al. Keratosis follicularis spinulosa decalvans is caused by mutations in MBTPS2. Hum Mutat. 2010;31(10):1125–33.
51. Alfadley A, et al. Two brothers with keratosis follicularis spinulosa decalvans. J Am Acad Dermatol. 2002;47(5 Suppl):S275–8.
52. Chauhan RK, et al. A rare presentation of keratosis follicularis spinulosa decalvans in female twins. Indian J Dermatol Venereol Leprol. 2018;84(5):645.
53. Tuzun Y, et al. Familial erythromelanosis follicularis and chromosomal instability. J Eur Acad Dermatol Venereol. 2001;15(2):150–2.
54. Acay MC. Erythromelanosis follicularis faciei et colli: a genetic disorder? Int J Dermatol. 1993;32(7):542.
55. Yanez S, Velasco JA, Gonzalez MP. Familial erythromelanosis follicularis faciei et colli--an autosomal recessive mode of inheritance. Clin Exp Dermatol. 1993;18(3):283–5.
56. Griffiths WA, Leigh IM. Disorders of keratinization. In: Champion RH, Burns DA, Breathnach SM, editors. Rook textbook of dermatology. Oxford: Blackwell; 1998. p. 1537–8.
57. Gerbig AW. Treating keratosis pilaris. J Am Acad Dermatol. 2002;47(3):457.
58. Alcantara Gonzalez J, et al. Keratosis pilaris rubra and keratosis pilaris atrophicans faciei treated with pulsed dye laser: report of 10 cases. J Eur Acad Dermatol Venereol. 2011;25(6):710–4.
59. Richard G, Harth W. Keratosis follicularis spinulosa decalvans. Therapy with isotretinoin and etretinate in the inflammatory stage. Hautarzt. 1993;44(8):529–34.

60. Al-Saif FM, et al. Erythromelanosis follicularis faciei et colli with reticulated hyperpigmentation of the extremities. Clin Case Rep. 2017;5(10):1576–9.
61. Kim WJ, et al. Topical tacalcitol ointment can be a good therapeutic choice in erythromelanosis follicularis faciei et colli. J Am Acad Dermatol. 2012;67(2):320–1.
62. Li YH, et al. Treatment of erythromelanosis follicularis faciei et colli using a dual-wavelength laser system: a split-face treatment. Dermatol Surg. 2010;36(8):1344–7.
63. Kurita T, et al. Very long-term outcome of non-surgically treated patients with temporal lobe epilepsy with hippocampal sclerosis: a retrospective study. PLoS One. 2016;11(7):e0159464.
64. Jang HS, Lee C, Cha JH, Kim SJ, Oh CK, Kwon KS. Clinicopathological study of 12 cases of erythromelanosis follicularis faciei et colli. Korean J Dermatol. 2001;39:574–80.

Cutaneous Collagenous Vasculopathy

Konstantinos-Antonios Kostopoulos-Kanitakis and Jean Kanitakis

Introduction

Cutaneous collagenous vasculopathy (CCV) is a rarely reported idiopathic cutaneous microangiopathy with characteristic clinicopathological features, first reported in 2000 [1]. A literature search performed until mid-March 2021 revealed 44 relevant articles [1–43] reporting a total of 60 patients, published as single case reports or small series. The precise incidence of CCV is unknown; despite the limited number of cases reported, the disease is probably underrecognized and therefore underreported; indeed, the clinical appearance of CCV is very similar, if not identical, to other conditions manifesting with telangiectasias (namely, generalized essential telangiectasia, GET), but the precise diagnosis of CCV requires histological examination which is not always performed. It is therefore possible that patients diagnosed with GET (or other dermatoses manifesting with acquired telangiectasias) had in fact CCV.

CCV predominantly affects women, who accounted for 65% (39/60) of all cases. The disease is usually diagnosed in late adulthood, during the 5th–7th life decade (mean age 61 years). Over 58% of patients are aged 60 years or older; however, younger adults can be affected, and the disease has been described in two adolescents [6, 29]. The delay between disease onset and diagnosis is long, ranging from several weeks or months up to 57 years [29]. Among the patients for whom ethnicity was explicitly mentioned, all patients were Caucasians with the exception of two Japanese ones [29, 31].

K.-A. Kostopoulos-Kanitakis
Department of Medicine, European Uiversity Cyprus, School of Medicine, Nicosia, Cyprus

J. Kanitakis (✉)
Department of Dermatology, Edouard Herriot Hospital, Lyon, France
e-mail: jean.kanitakis@univ-lyon1.fr

F. Rongioletti, B. R. Smoller (eds.), *New and Emerging Entities in Dermatology and Dermatopathology*, https://doi.org/10.1007/978-3-030-80027-7_15

Clinical Features

CCV has characteristic and rather stereotypical clinical features: it manifests with the progressive development of telangiectasias that usually start on the lower limbs (dorsal foot, ankles, shins, knees) and spread symmetrically upwards over the thighs, the trunk (abdomen, back, chest) and the arms (Fig. 1a,b). They spare the nails, mucous membranes and (as a rule) the head and neck area; two patients had lesions on the face/neck (chin, retro-auricular and glabellar areas) [5, 26]. In one case the disease started on the breasts before spreading to the back and the feet [17], and in another it started on the upper extremities [41]. In three cases the lesions were limited to one limb, including the thigh [2], the leg [9] or the arm/forearm [35], and in one case they were limited to both forearms [9]. One case each manifesting with annular [24] or papular [38] lesions has been reported. The telangiectasias are usually blanchable, although sometimes they were reportedly non-blanchable [21, 30, 32] and/or petechial [21, 33]. They are usually flat and bright red, but may become slightly raised and purplish over time [23]. There is no notable seasonal variation, although in some cases the lesions were reportedly more prominent during summertime [5, 9, 18]. The lesions are as a rule asymptomatic. Pruritus has

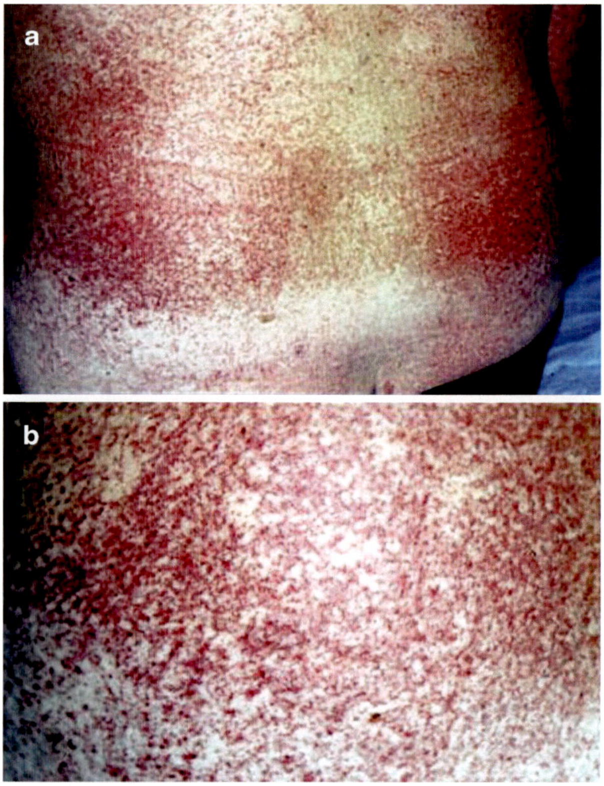

Fig. 1 (**a**): Diffuse acquired telangiectasias over the trunk of a 65-year-old male patient. (**b**): Closer view of the lesions. (Reprinted with permission from Ref. [3])

rarely been reported [5, 10, 22, 42], although the causative role of CCV lesions is unclear. In one case the lesions were hypothermic [17]. Dermatoscopic examination of early telangiectasias shows vascular features such as red dots, serpentine, comma-like, glomerular or linear, more or less branching red vessels [11, 27, 30, 35, 38]. The oldest lesions are violaceous vessels distributed in a tortuous, serpentine pattern [27].

The majority of patients with CCV have had concomitant diseases. The most common of them include arterial hypertension (43% of patients) [2, 4, 8–10, 13, 15, 17, 18, 22, 26–28, 30, 32, 33, 38, 39, 41, 43, 44]; diabetes mellitus, usually type II (20%) [2, 9, 10, 12, 16, 19, 21, 29, 33, 41]; various malignancies (15%) such as myelodysplastic syndrome [12]; carcinomas of the breast [20, 26, 35] lung [17], ovary [23], kidney [31] and skin [5, 43]; hypercholesterolaemia/hyperlipidaemia (13%) [2, 4, 9, 13, 22, 33, 41]; mood disorders/depression (8%) [1, 6, 8, 9, 41]; and coronary artery disease (7%) [3, 17, 32, 43]. Rarer associations include sleep apnoea [9, 26, 41], psoriasis [2, 5, 10], lupus erythematosus [8, 40] and rosacea [13]. The association with these comorbidities could well be fortuitous, explained by the age of patients. With very rare exceptions [11, 36], the patients do not mention a history of (personal or family) tendency for bleeding. One patient had thrombophilia due to a heterozygous prothrombin G20210A mutation [42]. Some patients have been explicitly reported as ‘otherwise healthy’ [7, 14, 16, 25].

Histopathologic Features

These are characteristic and allow the diagnosis to be made with confidence. Routinely stained sections show in the upper dermis several dilated capillary vessels with characteristic, thick walls containing an amorphous hyaline, eosinophilic material (Fig. 2a-c). This is positive with PAS [3–5, 13, 27, 31, 41, 44] and Masson’s trichrome stains [3, 27, 43] (Fig. 3a,b), but negative for amyloid stains (Congo red, crystal violet) [3, 6, 12, 38, 43]. By immunohistochemistry, the thickened wall of the affected capillaries is immunoreactive for type IV collagen (Fig. 2d) [1–3, 5, 8, 10, 15, 22, 25–29, 31, 34, 35, 37, 38, 42, 44]. The endothelial cells of the involved vessels express the CD31 and CD34 antigens [1, 3, 7, 12, 17, 36] but not D2–40/podoplanin [8, 12], showing they are blood, rather than lymphatic, vessels. As a rule there is no inflammation, vasculitis or haemorrhage; minimal perivascular inflammation [3, 17, 21, 25, 38] and red-blood cell extravasation [19, 34] have occasionally been reported. In one case the affected vessels contained occlusive fibrin thrombi [12]. Immunostaining for HHV-8 is negative [3, 12]. Direct immunofluorescence has been performed in eight cases [3, 12, 13, 17, 34, 36, 40]; six of them were negative, and two had vascular deposits of fibrinogen [12] or IgG [34]; however, these deposits were considered to be non-immunologically mediated, likely reflecting antibody trapping/nonspecific absorption in the thickened vessel walls [34].

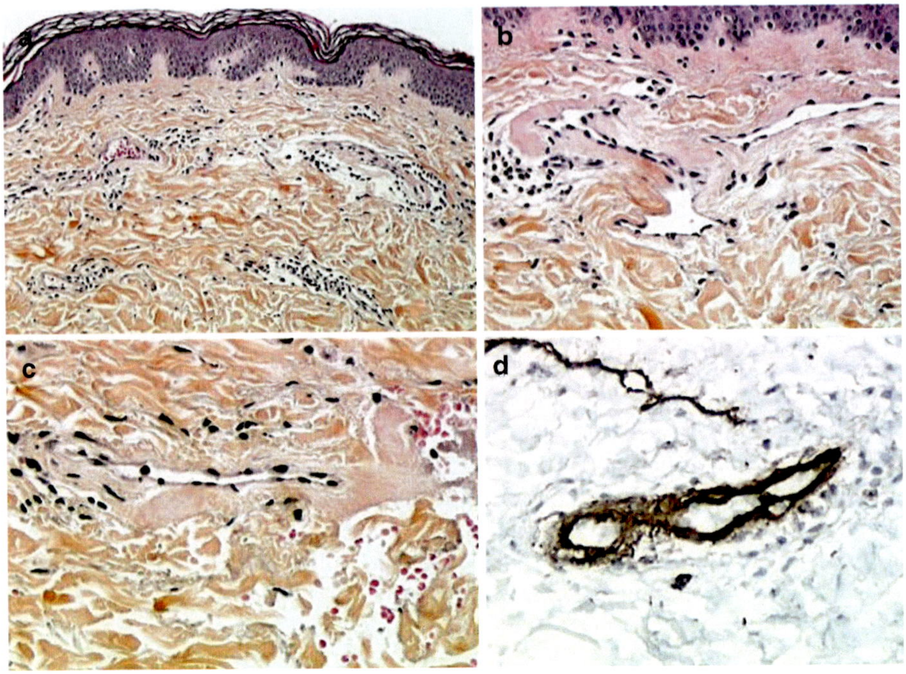

Fig. 2 (**a**). Histological examination of a skin biopsy shows in the papillary dermis several dilated blood capillaries with a thick wall. (**b**, **c**): At higher magnification, the thick hyaline wall of capillaries is well seen. (**d**): Immunolabelling with an antibody to type IV collagen highlights the thick capillary wall (immunoperoxidase revealed with aminoethylcarbazole). (Reprinted with permission from Ref. [3])

Transmission electron microscopy has been performed in some cases [1, 3, 16, 17, 22, 26, 27, 36] and has shown a multi-laminated basement membrane surrounding the affected vessels (post-capillary venules), with marked deposition of a granular material admixed with fine collagen fibres around the affected vessels (corresponding to the hyaline material seen by optical microscopy) (Fig. 4). In four cases [6, 14, 16, 26] Luse bodies (long-spacing collagen) were found within the thickened vessel walls. Pericytes are few and contain sparse cytoplasmic actin microfilaments [16].

Work-Up

Laboratory work-up (including hemogram, coagulation tests, liver and renal function, sedimentation rate, antinuclear antibodies, viral serologies) is usually negative or within normal limits. CCV seems therefore to be a purely cutaneous microangiopathy, so that no specific work-up is needed in the management of the patients. If necessary, blood tests will rule out a bleeding diathesis (which can be seen in

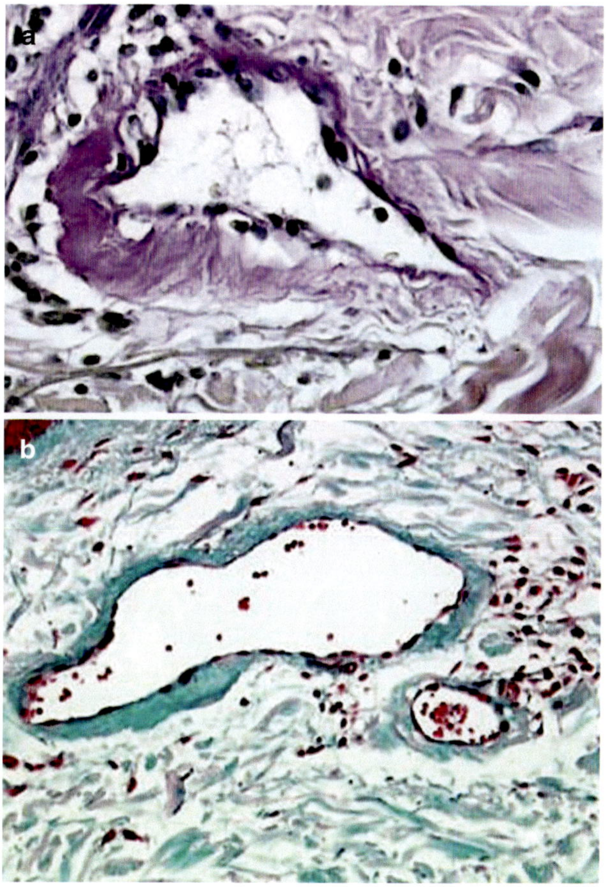

Fig. 3 The thick wall of telangiectatic vessels is positive for PAS (**a**) and Masson's trichrome stain (**b**). (Reprinted with permission from Ref. [3])

haemorrhagic hereditary telangiectasia, an autosomal dominant disorder manifesting with recurrent epistaxis, telangiectasias and visceral arteriovenous malformations, caused by mutations of the activin A receptor-like type 1 and endoglin genes) [44]. Of note, a unique patient with CCV thrombophilia due to heterozygous prothrombin mutation G20210A has been reported [42].

Differential Diagnosis

The clinical differential diagnosis of CCV includes diseases manifesting with acquired progressive telangiectasias, such as generalized essential telangiectasia (GET), telangiectatic mastocytosis (telangiectasia macularis eruptiva perstans, TMEP), unilateral naevoid telangiectasia, angioma serpiginosum and telangiectasias associated with administration of calcium blockers. Similar to CCV, GET shows a female predominance but starts earlier in life, usually during the fourth life

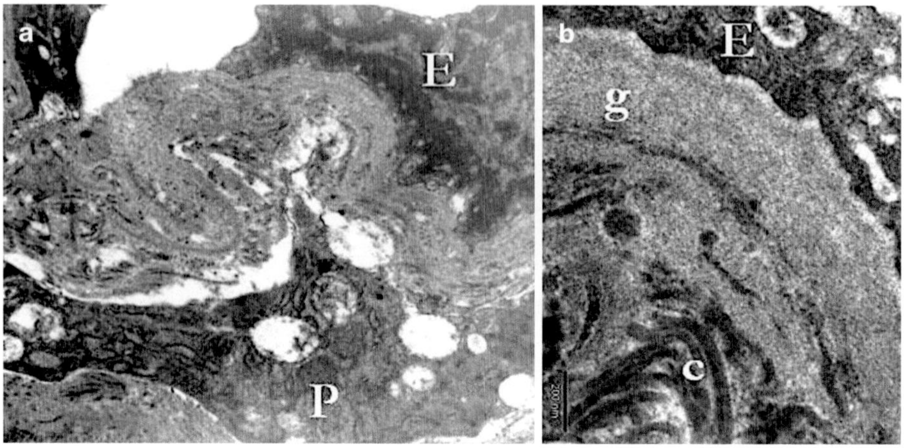

Fig. 4 Electron-microscopic examination shows the wall of affected capillaries to consist of a granular material (g) admixed with fine collagen fibres (c). E: Endothelial cells. P: Activated perivascular cells. Original magnifications: (**a**): ×13,000, (**b**): ×40,000

decade [45]. Telangiectasias associated with calcium blockers (such as felodipine, nifedipine and amlodipine) are photodistributed and predominate on the face and neck [46]. TMEP predominates on the trunk and shows the Darier's sign, which is absent in CCV. The rare cases of CCV with limited distribution over one limb [2, 9] should be differentiated from unilateral naevoid telangiectasia [47]. The exceptional papular form [38] should be differentiated from cherry angiomas. Hereditary diseases manifesting with widespread telangiectasias (such as hereditary haemorrhagic telangiectasia, hereditary benign telangiectasia and ataxia-telangiectasia) can be ruled out on the basis of their familial character, association with systemic (namely neurologic or haematologic) manifestations and/or dermatomal distribution. In case of doubt, histopathological examination clearly separates these entities, as the characteristic eosinophilic hyaline deposits on the vessel walls are distinctive and unique to CCV. From a microscopic point of view, some dermatoses (such as atrophie blanche, porphyrias/pseudoporphyrias, amyloidosis and lipoid proteinosis) may show some resemblance to CCV as they contain capillaries with thickened, occasionally hyaline, walls; however these entities have different clinical settings.

Etiopathogenesis

The etiopathogenesis of CCV is unknown. It has been speculated that the distinctive microscopic vascular changes of CCV could be triggered by repeated injury to the microvascular endothelium, which would lead to microthrombosis, endothelial cell hyperplasia, reduplication of vascular basement membrane, activation of veil (repair perivascular) cells and reparative perivascular fibrosis, producing the characteristic perivascular hyaline deposits; however, the initiating trigger of this injury remains unknown. Inciting factors could be genetic, infectious, metabolic/hormonal and chemical/environmental [16]. Patients with CCV have various comorbidities (namely hypertension, diabetes mellitus, hyperlipidaemia, coronary disease), but these could be fortuitous, accounted for by the age of patients. The majority of patients with CCV were taking medications for their comorbidities, and some of them (namely antihypertensive ones) could favour the development of telangiectasias through their vasodilating effects. Two cases developed following the administration of the VEGF-R inhibitor axitinib for renal cell carcinoma [31] and gemcitabine for breast cancer [20], and one case developed a few weeks after coronary bypass surgery [32]. However, the role of these factors, if any, seems anecdotal. Two cases associated with neurological disorders (multiple sclerosis and complex regional pain syndrome) were considered to be induced by these diseases via a neurologically induced endothelial damage [39], but this link remains unproven; similarly, the role of the heterozygous prothrombin mutation G20210A detected in one patient with hypercoagulability syndrome is unknown, although it has been hypothesized that the ensuing hypercoagulability syndrome could favour the development of CCV via the development of intravascular microthrombi [42].

Therapy

The most consistently effective treatment of CCV-associated telangiectasias is laser treatment, which has been so far tried in five patients. In one of them, treatment with KTP laser was discontinued because of poor tolerance and inefficiency [26]; however, the remaining four patients, treated with PDL or multiplex laser (associated with Nd:Yag), experienced very good results, with an almost complete clearing of the lesions [7, 23, 25, 40]. In one case, post-treatment skin biopsy showed a microscopic disappearance of the pathologic vessels [25]. An attempt to treat CCV with corticosteroids was unsuccessful [38]. Compression stockings were tried in one case [33], but the results were not mentioned.

Prognosis and Course

The prognosis of CCV is good as the disease is benign and causes mostly cosmetic discomfort. The course is chronic. In most cases the disease is slowly progressive over months or years, with telangiectasias spreading from the site of initial appearance (usually the legs) to other body zones, such as the abdomen and upper limbs. The lesions tend to become darker with time [3]. In one case allegedly triggered by gemcitabine, the lesions improved with supportive care [20].

Conclusions

Cutaneous collagenous vasculopathy is a rarely reported condition of unknown aetiopathogenesis, belonging to the group of microvasculopathic diseases manifesting with progressive, acquired telangiectasias. It is clinically very similar, if not identical, to generalized essential telangiectasia, but has distinctive microscopic findings which allow the diagnosis and differentiation from other diseases manifesting with acquired telangiectasias. Although benign, it may cause cosmetic burden. If desired by the patient, laser treatment can be attempted. Study of additional cases will hopefully help in the unravelling of the aetiology of this puzzling condition and proposing efficient preventive and therapeutic measures.

References

1. Salama S, Rosenthal D. Cutaneous collagenous vasculopathy with generalized telangiectasia: an immunohistochemical and ultrastructural study. J Cutan Pathol. 2000;27:40–8.
2. Davis T, Mandal R, Bevona C, Tsai Y, Moschella S, Staszewski R, Zembowicz A. Cutaneous collagenous vasculopathy: a report of three cases. J Cutan Pathol. 2008;35:967–70.
3. Kanitakis J, Faisant M, Wagschal D, Haftek M, Claudy A. Cutaneous collagenous vasculopathy: ultrastructural and immunohistochemical study of a new case. Am J Clin Dermatol. 2010;11:63–6.
4. Monteagudo B, Pérez-Valcárcel J, Ramírez-Santos A, Cabanillas M, Suárez-Amor O. Cutaneous collagenous vasculopathy: a case report and review of the literature. Actas Dermosifiliogr. 2010;101:444–7.
5. Perez A, Wain ME, Robson A, Groves RW, Stefanato CM. Cutaneous collagenous vasculopathy with generalized telangiectasia in two female patients. J Am Acad Dermatol. 2010;63:882–5.
6. Lloyd BM, Pruden SJ 2nd, Lind AC, Berk DR. Cutaneous collagenous vasculopathy: report of the first pediatric case. Pediatr Dermatol. 2011;28:598–9.
7. Echeverría B, Sanmartín O, Botella-Estrada R, Vitiello M. Cutaneous collagenous vasculopathy successfully treated with pulsed dye laser. Int J Dermatol. 2012;51:1359–62.
8. González Fernández D, Gómez Bernal S, Vivanco Allende B, Pérez ON. Cutaneous collagenous vasculopathy: description of two new cases in elderly women and review of the literature. Dermatology. 2012;225:1–8.
9. Burdick LM, Lohser S, Somach SC, Billings SD. Cutaneous collagenous vasculopathy: a rare cutaneous microangiopathy. J Cutan Pathol. 2012;39:741–6.
10. Bernard S, Cawet B, Theate Y, Bataille AC, Marot L. Cutaneous collagenous vasculopathy: a rare cause of generalized telangiectasia. Ann Dermatol Venereol. 2012;139:381–6.
11. Bardazzi F, Virdi A, Odorici G, Balestri R, Infusino S, Patrizi A. Cutaneous collagenous vasculopathy: report of a case. Clin Exp Dermatol. 2014;39:228–30.
12. Salama S, Chorneyko K, Belovic B. Cutaneous collagenous vasculopathy associated with intravascular occlusive fibrin thrombi. J Cutan Pathol. 2014;41:386–93.
13. Brady BG, Ortleb M, Boyd AS, Powers J. Cutaneous Collagenous Vasculopathy. J Clin Aesthet Dermatol. 2015;8:49–52.
14. Ma DL, Vano-Galvan S. Images in clinical medicine. Cutaneous collagenous vasculopathy. N Engl J Med. 2015;373:e14.
15. Toda-Brito H, Resende C, Catorze G, Viana I. Cutaneous collagenous vasculopathy: a rare cause of generalised cutaneous telangiectasia. BMJ Case Rep. 2015;2015 pii:bcr2015210635.

16. Salama SS. Cutaneous collagenous vasculopathy: a new case series with clinicopathologic and ultrastructural correlation, literature review, and insight into the pathogenesis. Am J Dermatopathol. 2015;37:368–75.
17. Borroni RG, Derlino F, Agozzino M, Concardi M, Arbustini E, Brazzelli V. Hypothermic cutaneous collagenous vasculopathy with centrifugal spreading. J Eur Acad Dermatol Venereol. 2015;29:1444–6.
18. Meah N, Khirwadkar N, Ellison J. A rare case of cutaneous collagenous vasculopathy. Australas J Dermatol. 2016;57:e97–9.
19. Heymann WR. Cutaneous collagenous vasculopathy-associated benign pigmented purpura. Skinmed. 2016;14:308–9.
20. Leone JP. Gemcitabine induced cutaneous collagenous vasculopathy in a breast cancer patient. Breast J. 2016;22:580.
21. Rambhia KD, Hadawale SD, Khopkar US. Cutaneous collagenous vasculopathy: A rare case report. Indian Dermatol Online J. 2016;7(1):40–2.
22. Castiñeiras-Mato I, Rodríguez-Lojo R, Fernández-Díaz ML, Bal-Nieves F. Cutaneous collagenous vasculopathy: a case report and review of the literature. Actas Dermosifiliogr. 2016;107:444–7.
23. Basso D, Ribero S, Blazek C, Dietrich N, Beltraminelli H, Ramelet AA, Borradori L, Adatto M. cutaneous collagenous vasculopathy: a rare form of microangiopathy successfully treated with a combination of multiplex laser and optimized pulsed light with a review of the literature. Dermatology. 2016;232:107–11.
24. García-Martínez P, Gomez-Martin I, Lloreta J, Pujol RM. Multiple progressive annular telangiectasias: A clinicopathological variant of cutaneous collagenous vasculopathy? J Cutan Pathol. 2017;44:982–5.
25. Mitteldorf C, Joest B, Tronnier M. Cutaneous collagenous vasculopathy – remission of perivascular deposits after pulsed dye laser therapy. J Dtsch Dermatol Ges. 2017;15:936–8.
26. Bondier L, Tardieu M, Leveque P, Challende I, Pinel N, Leccia MT. Cutaneous collagenous vasculopathy: report of two cases presenting as disseminated telangiectasias and review of the literature. Am J Dermatopathol. 2017;39:682–8.
27. Knöpfel N, Martín-Santiago A, Saus C, Escudero-Góngora MM, Del Pozo LJ, Gómez C. Extensive acquired telangiectasias: comparison of generalized essential telangiectasia and cutaneous collagenous vasculopathy. Actas Dermosifiliogr. 2017;108:e21–6.
28. Vázquez-Osorio I, Gonzalvo-Rodríguez P, Rodríguez-Díaz E. Cutaneous collagenous vasculopathy: A rare cause of generalized cutaneous telangiectasia. Med Clin (Barc). 2017;148(4):e23.
29. Motegi SI, Yasuda M, Yamanaka M, Amano H, Ishikawa O. Cutaneous collagenous vasculopathy: report of first Japanese case and review of the literature. Australas J Dermatol. 2017;58:145–9.
30. Vasava D, Mehta H. Dermoscopic features of cutaneous collagenous vasculopathy: a report of rare disorder. Indian Dermatol Online J. 2018;9:342–4.
31. Matsuzaki Y, Takahashi M, Minakawa S, Jin K, Nakano H, Sawamura D. Cutaneous collagenous vasculopathy induced by the vascular endothelial growth factor receptor inhibitor axitinib. Int J Dermatol. 2018;57:e167–9.
32. Rahnama-Moghadam S, Burgin C, Gilbert J, Warren S. Cutaneous collagenous vasculopathy: development after coronary artery bypass surgery. Dermatol Online J. 2018;24(5):13030/qt0k8258qw.
33. Roy SF, Ghazawi FM, Veilleux B, Bouffard D, Bélisle A. A rare cause of blanching red legs: cutaneous collagenous vasculopathy. Int J Dermatol. 2018;57:349–50.
34. Clark ML, McGuinness AE, Vidal CI. Cutaneous collagenous vasculopathy: a unique case with positive direct immunofluorescence findings. Am J Dermatopathol. 2019;41:77–9.
35. Sartori DS, Almeida HL Jr, Dorn TV, Ruas CP. Cutaneous collagenous vasculopathy: light and transmission electron microscopy. An Bras Dermatol. 2019;94:211–3.
36. Karimkhani C, Boyers LN, Olivere J, Smith C. Cutaneous collagenous vasculopathy. Cutis. 2019;103:E7–8.

37. Jaquinandi V, Stivalet O, Grabas M. Cutaneous collagenous vasculopathy: Differential diagnosis of primary telangiectasia as generalized essential telangiectasia, hereditary hemorrhagic telangiectasia, and hereditary benign telangiectasia. Vasc Med. 2019;24:261–2.
38. Conde-Ferreirós A, Roncero-Riesco M, Cañueto J, Román-Curto C, Santos-Briz Á. Cutaneous collagenous vasculopathy: papular form. Dermatol Online J. 2019;25(8):13030/qt4v5650m8.
39. Castillo B, Nelson G, Rodriguez-Waitkus P, Shenefelt P, Seminario-Vidal L. Two cases of cutaneous collagenous vasculopathy of neurologically induced etiology (abstr). J Am Acad Dermatol. 2017;76(supp. 1):AB271.
40. Bouvarel C, Chasseuil H, Chasseuil E, Boutin D, Frouin E, Hainault E. Vasculopathie cutanée collagénique traitée par laser vasculaire. Ann Dermatol Venereol. 2020;147(suppl):A205.
41. Lobo Y, Blake T, Herat A. Asymptomatic disseminated telangiectasias: a rare case of cutaneous collagenous vasculopathy. Dermatol Online J. 2020;26(10):13030/qt0s39g4tt.
42. Eldik H, Leisenring N, Al-Rohil R, Marano A. Cutaneous collagenous vasculopathy in a middle-aged woman with a history of prothrombin G20210A thrombophilia. J Cutan Pathol. 2021. doi: https://doi.org/10.1111/cup.13895. Online ahead of print.
43. Nelson G, Cameron M, Rodriguez-Waitkus P, Fenske N. Cutaneous collagenous vasculopathy. Cutis. 2020;105:e23–4.
44. Kim BG, Jung JH, Kim MJ, Moon EH, Oh JH, Park JW, Cha HE, Kim JH, Kim YJ, Chung JW, Hahm KB, Jin HR, Jang YJ, Kim SW, Chung SK, Kim DW, Lee YJ, Kim ST. Genetic variants and clinical phenotypes in Korean patients with hereditary hemorrhagic telangiectasia. Clin Exp Otorhinolaryngol. 2021. https://doi.org/10.21053/ceo.2020.02124. Epub ahead of print.
45. Gordon Spratt E, DeFelice T, O'Reilly K, Robinson M, Patel R, Sanchez M. Generalized essential telangiectasia. Dermatol Online J. 2012;18(12):13.
46. Bakkour W, Haylett AK, Gibbs NK, Chalmers R, Rhodes L. Photodistributed telangiectasia induced by calcium channel blockers: case report and review of the literature. Photodermatol Photoimmunol Photomed. 2013;29:272–5.
47. Micalizzi C, Astrid H, Cozzani E, Cabiddu F, Guadagno A, Parodi A. Unilateral nevoid telangiectasia: a rare and underdiagnosed skin disease. Eur J Dermatol. 2020;30:601–2.

Acquired Hyperpigmentation Disorders of Uncertain Etiology

Shital Poojary and Franco Rongioletti

Lichen Planus Pigmentosus

Introduction

Lichen planus pigmentosus (LPP) is an uncommon variant of lichen planus characterized by dark brown to grayish macular pigmentation predominantly seen on photo-exposed areas of the face, neck, and flexures, commonly described in skin types IV and V.

The first cases of LPP were described in 1935 as "lichens atypiques ou invisible pigmentogenes" and later in 1956 from Japan. The first comprehensive study on LPP was published by Bhutani et al. in 1974 [1] and later by Kanwar et al. in 2003 [2].

LPP is characterized by a lichenoid tissue reaction followed by pigmentary incontinence and is associated with lesions of lichen planus in a minimal proportion of patients [3]. Some authors consider LPP, erythema dyschromicum perstans (EDP), and ashy dermatosis (AD) as the same condition, whereas others consider them to be different [4, 5]. Recently, a global consensus has stated that LPP is a separate condition from EDP/AD with similar histopathological features [4]. LPP has been mostly reported from Asian and Latin American countries and very rarely from European countries. It is common in the age group of 30–50 years but has been reported in children and elderly as well. There is a general female preponderance, but the study by Al-Mutairi et al. suggests a male preponderance [6]. Bhutani et al. reported equal distribution in males and females in India [1].

S. Poojary
KJ Somaiya Medical College, Mumbai, India

F. Rongioletti (✉)
University Vita-Salute S.Raffaele, Milan, Italy

F. Rongioletti, B. R. Smoller (eds.), *New and Emerging Entities in Dermatology and Dermatopathology*, https://doi.org/10.1007/978-3-030-80027-7_16

Clinical Features

LPP is characterized by the insidious onset of acquired, large (>5 cm), and small (0.5–5 cm), brownish black to gray macules/patches on the face and neck, with or without present or past evidence of lichen planus elsewhere [4]. The facial areas which are predominantly involved are the preauricular, temporal, forehead, mental, and submental region. Morphological variants include diffuse (Fig.1a), patchy

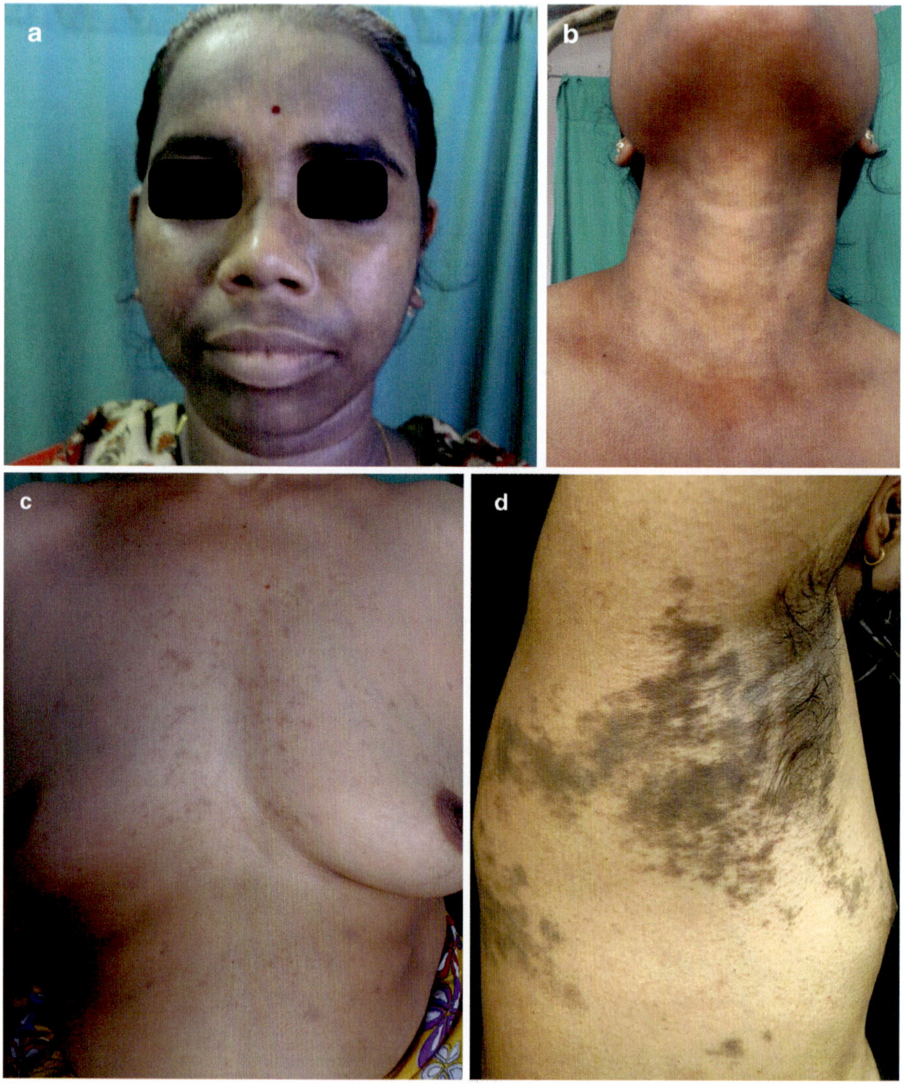

Fig. 1 Lichen planus pigmentosus (LPP). (**a**) Diffuse type. (**b**) Patchy type. (**c**) Follicular type. (**d**) Flexural type

(Fig.1b), reticular, and (peri)follicular (Fig.1c). Other variants include linear, blaschkoid, and zosteriform forms. The upper extremities are more commonly involved than lower extremities. Flexural areas are involved in 20–30% of cases and occasionally may be the only area involved (LPP inversus) (Fig.1d). Periorbital and perioral pigmentation may also be present. Occasionally LPP involves the entire body. Oral mucosa is rarely involved, with brownish black pigmentation of buccal mucosa and tongue. The lesions are mostly asymptomatic, but some patients may complain of mild pruritus and photosensitivity. Accompanying classical lesions of lichen planus may be seen in up to 10–30% of cases. LPP has been reported in association with lichen planopilaris and frontal fibrosing alopecia. Any association with atopy, chronic hepatitis, and autoimmune thyroiditis needs to be further studied. As for dermoscopy, Pirmez et al. described four patterns of pigmentation: (1) pseudonetwork, (2) dotted pattern, (3) speckled blue-gray dots, and (4) blue-gray dots arranged in circle [7] (Fig.2a).

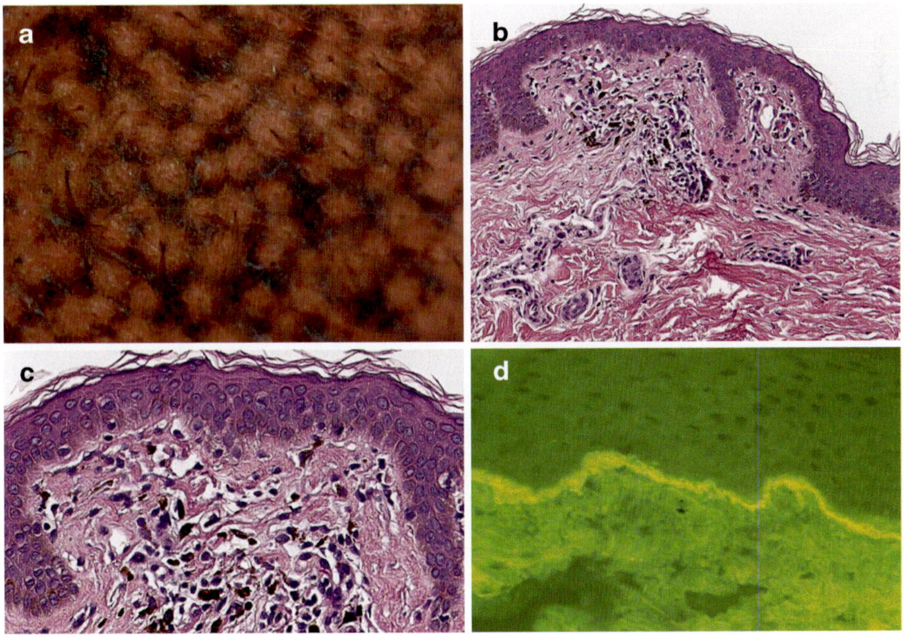

Fig. 2 Lichen planus pigmentosus. (**a**) Dermoscopy showing a pseudoreticular pattern. (**b**) Histopathology showing a slight basal cell vacuolization with perivascular infiltrate and melanophages. Epidermis is mostly atrophic with orthokeratosis. (**c**) Close-up of atrophic epidermis, slight basal cell vacuolization, perivascular infiltrate, and abundant melanophages (**d**). Linear deposit of fibrinogen at the dermoepidermal junction

Histopathologic Features

Lichenoid tissue reaction is the predominant feature in active lesions. It may be seen only as basal cell vacuolization with a perivascular infiltrate (Fig.2b,c) or a distinctive band-like infiltrate. The epidermis may be normal but often is atrophic. Acanthosis is not a prominent feature unlike lichen planus. There may be basket wave or orthokeratotic type of hyperkeratosis. The dermis shows a lymphocytic perivascular infiltrate and interstitial/perivascular melanophages which form clusters in older lesions. Late lesions may not show any infiltrate with only basal cell vacuolization and dense melanin incontinence. The immunopathology includes a population of helper/inducer (CD4+) and cytotoxic (CD8+) T cells and epidermal keratinocytes expressing HLA-DR+. Direct immunofluorescence may show linear deposition of IgM, C3, and fibrinogen (Fig.2d) at the dermoepidermal junction in about 15% of cases [2]. Occasionally there may be globular deposition of IgM in the papillary dermis [6].

Etiopathogenesis

The etiology of LPP is unclear. The association with hepatitis C infection has been outlined [6]. Patients of LPP with coexistent HCV infection tend to be older in age and also generally have persistent disease of longer duration. Application of mustard oil, amla oil, henna, and paraphenylenediamine in hair dyes has been implicated as triggers in several studies. Photo exposure is also implicated in the etiology as there is often predominant involvement of sun-exposed areas [2]. The pathogenesis of LPP is similar to LP and is characterized by a cellular immune response mediated by CD8 + T lymphocytes which mount a cytotoxic response against keratinocytes resulting in basal cell damage and pigmentary incontinence.

Differential Diagnoses

If the hyperpigmentation is strictly limited to known areas previously involved by lichen planus lesions, or by current visible and palpable lesions of lichen planus, such cases should be considered as lichen planus with post-inflammatory hyperpigmentation and not LPP [4].

Therapy

Treatment of LPP is often unsatisfactory, and various topical and systemic modalities have been tried with variable success. Avoidance of exacerbating factors such as mustard oil application and sun exposure is important. Moderate- to high-potency corticosteroids are helpful especially in active lesions. Tacrolimus ointment once or twice daily for 3 months showed 50% improvement in a study from Al-Mutairi [6]. Depigmenting agents such as 4% hydroquinone, kojic acid, and modified Kligman's formula (tretinoin 0.025% to 0.05%, hydroquinone 4%, 0.1% dexamethasone) are useful as adjuvant therapies. Q-switched (1064 nm Nd- YAG) laser can be used in addition to topical and systemic therapies [8].

Dexamethasone in weekly pulse dosage can be useful to stabilize active disease and can be given in conjunction with topical therapies up to 3 months [9].

Dapsone 100 mg daily in conjunction with topical tacrolimus for a period of 4 months was successful in a series of five patients [10]. Isotretinoin in a dose of 20 mg/day or 0.3 mg/kg/day was shown to stabilize the disease in 4–6 weeks in a study by Muthu et al. with improvement of pigmentation in 3 months [11]. Other systemic treatments which have been considered for LPP include mycophenolate mofetil, methotrexate and colchicine.

Prognosis and Course

LPP leads to significant esthetic concern and distress among affected patients, especially in females. Longer disease duration has been associated with widespread disease.

The course is chronic and unpredictable with an insidious onset, a gradual progressive diffusion, and occasional episodes of exacerbations and improvement. However, a complete clearance was rarely attained [12].

Erythema Dyschromicum Perstans and Ashy Dermatosis

Introduction

Ashy dermatosis (AD) was first described by Ramirez in 1957 as "dermatitis cenicienta [13]." The term "Erythema dyschromicum perstans" (EDP) was first used by Convit et al [14]. In this setting, AD and EDP are considered the same entity and the terms are used as synonyms.

EDP has been reported in all age groups and both sexes equally. Adult cases have been mostly of Hispanic lineage, while childhood cases have been mostly Caucasian [15, 16]. There is no clear gender predilection, but some authors report that EDP may be more common in females [15, 16].

Clinical Features

EDP/AD is characterized by the rapid onset of large, relatively well-defined, from oval or round to polycyclic, gray macules predominantly on the trunk and often distributed symmetrically (Fig.3a, b). Occasionally, some cases with unilateral distribution have been described. In the active stage, the macules have a characteristic erythematous, elevated border. The border eventually tends to disappear within several months. Although AD and EDP can be considered to be synonymous, a global consensus concluded that the presence of erythematous borders should be better labeled as EDP. The lesions are usually asymptomatic, but occasional itching has been reported. The trunk and proximal extremities are more commonly involved followed by the face and neck. The lesions can appear both on exposed and unexposed areas. The major axis of the lesions may follow the skin cleavage lines.

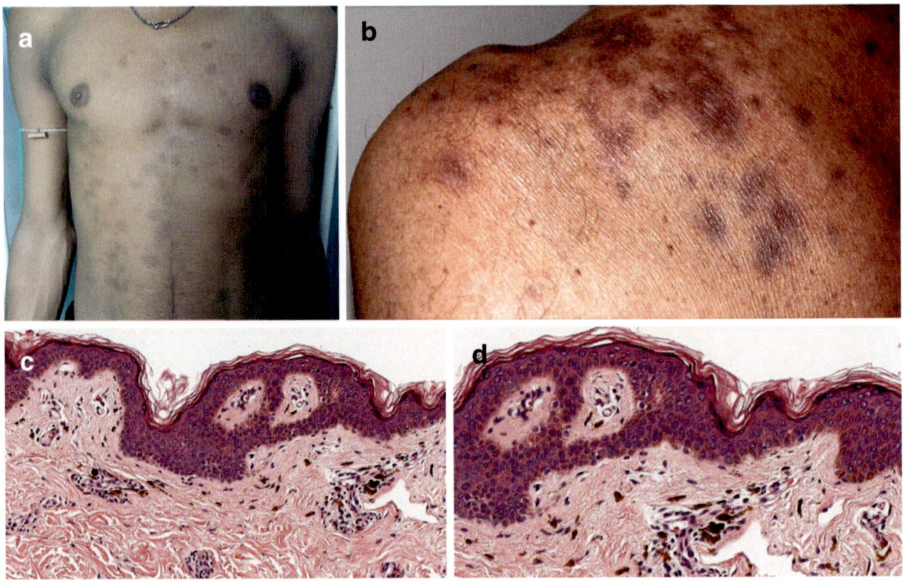

Fig. 3 Erythema dyschromicum perstans/ashy dermatosis (EDP/AD). (**a**) Rapid onset of large, well-defined, from oval or round to polycyclic, gray macules predominantly on the trunk and distributed symmetrically in Indian patient. (**b**) EDP/AD in a Caucasian skin. Some of the pigmented macules have a slight erythematous hue. (**c**) Slight perivascular lymphocytic infiltrate with melanophages. No apparent vacuolar degeneration is seen (**d**). Close-up of the infiltrate and melanophages with dilated capillaries

The palms, soles, nails, and mucous membranes are usually spared [15, 17, 18]. Dermoscopy may show gray-blue dots corresponding to melanophages in the dermis.

Histopathologic Features

Histology of EDP/AD is characterized by a vacuolar interface dermatitis with melanophages in the superficial dermis and a mild-to-moderate superficial perivascular lymphohistiocytic infiltrate (Fig.3c,d). The epidermis can appear as hyperkeratotic or atrophic, sometimes with apoptotic keratinocytes. According to Chang et al., EDP/AD can be subdivided into active, inflammatory lesions with prominent basal vacuolar degeneration and a focal, sometimes lichenoid lymphocytic infiltration and inactive lesions with only melanophages in the superficial dermis [19]. Thus, interface dermatitis is not a feature necessary to diagnose EDP/AD.

Etiopathogenesis

The cause is unknown. There have been reports attributing cause to intestinal parasites or drugs, but these causes have not garnered evidence. It has also been associated with enterovirus, hepatitis C, and HIV infection [20–22].

HLA-DR4 allele may be a risk factor for EDP in Mexican patients. Vasquez-Ochoa et al. demonstrated predominance of CD8+ T lymphocytes (cytotoxic) in the dermis and HLA-DR+ and ICAM-1+ keratinocytes in the epidermis possibly suggesting the role of antigenic stimulation in the etiology of EDP [23, 24].

Ingestion of ammonium nitrate, radio-contrast media, or chlorothalonil has been implicated invariably [25]. A relation with the intake of drugs such as omeprazole, ethambutol, hydroxyurea, benzodiazepines, and penicillin has been suggested, but this was questioned as these cases can be labeled as drug-induced hyperpigmentation rather than LPP/AD [4].

Differential Diagnoses

The differential diagnosis includes lichen planus pigmentosus, post-inflammatory pigmentation, multiple fixed drug eruption, acquired dermal melanocytosis, melasma, idiopathic eruptive macular pigmentation, macular amyloidosis, drug-induced melanodermas, mastocytosis, and infectious diseases (leprosy, pinta).

The most frequent cause of confusion and controversy is with LPP, which predominates in exposed areas and flexural folds. The presence of an erythematous, raised border favors EDP. Another important differential diagnosis is with pigmented contact dermatitis characterized by finely reticulated pigmented lesions on the face and neck region. Avoidance of the contact allergen may resolve the problem. The most common allergens are detected in fragrances and cosmetics [26]. The hyperpigmentation of LPP/AD is deeper than the epidermal pigmentary disorders seen in melasma.

Workout

Patch testing using the standard series with or without additional allergens, such as fragrances, cosmetics, and metals, may provide more valuable information to distinguish EDP from pigmented contact dermatitis.

Therapy

No treatment of choice is available at present. Topical and systemic corticosteroids, oral vitamin A, and pigment lasers have resulted in favorable outcomes [17]. Topical tacrolimus provides an alternative therapeutic option [27]. Interestingly, in a small number of patients with positive hepatitis C virus serology, a significant improvement was achieved after a year of antiviral medication [20]. It is unknown if these cases should be better labeled as LPP. A number of limited additional treatment modalities have been attempted, but all with uncertain responses including isotretinoin, dapsone, clofazimine, topical tacrolimus, and NBUVB [28, 29].

Prognosis and Course

EDP/AD is a cosmetically distressing dermatosis. The disease is slowly progressive and tends to be persistent. Spontaneous healing after months or years has been reported in children [15].

Idiopathic Eruptive Macular Pigmentation

Idiopathic eruptive macular pigmentation (IEMP) was initially described by Degos et al. [30] with a predilection for adolescents and young adults.

Clinical Features

Diagnostic criteria are characterized by well-defined small, brown macules (0.5–2 cm, < 5 cm) involving the neck, proximal extremities, and trunk [4, 31] (Fig.4). It is not preceded by any inflammatory skin disorder or any prior drug exposure.

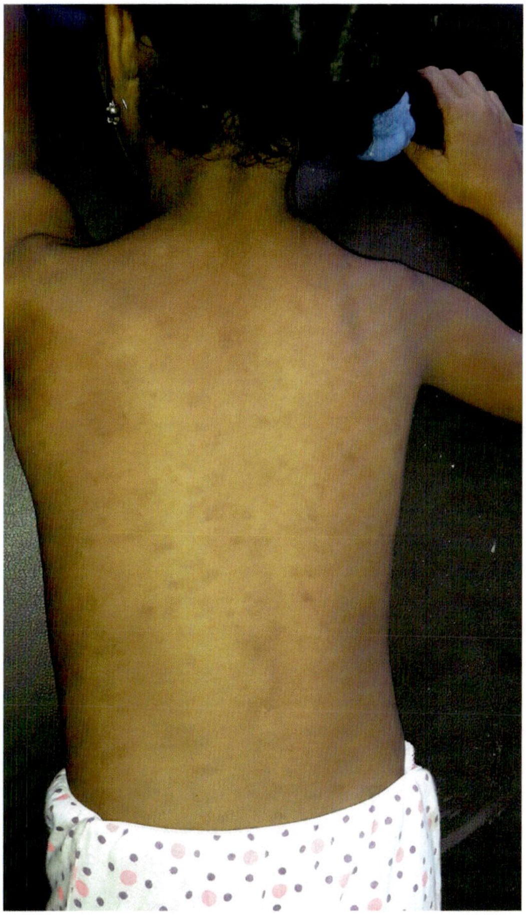

Fig. 4 Idiopathic eruptive macular pigmentation (IEMP). Brow, relatively small macules involving the back of a young Indian patient that was not preceded by any inflammatory skin disorder or any prior drug exposure

Histopathologic Features

Histopathology is characterized by hyperpigmentation of the basal layer of the epidermis, dermal melanophages, and absence of basal cell vacuolization/interface change/lichenoid inflammation. There is no increase in mast cell counts [4].

Differential Diagnoses

The pigmented macules are smaller in size (ranging from 5 to 25 mm) compared to the typical larger macules of EDP/AD. Joshi et al. proposed to classify IEMP to an eruptive form of acanthosis nigricans as they observed features of hyperkeratosis, epidermal pigmentation, and papillomatosis in some lesions [32].

Therapy

No treatment is required.

Prognosis and Course

The lesions typically resolve in several months or in a few years without any treatment.

Conclusions

The nosology of LPP, EDP, AD, and IEMP is controversial as these conditions have several overlapping clinical and histologic features. Some authors consider LPP, EDP, and AD as the same condition, whereas others consider them to be different [4, 5]. Recently, a global consensus has stated that LPP is a separate condition from EDP/AD with similar histopathological features, while EDP and AD are the same disease, and these two terms should be considered as synonyms [4]. If a difference can be highlighted between EDP and AD, this is due to the presence of an erythematous, raised border in EDP. Acquired large (e.g., >5 cm) and small (e.g., 0.5–5 cm) macules of pigmentation of uncertain etiology involving predominantly the head and neck, with or without present or past evidence of lichen planus in Asian/African patients, may be termed LPP. Acquired large (>5 cm) hyperpigmented macules predominantly on the trunk and often distributed symmetrically are characteristic in EDP/AD. Small macules (0.5–2 cm) of acquired pigmentation, occurring predominantly in adolescents and young adults, can be termed IEMP, provided that the pigmented macules did not appear following a known disease episode such as a viral exanthem, a lichenoid drug eruption, or pityriasis rosea, etc. (Table 1). The umbrella term of "acquired macular pigmentation of uncertain etiology" has been proposed for all these conditions. Histology may be similar in LPP and EDP/AD with the presence of dermal melanophages with or without interface dermatitis at some stage. In IEMP, on the other hand, signs of interface dermatitis are lacking and only epidermal hypermelanosis with melanophages with or without papillomatosis is seen. While LPP and EDP/AD run a chronic course and are sometimes difficult to treat, spontaneous recovery in a few months to years is expected for IEMP.

Table 1 Main clinical and histological differences of "acquired macular pigmentations of uncertain etiology"

Findings	EDP/AD	LPP	IEMP
Age at onset	Young adult	30–50 y	Children/adolescent
Sex	No predilection (>female?)	No predilection	No predilection
Skin type	Darker	Darker	Lighter
Symptoms	Asymptomatic/mild pruritus	Mild pruritus	Asymptomatic
Color	Blue-gray	Brownish-gray	Dark brown
Size and border	Large patches, can be diffuse or well defined with raised erythematous border	Few centimeters, diffuse	Smallest 0.5–2 cm, well defined
Distribution	Trunk most common, followed by face and neck	Face and neck most common, followed by trunk; can be on flexures	Trunk and extremities
Mucosal involvement	None	Rare	None
Association	Not proven	Lichen planus in 9–27%, lichen planopilaris, hepatitis C infection	None
Clinical course	Chronic, refractory to treatment	Chronic, refractory to treatment	Spontaneous healing in a few months to years
Histology	Basal vacuolization, melanophages, perivascular lymphocytic infiltrate	Basal vacuolization, melanophages, perivascular lymphocytic infiltrate, sometimes lichenoid	Mainly increased pigmentation of the basal cell layer (epidermal hypermelanosis), dermal melanophages

EDP/AD erythema dyschrormicum perstans/ashy dermatoses, *LPP* lichen planus pigmentosus, *IEMP* idiopathic eruptive macular pigmentation

Acquired Brachial Cutaneous Dyschromatosis (ABCD)

Introduction

Acquired brachial cutaneous dyschromatosis (ABCD*)* is a newly defined acquired pigmentary disorder that was first described in 2000 [33]. It is probably more underestimated than uncommon. ABCD was initially observed in 20 patients who were middle-aged postmenopausal women with Fitzpatrick skin types III–IV and in one man [33].

Clinical Features

ABCD presents as chronic, asymptomatic, gray-brown, geographic-shaped hyperpigmented patches intermingled with hypopigmented, atrophic macules on the dorsal aspect of the forearms, usually bilaterally and distally located (Fig.5a). Nine out of 20 patients showed poikiloderma of Civatte on their neck, and 13 out of 20 patients had arterial hypertension which had been treated with antihypertensive

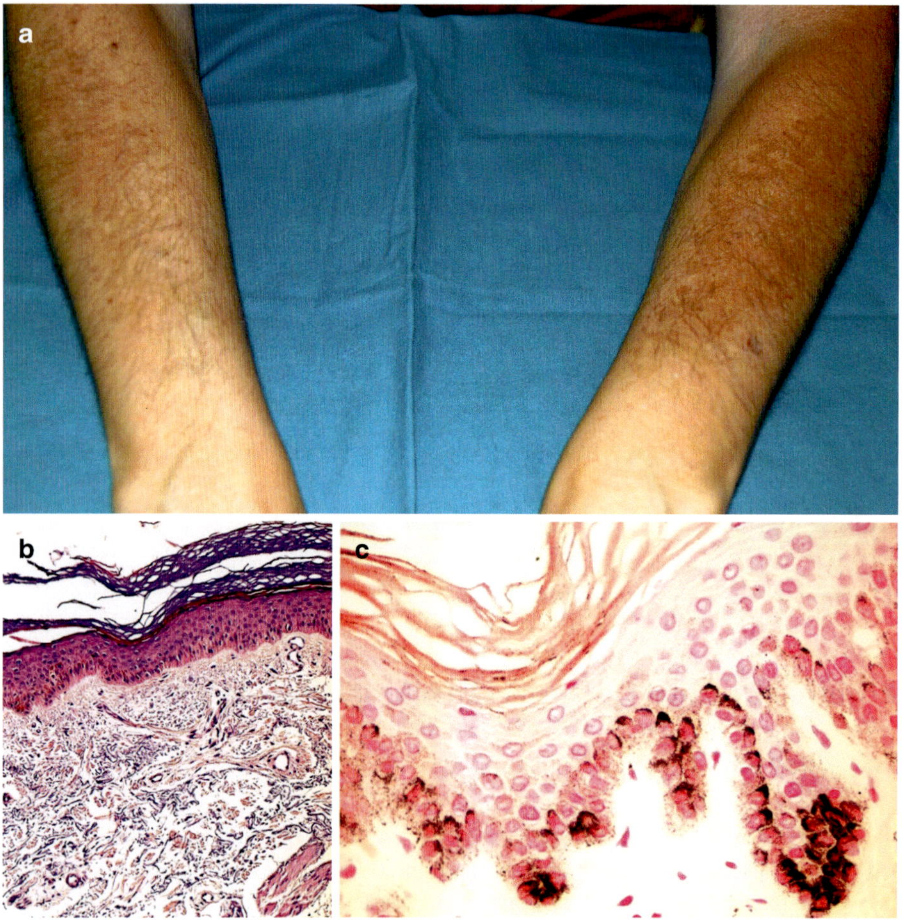

Fig. 5 Acquired brachial cutaneous dyschromatosis (ABCD). (**a**) Chronic, asymptomatic, gray-brown, geographic-shaped hyperpigmented patches intermingled with hypopigmented, atrophic macules on the dorsal aspect of the forearms in a bilaterally way. (**b**) Histopathology showing epidermal atrophy with basal layer hyperpigmentation, solar elastosis, and dilated capillaries. No melanophages nor inflammatory infiltrates are apparently seen (H-E stain). (**c**) Caplike disposition of melanin on the top of the nuclei of keratinocytes highlighted by Fontana-Masson stain for melanin

drugs for several years prior to the onset of pigmentation. In particular, 10 out of these 13 patients had been taking ACE inhibitors [33].

Histopathologic Features

Microscopic features show epidermal atrophy with blunted rete ridges (Fig.5b). Basal layer hyperpigmentation is present, especially with a caplike disposition of melanin on the top of the nucleus that is highlighted by Fontana-Masson stain for melanin (Fig.5c). No increased number of melanocytes is observed with immunostains for melanocytes such as Melan-A. Several dilated vessels are seen in the upper portion of the dermis as well as a slight perivascular inflammatory infiltrate in the superficial portion of the dermis. Solar elastosis can be a finding (Fig.5b). There is usually no pigmentary incontinence. Histopathology of the hypopigmented, atrophic macules stained with Congo red does not demonstrate amyloid deposition, and periodic acid-Schiff stain does not show any fungal organism.

Etiopathogenesis

The etiopathogenesis of ABCD is still unclear. Exposure to ultraviolet light, pregnancy, oral contraceptives, hormone replacement therapy, thyroid autoimmunity, cosmetic ingredients, and phototoxic drugs have been suggested as triggering factors. Two main controversial hypotheses have been considered. The first suggests a relationship between hypertension and antihypertensive medication, specifically ACE inhibitors. Another hypothesis suggests that ABCD is due to cumulative sun damage [34, 35]. However, in the last patient reported in 2018, no history of hypertension and chronic sun exposure was recorded [36].

Differential Diagnosis

The main differential diagnosis involves extrafacial melasma appearing as hyperchromic symmetrical patches on the forearms with irregular borders, affecting menopausal women in the fifth decade of life [37]. The two conditions look similar, although in extrafacial melasma hypopigmented atrophic macules are lacking. Additional sites, especially the face and neck, plus the sternum and rarely the back, can be involved in extrafacial melasma that is often associated with a positive family history. A relationship with hormone replacement therapy has also been suggested [38]. The absence of any relation to estrogens, pregnancy, or hormone replacement therapy further helps to distinguish ABCD from melasma.

Acquired bilateral telangiectatic macules or acquired bilateral telangiectasia macularis eruptiva perstans is a newly described acquired pigmentary disorder characterized by irregular dark to brown telangiectatic macules without hypopigmented atrophic macules on both arms, mostly in middle-aged men opposed to ABCD [39]. However, it is unclear if this condition is a variant of cutaneous mastocytosis or is a photoaging-related reactive process of chronic sun exposure. Medical history is helpful to rule out specific hyperpigmentation induced by drugs such as antimalarials, amiodarone, cytotoxic drugs, tetracycline, heavy metals, and psychotropic drugs; in this setting, histologic findings often show the presence of pigment-laden macrophages around blood vessels and eccrine glands. The pigment may be positive with Fontana-Masson stain for melanin, or with Perls stain, indicating the presence of iron [40]. LPP presents with mottled gray-brown macules on the sun-exposed areas such as the face, neck, trunk, limbs, and flexural folds with microscopic findings of an interface dermatitis and melanophages [3]. Dyschromatosis symmetrica (acropigmentation of Dohi) is a rare autosomal dominant genodermatosis mainly seen in Japanese patients characterized by hyperpigmented and hypopigmented macules, on the extremities appearing during early childhood, due to a mutation adenosine deaminase (ADAR) gene [41]. Another important differential diagnosis is with pigmented contact dermatitis characterized by finely reticulated pigmented lesions on the face and neck region due to allergens such as fragrances and cosmetics [26].

Therapy

No treatment is strongly effective. Topical depigmenting agents such as hydroquinone, topical retinoids, chemical peels, and laser therapy can be considered as well as sun protection [42]. A significant improvement in skin pigmentary disorders with treatment using non-ablative and ablative fractional photothermolysis in comparison to treatment with other resurfacing devices has been reported [43] .

Prognosis and Course

The condition is benign and asymptomatic and constitutes only a reason of aesthetic concern.

Conclusions

ABCD is a relatively newly described, acquired disorder of pigmentation characterized by geographic-shaped, gray brown hyperpigmented patches, interspersed with hypopigmented macules that involve the dorsal aspects of the forearms in postmenopausal women. The condition is probably underreported as it is asymptomatic, and many patients do not seek advice, or the condition goes unnoticed. A possible association with arterial hypertension and ACE inhibitors has been suggested, but also cumulative UV damage could play a role. Additional reports are needed to better clarify both its etiopathogenesis and an effective management for this disorder.

References

1. Bhutani LK, Bedi TR, Pandhi RK, Nayak NC. Lichen planus pigmentosus. Dermatologica. 1974;149(1):43–50. https://doi.org/10.1159/000251470. PMID: 4154221.
2. Kanwar AJ, Dogra S, Handa S, Parsad D, Radotra BD. A study of 124 Indian patients with lichen planus pigmentosus. Clin Exp Dermatol. 2003;28(5):481–5. https://doi.org/10.1046/j.1365-2230.2003.01367.x. PMID: 12950331.
3. Robles-Méndez JC, Rizo-Frías P, Herz-Ruelas ME, Pandya AG, Ocampo CJ. Lichen planus pigmentosus and its variants: review and update. Int J Dermatol. 2018;57(5):505–14.
4. Kumarasinghe SPW, Pandya A, Chandran V, Rodrigues M, Dlova NC, Kang HY, Ramam M, Dayrit JF, Goh BK, Parsad D. A global consensus statement on ashy dermatosis, erythema dyschromicum perstans, lichen planus pigmentosus, idiopathic eruptive macular pigmentation, and Riehl's melanosis. Int J Dermatol. 2019;58(3):263–72.
5. Mendiratta V, Sanke S, Chander R. Lichen planus Pigmentosus: a Clinico-etiological study. Indian Dermatol Online J. 2019;10(3):288–92.
6. Al-Mutairi N, El-Khalawany M. Clinicopathological characteristics of lichen planus pigmentosus and its response to tacrolimus ointment: an open label, non-randomized, prospective study. J Eur Acad Dermatol Venereol. 2010;24(5):535–40. https://doi.org/10.1111/j.1468-3083.2009.03460.x. Epub 2009 Oct 15. PMID: 19840200.
7. Pirmez R, Duque-Estrada B, Donati A, Campos-do-Carmo G, Valente NS, Romiti R, Sodré CT, Tosti A. Clinical and dermoscopic features of lichen planus pigmentosus in 37 patients with frontal fibrosing alopecia. Br J Dermatol. 2016;175(6):1387–90. https://doi.org/10.1111/bjd.14722. Epub 2016 Oct 23. PMID: 27233640.
8. Kim JE, Won CH, Chang S, et al. Linear lichen planus pigmentosus of the forehead treated by neodymium: yttrium aluminum- garnet laser and topical tacrolimus. J Dermatol. 2012;39:189–91.
9. Sindhura KB, Vinay K, Kumaran MS, et al. Lichen planus pigmentosus: a retrospective clinico-epidemiologic study with emphasis on the rare follicular variant. J Eur Acad Dermatol Venereol. 2015;30:e142–4.
10. Verma P, Pandhi D. Topical tacrolimus and oral dapsone combination regimen in lichen planus pigmentosus. Skinmed. 2015;13:351–4.

11. Muthu SK, Narang T, Saikia UN, et al. Low-dose oral isotretinoin therapy in lichen planus pigmentosus: an open-label non-randomized prospective pilot study. Int J Dermatol. 2016;55:1048–54.
12. Vinay K, Kumar S, Bishnoi A, Aggarwal D, Radotra BD, Parsad D, Sendhil KM. A clinico-demographic study of 344 patients with lichen planus pigmentosus seen in a tertiary care center in India over an 8-year period. Int J Dermatol. 2020;59(2):245–52. https://doi.org/10.1111/ijd.14540. Epub 2019 Jun 23. PMID: 31231800.
13. Ramirez CO. The ashy dermatosis (erythema dyschromicum perstans). Epidemiological study and report of 139 cases. Cutis. 1967;3:244–7.
14. Convit J, Kerdel-Vegas F, Rodriguez G. Erythema dyschromicum perstans. A hitherto undescribed skin disease. J Invest Dermatol. 1961;36:457–65.
15. Torrelo A, Zaballos P, Colmenero I, et al. Erythema dyschromicum perstans in children: a report of 14 cases. J Eur Acad Dermatol Venereol. 2005;19:422–6.
16. Pandya AG, Guevara IL. Disorders of hyperpigmentation. Dermatol Clin. 2000;18:91–8.
17. Udompanich S, Vachiramon V. Acquired macular pigmentation of unknown etiology. J Clin Aesthet Dermatol. 2019;12(1):38–46. Epub 2019 Jan 1. PMID: 30881577; PMCID: PMC6405250.
18. Imanishi H, Tsuruta D, Kobayashi H, et al. Two cases of unilateral ashy dermatosis. Case Rep Dermatol. 2011;3:1–4. 38
19. Chang SE, Kim HW, Shin JM, Lee JH, Na JI, Roh MR, Lee JH, Lee GY, Ko JY. Clinical and histological aspect of erythema dyschromicum perstans in Korea: a review of 68 cases. J Dermatol. 2015;42(11):1053–7. https://doi.org/10.1111/1346-8138.13002. Epub 2015 Jun 29. PMID: 26118942.
20. Kontochristopoulos GJ, Aroni K, Anagnostopoulos G, et al. Erythema dyschromicum perstans and hepatitis C virus infection. Int J Dermatol. 2001;40:346–8.
21. Melo CRF, Sa MC, Carvalho S. Erythema dyschromicum perstans in a child following an enteroviral meningitis. An Bras Dermatol. 2017;92:137–8.
22. Venencie PY, Lemay D, Verroust F. Erythema dyschromicum perstans following human immunodeficiency virus seroconversion in a child with hemophilia B. Arch Dermatol. 1988;124:1013–4.
23. Correa MC, Memije EV, Vargas-Alarcon G, et al. HLA-DR association with the genetic susceptibility to develop ashy dermatosis in Mexican mestizo patients. J Am Acad Dermatol. 2007;56:617–20.
24. Vasquez-Ochoa LA, Isaza-Guzman DM, Orozco-Mora B, et al. Immunopathologic study of erythema dyschromicum perstans (ashy dermatosis). Int J Dermatol. 2006;45:937–41.
25. Li S, Arvisais-Anhalt S, Vandergriff T, Le LQ. Ashy dermatosis-like hyperpigmentation in a patient taking hydroxyurea. JAAD Case Rep. 2020;6(9):797–800. https://doi.org/10.1016/j.jdcr.2020.06.030. PMID: 32875022; PMCID: PMC7452229.
26. Tienthavorn T, Tresukosol P, Sudtikoonaseth P. Patch testing and histopathology in Thai patients with hyperpigmentation due to erythema dyschromicum perstans, lichen planus pigmentosus, and pigmented contact dermatitis. Asian Pac J Allergy Immunol. 2014;32:185–92.
27. Mahajan VK, Chauhan PS, Mehta KS, et al. Erythema dyschromicum perstans: response to topical tacrolimus. Indian J Dermatol. 2015;60:525.
28. Bahadir S, Cobanoglu U, Cimsit G, et al. Erythema dyschromicum perstans: response to dapsone therapy. Int J Dermatol. 2004;43:220–2.
29. Wang F, Zhao YK, Wang Z, et al. Erythema dyschromicum perstans: response to isotretinoin. JAMA Dermatol. 2016;152:841–2.
30. Degos R, Civatte J, Belaich S. La pigmentation maculeuse eruptive idiopathique. Ann Dermatol Venereol. 1978;105:177–82.
31. Sanz de Galdeano C, Leaute-Labreze C, Bioulac-Sage P, et al. Idiopathic eruptive macular pigmentation: report of 5 patients. Pediatr Dermatol. 1996;13:274–7.
32. Joshi R, Palwade PK. Idiopathic eruptive macular pigmentation or acanthosis nigricans? Indian J Dermatol Venereol Leprol. 2010;76:591.

33. Rongioletti F, Rebora A. Acquired brachial cutaneous dyschromatosis: a common pigmentary disorder of the arm in middle-aged women. J Am Acad Dermatol. 2000;42:680–4.
34. Hu SW, Chu J, Meehan S, Kamino H, et al. Acquired brachial cutaneous dyschromatosis. Dermatol Online J. 2011;17:16.
35. Abidi N, Foering K, Sahu J. Acquired brachial cutaneous dyschromatosis in a 60-year-old male: a case report and review of the literature. Case Rep Dermatol Med. 2014;2014:452720.
36. Choi MJ, Byun JY, Choi HY, et al. Acquired brachial cutaneous Dyschromatosis in a middle aged Malle. Ann Dermatol. 2018;30(3):342–4.
37. Ritter CG, Fiss DVC, da Borges Costa JAT, et al. Extra-facial melasma: clinical, histopathological, and Immunohistochemical Case-Control Study. J Eur Acad Dermatol Venereol. 2013;27(9):1088–94.
38. O'brien TJ, Dyall-Smith D, Hall AP. Melasma of the forearms. Austr J Dermatol. 1997;38:35–7.
39. Park JH, Lee DJ, Lee YJ, et al. Acquired bilateral telangiectatic macules: a distinct clinical entity. JAMA Dermatol. 2014;150:974–7.
40. Dereure O. Drug-induced skin pigmentation. Epidemiology, diagnosis and treatment. Am J Clin Dermatol. 2001;2:253–62.
41. Hayashi M, Suzuki T. Dyschromatosis symmetrica hereditaria. J Dermatol. 2013;40(5):336–43.
42. Picardo M, Carrera M. New and experimental treatments of cloasma and other hypermelanoses. Dermatol Clin. 2007;25(3):353–ix. https://doi.org/10.1016/j.det.2007.04.012.
43. Tierney EP, Hanke CW. Review of the literature: treatment of dyspigmentation with fractionated resurfacing. Dermatol Surg. 2010;36(10):1499–508.

Eruptive Pseudoangiomatosis, Eruptive Hypomelanosis and Paraviral Exanthems

Francesco Drago and Giulia Ciccarese

Eruptive Pseudoangiomatosis

Introduction Eruptive pseudoangiomatosis (EP) is a rare, self-limiting exanthem occurring mainly in children. Cherry et al. described in 1969 four children between the ages of 8 and 11 months with acute, transitory haemangioma-like skin lesions during Echovirus infections [1]. More than 20 years later, Prose et al. observed three children with acute onset and spontaneous regression of angioma-like papules in the context of upper respiratory infections; based on the natural history and histopathological features of these exanthems, they coined the term “EP” [2]. The first case in adulthood was described in 2000 by Guillot et al. [3] In adult patients with EP, some peculiar features have been observed: female predominance, absence of prodromal symptoms and longer duration than in childhood [4].

Clinical features The elementary lesions of EP are asymptomatic or slightly itchy, round, bright red macules and/or papules of 2–5 mm diameter, very similar to haemangiomas but surrounded by a perilesional blanched halo ranging from 1 to 4 mm. The number of the lesions may vary from few to many elements involving the face (especially the cheeks), neck, trunk and extremities (Fig. 1a). Pressure on the centre of the lesions resulted in their complete blanching [1–5]. An annular configuration has been described in two patients [6]. The lesions are asymptomatic or mildly symptomatic and spontaneously recovered in about 2 weeks in children and 4 weeks in adults.

Histopathologic features EP skin lesions reveal an intact epidermis; the upper reticular dermis and, mainly, the papillary dermis are characterized by dilated small

F. Drago · G. Ciccarese (✉)
Department of Specialized Medicine, Dermatology Unit, Ospedale Policlinico San Martino, Genoa, Italy

F. Rongioletti, B. R. Smoller (eds.), *New and Emerging Entities in Dermatology and Dermatopathology*, https://doi.org/10.1007/978-3-030-80027-7_17

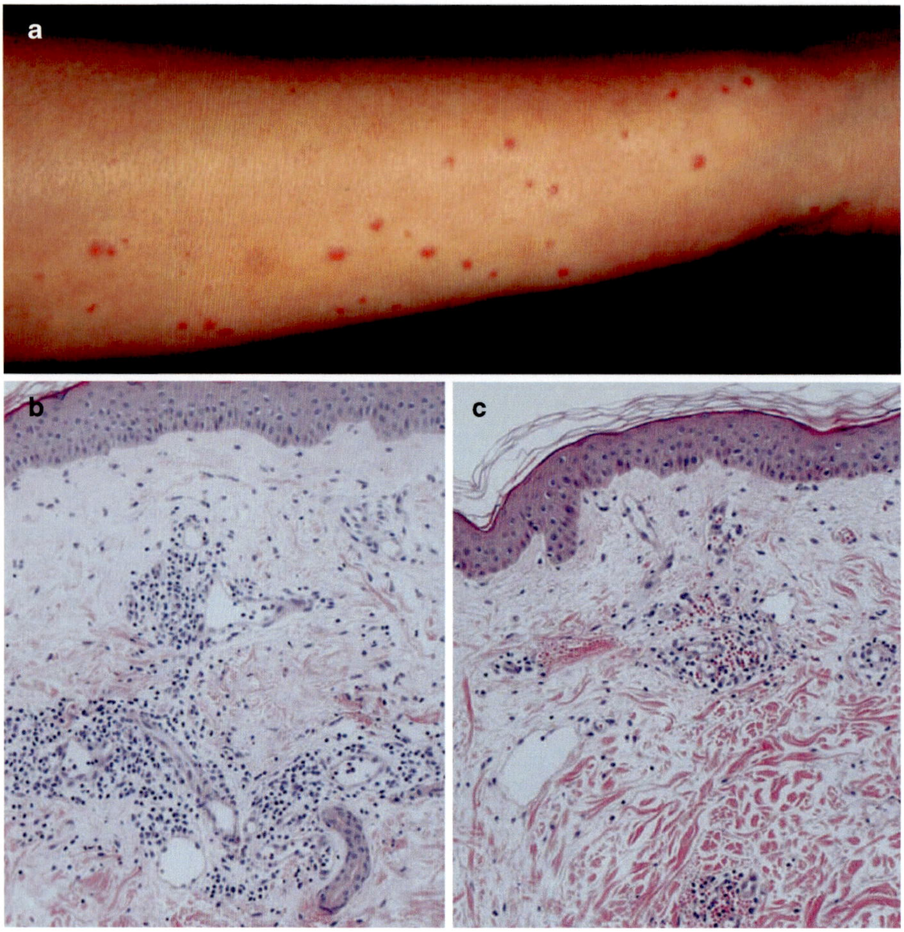

Fig. 1 Eruptive pseudoangiomatosis: (**a**) erythematous macules and/or papules of 2-5 mm diameter surrounded by a perilesional 1-4 mm blanched halo on the dorsum of an arm; (**b**) biopsy of skin lesions shows an intact epidermis while the upper dermis is characterized by oedema, lymphocytic infiltration around the dilated capillaries; (**c**) extravasated erythrocytes. (Courtesy of Prof. Soo-Chan Kim)

blood vessels and capillaries with plump endothelial cells protruding into the lumen; these cells have slightly enlarged nuclei, some of them being in mitosis and may have a hobnail appearance. Such features are considered quite specific, though not pathognomonic, of EP. In addition, a mild lympho-histiocytic perivascular infiltrate, extravasated erythrocytes and melanophages around the vessels [1, 2, 6] (Fig. 1b) and intravascular neutrophil infiltration [7] can be other findings helpful in diagnosing EP. Notably, the number of vessels in the dermis is not increased in EP lesions, differently from true angiomas [1, 2, 6].

Etiopathogenesis Etiopathogenesis is still unknown; however, EP occurrence after prodromal symptoms, such as fever, malaise, diarrhoea, headache and cough, and spontaneous resolution after 2–18 days, suggests the role of a viral infection [1, 2, 5]. Furthermore, reports of EP cases within families [8, 9] and in patients receiving immunosuppressive treatments support this hypothesis [10, 11]. Cherry et al. isolated Echovirus 25 RNA from the oropharynx of two children with EP and Echovirus 32 RNA from the oropharynx and the rectum of two other children with EP; they also found neutralizing antibodies to these viruses in the patient's serum. The authors speculated that the capillary dilatation of the lesions may result from a direct viral effect in the endothelial cells or from the antigen-antibody complexes binding to the endothelium and that the papular component may be related to the concomitant perivascular oedema [1]. Later, the white halo has been explained with a reactive vasoconstriction around papular EP lesions, similar to that observed around pyogenic granuloma or nevoid teleangectasia [5]. However, Echoviruses have never been detected in the skin lesions. Other authors suggested an association with Epstein-Barr virus (EBV) [10] and adenovirus [6] since they have found positive serology for these viruses in patients with EP. Unfortunately, viral DNA detection in the serum and/or in the skin lesions by polymerase chain reaction (PCR) was not performed in such cases [6, 10], and serology alone does not represent an evidence of an active viral infection. Several Japanese authors described outbreaks or single cases of EP-like lesions which they assumed to be caused by mosquito bites, calling this eruption "Erythema punctatum Higuchi" [12]. Ban et al. reported that when a great number of *Culex pipiens pallens,* very common mosquitos in Japan, attacked the Hashima City Hospital, they found many inpatients with erythema punctatum Higuchi. The authors suggested that a viral agent may be transmitted by mosquitos and that EP and erythema punctatum Higuchi, showing the same clinical features and evolution, belong to the same entitiy [12]. A few years later, also Italian authors described EP-like lesions on the exposed skin of bedridden or immunosuppressed patients that were presumably bitten by the numerous mosquitos infesting their hospital wards [13].

Differential diagnosis Differential diagnoses include spider angiomas, multiple capillary haemangiomas, multiple pyogenic granulomas and bacillary angiomatosis. However, in all these skin disorders, spontaneous resolution does not occur. Spider angiomas and cherry angiomas do not blanch completely with pressure and refill from the centre on release. Bacillary angiomatosis and pyogenic granuloma appear with larger lesions lasting longer than the 7- to 15-day duration as observed in EP. Moreover, the occurrence of multiple pyogenic granulomas is rare. In doubtful cases, differential diagnoses could be ruled out with histological examination [1–5].

Prognosis Prognosis is excellent because EP is a self-limiting condition and spontaneous regression of the lesions is the rule.

Therapy Treatment with topical/oral corticosteroids and oral antihistamine does not affect the natural course of the eruption. Since the lesions are asymptomatic or mildly symptomatic and spontaneously resolve, no treatment is necessary.

Eruptive Hypomelanosis

Introduction The definition "eruptive hypomelanosis" (EH) applies to the sudden onset of asymptomatic, hypopigmented macules, symmetrically distributed on the extremities of children, that appear about 8 days after constitutional symptoms. The lesions have a spontaneous resolution in 3–4 weeks without scarring. EH was first described by Zawar et al. in 2014 as a novel exanthem [1], and, to date, about 20 cases have been described [14–17], all but one [18] from Asian countries.

Clinical features EH occurs in children aged 3–11 years, usually 5 to 14 days after prodromal symptoms concerning upper respiratory tract infection (usually rhinitis). The eruption is characterized by monomorphic, hypopigmented, macular lesions with a circular/oval shape, 2–8 mm in diameter and rather distinct margins. Sometimes fine scales are present. The macules appear in single or successive crops with a symmetrical distribution on the upper and/or lower extremities sometimes involving the face [14–17] and trunk [18] (Fig. 2). The skin lesions are asymptomatic or only slightly itchy. Systemic signs and symptoms may be observed during the skin eruption such as sore throat and enlarged lymph nodes [14].

Histopathologic features Histopathology is not specific showing orthokeratosis, mild epidermal spongiosis and inflammatory lymphocytic infiltrates in the upper dermis [14, 18].

Etiopathogenesis The etiopathogenesis of EH is unknown. However, several factors suggest a viral etiology: the prodromal symptoms like coryza, the predictable clinical course with possible successive crops of monomorphic lesions [14, 16–18],

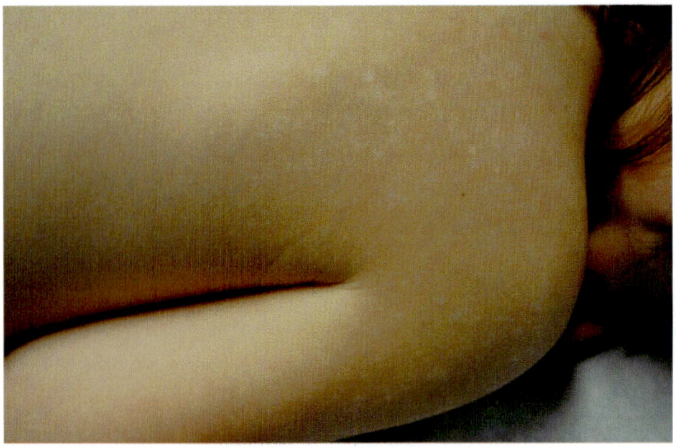

Fig. 2 Eruptive hypomelanosis: monomorphic, hypopigmented, macular lesions with a circular/oval shape, 2-8 mm in diameter on the back. (Courtesy of Prof. Dirk Van Gysel)

the spontaneous remission and the occurrence in family clustering [14–18]. Rhinovirus was detected by polymerase chain reaction (PCR) from patients' nasopharyngeal aspirate suggesting that the virus may play a role in the pathogenesis [18]. However, viral genomic content detection by PCR in plasma, peripheral blood mononuclear cells and lesional skin and serological examinations (demonstrating seroconversion) have never been demonstrated. Potassium hydroxide examination of skin scrapings from EH lesions, performed in most of the cases described in the literature, resulted negative and Wood's light examination did not reveal fluorescence [14]; these results allow to exclude a fungal or yeast infection associated with EH.

Differential diagnosis Differential diagnoses include pityriasis versicolor, pityriasis alba, progressive macular hypomelanosis and post-inflammatory hypopigmentation. Pityriasis versicolor is uncommon before puberty, when the function of the sebaceous glans initiates and manifests with sharply demarcated, hypopigmented macules that tend to persist for months even after treatment. In addition, potassium hydroxide examination of skin scrapings from scaly lesions reveals the typical thick-walled spherical yeast in clusters, characteristic of *Malassezia furfur*, and examination under Wood's light evidences a yellowish or orange glow. Pityriasis alba usually occurs in patients with history of atopy and is characterized by large (2–3 cm diameter), hypopigmented, scaly macules preceeded by erythematous lesions; these changes may persist for months [14–18]. Progressive macular hypomelanosis occurs in adults (more often in people living in tropical countries) with asymptomatic, ill-defined, nummular, hypopigmented spots on the trunk, confluent in and around the midline, rarely extended to the extremities and neck/head region. The hypopigmented lesions demonstrate a punctiform orange-red follicular fluorescence with a Wood's lamp, probably due to the presence of Gram-positive bacteria (*Propionibacterium acnes*) in follicles of the hypopigmented spots [19]. Post-inflammatory hypopigmentation happens after a preceding eruption in the involved skin area; lesions have fairly distinct margins and a rapid disappearance [14].

Prognosis Prognosis is excellent since EH has a predictable time course with complete resolution in 2–4 weeks.

Therapy Treatment is not necessary since this condition is usually asymptomatic and self-limiting.

Paraviral Exanthems

An exanthem is defined as any eruptive skin rash that may be associated with lesions of the mucous membranes (enanthem), fever or systemic symptoms. It may be the manifestation of an infectious disease or an adverse reaction to drugs and is among the most frequent reasons for consultation of a dermatologist. Six exanthems have been classified as classic (measles, scarlet fever, chickenpox, rubella, erythema infectiosum, exanthem subitum). Other exanthems with different morphologies have been described over time and then defined as "atypical exanthems" [20, 21]. In 2005, Lipsker and Saurat coined the term "paraviral eruptions" to define some of these "atypical exanthems" dividing them into two main categories [22]. The first includes skin eruptions that are clinically well-defined and in which at least one identified viral agent has been well established. It embraces eruptions such as pityriasis rosea (PR), papular acrodermatitis of childhood (Gianotti-Crosti syndrome, GCS) and papular-purpuric gloves and socks syndrome (PPGSS). In the latter category, typical and easily identifiable eruptions (such as asymmetric periflexural exanthem or eruptive psudoangiomatosis) have been included, in which, however, a viral infection is suspected but not yet proven. Lipsker and Saurat should be commended for their effort to shed light on a controversial issue, but "paraviral eruption" is a definition that may open the door to many bold uses. For example, authors included in the group several eruptions such as pityriasis lichenoides et varioliformis acuta and pityriasis lichenoides chronica, whose infectious aetiology has been suspected but is far from being ascertained [23]. Indeed, if a rash is clinically monomorphic and a viral cause is well established, it should simply be called "viral eruption". This applies, for example, to PR in which only two viruses, namely, human herpesvirus (HHV)-6 and HHV-7, have been well proven in its aetiology. The same can be said for PPGSS caused by parvovirus B19 (PVB19) and hand-foot-and-mouth disease, which, even in its atypical form, is invariably caused by enteroviruses [20, 21]. Other eruptions resembling PR, as those caused by drugs, should be defined as PR-like eruptions having clinical, histopathologic and virologic features that may distinguish them from typical PR. In this meaning, PR-like eruptions can be compared to drug morbilliform eruptions and arranged in a different group [24]. Therefore, it is better to include under the term "Paraviral Eruptions" only those eruptions waiting for a more definite viral aetiology.

Pityriasis Rosea

Introduction Pityriasis rosea (PR) is an acute, self-limiting exanthematous disease associated with the endogenous systemic reactivation of HHV-6 and/or HHV-7 and characterized by oval erythematous-squamous lesions on the trunk and limbs, usually sparing the face, scalp, palms and soles. The eruption follows a distinctive and constant pattern and course in most of the cases. Mild prodromal symptoms may be present. Numerous studies have tried to establish PR prevalence estimating it at 1–2% of new patients attending dermatological departments, but taking into account the atypical forms and the forms that non-dermatologists fail to diagnose, this figure is probably underestimated [25]. PR affects mainly young adults (age of maximum incidence between 10 and 35 years), immunosuppressed patients or subjects undergoing stress or recent surgical procedures [26].

Clinical features Constitutional symptoms of infection such as fatigue, headache, sore throat, nausea, loss of appetite, difficulty in concentration, irritability and gastrointestinal and upper respiratory symptoms may precede or accompany the skin eruption, but they are frequently mild and neglected [27]. Typically, the disease begins with a solitary patch, the so-called herald patch (HP) or mother patch. The patch is a sharply defined, oval plaque, with a paler central, wrinkled area and a darker red peripheral zone, covered by fine scale resembling bran and with a marginal collarette of pityriasiform scale. It usually occurs on the trunk, the thigh, the upper arm or the neck and progressively enlarges, reaching 3–5 cm or more in diameter. The HP is absent or undetected in 20% of cases. Usually, it remains solitary for about 2 weeks, after which the generalized eruption abruptly develops, but rarely the primary plaque may be the sole manifestation of the disease. This secondary eruption, localized mainly on the trunk, appears in crops, at intervals of a few days, characterized by symmetrical patches that are similar to the initial one but smaller and symmetrically oriented with their long axes along the cleavage lines (Christmas tree or theatre curtain distribution) (Fig. 3a). Pruritus is usually moderate or absent

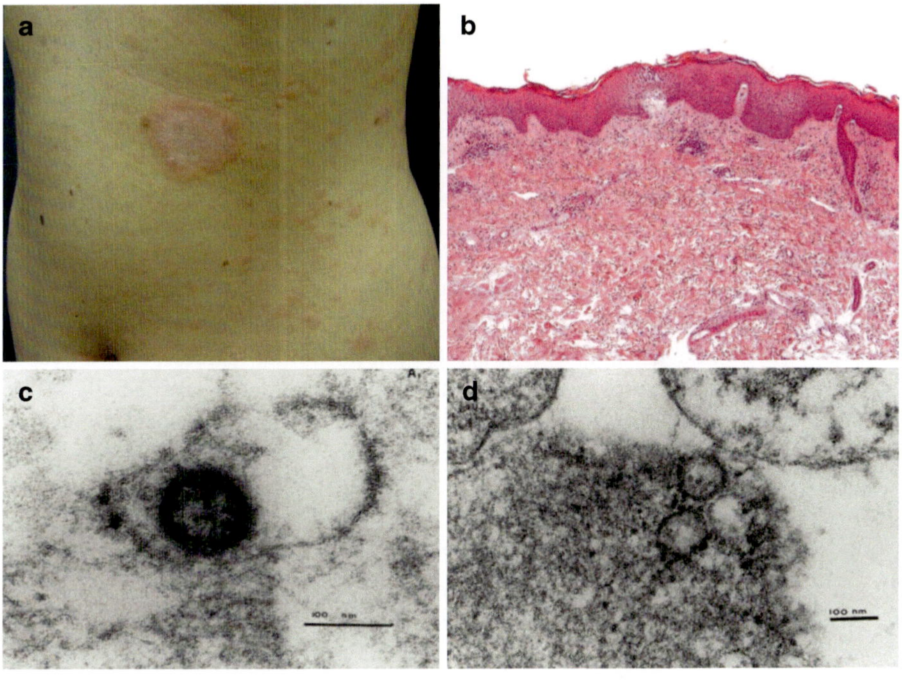

Fig. 3 Pityriasis rosea: (**a**) erythematous, sharply defined, oval plaque, with a paler centre covered by fine scale (herald patch) on the trunk; similar smaller patches symmetrically oriented with their long axes along the cleavage lines of the trunk constitute the secondary eruption; (**b**) PR epidermis shows mild acanthosis, parakeratosis in mounds and foci of spongiosis; in the dermis, extravasated red blood cells are accompanied by capillary dilatation and perivascular infiltrate of lymphocytes, monocytes and eosinophils (courtesy of Prof. Carlo Tomasini); (**c**) Electron microscopy of skin specimens of PR patients shows in both epidermis and dermis herpes virus-like particles in various stages of morphogenesis: these virions contain a capside, an electrodense cylindrical core, a tegument and an envelope with spikes; (**d**) virions are also interspersed among keratinocytes in the vicinity of the dermal–epidermal junction; keratinocytes exhibited gross cytolytic degeneration and are even disintegrated

but following topical remedy may be more severe [26, 27]. Oral involvement may be present and is probably largely underestimated because examination of the mucous membranes during PR is often neglected. Petechial and maculopapular lesions are the most frequent and strongly associated with systemic symptoms and PR atypical forms [28]. The exanthem fades slowly and the duration may vary from 3 to 6 weeks [26, 27]. Besides the typical presentation of PR, atypical forms have been described. They may be atypical in the morphology, distribution, number, severity of symptoms and course [29–33]. Among the PR atypical forms, the relapsing and persistent ones may be included. Relapsing PR is a variant that recurs usually within 1 year from the initial presentation and occurs in 2.8% of the patients [25, 31]; it consists mostly of a single episode of relapse, though multiple cases have been reported [34, 35]. The persistent PR is an atypical form that lasts for over 12 weeks without interruption [32]; systemic symptoms (especially fatigue and impaired concentration) are almost constantly reported and oral lesions are more common than in classic PR [28]. PR in children younger than 10 years of age is uncommon, and only 6% of cases are seen in children below that age. However, PR in children may be considered a distinct form due to its peculiar clinical and laboratory features. Indeed, the mean time lapse between HP and generalized eruption and the duration of the exanthem is shorter than in adults [33]; oral involvement is commoner than in adults [28].

Histopathologic features The histopathologic features, as it occurs in most exanthems, are largely not specific. However, classic PR shows in the epidermis mild acanthosis, parakeratosis in mounds, a thinned granular layer and foci of spongiosis with variable amount of lymphocytic exocytosis. In the dermis, extravasated red blood cells are accompanied by capillary dilatation and perivascular infiltrate of lymphocytes, monocytes and eosinophils. HP shows similar features, with a deeper infiltrate and more acanthosis. Dyskeratotic cells may be present, especially in the HP, and exhibit an aggregation of tonofilaments, many vacuoles, intracytoplasmic desmosomes and viral-like particles [36, 37]. Multinucleated giant cells and acantholysis have also been observed and related to a viral infection [38].

Etiopathogenesis The monomorphous clinical features frequently preceded by prodromal symptoms and self-limiting course of PR reproduce those of other known exanthems. Therefore, an infectious etiology has long been suspected. A viral origin has been suggested decades ago by the light and electron microscopy observation of intranuclear and intracytoplasmic virus-like particles and by the detection of cytolytic degeneration of keratinocytes [36–38]. More recently, a large body of evidence using the most modern biological techniques supports a lead role for endogenous systemic reactivation of HHV-6 and/or HHV-7 in PR [39–43]. Several studies detected HHV-6 and HHV-7 DNA by PCR and calibrate quantitative real-time PCR in plasma, peripheral blood mononuclear cells (PBMCs) and skin samples of patients with PR. Furthermore, cytopathic effects specific for herpesviruses were observed in co-cultured mononuclear PBMCs from PR patients. High levels of interferon α and γ were detected in sera of patients with PR, and virions resembling herpesviruses were shown by electron microscopy in the cell-free supernatants of their co-cultured PBMCs and also in their skin specimens (Fig. 3c, d) [39, 41]. Furthermore, HHV-6 viral messenger RNA (mRNA) expression by in situ hybridization and HHV-6 and HHV-7 antigens were observed in PR skin lesions [40, 42]. The cytopathic effects found in culture, the detection of cell-free circulating viral DNA in plasma, the presence in PR skin lesions of the specific HHV-6 and HHV-7 antigens involved in the late stages of the infection as well as their mRNA expressions are all markers of active viral replication and emphasize the role of both viruses in the pathogenesis of the disease [40–42]. Neutralizing antibodies and high-avidity IgG antibodies against HHV-6 and HHV-7 have been demonstrated in patients with PR, indicating a viral endogenous reactivation [40]. The inverse correlation described between titre of anti-HHV-7 neutralizing antibodies and detection of HHV-7 DNA in plasma of PR patients suggest that humoral response acts limiting the systemic reactivation and dissemination of the virus. The etiopathogenesis of PR as the consequence of HHV-6 and/or HHV-7 reactivation (the viruses may be reactivated independently or simultaneously) can fit the few familiar cases, the poor/absent contagiousness, the age of onset, the recurrent or persistent cases of PR and the occurrence after or during stressful events or in moderately immunocompromised condition with altered immune response such as the pregnancy. In this regard, PR developing during pregnancy may rarely be followed by complications such as premature delivery and even foetal death due to HHV-6 systemic active infection [44, 45]. The onset of PR before week 15 of gestation, the presence of constitutional symptoms and enanthem are major risk factors for complications [45].

Differential diagnosis In the typical cases the diagnosis presents little difficulty. The distribution, morphology, presence of HP and predictable course are enough distinctive. Several patterns of drug eruption must be ruled out. The acute onset without a HP, pruritus and the tendency to confluence of the lesions can help in the diagnosis. PR-like eruption is a drug-induced skin rash with clinical features that remarkably resemble genuine PR. Recently, criteria have been proposed for distinguishing between the two forms [24, 27]. In PR-like eruptions, prodromal systemic symptoms are absent, and the lesions are more confluent and itchy usually involving the limbs more extensively. Laboratory results in PR-like patients frequently show blood eosinophilia and lack of HHV-6/7 systemic active infection. Histopathology often reveals necrotic keratinocytes within the epidermis, dermal eosinophil infiltrate, perivascular infiltrate and signs of junctional vacuolar degeneration. Lastly, patients with PR-like eruptions quickly recovered after discontinuing the drug. Other diseases which can mimic PR are seborrhoeic dermatitis (no HP, eruption more persistent, recurrent and involving scalp, scales greasy and thicker), secondary syphilis (papules usually more infiltrated, involving frequently palms and soles, lymphadenopathy constant), guttate psoriasis and pityriasis lichenoides (in both diseases, the lesions are papular and persistent, surmounted by silvery scales in the first and more polymorphic in the latter) [24, 27].

Prognosis The course is usually self-limiting and predictable.

Treatment No treatment is usually necessary. Itching, when present, is usually mild and bearable. Topical medications may exacerbate or cause itching. Evidence has been found inadequate for the efficacy of emollients, topical and systemic antihistamines and corticosteroids, sunlight and artificial ultraviolet therapy [46]. Acyclovir treatment (800 mg orally 5 times a day) accelerated the clearance of the lesions in a placebo-controlled study, but it is generally not necessary [47]. When PR develops during the first 15 weeks of gestation with constitutional symptoms, unusual extension and long duration of the lesions, a course of therapy with acyclovir may be considered. However, no treatment can be recommended on the basis of evidence-based medicine and rest and reassurance are probably the best cure. Importantly, it is mandatory to perform a careful follow-up with available instrumental techniques such as ultrasound scans that can promptly detect pregnancy or foetal complications [45].

Gianotti-Crosti Syndrome (Papular Acrodermatitis of Childhood)

Introduction Gianotti-Crosti syndrome (GCS) is a distinctive self-limiting infectious exanthem of childhood characterized by papulovesicular lesions affecting mainly the face, buttocks and limbs [48].

Clinical features GCS is characterized by symmetric monomorphic pink to red-brown papular or papulovesicular lesions that are a few millimetres in diameter, distributed on the face, buttocks and limbs (Fig. 4a). In newborns several lesions may be oedematous. GCS usually begins on the thighs and buttocks, then spreading

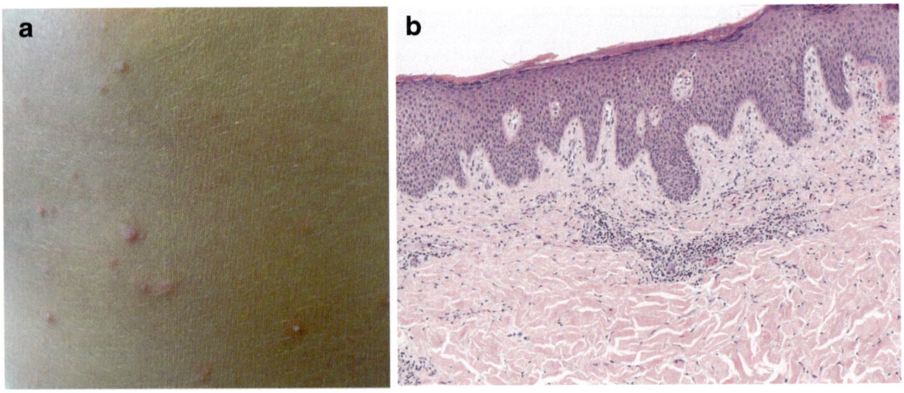

Fig. 4 Gianotti-Crosti syndrome. (**a**) Detail of pink papulovesicular lesions that are few millimetres in diameter, distributed on the legs; (**b**) biopsy shows non-specific histological features: irregular acanthosis, focal spongiosis and parakeratosis of the epidermis and a chronic lymphohistiocytic inflammatory infiltrate with few eosinophils in the superficial dermis. (Courtesy of Dr. Antonio Guadagno)

to the extensor surfaces of the limbs and lastly involving the face. The rash develops over the course of 3–5 days and the colour may be changed by purpuric staining especially on the legs, buttocks and areas of trauma. The eruption fades in about 3 weeks with mild desquamation. The mucous membranes usually are spared. Low-grade fever may occur but constitutional symptoms and pruritus are usually lacking. Axillary and inguinal lymphadenopathy is common and may persist after the resolution of the eruption. Laboratory findings are usually inconclusive, but in cases associated with hepatitis B or Epstein-Barr virus infections, elevated levels of liver enzymes can be found [20, 21].

Histopathologic features The histopathological findings are rather nonspecific. The skin lesions show mild acanthosis and hyperkeratosis with focal spongiosis and papillary oedema with an infiltrate of lymphocytes and histiocytes around dilated capillaries in the dermis (Fig. 4b). There may be scale crusts in later lesions [49, 50].

Etiopathogenesis GCS is considered a unique cutaneous response to viral infection, mostly associated with hepatitis B virus and EBV. Worldwide, with the advent of more universal hepatitis B immunization, EBV is now the most common cause of GCS. Other viral infections have rarely been associated with GCS such as Coxsackievirus A16, B4 and 5, Echovirus 7 and 9, cytomegalovirus, respiratory syncytial virus, parainfluenza virus and hepatitis A virus [51–53]. Bacterial infections and recent immunizations may be other inciting factors. However, the association between these cases and GCS is inconclusive: the cited articles are quite old whereby methods to detect viral sequences or antigens in tissues were not yet available. Their evidence was based mainly on serology which, if used alone, rarely provides conclusive evidence for an aetiologic link. Immunohistochemical findings of the cutaneous inflammatory infiltrate suggest a type IV hypersensitivity reaction to viral or bacterial antigens within the dermis, which happens when the infection has usually subsided. However, electron microscopy has never revealed virus particles. Increased human beta-defensin-4 activity in the epidermis has recently been reported, indicating viral antigenemia rather than a type IV hypersensitivity reaction, as a possible cause of GCS in some viral cases [54].

Differential diagnosis Conditions to be differentiated are Henoch-Schonlein purpura (purpuric lesions not infiltrated, systemic involvement), erythema multiforme (target lesions with central blistering, mucous membrane involvement), pityriasis lichenoides acuta (more prolonged course, ulcerated lesions that resolve with varioliform scars) and gloves and socks syndrome (lesions demarcated at the wrists and ankles).

Prognosis GCS is self-limited eruption with a good prognosis.

Therapy There is no specific treatment. Rarely, oral antihistamines may be prescribed for itching. The use of topical products is not recommended [52, 53].

Asymmetric Periflexural Exanthem of Childhood (APEC)

Introduction APEC, also known as unilateral laterothoracic exanthem, is a distinctive and a self-limited exanthem which typically affects children and less frequently adults. It is usually characterized by its asymmetric localization and unilateral onset and by its stereotypical morphology and distribution [55, 56].

Clinical features APEC typically affects children mostly between the ages of 2 and 3 years but can also affect adults. The initial presentation is classically unilateral and presents as an erythematous macular-papular exanthem (defined as scarlet or morbilliform) starting from an axillary fold. It can rarely begin in other flexures, such as the thigh, flank or inguinal fold. Later, after a few days, the exanthem may spread centrifugally to involve the thorax, the corresponding arm and the contralateral side. In almost all patients, at the time of consultation, is bilateral, although one side was usually more involved. The papules may coalesce in reticular and annular plaque. The eruption spares the face, palms, soles and mucous membranes. Mild prodromal symptoms may be present. Pruritus is usually mild. The lesions may develop central dusky grey discolouration and resolve in 4–6 weeks with a fine desquamation [55, 56].

Histopathologic features The findings are largely not specific. The epidermis shows mild exocytosis and spongiosis without associated hyperparakeratosis or parakeratosis. In the dermis there is a mild to moderate, perivascular, predominantly lymphocytic infiltrate. Characteristically, the infiltrate clustered around the dermal eccrine ducts, though the secretory coils were generally undamaged [55, 56].

Etiopathogenesis The aetiology of APEC remains unknown. A viral etiology is suggested by the clinical appearance of the eruption, the possible prodromal symptoms and the clinical course but never demonstrated. It has been suggested that many forms of APEC are actually forms of PR that remains localized to the axilla or involves mainly the trunk in a unilateral pattern [57].

Differential diagnosis Differential diagnosis of APEC includes drug reactions, nonspecific viral eruption, scarlet fever, Gianotti-Crosti syndrome, atypical pityriasis rosea, contact dermatitis and tinea corporis.

Prognosis APEC is a self-limiting disease that spontaneously resolves within 4–6 weeks.

Therapy No treatment is usually required [55–57].

Papular-Purpuric Gloves-and-Socks Syndrome

Introduction Papular-purpuric gloves-and-socks syndrome (PPGSS) is a rare exanthem affecting the distal part of the extremities in children and adults [58].

Clinical features Mild prodromal symptoms such as asthenia, low-grade fever, arthralgias and myalgias recall a viral infection. Later, itchy, painful, symmetrical oedema and erythematous purpuric papules on the hands and feet, sharply marginated on the wrists and ankles, occur. Mucous membranes may rarely be involved with petechiae, vesico-pustules and erosions on the hard and soft palate.

Histopathologic features Nonspecific findings such as slight acanthosis of the epidermis, inflammatory perivascular lymphocytic infiltrate with neutrophils and eosinophils and abundant extravasated erythrocytes in the papillary dermis recall a viral infection. Vacuolar degeneration of the basal layer of the epidermis and a lichenoid inflammatory infiltrate are rarely described [58].

Etiopathogenesis Although several viruses have been involved as causative agent for PPGSS, only acute infection by parvovirus B19 (PVB19) has been proven to cause the syndrome. Indeed, primary infection by PVB19 was demonstrated by seroconversion against this virus and by detection of its DNA by PCR in the sera and in the skin and by detection of PVB19 VP2 structural protein in the dermal blood vessels [59, 60].

Differential diagnosis Gianotti-Crosti syndrome (different distribution of the lesions), atypical measles (possible onset on limbs but different final cutaneous involvement, more severe prodromal symptoms and Koplik's spots), various forms of rickettsiosis (involvement of palms, soles and trunk, severe systemic symptoms) and Kawasaki disease (conjunctival, lips, oral cavity and visceral involvement, diffuse lymph node enlargement, lamellar desquamation of hands and feet) should be excluded.

Prognosis The exanthem usually resolves spontaneously within 1 to 2 weeks.

Therapy. No treatment is required [61–63].

Pityriasis Lichenoides

Introduction Pityriasis lichenoides (PL) is an uncommon disease of unknown aetiology with a clinical and histopathologic spectrum ranging from acute to chronic (PLC) forms. The acute form, commoner in the young, includes pityriasis lichenoides et varioliformis acuta (PLEVA) and Mucha-Habermann disease [64].

Clinical features The skin eruption is usually the first manifestation of PLEVA, but it may be preceded by fever and nonspecific constitutional symptoms lasting a few days. The eruptions develop in crops and, therefore, lesions may be present in all stages of development. Patients show erythematous/edematous papules which may evolve into vesicles and pustules that in turn evolve into crusted erosions leaving superficial scars. If necrosis is severe, it can determine ulcers which result in varioliform scars. The patients may complain of mild itching or burning sensation. PLEVA most often occurs on the trunk, limbs and flexural areas, but diffuse and generalized eruptions may also occur (Fig. 5a, b). PLEVA can lasts from a few weeks to several months. Mucha-Habermann disease is a variant of PLEVA characterized by severe malaise, high fever, myalgias, arthralgias and visceral involvement. Necrotic papules evolve quickly into large painful coalescent ulcers with necrotic crusts. Mucous membranes may be affected. PLC has a much more indolent clinical course characterized by the presence of reddish brown papules with an adherent central micaceous scale which tends to detach spontaneously or by mild scraping leaving pigmented macules that slowly resolve without scarring. The disease can last from weeks to several months.

Histopathologic features The findings of PL are similar in both forms though in the acute one the epidermal and dermal alterations are more severe. In PLC, the epidermis shows focal parakeratosis, acanthosis, spongiosis, small amounts of necrotic keratinocytes and low vacuolar interface dermatitis with lymphocyte exocytosis. The dermis shows oedema, sparse superficial perivascular infiltrate composed of lymphocytes and macrophages that only focally impinge on the dermoepidermal junction. Extravasated erythrocytes can be present in the epidermis

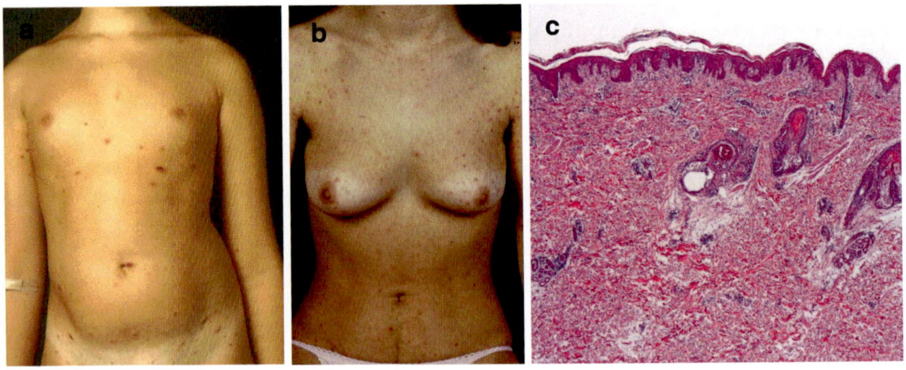

Fig. 5 Pityriasis lichenoides. (**a**, **b**) The eruption develops in crops; therefore, lesions in various stages of development may be simultaneously present: erythematous/edematous papules, vesicles, pustules and crusted erosions; (**c**) biopsy shows broad parakeratosis, basal vacuolar changes and a prominent lymphocytic exocytosis in the epidermis; hemorrhage in the papillary dermis with extension of extravasated erythrocytes into the epidermis is also present. The lymphohistiocytic inflammatory infiltrate is moderate and involves the superficial and deep dermal plexus. (Courtesy of Prof. Carlo Tomasini and Dr. Antonio Guadagno)

and dermis. PLEVA shows similar epidermal changes, but more severe and keratinocyte necrosis may result in erosions and ulcerations. The dermal perivascular infiltrate is heavier, diffusely obscuring the dermoepidermal junction and extending deeply into the reticular dermis often exhibiting a wedge-shape appearance (Fig. 5c). Inflammatory cells may invade vessel walls but true fibrinoid necrosis and leucocytoclasia is rare [64].

Etiopathogenesis PL affects both children and young adults without racial predilection. Overall, the chronic form is more common than the acute. The cause of PL remains unknown. A hypersensitive reaction to viral antigen or drugs has been suggested. However, all attempts to detect a viral agent have failed. Authors found positive results of serologic tests for acute toxoplasmosis during PL [65, 66]. Furthermore, specific treatment against *Toxoplasma gondii* achieved prompt improvement of PL. PL is also regarded as a primary lymphoproliferative process because monoclonal T-cell population was discovered in the skin lesions. The concept that PL should be included in the lymphoproliferative disorders is still debated.

Differential diagnosis PLC may recall PR (HP, shorter course and "theatre curtain" pattern of eruption), guttate psoriasis (scale less cohesive and more uniform pattern of lesions) and secondary papulosquamous syphilis (involvement of palms and soles, positivity of serologic tests). GCS and varicella need to be differentiated from PLEVA.

Prognosis PL has a chronic indolent course and may regress in a few weeks or last for months. PLEVA usually has a shorter duration than PLC.

Therapy The unknown aetiology obliges to empirical drugs and regimens. Several topical and systemic treatments are used ranging from topical and systemic steroids to oral antibiotics (tetracycline, erythromycin). Probably, phototherapy achieves the best therapeutic response, especially in PLC. For more severe forms methotrexate may be tried. The effectiveness of topical tacrolimus is doubtful [65, 66].

Bibliography

1. Cherry JD, Bobinski JE, Horvath FL, Comerci GD. Acute hemangioma-like lesions associated with ECHO viral infections. Pediatrics. 1969;44:498–502.
2. Prose NS, Tope W, Miller SE, Kamino H. Eruptive pseudoangiomatosis: a unique childhood exanthem? J Am Acad Dermatol. 1993;29:857–9.
3. Guillot B, Dandurand M. Eruptive pseudoangiomatosis arising in adulthood: 9 cases. Eur J Dermatol. 2000;10:455–8.
4. Jung J, Kim SC. Eruptive pseudoangiomatosis: three cases in Korean middle-aged women. Acta Derm Venereol. 2004;84:241–2.
5. Neri I, Patrizi A, Guerrini V, Ricci G, Cevenini R. Eruptive pseudoangiomatosis. Br J Dermatol. 2000;143:435–8.

6. Chuh A, Panzer R, Rosenthal AC, et al. Annular Eruptive Pseudoangiomatosis and Adenovirus Infection: A Novel Clinical Variant of Paraviral Exanthems and a Novel Virus Association. Acta Derm Venereol. 2017;97:354–7.
7. Kim JE, Kim BJ, Park HJ, et al. Clinicopathologic review of eruptive pseudoangiomatosis in Korean adults: report of 32 cases. Int J Dermatol. 2013;52:41–5.
8. Calza AM, Saurat JH. Eruptive pseudoangiomatosis: a unique childhood exanthem? J Am Acad Dermatol. 1994;31:517–8.
9. Stoebner PE, Templier I, Ligeron C, Meynadier J, Meunier L. Familial eruptive pseudoangiomatosis. Dermatology. 2002;205:306–7.
10. Navarro V, Molina I, Montesinos E, Calduch L, Jordá E. Eruptive pseudoangiomatosis in an adult. Int J Dermatol. 2000;39:237–8.
11. Chaniotakis I, Nomikos K, Gamvroulia C, Zioga A, Stergiopoulou C, Bassukas ID. Eruptive pseudoangiomatosis: report of an adult case and unifying hypothesis of the pathogenesis of paediatric and adult cases. Dermatology. 2007;215:59–62.
12. Ban M, Ichiki Y, Kitajima Y. An outbreak of eruptive pseudoangiomatosis-like lesions due to mosquito bites: erythema punctatum Higuchi. Dermatology. 2004;208:356–9.
13. Restano L, Cavalli R, Colonna C, Cambiaghi S, Alessi E, Caputo R. Eruptive pseudoangiomatosis caused by an insect bite. J Am Acad Dermatol. 2005;52:174–5.
14. Zawar V, Bharatia P, Chuh A. Eruptive hypomelanosis: a novel exanthem associated with viral symptoms in children. JAMA Dermatol. 2014;150:1197–201.
15. Chuh A, Zawar V, Maheshwari A, Bharatia P. A mini-epidemic of eruptive hypomelanosis in three children of the same family; the first piece of epidemiological evidence for an infectious cause of a novel paraviral exanthem. Clin Exp Dermatol. 2016;41:680–1.
16. Chuh A, Bharatia P, Zawar V. Eruptive Hypomelanosis in a Young Child as a "Paraviral Exanthem". Pediatr Dermatol. 2016;33:e38–9.
17. Zawar V, Bharatia P, Chuh A. Eruptive hypomelanosis in a child, a new viral exanthem. Indian J Dermatol Venereol Leprol. 2016;82:85–6.
18. Donné M, Fölster-Holst R, Van Gysel D. Eruptive hypomelanosis - First case reported outside Asia. J Dtsch Dermatol Ges. 2018;16:1260–2.
19. Relyveld GN, Menke HE, Westerhof W. Progressive macular hypomelanosis: an overview. Am J Clin Dermatol. 2007;8:13–9.
20. Drago F, Paolino S, Rebora A, et al. The challenge of diagnosing atypical exanthems: a clinico-laboratory study. J Am Acad Dermatol. 2012;67:1282–8.
21. Drago F, Ciccarese G, Gasparini G, et al. Contemporary infectious exanthems: an update. Future Microbiol. 2017;12:171–93.
22. Lipsker D, Saurat J-H. A new concept: paraviral eruptions. Dermatology. 2005;211:309–11.
23. Fölster-Holst R, Zawar VP, Chuh A. Paraviral exanthems. Expert Rev Anti Infect Ther. 2016;14:601–11.
24. Drago F, Ciccarese G, Parodi A. Pityriasis rosea and pityriasis rosea-like eruptions: How to distinguish them? JAAD Case Rep. 2018;4:800–1.
25. Bjornberg A, Hellgren L. Pityriasis rosea: a statistical, clinical, and laboratory investigation of 826 patients and matched healthy controls. Acta Derm Venereol Suppl (Stockh). 1962;42(Suppl):1–68.
26. Drago F, Broccolo F, Rebora A. Pityriasis rosea: an update with a critical appraisal of its possible herpesviral etiology. J Am Acad Dermatol. 2009;61:303–18.
27. Drago F, Ciccarese G, Rebora A, Broccolo F, Parodi A. Pityriasis Rosea: A Comprehensive Classification. Dermatology. 2016;232:431–7.
28. Ciccarese G, Broccolo F, Rebora A, Parodi A, Drago F. Oropharyngeal lesions in pityriasis rosea. J Am Acad Dermatol. 2017;77:833–837.e4.
29. Chuh A, Zawar V, Lee A. Atypical presentations of pityriasis rosea: case presentations. J Eur Acad Dermatol Venereol. 2005;19:120–6.
30. Drago F, Ciccarese G, Rebora A, Parodi A. Pityriasis rosea and pityriasis rosea-like eruption: can they be distinguished? J Dermatol. 2014;41:864–5.

31. Drago F, Ciccarese G, Rebora A, Parodi A. Relapsing pityriasis rosea. Dermatology. 2014;229:316–8.
32. Drago F, Broccolo F, Ciccarese G, Rebora A, Parodi A. Persistent pityriasis rosea: an unusual form of pityriasis rosea with persistent active HHV-6 and HHV-7 infection. Dermatology. 2015;230:23–6.
33. Drago F, Ciccarese G, Broccolo F, Cozzani E, Parodi A. Pityriasis rosea in children: clinical features and laboratory investigations. Dermatology. 2015;231:9–14.
34. Halkier-Sørensen L. Recurrent pityriasis rosea. New episodes every year for five years. A case report. Acta Derm Venereol. 1990;70:179–80.
35. Zawar V, Kumar R. Multiple recurrences of pityriasis rosea of Vidal: a novel presentation. Clin Exp Dermatol. 2009;34:e114–6.
36. Metz J. An electron microscopic investigation of the pityriasis rosea. J Cutan Pathol. 1977;4:228.
37. Aoshima T, Komura J, Ofuji S. Virus-like particles in the herald patch of pityriasis rosea. Dermatologica. 1981;162:64–5.
38. El-Shiemy S, Nassar A, Mokhtar M, Mabrouk D. Light and electron microscopic studies of pityriasis rosea. Int J Dermatol. 1987;26:237–9.
39. Drago F, Ranieri E, Malaguti F, Battifoglio ML, Losi E, Rebora A. Human herpesvirus 7 in patients with pityriasis rosea. Electron microscopy investigations and polymerase chain reaction in mononuclear cells, plasma and skin. Dermatology. 1997;195:374–8.
40. Broccolo F, Drago F, Careddu AM, et al. Additional evidence that pityriasis rosea is associated with reactivation of human herpesvirus-6 and -7. J Invest Dermatol. 2005;124:1234–40.
41. Drago F, Malaguti F, Ranieri E, Losi E, Rebora A. Human herpesvirus-like particles in pityriasis rosea lesions: an electron microscopy study. J Cutan Pathol. 2002;29:359–6.
42. Watanabe T, Kawamura T, Jacob SE, et al. Pityriasis rosea is associated with systemic active infection with both human herpesvirus-7 and human herpesvirus-6. J Invest Dermatol. 2002;119:793–7.
43. Kosuge H, Tanaka-Taya K, Miyoshi H, et al. Epidemiological study of human herpesvirus-6 and human herpesvirus-7 in pityriasis rosea. Br J Dermatol. 2000;143:795–8.
44. Drago F, Broccolo F, Javor S, Drago F, Rebora A, Parodi A. Evidence of human herpesvirus- 6 and -7 reactivation in miscarrying women with pityriasis rosea. J Am Acad Dermatol. 2014;71:198–9.
45. Drago F, Ciccarese G, Herzum A, Rebora A, Parodi A. Pityriasis Rosea during Pregnancy: Major and Minor Alarming Signs. Dermatology. 2018;234:31–6.
46. Chuh AA, Dofitas BL, Comisel GG, Reveiz L, Sharma V, Garner SE, et al. Interventions for pityriasis rosea. Cochrane Database Syst Rev. 2007;2:CD005068.
47. Drago F, Vecchio F, Rebora A. Use of high-dose acyclovir in pityriasis rosea. J Am Acad Dermatol. 2006;54:82–5.
48. Gianotti F. Papular acrodermatitis of childhood: an Australia antigen disease. Arch Dis Child. 1973;48:794–5.
49. Caputo R, Ackerman AB, Sison-Torre EQ. Gianotti-Crosti syndrome. In: Pediatric Dermatology and Dermatopathology. PhiladelfiaLea & Febiger; 1993. p. 399–410.
50. Gianotti F. Papular acrodermatitis of childhood and other papulovesicular acrolocated syndromes. Br J Dermatol. 1979;100:49–59.
51. Taieb A, Plantin P, du Pasquier P, Guillet G, Maleville J. Gianotti-Crosti syndrome a study of 26 cases. Br J Dermatol. 1986;115:49–59.
52. Caputo R, Gelmetti C, Ermacora E, Gianni E, Silvestri A. Gianotti-Crosti syndrome: a retrospective analysis of 308 cases. J Am Acad Dermatol. 1992;26:207–10.
53. Drago F, Javor S, Ciccarese G, Parodi A. Gianotti-Crosti syndrome as presenting sign of cytomegalovirus infection: A case report and a critical appraisal of its possible cytomegalovirus etiology. J Clin Virol. 2016 May;78:120–2.
54. Caltabiano R, Vecchio GM, De Pasquale R, Loreto C, Leonardi R, Vasquez E. Human ß-defensin 4 expression in Gianotti-Crosti. Acta Dermatovenerol Croat. 2013;21:43–7.

55. McCuaig CC, Russo P, Powell J, Pedneault L, Lebel P, Marcoux D. Unilateral laterothoracic exanthem. A clinicopathologic study of forty-eight patients. J Am Acad Dermatol. 1996;34:979–84.
56. Taïeb A, Mégraud F, Legrain V, Mortureux P, Maleville J. Asymmetric periflexural exanthem of childhood. J Am Acad Dermatol. 1993;29:391–3.
57. Drago F, Ciccarese G, Parodi A. Can unilateral pityriasis rosea be considered a form of superimposed lateralized exanthem? J Clin Diagn Res. 2017;11:WL01.
58. Harms M, Feldmann R. JH Saurat. Papular-purpuric "gloves and socks" syndrome. J Am Acad Dermatol. 1990;23:850–4.
59. Grilli R, Izquierdo MJ, Fariña MC, et al. Papular purpuric "gloves and socks" syndrome: polymerase chain reaction demonstration of parvovirus B19 DNA in cutaneous lesions and sera. J Am Acad Dermatol. 1999;41:793–6.
60. Santonja C, Nieto-González G, Santos-Briz Á, et al. Immunohistochemical detection of parvovirus B19 in "gloves and socks" papular purpuric syndrome: direct evidence for viral endothelial involvement. Report of three cases and review of the literature. Am J Dermatopathol. 2011;33:790–5.
61. Harms M, Feldmann R. JH Saurat. Papular-purpuric "gloves and socks" syndrome. J Am Acad Dermatol. 1990;23:850–4.
62. Grilli R, Izquierdo MJ, Fariña MC, et al. Papular purpuric "gloves and socks" syndrome: polymerase chain reaction demonstration of parvovirus B19 DNA in cutaneous lesions and sera. J Am Acad Dermatol. 1999;41:793–6.
63. Santonja C, Nieto-González G, Santos-Briz Á, et al. Immunohistochemical detection of parvovirus B19 in "gloves and socks" papular purpuric syndrome: direct evidence for viral endothelial involvement. Report of three cases and review of the literature. Am J Dermatopathol. 2011;33:790–5.
64. Bowers S. EM Warsha. Pityriasis lichenoides and its subtypes. J Am Acad Dermatol. 2006;55:557–72.
65. Rongioletti F, Rivara G, Rebora A. Pityriasis lichenoides et varioliformis acuta and acquired toxoplasmosis. Dermatologica. 1987;175:41–4.
66. Zlatkov NB, Andreev VC. Toxoplasmosis and pityriasis lichenoides. Br J Dermatol. 1972;87:114–6.

Morbihan Disease

WenChieh Chen, Bodo Melnik, and Gerd Plewig

Introduction

In 1973, Degos and coauthors reported chronic facial erythema and edema in a 64-year-old man, and with their previous case from Vannes in the Morbihan Department of Brittany, France, they described features of what is today known as Morbihan disease [1]. Earlier, in 1966, Carney presented probably the first case of acne-associated facial edema at the Los Angeles Dermatological Society with a mistaken diagnosis of lymphoma and discussed the presence of mast cells in histology and treatment with X-ray irradiation [2]. In 1981, Laugier and Gilardi from France made the first comprehensive review of Morbihan disease, introducing this terminology [3]. In 1985, Connelly and Winkelmann from the Mayo Clinic used *solid facial edema* to describe this situation in a 17-year-old boy with moderate acne [4]. In 1993, Plewig and Kligman mentioned persistent edema of rosacea as a variant of rosacea [5]. Association between lymphedema and rosacea was proposed as early as 1976 [6] and expressed in different related terms, such as persistent facial lymphedema [7], lymphedematous rosacea, rosaceous, or rosacea lymphedema [8]. This brief historical review of literature signifies persistent solid facial edema as the cardinal feature of Morbihan disease and raises questions about the strength of its association with acne or rosacea in concurrence.

W. Chen
Department of Dermatology and Allergy, Technical University of Munich, Munich, Bavaria, Germany

B. Melnik
Department of Dermatology, Environmental Medicine and Health Theory, University of Osnabrueck, Osnabrueck, Lower Saxony, Germany

G. Plewig (✉)
Department of Dermatology and Allergy, University of Munich, Munich, Bavaria, Germany
e-mail: gerd.plewig@med.uni-muenchen.de

F. Rongioletti, B. R. Smoller (eds.), *New and Emerging Entities in Dermatology and Dermatopathology*, https://doi.org/10.1007/978-3-030-80027-7_18

Epidemiology

The true prevalence is unknown. It is generally considered as a rare disease, which can be underestimated due to underreporting, underdiagnosis, or misdiagnosis. Most of the reports come from Western countries, showing a predominance in Caucasians and rarity in people of color. Association with acne occurs predominantly in men under 20 years of age [9]. The disease itself or association with rosacea is more commonly seen in people beyond 40 years of age. Gender difference varies in different studies, while male predominance was observed in our own experience.

Clinical Manifestations

The solid woody-hard nonpitting edema develops predominantly in the mid third of the face, involving the glabella, eyelids, nasal bridge, nasolabial folds, and cheeks, without scaling or *peau d'orange* phenomenon (Fig. 1). Lower eyelids are usually

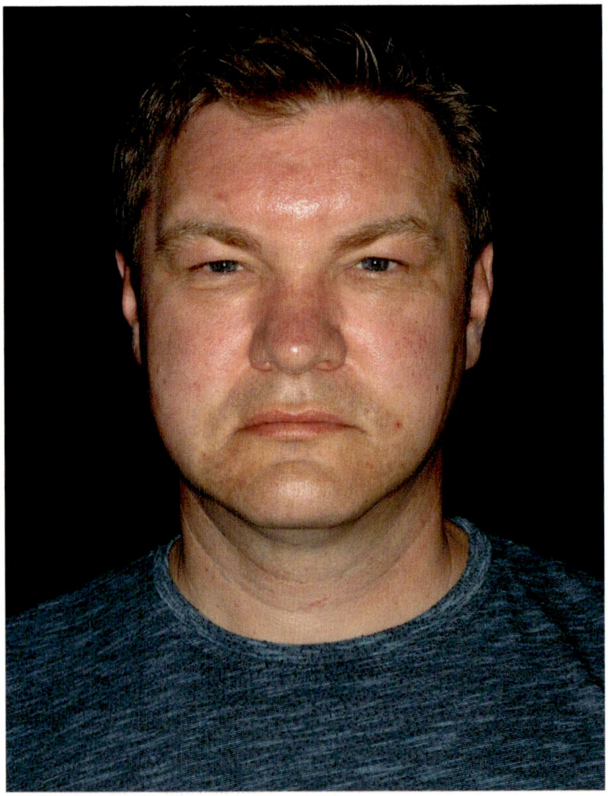

Fig. 1 Morbihan disease. Adult patient. It is a clinical *prima vista* diagnosis. Bilateral distribution of edema-looking erythematous, nonpitting fibrosis. Typical infiltrations on the forehead, upper and lower eyelids and cheeks. Written consent of patient for photography and publication without eye cover. (Copyright Department of Dermatology and Allergy, University of Munich, Germany)

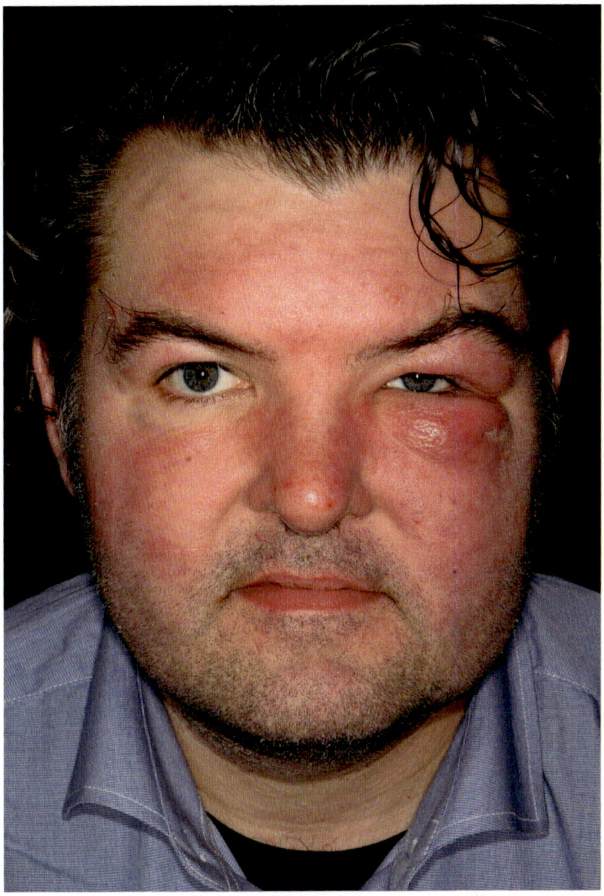

Fig. 2 Morbihan disease, progressive advanced stage, *prima vista* diagnosis. The patient was seen and treated *alio loco* by general practitioner, dermatologist, and plastic surgeon. Previous treatment with oral antibiotics, isotretinoin, and autologist abdominal lymph node transplantation to left lower and upper eyelid (2018). Postoperative unspecific non-viral ulceration. Characteristic nonpitting edematous fibrosis of central face. Written consent of patient for photography and publication without eye cover. (Copyright Department of Dermatology and Allergy, University of Munich, Germany)

more affected than the upper ones, with infraorbital swelling as a characteristic appearance (Fig. 2). Localized, asymmetric [10], or unilateral occurrence has been described [11, 12], with unknown long-term development. The skin does not indent by finger pressure. It persists ad infinitum, often increasing in severity with time, with little day-to-day variation (Fig. 3). Spontaneous involution is unlikely. Subjective complaints are slight, except for deformed facial contours. The appearance may be grotesque, presenting a grave threat to self-esteem. Cosmetic concerns are usually distressful. Otherwise, complications are rare and may include visual disturbance, excessive tearing, and headache. The disease has a chronic progressive course and is often refractory to treatment, sometimes evolving into severe forms.

Edema associated with fibrosis is not a typical expression of acne, but association of Morbihan disease with acne has been described mainly in adolescence or early adulthood. It is normally a low-grade papulopustular acne, but no severe acne with strong inflammation or acne conglobata. Most patients have a history of acne

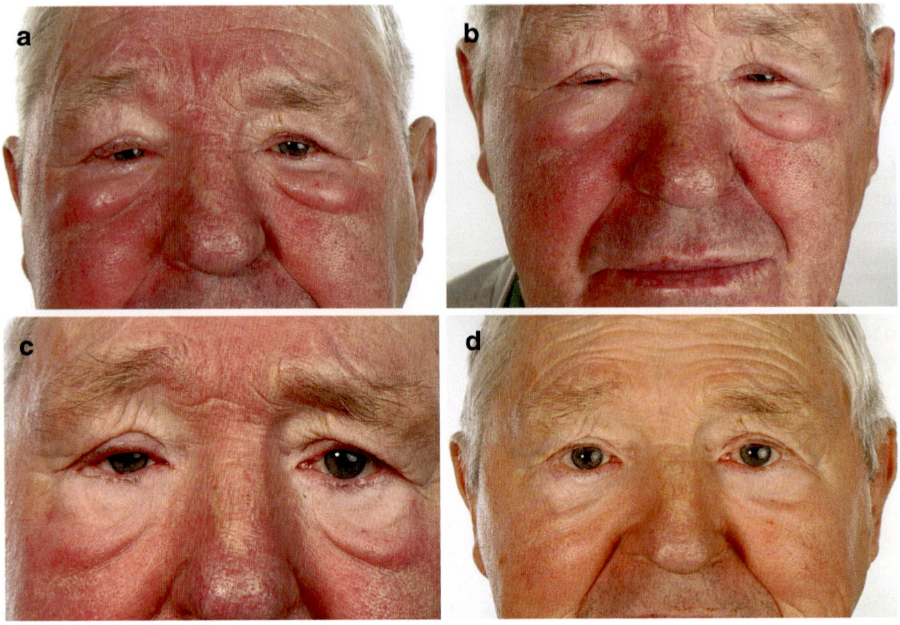

Fig. 3 Morbihan disease, much advanced stage. Photographic documentation four times. (**a**) 20.03.2021; (**b**) 02.06.2017; (**c**) 06.12.2017; (**d**) 12.03.2020. Treatment with 10 mg/day isotretinoin and 5 mg /day desloratadine for 18 months with striking results. Written consent of patient for photography and publication without eye cover. (Copyright Professor Dr. Martin Schaller, Department of Dermatology, University of Tubingen, Germany)

which predates the edema by 2–5 years or even longer [5]. This metachronous occurrence casts doubt on a causal relation.

Classical rosacea can be accompanied by varying degrees of transient or long-lasting edema in the presence of flushing and blushing, which is more pronounced during the early morning hours or after a whole-day outdoor activity. Subjective complaints are more related to rosacea, but not the edema. The classical Morbihan disease normally displays persistent edema without or with mild features of rosacea. To view Morbihan disease as a special form or variant of rosacea is questionable [5, 13] and not our view. Like acne, rosacea is either a synchronous or metachronous comorbidity, while distinction of Morbihan disease from rosacea lymphedema/ lymphedematous rosacea should be made.

Histopathology

The diagnosis is usually made clinically. There is no accepted classification correlating clinical features and histopathological findings. The histopathology is non-specific but compatible and may be necessary in atypical cases to exclude other rare

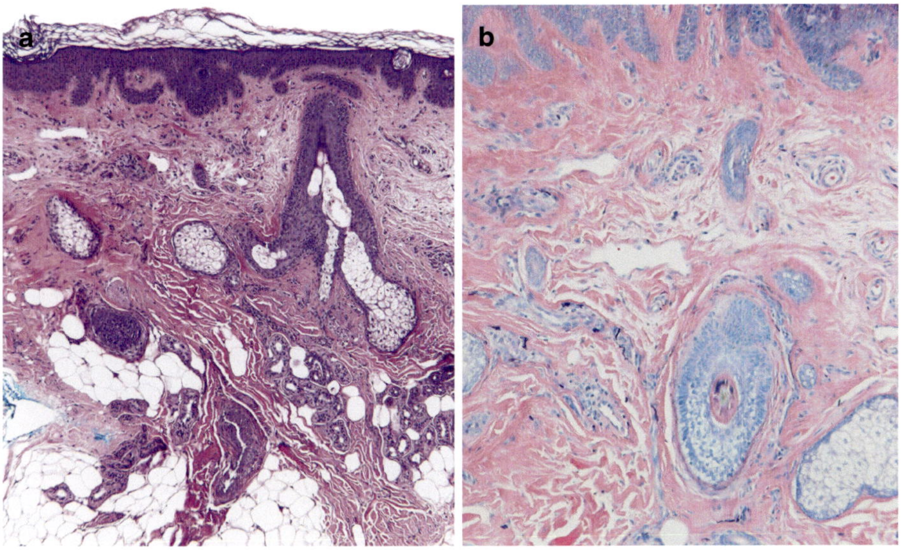

Fig. 4 (**a**) Morbihan disease. Biopsy from cheek. Ectatic lymph vessels and telangiectasias in upper corium. Dense fibrosis in mid and deep corium. H & H × 100. (**b**) Ectatic lymph vessels, dense fibrosis, and sparse mast cells. Giemsa × 200. (Copyright Professor Dr. Peter Kind, Offenbach, Germany)

causes. There is mild edema in the mid to deep dermis, conspicuous and often pronounced deep reaching fibrosis, dilated lymph vessels, and variously dense perivascular lymphohistiocytic infiltrate [5, 14] (Fig. 4). An increased number of mast cells in the lesion sites were observed in typical cases (Fig. 5), but a recent study found the mean number per 10 high-power field to be much lower than previously reported in telangiectatic rosacea or rhinophyma and within previously reported limits in healthy skin [14]. Evidently the amount of mast cells correlates with the amount of fibrosis and duration of the disease (Fig. 6).

The key feature is fibrosis with thickening of the connective tissue up to two to four times its normal size, extending into the subcutaneous fat in fibrous strands (Fig. 6). Perifollicular fibrosis and peri- or intralymphatic granuloma have been observed in up to 50% of the patients [5, 14], but their correlation with the disease severity is unknown. It is unclear whether these are the primary process or later findings in advanced disease. Differential diagnosis in histopathology may include Melkersson-Rosenthal syndrome with pareiitis granulomatosa, granulomatous rosacea, lupus miliaris disseminatus faciei, and sarcoidosis, but all of them differ from genuine Morbihan disease, in conjunction with clinical features.

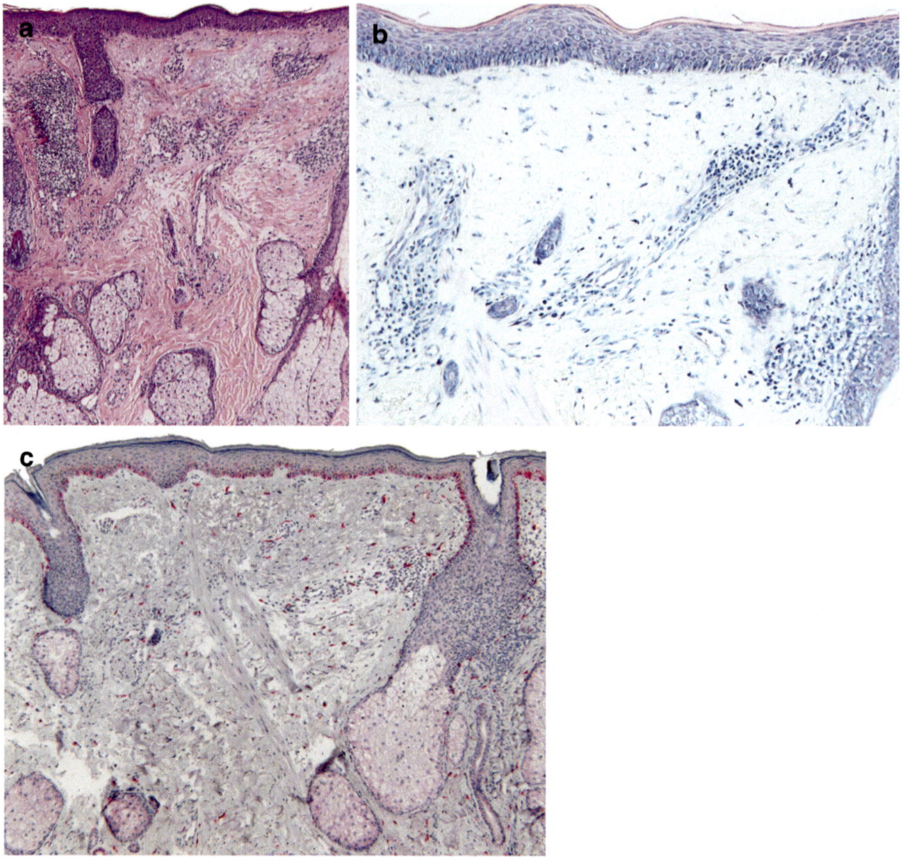

Fig. 5 (**a**) Morbihan disease. Biopsy from cheek. Actinic damage of upper corium. Dilated lymph vessels and venous vasculature. Perivascular and perisebaceous follicle round cell infiltrates. Dense fibrosis of mid-corium (and deeper corium, not shown here). H & E × 100. (**b**) Morbihan disease. Mast cells around vascular structures and dispersed in the corium. Giemsa × 200. (**c**) Morbihan disease. Same biopsy as (**a, b**). CD117 stain for better visualization of mast cells. Actinic elastosis above, fibrosis below. (Copyright Professor Dr. Michael Flaig, Department of Dermatology and Allergy, University of Munich, Germany)

Etiopathogenesis

Pathogenesis remains largely unknown, while clinical evidence indicates a disease sui generis. Because Morbihan disease is rare while acne and rosacea are common, their coexistence is probably coincidental rather than correlated. Simultaneous appearance has been observed only in single cases, and there is no correlation between development of the solid facial edema and the severity of acne or the subtypes/stages of rosacea. In comparison to acne or rosacea, Morbihan disease shows a very refractory response to oral isotretinoin. This relatively scarce mast cell

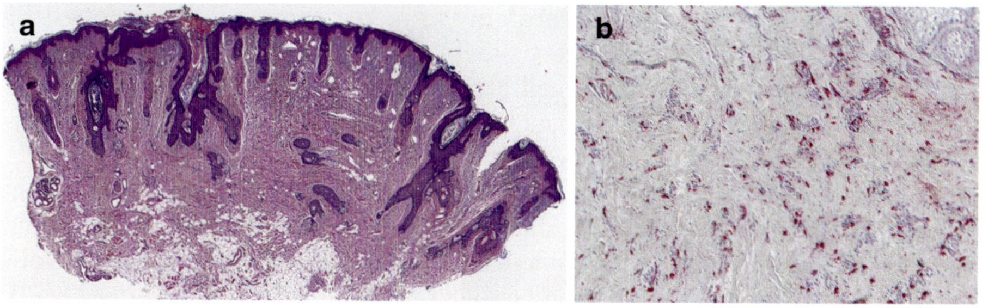

Fig. 6 (**a**) Morbihan disease. Advanced stage. Facial biopsy. Ectatic vasculature subepidermal, upper and mid-corium. Striking fibrosis extending deep into corium and subcutaneous fat. Regression of sebaceous lobules of sebaceous and vellus hair follicles, replace by fibrosis. H & E, panoramic view. (**b**) Same biopsy as (**a**). Numerous mast cells throughout the densely fibrosed corium. CD117 stain for better demonstration of mast cells. (Copyright of Professor Dr. Gerd Plewig, Department of Dermatology and Allergy, University of Munich, Germany)

infiltrate in histology as compared to that in rosacea further supports the distinction of Morbihan disease from rosacea, according to Ramirez-Bellver et al. [14].

The original assumption that intense UV irradiation is responsible for the facial edema is not corroborated in other reports, especially for a few cases with exclusive or predominant involvement of the upper eyelids [15]. It is unclear why the persistent solid edema/fibrosis affects mainly the midface but no other extra-facial areas. There is generally no evidence for an allergic or autoimmune etiology. Contact urticaria associated with various cosmetic ingredients was found in a series of six patients [16], in whom photosensitivity was not confirmed and photocontact sensitization unclear. The role of smoking in inducing or exacerbating the edema remains to be determined. Some of our patients were non-smokers, and we do not believe in this context. There is no indication of a genetic predisposition to Morbihan disease, although an association with acne in twins was described [17].

The characteristic edema/fibrosis in the mid third of the face may be explained in consideration of the anatomy of the facial lymph drainage. Swelling in the eyelids and palpebromalar grooves is mainly caused by lymph stasis in the lateral 2/3 of the upper and lower eyelids draining to superficial lymph nodes in the preauricular/parotid basin. Disturbance in the medial 1/3 of the orbital lymphatic drainage directing to superficial lymph nodes in the submandibular basin is associated with swelling in the nasolabial grooves. The lymphatics in the frontal region begin from the superior edge of the eyebrow and drain into nasolabial, preauricular/parotid, and retroauricular lymph nodes, whereas an impairment can lead to frontal swelling. Therapeutically autologous lymph node transplantation, e.g., from the abdomen to periorbital location, is rarely propagated by plastic surgeons. We cannot follow this concept.

Histological and translational evidence indicates that increased mast cell activity may be an important driver in the pathogenesis of persistent solid facial edema/fibrosis in Morbihan disease [10, 14]. Mast cells are preferentially located in close proximity to both vascular and lymphatic vessels in normal state and on activation can regulate vascular flow and permeability to recruit various inflammatory cells from the vasculature into inflammatory sites [18, 19]. Among the multiple cytokines and signaling molecules, the mast cell-derived vascular endothelial growth factor (VEGF) can promote angiogenesis and lymphangiogenesis [20] and increase endothelial cell permeability, leading to edema, lymphedema, and lymphatic vessel dilations [14, 19]. Mast cells are often involved in skin fibrosis [21], another important histological feature of advanced Morbihan disease [21]. Isotretinoin, ketotifen, and desloratadine all affect mast cell function. In vitro and animal studies show all-trans-retinoic acid, the isomerization product of isotretinoin (13-cis-retinoic acid), inhibits mast cell proliferation [22], whereas ketotifen and desloratadine impair mast cell degranulation [23, 24], which provide potential explanations for their synergistic pharmacological effects [25–27].

As the density of mast cells is elevated in the mid- and late phase of many inflammatory processes, it remains to be determined whether their presence in Morbihan disease is disease specific or not. It is to note that the property and course of edema or fibrosis differ in diverse diseases associated with mast cells, such as angioedema, scleroderma, and lymphedema. It is crucial to demonstrate the expression of VEGF in the lesion sites of Morbihan disease. Lymphatic dysplasia is not confirmed in Morbihan disease [28]. Direct evidence is lacking in terms of lymphatic obstruction and vascular dilatation caused by marked peri- /intralymphatic granulomas and chronic inflammation [29]. Discrepancies between in vitro and in vivo findings must be kept in mind, especially in the clinical application of translational evidence [22, 23]. Superiority of levocetirizine to other antihistamines remains to be verified, based on the remarkable therapeutic effect demonstrated by Welsch and Schaller in their case report [27]. Studies are required to demonstrate the long-term effects of low-dose isotretinoin, tetracyclines, or antihistamines in reduction of the number and activity of mast cells.

Treatment

There is no standard treatment, while controlled studies are lacking. We have used in the past 25 years low-dose isotretinoin, 0.1–0.2 mg/kg body wt. daily, combined with 2 mg ketotifen daily, instead of desloratadine, over a period of 6–12 months or even longer [5, 25]. The efficacy of this combination is partly explained by the anti-inflammatory effect and tissue remodeling of isotretinoin in the regulation of fibroblast and extracellular matrix proteins [30]. Isotretinoin, ketotifen, and desloratadine show inhibitory effect on mast cells. The daily and cumulative doses of an effective isotretinoin treatment vary in different reports [9, 25, 26, 31, 32], which are difficult to compare based on the available data. A long period of treatment seems essential for a substantial persisting improvement in most treated patients. Combination of isotretinoin with desloratadine has displayed dramatic results in four patients [27] (Fig. 3). Recalcitrance or failure to treatment is not uncommon, while prediction of treatment response is difficult. Long-term follow-up over years after treatment cessation is mostly lacking [32].

In countries where oral isotretinoin is not available, both doxycycline (200 mg daily) and minocycline (100 mg daily), alone or in combination with initial low-dose systemic steroids, have been demonstrated to be effective [10, 29, 33, 34]. Due to the concerns of long-term use of antibiotics, it is not recommended by us.

Successful treatment in single case reports as monotherapy or supplements may include systemic prednisolone, thalidomide, diuretics (furosemide or spironolactone) [35], metronidazole, clofazimine, and omalizumab [36]. Local steroid injection and surgical intervention, including debulking, blepharoplasty, or autologous lymph node transplantation, have also been described [37, 38], but the therapeutic benefit-risk ratio is not convincing.

Differential Diagnosis

The primary pitfall is Melkersson-Rosenthal syndrome. In 1956 and the ensuing years, Schimpf termed dermatitis granulomatosa frontalis/periorbitalis to describe three men of middle to old age exhibiting long-lasting localized swelling in the fronto-glabella areas, with or without lingua plicata or rosacea, and histologic pictures of cheilitis granulomatosa [39]. In our view, they represented variants of Melkersson-Rosenthal syndrome but not Morbihan disease [40].

Conclusions

Morbihan disease remains enigmatic. An enhanced awareness of its characteristic manifestation helps to explore the true prevalence of this disease sui generis. The comorbidity with acne or rosacea appears coincidentally. Comparison of histopathology in different stages of the disease combined with investigation of mast cell density with computer-assisted techniques and molecular biology of mast activation may provide further clues to the pathogenesis. Long-term observation is required to better define the treatment response and disease course.

Acknowledgments Dr. Katharina Welsh and Prof. Dr. med. Martin Schaller from the Department of Dermatology and Allergy, Eberhard Karls University of Tubingen, Germany, kindly contributed the clinical pictures (Fig. 3). We thank Prof. Dr. Peter Kind, Histologielabor Offenbach, for the histologic figures. Professor Dr. Michael Flaig, Department of Dermatology and Allergy, University of Munich, Germany, kindly assisted with the production of histological illustrations.

References

1. Degos R, Civatte J, Beuve-Mery M. Nouveau cas d'oedeme erythemateux facial chronique. Bull Soc Fr Dermatol Sypiligr. 1973;80:257.
2. Carney JW. Solid edema of face (??). Arch Dermatol. 1966;94:664–6.
3. Laugier P, Gilardi S. L'cedème érythémateux chronique facial supérieur (Degos) [chronic erythematous oedema of the upper face (Degos). Morbihan disease (author's transl)]. Ann Dermatol Venereol. 1981;108:507–13.
4. Connelly MG, Winkelmann RK. Solid facial edema as a complication of acne vulgaris. Arch Dermatol. 1985;121:87–90.
5. Plewig G, Melnik B, Chen W. Acne and Rosacea. 4th ed. Cham: Springer; 2019. p. 72, 552, 563, 566.
6. Marks R. Common facial dermatoses. Bristol: Wright; 1976. p. 12.
7. Wilkin JK. Rosacea. Int J Dermatol. 1983;22:393–400.
8. Scerri L, Saihan EM. Persistent facial swelling in a patient with rosacea. Rosacea lymphedema. Arch Dermatol. 1995;131:1071–4.
9. Kuhn-Régnier S, Mangana J, Kerl K, Kamarachev J, French LE, Cozzio A, et al. Dermatol Ther (Heidelb). 2017;7:167–74.
10. Fujimoto N, Mitsuru M, Tanaka T. Successful treatment of Morbihan disease with long-term minocycline and its association with mast cell infiltration. Acta Derm Venereol. 2015;95:368–9.
11. Weeraman S, Birnie A. Rosacea causing unilateral Morbihan syndrome. BMJ Case Rep. 2019;12:e231074.
12. Heibel HD, Heibel MD, Cockerell CJ. Successful treatment of solid persistent facial edema with isotretinoin and compression therapy. JAAD Case Rep. 2020;6:755–7.
13. Balakirski G, Baron JM, Megahed M. Morbus Morbihan als Sonderform der Rosazea: Einblick in die Pathogenese und neue Therapieoptionen [Morbihan disease as a special form of rosacea: review of pathogenesis and new therapeutic options]. Hautarzt. 2013;64(12):884–6.
14. Ramirez-Bellver JL, Pérez-González YC, Chen KR, Díaz-Recuero JL, Requena L, Carlson JA, et al. Clinicopathological and immunohistochemical study of 14 cases of Morbihan disease: an insight into its pathogenesis. Am J Dermatopathol. 2019;41:701–7.
15. de Vasconcelos RCF, Eid NT, Eid RT, Moriya FS, Braga BB, Michalany AO. Morbihan syndrome: a case report and literature review. An Bras Dermatol. 2016;91(5 Supl 1):S157–9.
16. Wohlrab J, Lueftl M, Marsch WC. Persistent erythema and edema of the mid third and upper aspect of the face (morbus Morbihan): evidence of hidden immunologic contact urticaria and impaired lymphatic drainage. J Am Acad Dermatol. 2005;52:595–602.
17. Tosti A, Guerra L, Bettoli V, Bonelli U. Solid facial edema as a complication of acne vulgaris in twins. J Am Acad Dermatol. 1987;17(5 Pt 1):843–4.
18. Kunder CA, St John AL, Abraham SN. Mast cell modulation of the vascular and lymphatic endothelium. Blood. 2011;118:5383–93.
19. Pal S, Nath S, Meininger CJ, Gashev AA. Emerging roles of mast cells in the regulation of lymphatic immuno-physiology. Front Immunol. 2020;11:1234.
20. Varricchi G, Granata F, Loffredo S, Genovese A, Marone G. Angiogenesis and lymphangiogenesis in inflammatory skin disorders. J Am Acad Dermatol. 2015;73:144–53.
21. Strattan E, Palaniyandi S, Kumari R, Du J, Hakim N, Huamg T, et al. Mast cells are mediators of fibrosis and effector cell recruitment in dermal chronic graft-vs.-host disease. Front Immunol. 2019;10:2470.
22. Babina M, Artuc M, Guhl S, Zuberbier T. Retinoic acid negatively impacts proliferation and MC_{TC} specific attributes of human skin derived mast cells, but reinforces allergic stimulability. Int J Mol Sci. 2017;18:525.
23. Wang YH, Taché Y, Harris AG, Kreutner W, Daly AF, Wei JY. Desloratadine prevents compound 48/80-induced mast cell degranulation: visualization using a vital fluorescent dye technique. Allergy. 2005;60:117–24.

24. Iuvone T, Den Bossche RV, D'Acquisto F, Carnuccio R, Herman AG. Evidence that mast cell degranulation, histamine and tumour necrosis factor alpha release occur in LPS-induced plasma leakage in rat skin. Br J Pharmacol. 1999;128:700–4.
25. Jungfer B, Jansen T, Prybilla B, Plewig G. Solid persistent facial edema in acne: successful treatment with isotretinoin and ketotifen. Dermatology. 1993;187:34–7.
26. Mazzatenta C, Giorgino G, Rubegni P, de Aloe G, Fimiani M. Solid persistent facial oedema (Morbihan's disease) following rosacea, successfully treated with isotretinoin and ketotifen. Br J Dermatol. 1997;137:1020–1.
27. Welsch K, Schaller M. Combination of ultra-low-dose isotretinoin and antihistamines in treating Morbihan disease – a new long-term approach with excellent results and a minimum of side effects. J Dermatolog Treat. 2020:1–4.
28. Jansen T, Regele D, Schirren CG, Trautner B, Plewig G. Persistierendes Erythem und Odem des Gesichts bei Rosazea und Lymphgefässdysplasie [Persistent erythema and edema of the face associated with rosacea and lymph vessel dysplasia]. Hautarzt. 1998;49:932–5.
29. Nagasaka T, Koyama T, Matsumura K, Chen KR. Persistent lymphoedema in Morbihan disease: formation of perilymphatic epithelioid cell granulomas as a possible pathogenesis. Clin Exp Dermatol. 2008;33:764–7.
30. Bravo BSF, Azulay DR, Raggio Luiz R, Mandarim-De-Lacerda CA, Cuzzi T, Azulay MM. Oral isotretinoin in photoaging: objective histological evidence of efficacy and durability. An Bras Dermatol. 2015;90:479–86.
31. Smith LA, Cohen DE. Successful long-term use of oral isotretinoin for the management of Morbihan disease: a case series report and review of the literature. Arch Dermatol. 2012;148:1395–8.
32. Olvera-Cortés V, Pulido-Díaz N. Effective treatment of Morbihan's disease with long-term isotretinoin: a report of three cases. J Clin Aesthet Dermatol. 2019;12:32–4.
33. Ranu H, Lee J, Hee TH. Successful treatment of Morbihan's disease with oral prednisolone and doxycycline. Dermatol Ther. 2010;23:682–5.
34. Okubo A, Takahashi K, Akasaka T, Amano H. Four cases of Morbihan disease successfully treated with doxycycline. J Dermatol. 2017;44:713–6.
35. Messikh R, Try C, Bennani B, Humbert P. Maladie du Morbihan Œdème facial persistant solide Rosacée lymphœdémateuse Diurétiques Furosémide Traitement. Ann Dermatol Venereol. 2012;139:559–63.
36. Kafi P, Edén I, Swartling C. Morbihan syndrome successfully treated with Omalizumab. Acta Derm Venereol. 2019;99:677–8.
37. Renieri G. Chronisches Lidödem assoziiert mit Rosazea (Morbus Morbihan): Differenzialdiagnostische Schwierigkeiten und Therapieoptionen. Klin Monatsbl Augenheilkd. 2011;228:19–24.
38. Carruth BP, Meyer DR, Wladis EJ, Bradley EA, Al-Rohil R, Jones DM, et al. Extreme eyelid lymphedema associated with rosacea (Morbihan disease): case series, literature review, and therapeutic considerations. Ophthalm Plast Reconstr Surg. 2017;33(3S Suppl 1):S34–8.
39. Schimpf A. Dermatitis frontalis granulomatosa. Derm Wschr. 1956;133:120.
40. Veraldi S, Persico MC, Francia C. Morbihan syndrome. Indian Dermatol Online J. 2013;4:122–4.

Part II
Entities with Systemic Implications

Aquagenic (Pseudo)keratoderma

Laura Atzori, Caterina Ferreli, and Franco Rongioletti

Introduction

Aquagenic palmoplantar keratoderma (APK) is a rare skin disease, coded 498,359 in the Orphanet portal, whose pathogenesis remains undermined, but characterized by the exaggerate skin wrinkling of the palms, less frequently the soles in response to immersion or contact with water [1].

Other synonyms are aquagenic pseudo-keratoderma, aquagenic syringeal acrokeratoderma, aquagenic wrinkling of the palms, transient aquagenic palmar hyperwrinkling, and aquagenic (pseudo)keratoderma.

The condition was firstly described in two sisters in 1996 by English and McCollough, suggesting an autosomal recessive pattern of inheritance [2]. Because of the characteristic spontaneous healing after skin drying, they coined the term "transient reactive papulotranslucent acrokeratoderma," in contraposition to the "hereditary papulotranslucent acrokeratoderma," described by Onwukwe et al. [3], which is characterized by an autosomal-dominant transmission and persistent, yellowish to white papules and plaques, associated with fine-textured scalp hair and an atopic diathesis. With time, the more sporadic occurrence of APK has been outlined [4–15], with a predilection for women, age ranging from 8 to 65 years, with a mean of 27 years in a large case series [13].

Prevalence of the diseases is unknown and probably underestimated due to the mildness of symptoms and a very variable course during lifetime, with period of remission and different seasonal exacerbation, as well as complete recovery [16]. However, APK can represent the alerting sign of the occurrence of internal

L. Atzori (✉) · C. Ferreli
Dermatology Clinic, Department of Medical Sciences and Public Health, University of Cagliari, Cagliari, Italy
e-mail: atzoril@unica.it; ferreli@unica.it

F. Rongioletti
Dermatology Clinic, Vita-Salute S.Raffaele University, Milan, Italy

F. Rongioletti, B. R. Smoller (eds.), *New and Emerging Entities in Dermatology and Dermatopathology*, https://doi.org/10.1007/978-3-030-80027-7_19

pathologies. Already in 1974, Elliott RB [17], before formal characterization of the disorder, described the water-induced skin wrinkling among children affected with cystic fibrosis (CF), often as a presenting sign. This association has been increasingly confirmed in the following years [18–25], leading to the mutation discovery on the cystic fibrosis transmembrane conductance regulator gene (CFTR), usually the ΔF508, either homozygous or heterozygous. A prevalence of 41–84% of APK in patients with CF has been described [26–30].

Other acquired conditions associated with APK include cardiac diseases, nephrotic syndrome, Raynaud phenomenon, marasmus, and therapeutic drug intake [13, 31–33]. Especially nonsteroidal anti-inflammatory drugs, from acetylsalicylic acid to selective cyclooxygenase-2 enzyme inhibitors celecoxib and rofecoxib, have been found able to induce this anomalous hyperwrinkling of the skin in response to water contact [34–36]. Association with gabapentin, tobramycin, isotretinoin, and spironolactone has also been reported [37–39].

Clinical Features

Morphological changes develop characteristically 3–5 minutes after contact with water and consist of symmetrical hypopigmented, translucent, flat-topped, edematous papules and plaques, confluent to occupy normal folds, as well as exaggerating the roughness of the skin surface (hyperwrinkling) on palms (Figs. 1 and 2), fingers, and, rarely, on soles [4–14]. Lesions last from 10 minutes to 1 hour, resolving with skin drying. A duration of 2 hours has been reported [35]. Erythema is uncommon [40], and desquamation is also variable. Unilateral involvement has been reported [36, 41], as well as the uncommon presentation on the dorsum of hands and fingers, anterior face of the wrist, ankles, and medial aspect of heel [25, 42–45]. Both

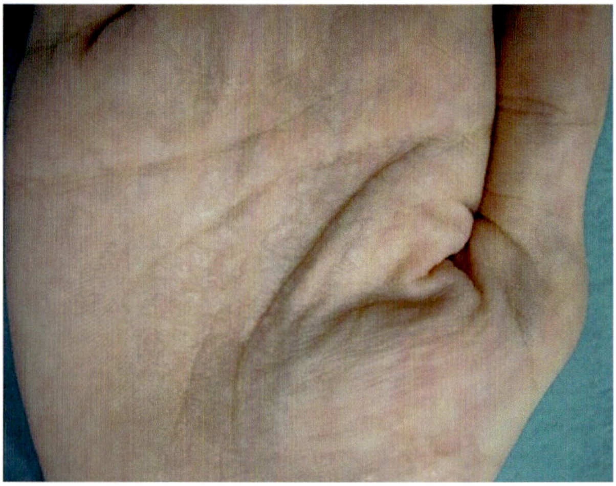

Fig. 1 Aquagenic keratoderma: hypopigmented, translucent, flat-topped, edematous papules and exaggerate roughness of the skin surface (hyperwrinkling) on the left palm

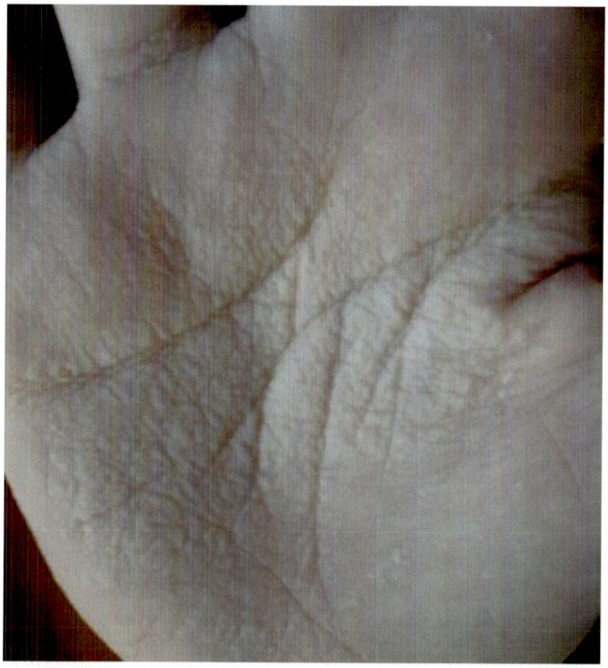

Fig. 2 Aquagenic keratoderma: closer view of the palmar lesions

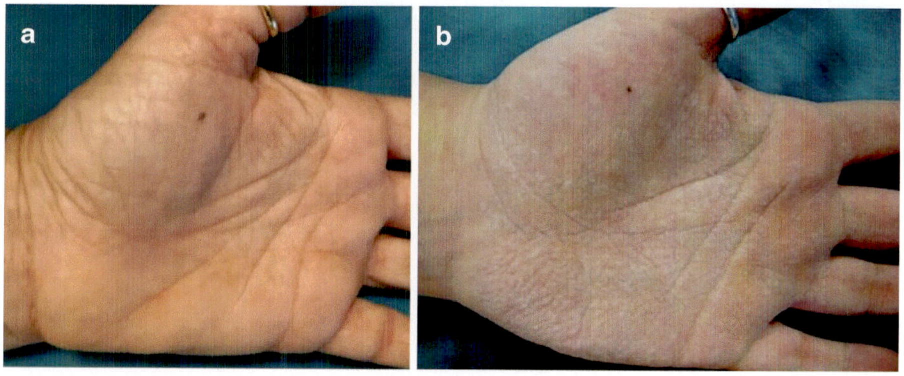

Fig. 3 Palmar surface before (**a**) and after hand immersion (**b**) into warm water for 5 minutes ("hands in the bucket" sign)

asymptomatic disease and variable pruritus to burning or painful lesions are reported. Associated palmoplantar hyperhidrosis is frequent [6, 13, 15]. Duration of water exposure and warm temperature influence the rapidity and intensity of the presentation. A diagnostic test (Fig. 3) to reproduce the lesions can be performed by plunging the patient's hands into warm or cold water for a few minutes ("hands in the bucket" sign) [6, 13, 30].

In patients with associated CF, a very rapid response to water contact (within 2–3 minutes) is characteristic of homozygous patients, while in CF carriers (9–25% of patients), the reaction typically takes 5–7 min to develop [30].

Histopathologic Features

Diagnosis is usually made on a clinical basis, and histopathologic studies are seldom performed due to the limited differential diagnosis options [13, 46]. However, it is important to perform the skin biopsy immediately after water immersion to preserve the pathologic findings, which completely disappear in the dry skin [7, 13, 47]. Most prevalent changes involve the epidermis (Fig. 4), showing ortho-hyperkeratosis, hyper-granulosis, and acanthosis. A remarkable increase of the stratum corneum thickness is associated with characteristic abnormal tinctorial affinity, related to the imbibition and increased water content, causing hydropic changes [13]. An abnormal pallor, or metachromasia of the corneum, is seen, with various shades of basophilic and eosinophilic staining reactions, associated with dilated sweat glands, acrosyringia, and dermal eccrine ducts, showing hyperplasia, clear cell changes, and vacuolation (Fig. 5). Sometimes, the lumen of the eccrine ductal structures shows an irregular-shaped lumen, with papillary projections and fluid eosinophilic secretion. Increased capillaries around the eccrine coils at the dermo-epidermal junction are other typical findings [13].

Histopathologic findings are noteworthy to exclude a true keratoderma, whose hyperkeratosis is due to an increased turnover of the keratinocytes or defect in cornification [48]. Thus, the name of "pseudo-keratoderma" should apply to APK.

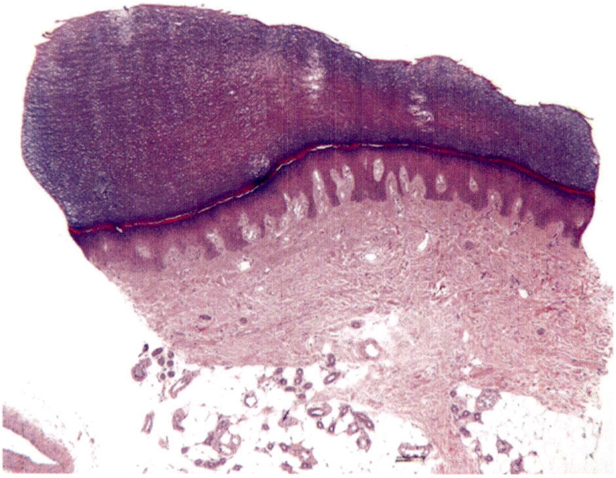

Fig. 4 Histopathology of palmar skin biopsy after water immersion: prominent epidermal changes, with ortho-hyperkeratosis, hyper-granulosis, and acanthosis. Characteristic metachromasia of the thickened stratum corneum, with various shades of basophilic and eosinophilic staining reaction (hematoxylin and eosin, magnification 4×)

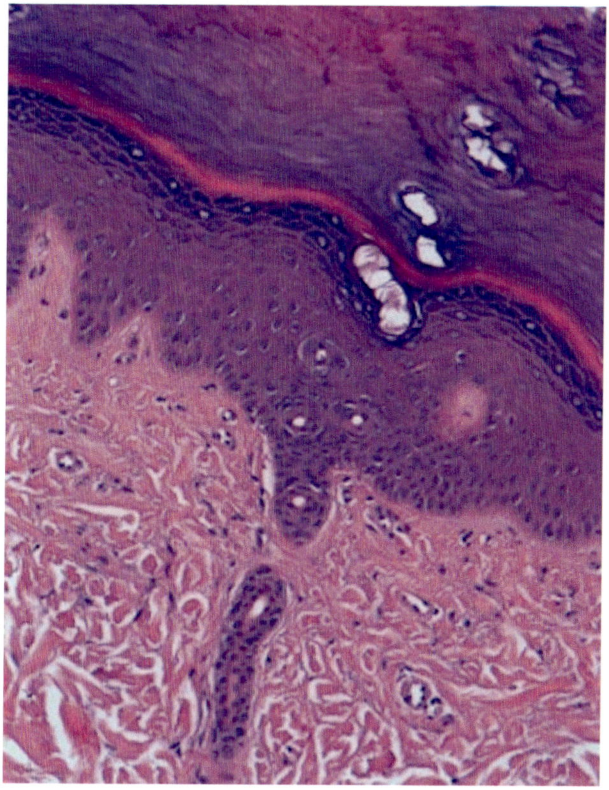

Fig. 5 Closer view of the stratum corneum metachromasia, hydropic changes, with associated dilated acrosyringia, and dermal eccrine ducts (H&E, 10×)

Work-Up

The diagnosis of APK is primarily based on clinical features and a careful anamnesis conveying all essential information. Although there are not standardized parameters for the "hands in the bucket test" (Fig. 3), usually it is performed asking the patient to immerse the hands in warm water (15 °C) for 5 minutes to replicate symptoms [5, 12, 13].

Dermoscopy soon after water immersion has been suggested as a noninvasive assessment to confirm the diagnosis, showing the stratum corneum hypertrophy and dilation of the eccrine ducts of the affected areas in respect to the surrounding skin [49, 50]. Histopathologic examination may be relevant to exclude other conditions.

Another important issue is to rule out associated pathology, especially asymptomatic CF, internal organ diseases, and drug intake. Complete screening of the CFTR gene should be recommended, because rare mutations, especially in heterozygosity, could be missed with panel screening [29, 51, 52].

Differential Diagnosis

The main differential diagnosis of APK is with the hereditary papulotranslucent acrokeratoderma, which appears soon after puberty, persists throughout the patient's life, and cannot be induced by water immersion or resolve by drying [3]. Histopathology is characterized by focal hyperkeratosis, acanthosis, and normal eccrine ducts [13].

A histopathological differential diagnosis is with the eccrine angiomatous nevus, which is a hamartomatous hyperplasia of the capillary vessels around dilated eccrine glands [53]. However, a hyperplasia of other dermal components is usually present, involving follicular structures, fat tissue, and nerve fibers. Mucin deposition is an additional finding. Clinical presentation is also different from APK, characterized by persistent brownish-yellow hyperhidrotic papules or plaque.

From a clinical point of view, other disorders triggered by a brief contact with water, such as aquagenic urticaria and aquagenic pruritus, consist of more generalized manifestations [54].

Etiopathogenesis

Hereditary transmission seems rare in respect to sporadic observations [2, 11, 13, 14, 55, 56]. Although the role of water as a trigger for the skin manifestations is well known, the exact APK pathogenesis remains unclear. Two events are characteristic and reproducible in this condition: an abnormal concentration of electrolytes in the sweat, and thus into keratinocytes of the epidermal layers, and an increased ability of the stratum corneum to absorb and retain water, similar to what happens in the defective atopic skin barrier [13]. Whether the primary culprit relies on a sweat glands' alteration or a structural defect of the stratum corneum keratinocytes remains uncovered. Insights are suggested by the frequent association with CF, whose mutations of the CFTR gene encode for an ion channel, involved in the regulation of intracellular electrolyte transport and consequent sweat salt concentration [16, 21, 26–29]. The loss of function of this gene may compromise the electrolyte reabsorption in the eccrine ducts and increase the osmotic influx water gradient from the epidermal cells. Another recent hypothesis [57] proposed an aberrant expression of the transient vanilloid receptor type 1 (TVRT-1), which is an osmosensitive receptor, whose expression is enhanced by temperature and acidity. Its activation results in an increased calcium influx and cell swelling [58]. A concomitant overexpression of selective aquaporins (AQPs), especially the AQP3, AQP5, and AQP10 which have the ability to rapidly open water channels, can play a role in the sweating dysregulation [59]. The involvement of the TVRT-1 also explains the characteristic worsening and more rapid occurrence of lesions with higher water temperature and salt concentration. Other potential pathogenetic mechanisms include a weakness of the eccrine duct wall, occlusion of the eccrine duct ostia, or an autonomic nervous system dysfunction [13]. A further confirmation of the role of the electrolytes in sweat is the ability of several drugs to induce AK, including cyclooxygenase 2 inhibitors and spironolactone, which are able to affect cell sodium reabsorption and retention [34–36, 40].

Therapy

Although often asymptomatic, APK can cause a relevant physical and psychological discomfort, especially in daily activities, as water contact cannot easily avoided. Discontinuation of suspect drugs to induce APK should be encouraged. Oral antihistamines may be useful in selected cases with prominent itching [40]. There is not a consensus recommendation, but several topical treatments have been proposed, with variable results. Aluminum chloride hexahydrate 20% is among most prescribed medications, followed by topical corticosteroids, salicylic acid 5% or 12% ointment, formalin in alcohol, urea ointment, barrier agents, and topical antibiotics [2, 13, 40, 60]. Ammonium lactate 12% cream applications or the use of gloves seems not to be effective [40].

Tap water iontophoresis has been effective in several cases [61, 62], targeting areas with high levels of electrolytes and producing a local electrochemical coagulation of proteins or interrupting the stimulus-secretion coupling essential to the sweat secretion.

Botulinum toxin injection is an option for poor response to topics [41, 63, 64], but patients should be very motivated due to the relative costs and temporary effects.

Oral oxybutynin chloride (2.5 mg twice daily), an anticholinergic agent effective on hyperhidrosis, has been suggested [44], but further experiences are lacking. Surgery, based on endoscopic thoracic sympathectomy, has been reported as efficacious in a 31-year-old man with long-term remission [65] and might be considered as a permanent solution for severe cases, especially when palmar hyperhidrosis is associated.

Prognosis and Course

Spontaneous remission has been described [16], and variations during patients' lifetimes are also frequently reported, with periods during which water exposure does not cause skin changes. Probably, the disease often goes unrecognized, as patients do not seek medical advice for symptoms that rapidly resolve with drying of the skin. A more severe course is characteristic of patients with associated homozygous CF, causing physical and psychologic discomfort.

Conclusions

Rare disorders, with a peculiar clinical presentation, such as APK are easily recognized if faced at least once. Although an autosomal recessive inheritance has been advocated, sporadic occurrence is much more frequent, affecting the palms and occasionally the soles of adolescent females. Lesions are reproducible by immersing the patient's hands into warm or cold water for a few minutes. Association with cystic fibrosis should be evaluated with genetic or sweat test, to exclude asymptomatic and late-onset cases. Other comorbidities and drug intake should also be investigated. Despite multiple hypotheses, etiopathogenetic understanding is incomplete. Histopathology supports the role of eccrine gland alterations, with dilated dermal ducts and ostia, as well as an exaggerated water retention in the stratum corneum. Treatment remains a challenge, especially for patients complaining severe discomfort in daily activity, requiring contact with water. Further investigations are warrant to elucidate fine pathogenetic mechanisms and indicate best treatments, targeting the causative factors.

References

1. Orphanet version 5.41.0 - Last updated: 2020-11-28. www.orpha.net
2. English JC, McCollough ML. Transient reactive papulotranslucent acrokeratoderma. J Am Acad Dermatol. 1996;34:686–7.
3. Onwukwe MF, Mihm MC Jr, Toda K. Hereditary papulotranslucent acrokeratoderma. A new variant of familial punctate keratoderma? Arch Dermatol. 1973;108:108–10.
4. MacCormack MA, Wiss K, Malhotra R. Aquagenic syringeal acrokeratoderma: report of two teenage cases. J Am Acad Dermatol. 2001;45:124–6.
5. Yan AC, Sumaira ZA, Alms WJ, et al. Aquagenic palmoplantar keratoderma. J Am Acad Dermatol. 2001;44:696–9.
6. Itin PH, Lautenschlager S. Aquagenic syringeal acrokeratoderma (transient reactive papulotranslucent acrokeratoderma). Dermatology. 2002;204:8–11.
7. Belloch I, Vergara G, Albares MP, et al. Aquagenic keratoderma. J Eur Acad Dermatol Venereol. 2003;17:306–7.
8. Schmults C, Sidhu G, Urbanek W. Aquagenic syringeal acrokeratoderma. Dermatol Online J. 2003;9:27.
9. Davis LS, Woody CM. Idiopathic aquagenic wrinkling of the palms. Pediatr Dermatol. 2004;21:180.
10. Yalcin B, Artuz F, Toy GG, et al. Acquired aquagenic papulotranslucent acrokeratoderma. J Eur Acad Dermatol Venereol. 2005;19:638–59.
11. Saray Y, Seçkin D. Familial aquagenic acrokeratoderma: case reports and review of the literature. Int J Dermatol. 2005;44:906–9.
12. Xia Y, Gunning ST, Schulz-Butulis BA. Aquagenic syringeal acrokeratoderma. Cutis. 2006;78:304.
13. Rongioletti F, Tomasini C, Crovato F, Marchesi L. Aquagenic (pseudo) keratoderma: a clinical series with new pathological insights. Br J Dermatol. 2012;167:575–82.
14. Nazik H, Nazik S, Çoban FG, Demir B. Sporadic and familial cases of aquagenic keratoderma. J Dermatol Case Rep. 2016;10:10–3.

15. Montoya C, Arias LM, Salazar M, Restrepo R. Water-induced dermatosis: Aquagenic keratoderma. A case report. Biomedica. 2019;39:247–51.
16. Coelho-Macias V, Fernandes S, Lamarão P, et al. Aquagenic keratoderma associated with a mutation of the cystic fibrosis gene. Rev Port Pneumol. 2013;19:125–8.
17. Elliott RB. Letter: skin wrinkling in cystic fibrosis. Lancet. 1974;2(7872):108.
18. Lowes MA, Khaira GS, Holt D. Transient reactive papulotranslucent acrokeratoderma associated with cystic fibrosis. Australas J Dermatol. 2000;41:172–4.
19. Gild R, Clay CD. Aquagenic wrinkling of the palms in a cystic fibrosis carrier. Australas J Dermatol. 2008;49:19–20.
20. Misery L, Garçon N, Roguedas AM. Aquagenic palmoplantar keratoderma and cystic fibrosis. Ann Dermatol Venereol. 2009;136:491–2.
21. Berk DR, Ciliberto HM, Sweet SC, et al. Aquagenic wrinkling of the palms in cystic fibrosis: comparison with controls and genotype–phenotype correlations. Arch Dermatol. 2009;145:1296–9.
22. Tolland JP, Boyle J, Hall V, et al. Aquagenic wrinkling of the palms in an adult cystic fibrosis population. Dermatology. 2010;221:326–30.
23. Garçon-Michel N, Roguedas-Contios AM, Rault G, et al. Frequency of aquagenic palmoplantar keratoderma in cystic fibrosis: a new sign of cystic fibrosis? Br J Dermatol. 2010;163:162–6.
24. Stewart LC, Doe SJ, Bourke SJ, Leech S. Aquagenic palmar wrinkling as a presenting feature of cystic fibrosis gene dysfunction. Clin Exp Dermatol. 2009;34:e647–9.
25. Weil B, Chaillou E, Troussier F, et al. Aquagenic palmoplantar keratoderma in children with cystic fibrosis. Arch Pediatr. 2013;20:1306–9.
26. Raynal C, Girodon E, Audrezet MP, et al. CFTR gene variants: a predisposition factor to aquagenic palmoplantar keratoderma. Br J Dermatol. 2019;181:1097–9.
27. Nadal M, Laudier B, Malinge MC, et al. Aquagenic palmar keratoderma in a patient heterozygous for the mutation c.3197G>C in the CFTR gene. Ann Dermatol Venereol. 2015;142:201–5.
28. Katz KA, Yan AC, Turner ML. Aquagenic wrinkling of the palms in patients with cystic fibrosis homozygous for the delta F508 CFTR mutation. Arch Dermatol. 2005;141:621–4.
29. Thomas JM, Durack A, Sterling A, et al. Aquagenic wrinkling of the palms: a diagnostic clue to cystic fibrosis carrier status and non-classic disease. Lancet. 2017;389(10071):846.
30. Chinazzo C, De Alessandri A, Menoni S, et al. Aquagenic wrinkling of the palms and cystic fibrosis: an Italian study with controls and genotype-phenotype correlations. Dermatology. 2014;228:60–5.
31. Lim KS, Ng SK. Aquagenic wrinkling of the palms in a boy with a congenital cardiac anomaly. J Eur Acad Dermatol Venereol. 2007;21:985–6.
32. Gild R, Clay CD, Morey S. Aquagenic wrinkling of the palms in cystic fibrosis and the cystic fibrosis carrier state: a case–control study. Br J Dermatol. 2010;163:1082–4.
33. Schmutz JL, Barbaud A, Trechot P. Rofecoxib-induced aquagenic edema with puckering of the palms of the hands: the first case. Ann Dermatol Venereol. 2003;130:813.
34. Vildósola S, Ugalde A. Celecoxib-induced aquagenic keratoderma. Actas Dermosifiliogr. 2005;96:537–9.
35. Carder KR, Weston WL. Rofecoxib-induced instant aquagenic wrinkling of the palms. Pediatr Dermatol. 2002;19:353–5.
36. Khuu PT, Duncan KO, Kwan A, et al. Unilateral aquagenic wrinkling of the palms associated with aspirin intake. Arch Dermatol. 2006;142:1661–2.
37. Ludgate MW, Patel D, Lamb S. Tobramycin-induced aquagenic wrinkling of the palms in a patient with cystic fibrosis. Clin Exp Dermatol. 2009;34:e75–7.
38. Emiroglu N, Cengiz FP, Su O, Onsun N. Gabapentin-induced aquagenic wrinkling of the palms. Dermatol Online J. 2017;23:13030/qt64k739q5.
39. Aktaş H. A new trigger for aquagenic wrinkling: isotretinoin. Indian Dermatol Online J. 2019;10:593–4.
40. Luo DQ. Aquagenic acrokeratoderma: a case with family history and unusual involvements of the palms and soles, and the dorsum of fingers and toes. J Dermatol. 2011;38:612–5.

41. Houle MC, Al Dhaybi R, Benohanian A. Unilateral aquagenic keratoderma treated with botulinum toxin A. J Dermatol Case Rep. 2010;4:1–5.
42. Angra D, Angra K, Rodney IJ. Aquagenic palmoplantar keratoderma with dorsal hand involvement in an adolescent female. JAAD Case Rep. 2016;2:239–40.
43. Pardo J, Sánchez-Motilla JM, Latasa JM. Queratodermia acuagénica de características atípicas [Atypical aquagenic keratoderma]. Actas Dermosifiliogr. 2005;96:540–2.
44. Dixit N, Sardana K, Tandon S, Singh Y. Atypical aquagenic keratoderma treated with oxybutynin chloride. An Bras Dermatol. 2018;93:308–9.
45. Flann S, Pembroke A. A localized form of aquagenic syringeal acrokeratoderma. Clin Exp Dermatol. 2010;35:e147–8.
46. Baldwin BT, Prakash A, Fenske NA, Messina JL. Aquagenic syringeal acrokeratoderma: report of a case with histologic findings. J Am Acad Dermatol. 2006;54:899–902.
47. Bardazzi F, Savoia F, Dika E, et al. Acquired aquagenic keratoderma. Pediatr Dermatol. 2007;24:197–8.
48. Hannah-Shmouni F, MacNeil L, Lara-Corrales I, et al. Whole-exome sequencing identifies a homozygous pathogenic variant in TAT in a girl with palmoplantar keratoderma. Mol Genet Metab Rep. 2019;21:100534.
49. Sezer E, Erkek E, Duman D, et al. Dermatoscopy as an adjunctive diagnostic tool in aquagenic syringeal acrokeratoderma. Dermatology. 2012;225:97–9.
50. Ghosh SK, Agarwal M, Ghosh S, Dey AK. Aquagenic palmar wrinkling in two Indian patients with special reference to its dermoscopic pattern. Dermatol Online J. 2015;21:1303.
51. Cabrol C, Bienvenu T, Ruaud L, Girodon E, Noacco G, Delobeau M, Fanian F, Richaud-Thiriez B, Van Maldergem L, Aubin F. Aquagenic palmoplantar keratoderma as a CFTR-related disorder. Acta Derm Venereol. 2016;96:848–9.
52. Martín Carmona J, Gómez Moyano E, Gómez Huelgas R, Martínez PL. Aquagenic keratoderma and cystic fibrosis screening. Med Clin (Barc). 2020;S0025-7753(20):30509–1.
53. Butler EG, Derienzo DP, Harford R. Painful plaque on a young man. Eccrine angiomatous hamartoma. Arch Dermatol. 2006;142:1351–6.
54. Wang F, Zhao YK, Luo ZY, Gao Q, Wu W, Sarkar R, Luo DQ. Aquagenic cutaneous disorders. J Dtsch Dermatol Ges. 2017;15(6):602–8.
55. Vale R, Adam DN. Idiopathic aquagenic wrinkling of the palms in sisters. J Dermatol. 2012;39:471–2.
56. Neri I, Bianchi F, Patrizi A. Transient aquagenic palmar hyperwrinkling: the first instance reported in a young boy. Pediatr Dermatol. 2006;23:39–42.
57. Tchernev G, Semkova K, Cardoso JC, Ananiev JJ, Wollina U. Aquagenic keratoderma. Two new case reports and a new hypothesis. Indian Dermatol Online J. 2014;5:30–3.
58. Nishihara E, Hiyama TY, Noda M. Osmosensitivity of transient receptor potential vanilloid 1 is synergistically enhanced by distinct activating stimuli such as temperature and protons. PLoS One. 2011;6:e22246.
59. Gironi LC, Colombo E, Zottarelli F, et al. Aberrant expression of aquaporin-3 in hereditary papulotranslucent acrokeratoderma and aquagenic palmoplantar keratoderma. Eur J Dermatol. 2018;28:262–3.
60. Denos C, Dreyfus I, Chiaverini C, et al. Clinical and evolutionary characteristics of a child with aquagenic keratoderma: a retrospective study of 12 patients. Ann Dermatol Venereol. 2018;145:250–6.
61. Errichetti E, Piccirillo A. Aquagenic keratoderma treated with tap water iontophoresis. Indian J Dermatol. 2015;60:212.
62. Siah TW, Hampton PJ. The effectiveness of tap water iontophoresis for palmoplantar hyperhidrosis using a Monday, Wednesday, and Friday treatment regime. Dermatol Online J. 2013;19:14.

63. Bagazgoitia L, Perez-Carmona L, Salguero I, et al. Aquagenic keratoderma: successful treatment with botulinum toxin. Dermatol Surg. 2010;36:434–6.
64. Garayar Cantero M, Delgado Mucientes C, Muñoz F-LC. Use of botulinum toxin in the treatment of aquagenic keratoderma: one case report. Dermatol Ther. 2018;31:e12689.
65. Garçon-Michel N, Roguedas-Contios AM, Rault G, Le Bihan J, Ramel S, Revert K, et al. Frequency of aquagenic palmoplantar keratoderma in cystic fibrosis: a new sign of cystic fibrosis? Br J Dermatol. 2010;163:162–6.

New or Unusual Skin Manifestations in Monoclonal Gammopathies

Nicolas Ortonne and Saskia Ingen-Housz-Oro

Introduction

Monoclonal gammopathies (MG) are characterized by a clonal proliferation of cells of the B lineage producing immunoglobulin which accumulates in the blood and/or tissues. MG are frequent and can be diagnosed in up to 3% of subjects over 70 years of age and are of "undetermined significance" (monoclonal gammopathy of unknown significance, MGUS) in more than 80% of cases.

Some dermatoses are strongly associated with the presence of a MG [1, 2]. They may be referred to as monoclonal gammopathy of cutaneous significance (MGCS), broadening the concept of monoclonal gammopathies of renal significance [3]. They arise from three main pathophysiological mechanisms:

1. Direct skin infiltration by the monoclonal population of plasma cells
2. Induction of secondary lesions by deposits of immunoglobulins
3. Skin lesions induced by the biological activity of monoclonal immunoglobulins

Dermatologists and dermatopathologists can thus play a key role in the early diagnosis of MG and MG-associated hemopathies when skin manifestations are the first manifestation of the disease.

N. Ortonne (✉)
Department of Pathology, Hopital Henri Mondor, Assistance-Publique – Hopitaux de Paris, Creteil, France
e-mail: nicolas.ortonne@aphp.fr

S. Ingen-Housz-Oro
Department of Dermatology, Hopital Henri Mondor, Assistance-Publique – Hopitaux de Paris, Creteil, France

F. Rongioletti, B. R. Smoller (eds.), *New and Emerging Entities in Dermatology and Dermatopathology*, https://doi.org/10.1007/978-3-030-80027-7_20

Clinical and Histopathologic Features

Specific Lymphocytic and Plasma Cell Infiltrations of the Skin

Specific cutaneous involvement in patients with multiple myeloma (MM) and Waldenström's disease (WD) is very uncommon [4]. In WD, skin involvement may be inaugural and can show large cell transformation. Clinically, lesions are infiltrated violaceous plaques, papules, or nodules. Ulcerated tumors can be seen in transformed cases of WD. While molecular alterations associated with MM, solitary plasmacytoma, and MGUS are heterogeneous, most WD are associated with a *MYD88* L265P hot spot mutation, which can be used for the diagnosis in skin-specific localizations [5].

Deposition of Immunoglobulins

Deposition of Ig mostly occurs in the clinical setting of AL amyloidosis or Waldenström's disease (WD). The deposits can be intra- or extravascular and composed of the whole Ig or part of it (light chain).

- Amyloidosis. Skin and mucous membrane lesions are observed in 29 to 40% of patients suffering from AL amyloidosis. The most common presentation is a non-infiltrated ecchymotic purpura, described in 15% of patients [6], usually affecting the eyelids, armpits, the umbilicus, and the anogenital regions, spontaneously or after a minor trauma (friction, hyperpression, etc.) [7]. It reflects capillary fragility due to deposition of amyloid material in the vessel walls. Papules, nodules, and patches of waxy appearance, sometimes hemorrhagic, are also frequent and reflect accumulation of the amyloid material in the dermis. On the face, the plaques may coalesce and give a "leonine facies" appearance. Perianal and vulvar lesions resembling condylomas have also been described. Sometimes the lesions have a yellowish appearance, reminiscent of xanthomas. Other rare manifestations are scleroderma-like appearances, hemorrhagic bullae due to skin fragility, diffuse or localized alopecia, nail fragility or total onycholysis, a cutis laxa appearance, or even induration of the blood vessels producing a "rope" appearance. In mucosae, the tongue is often affected. It may be smooth, covered with papules or waxy nodules, sometimes ulcerated. Macroglossia with dental impressions on the lateral edges is a classical feature and may be the cause of dysphagia or dysarthria. Petechial or ecchymotic lesions are possible, as is xerostomia related to salivary gland infiltration. Histology usually allows identification of the eosinophilic amorphous material which is stained by Congo red and thioflavin (Fig. 1a, b). In addition to deposits in the basal lamina of the epidermis, vessels, and cutaneous adnexae, subcutaneous fat involvement with rimming around adipocytes is a classical feature. Subcutaneous

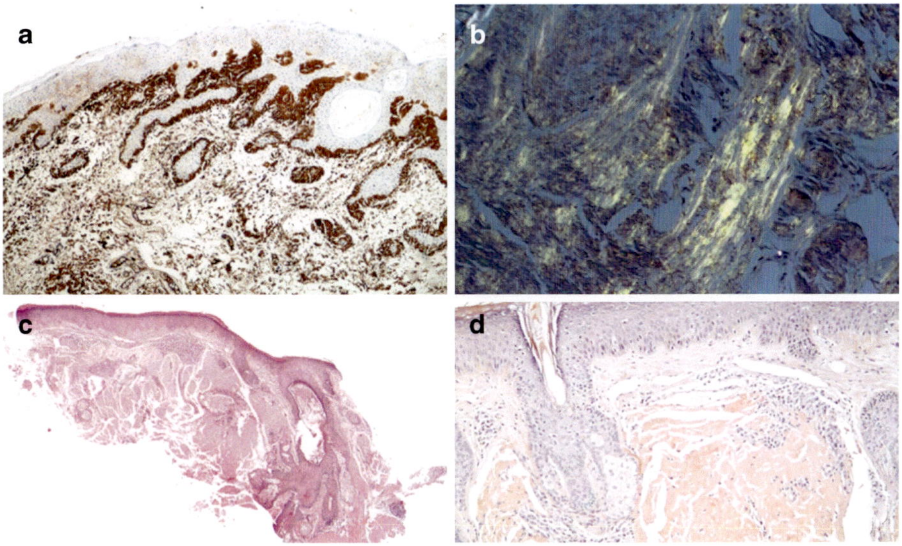

Fig. 1 AL amyloidosis
(**a**) Immunostaining of Lambda light-chain AL amyloidosis showing deposits on the basement membranes of the epidermis and dermal capillaries and in the dermis (anti-Lambda light chain, original magnification ×100). (**b**) Birefringence of the dermal deposits after Congo red staining under polarized light (Congo red stain, original magnification ×400). (**c**) Nodular amyloidosis showing diffuse dermal eosinophilic material throughout the dermis (hematoxylin, eosin, and saffron (HES), original magnification ×25). (**d**) Positive Congo red staining of the dermal deposits (Congo red stain, original magnification ×200)

fat biopsy or aspirate is therefore useful for diagnosis [8]. Nodular amyloidosis presents as a localized gum tumor of elastic consistency, while infiltration by amyloid deposits is massive on histological examination (Fig. 1c, d). This rare peculiar variant is usually not associated with systemic involvement [9].

- Monoclonal (type I) cryoglobulins are most often of the IgM kappa type. Clinically, lesions present as a stellar or retiform purpura which can evolve toward necrosis (Fig. 2a). They usually affect extremities, i.e., cold exposed areas (fingers, toes, nose, and helix). They actually cause a thrombotic vasculopathy (Fig. 2b, c) leading to necrotic lesions.

Three other very rare skin manifestations may be secondary to deposits of whole immunoglobulins in the skin.

- Cutaneous macroglobulinosis, due to IgM storage in the dermis, is one of the specific skin manifestations of WD [10, 11], with no prognostic significance. These skin lesions are clinically flesh-colored papules which are sometimes umbilicated (Fig. 2d). They can coalesce to form necrotic-looking plaques, sometimes with transepidermal elimination of the storage material. Histologically, intradermal collections of an eosinophilic hyaline PAS+ Congo red-negative material are seen (Fig. 2e). Accumulation of a monoclonal IgM can be evidenced

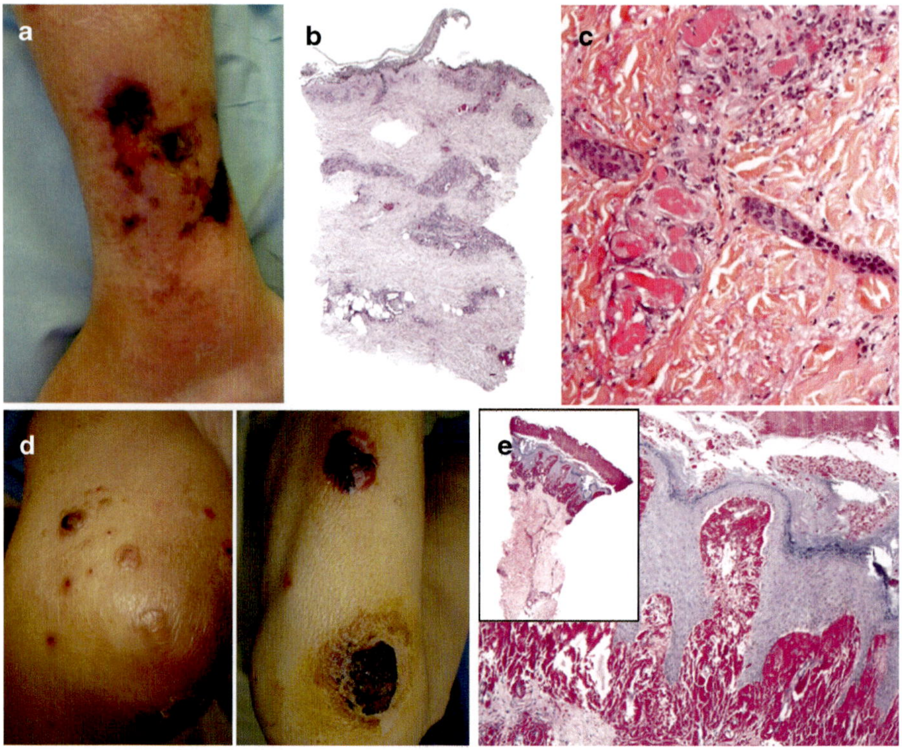

Fig. 2 Type I cryoglobulin and dermal macroglobulinosis
(**a**) Large ill-defined areas of cutaneous necrosis on the left ankle of a patient with IgM-λ cryoglobulin associated with a B-cell lymphoma. (**b**) Thrombosing vasculopathy due to type I cryoglobulin, with scattered periodic acid-Schiff (PAS)-positive thrombi in dermal capillaries, together with epidermal ischemic necrosis and detachment (PAS stain, original magnification ×25). (**c**) High magnification view of dermal thromboses (HES, original magnification ×200). (**d**) Clinical manifestations of cutaneous dermal macroglobulinosis, with scattered skin-colored or necrotic papules and large areas of skin necrosis on the elbows of two patients with WD. (**e**) Dermal macroglobulinosis showing PAS-positive amorphous material with transepidermal elimination (PAS stain, original magnifications: ×100 and ×25[inset])

using immunofluorescent studies, while electron microscopy shows an extracellular granular material, contrasting with the fibrillar deposits seen in amyloidosis [12].

- Follicular spicules of the nose are rare lesions of patients with MM [13, 14]. Clinically, they manifest as multiple follicular keratoses, with sometimes a filiform aspect. Histologically, homogeneous eosinophilic deposits of monoclonal immunoglobulin can be observed in the inter-keratinocytic spaces of the superficial layers of the follicular infundibulum [15].
- IgM bullous disease is a very rare disorder described in a context of WD [16, 17]. Clinically, it presents as a more or less diffuse and chronic vesiculo-bullous rash with pronounced skin fragility. The disease is characterized by deposits of monoclonal IgM kappa immunoglobulins at the dermal-epidermal junction.

Vascular Disorders

Besides leukoclastic vasculitis, other rare complications involving dermal vessels can develop in patients with MG.

- Various skin manifestations (70–90% of cases) have been described in POEMS: localized or diffuse hyperpigmentation, hypertrichosis, acrosyndrome with Raynaud's syndrome and digital hippocratism, diffuse or localized skin sclerosis, and ruby spots, but glomeruloid angioma is the most specific lesion (Fig. 3). The latter has a very specific histological appearance, showing vascular spaces containing a conglomerate of vascular loops resembling the renal glomerulus (Fig. 3b). Eosinophil globules corresponding to deposits of immunoglobulins are often found within the lesion.
- AESOP (adenopathy and extensive skin patch overlying a plasmacytoma) is a rare syndrome characterized by purple or erythematous-purplish macules, smooth and shiny with blunt but sharp edges. The lesions are next to an underlying bone solitary plasmacytoma and are associated with regional lymphadenopathies. The histology shows a vascular proliferation made up of mature capillaries [18].

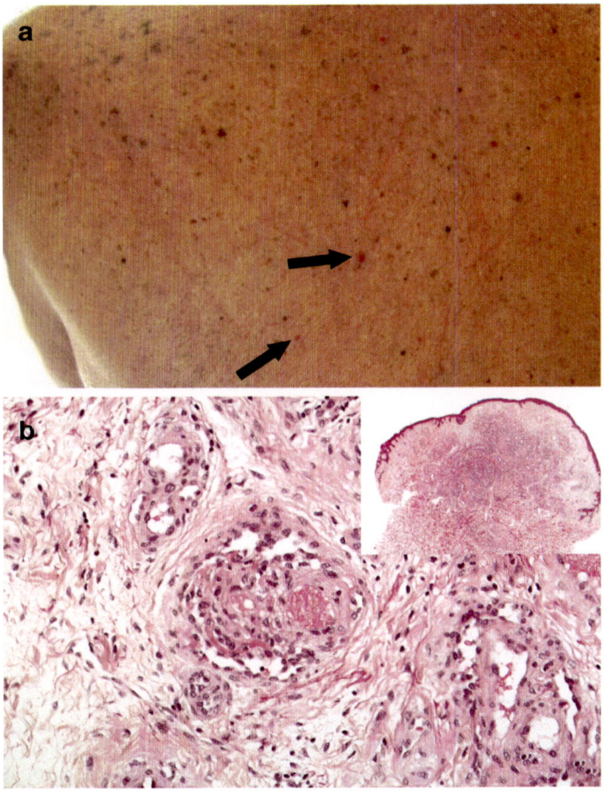

Fig. 3 POEMS syndrome (**a**) Melanoderma with small angiomatous macules on the back. (**b**) Histological aspect of one of the angiomatous macules shows a glomeruloid angioma with a vascular proliferation made of aggregates of capillaries with often a pseudo-Bowman capsule at their periphery (HES, original magnifications: ×200 and ×25[inset])

– MG-associated systemic capillary leak syndrome, also known as Clarkson's disease, is a rare condition characterized by edematous and recurrent outbreaks, linked to an exaggeration of capillary permeability, with leakage of proteins whose molecular weight is less than 350–700 kDa. During relapses, massive extravasation of fluid out of the vessels results in hypovolemic shock that can lead to death. In 90% of cases, a monoclonal immunoglobulin is found [19].

Schnitzler's Syndrome and Cutaneous Neutrophilic Infiltrates

On pathophysiological grounds, Schnitzler's syndrome (SS) belongs to the group of auto-inflammatory disorders and clinically to the "neutrophilic urticarial dermatoses" [20]. SS is usually associated with monoclonal IgM kappa. It manifests as urticarial lesions which histologically are rich in neutrophils (Fig. 4a). SS is defined by the association of a chronic urticaria with flares of fever, arthralgia, bone pain, deterioration of general condition, and a high amount of monoclonal IgM immunoglobulins outside the context of WD. Histopathologically, the infiltrates are made of a perivascular and interstitial neutrophils scattered in the mid-dermis without evidence of vasculitis [21, 22].

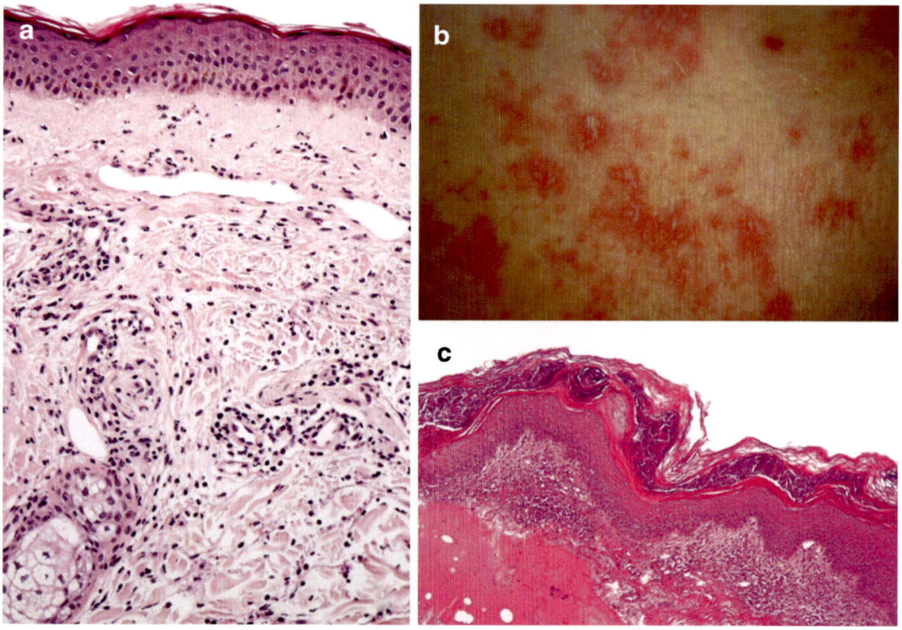

Fig. 4 Neutrophilic urticaria in Schnitzler's syndrome and subcorneal pustulosis
(**a**) Neutrophilic urticaria with scattered neutrophils in the dermis and slight dermal edema (HES original magnification: ×100). (**b**) Subcorneal pustulosis with multiple large pustules on the back. (**c**) Histology shows a unilocular pustule superficially located within the stratum corneum (HES original magnification: ×100)

Besides SS, other neutrophilic dermatoses have been described in association with an MG. They include subcorneal pustulosis (Fig. 4b, c) [23], erythema elevatum diutinum, Sweet's syndrome (classical and "lympho-histiocytic/histiocytic" variants), and pyoderma gangrenosum.

Cutaneous Lipid-Storage Disorders: Xanthomas and Xanthogranulomas

Normolipemic plane xanthomas, non-necrobiotic xanthogranulomas [24], and necrobiotic xanthogranulomas can develop in the context of MG (Fig. 5). While the histological appearance of normolipemic xanthoma is not different from hyperlipemic xanthomas, necrobiotic xanthogranuloma has a particular histological appearance [25]. In the latter, the lesions are infiltrated, slowly evolving xanthomatous plaques, most often on the periorbital region, but other face areas, trunk, arms, and upper thighs can all be affected. Histologically, trays of foamy histiocytes can be seen in the dermis infiltrating the middle dermis up to the hypodermis. There are multinucleated cells, in particular of the "Touton" type and more characteristically

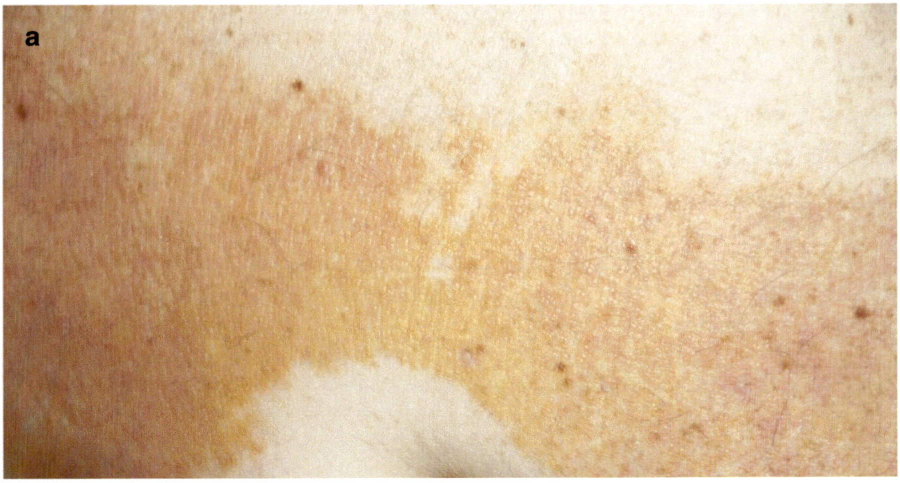

Fig. 5 Plane xanthoma and xanthogranulomas
(**a**) Large slightly infiltrated yellowish area on the posterior aspect of the right shoulder and scapula. (**b**) Multiple xanthogranulomas in patients with MGUS, in the form of mutinodular yellowish lesions on the face. (**c**, **d**) Histology of one of these xanthogranulomas showing a dense dermal infiltrate made of mononuclear and mulinucleated histiocytes, with numerous foamy cells, including Touton cells (HES, original magnifications: ×25 and ×200). (**e**, **f**) Necrobiotic xanthogranuloma: diffuse dermal infiltrate in the dermis, with areas of necrosis containing lipid crystals and surrounded by some bizarre multinucleated histiocytes with irregular and hyperchromatic nuclei (HES, original magnifications: ×25 and ×200)

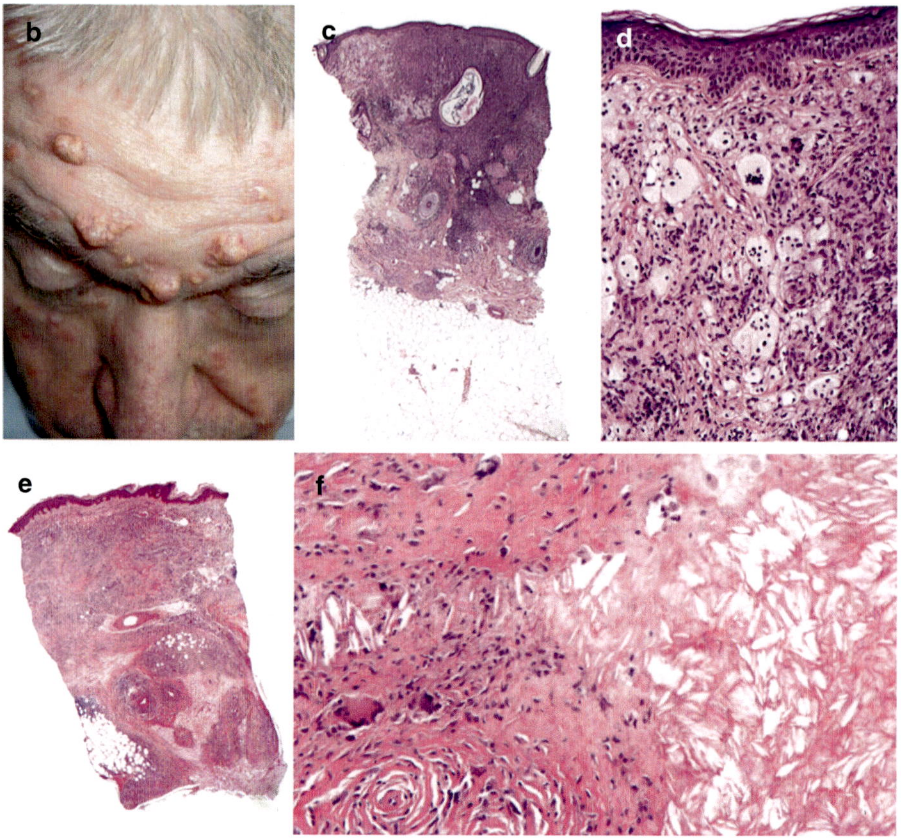

Fig. 5 (continued)

"bizarre" giant cells, with dystrophic and hyperchromatic nuclei (Fig. 5e, f). There are frequently areas of "necrobiosis" of the dermal support tissue in which lipid crystals are often noted.

Cutaneous Mucinoses

Localized papular mucinosis or lichen myxedematosus is characterized by waxy or whitish papules of 2–3 mm, isolated or coalescent located on the hands, forearms, trunk, head, and neck. The histological appearance would be less characteristic than in the diffuse form, showing deposits of mucin in the superficial and middle dermis with variable fibroblast proliferation but without fibrosis.

Scleromyxedema (papulosclerotic mucinosis, or Arndt-Gottron disease), is the generalized form of papular mucinosis (Fig. 6a, b). It manifests as a progressive

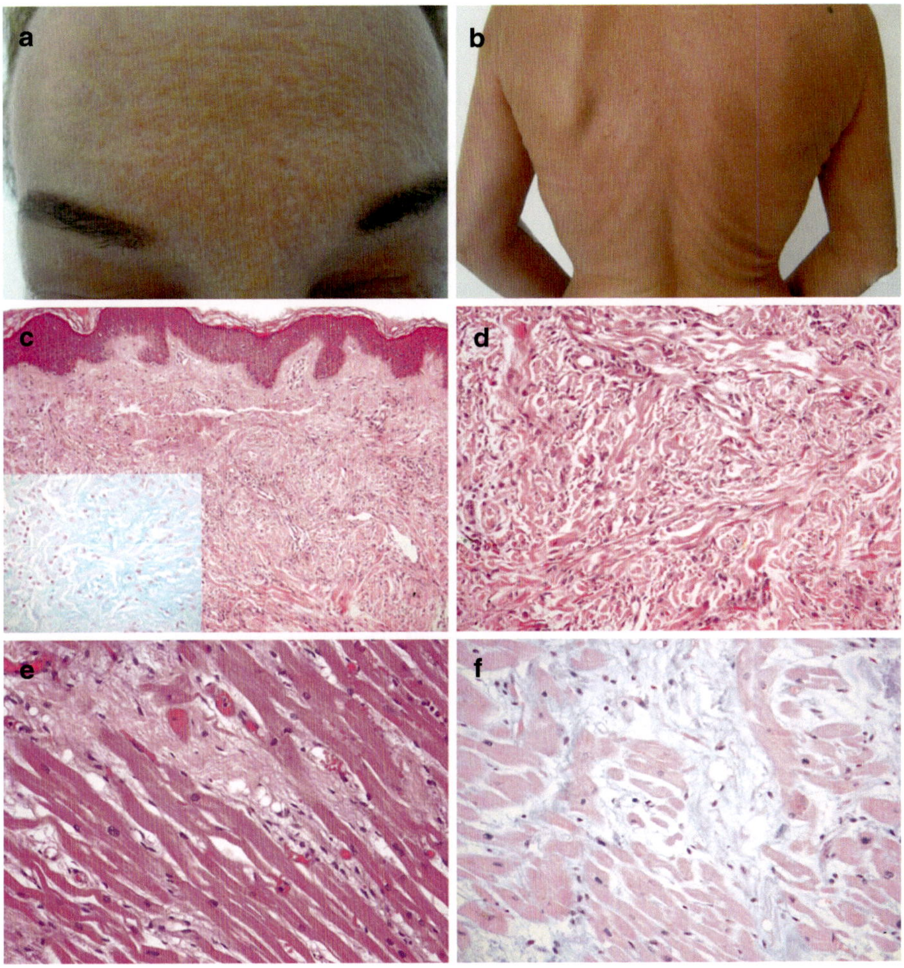

Fig. 6 Scleromyxedema with cardiac involvement
(**a**) Coalescing infiltrated papules on the forehead. (**b**) Diffuse skin infiltration with an aspect of "drappé" on the back. (**c**, **d**) Dermal interstitial infiltrate made of scattered spindle fibroblasts with dermal mucinosis (inset) and fibrosis (HES, original magnifications: ×100 and ×200, and Alcian blue stain, original magnification: ×400 [inset]).
(**e**, **f**) Autopsy specimen showing dissociation of the cardiac muscle fibers with mucin deposition (HES and Alcian blue stain, original magnifications: ×100 and ×200)

induration of the skin, sometimes with papules, which can be diffuse [26]. It may cause significant disability (microstomy, limitation of joint amplitudes) as well as aesthetic damage, but the prognosis is linked to visceral (especially cardiac) involvement. Histopathologically, scleromyxedema shows mucin deposits in the reticular dermis (Alcian blue positive), with fibroblast proliferation and fibrosis (Fig. 6b–d). In some cases, interstitial histiocytic/fibroblastic infiltrate reminiscent of granuloma annulare [27], or granulomatous aspects [28], can be seen.

Other Rare Complications

- Cutis laxa can affect the skin, lungs, cardiovascular system, digestive system, and urinary tract. It can be congenital or acquired, localized or generalized. Acquired forms occur in an acute setting, combining fever, inflammatory syndrome, and rash, or are associated with autoimmune disease or MG [29]. Microscopically, it is characterized by a disappearance of the elastic network of the papillary dermis and a decrease in elastic fibers on the rest of the dermis. There may be an infiltrate of large vacuolated macrophage cells. The main differential diagnosis histologically is elastolysis of the middle dermis, which as the name suggests is characterized by a disappearance of the elastic network of the reticular middle dermis.
- Acquired angioneurotic edema most often begins after 40 years old without a family background, unlike the hereditary form [30]. The disease progresses in flare-ups lasting 2–8 days, responsible for segmental edemas which are essentially subcutaneous, especially located in the extremities and on the face. The association with abdominal pain is very suggestive, and laryngeal edema makes the disease serious and life-threatening. The diagnosis is provided by the study of complement proteins during flare-ups, which shows in all cases a lowering of the C2 and C4 fractions while C3 is normal. The functional dosage of C1-INH is always lowered, but its antigenic activity is sometimes retained.
- Xanthoderma and xanthotrichia (yellow skin and hairs) have been described in patients with MM producing an anti-riboflavin (vitamin B2) IgGλ leading to skin accumulation [31] (Table 1).

Table 1 Main characteristics of skin manifestations of MG

Skin manifestation	Association to a MG/HD	MG class	Distinctive dermatological features (typical locations)	Histopathological features
AL amyloidosis	Almost constant	κ or λ	Minor trauma-induced purpura, papules/nodules, macroglossia	Dermal PAS- CR+ deposits
Type 1 cryoglobulin	Constant	IgM-κ	Reticulate purpura to necrosis (extremities)	Dermal PAS+ thromboses
Macroglobulinosis	Constant/ WD	IgM-- κ/λ	Skin-colored papules to large necrotic areas	Dermal PAS+ CR- deposits
Follicular spicules of the nose	Constant/ MM	IgG	Filiform follicular keratoses (nose)	Eosinophilic inter-keratinocytic deposits
IgM bullous disease	Constant/ WD	IgM-κ	Vesiculo-bullous rash and skin fragility	Subepidermal detachment
POEMS	Constant	IgM/ G/A	Hyperpigmentation, hypertrichosis, acrosyndrome skin sclerosis, and ruby spots	Glomeruloid vascular proliferation

Table 1 (continued)

Skin manifestation	Association to a MG/HD	MG class	Distinctive dermatological features (typical locations)	Histopathological features
AESOP	Constant	IgM/G/A	Erythematous plaque	Vascular proliferation
Capillary leak syndrome	Frequent	IgG κ/λ	Recurrent edema	Clinical/biological diagnosis
Schnitzler's syndrome	Constant	IgM-κ	Chronic urticaria	Scattered dermal neutrophils
Subcorneal pustulosis	Frequent	IgA	Large superficial pustules (trunk)	Unilocular subcorneal pustules
EED/Sweet/PG	Rare	IgA	Identical to non-MG-associated forms	Identical to non-MG-associated forms
Normolipemic plane xanthoma	Frequent	IgG	Slightly infiltrated yellowish plaques	Dermal xanthomized histiocytes
Necrobiotic xanthogranuloma	Frequent	IgG-κ	Yellowish plaque (periorbital area)	Dermal necrosis with lipid crystals and bizarre histiocytes
Papular mucinosis	Frequent	IgG-λ	Papules (head, trunk, extremities)	Dermal mucinosis
Scleromyxedema	Frequent	IgG-λ	Widespread papules and skin thickening	Dermal mucin, fibroblast proliferation, and fibrosis
Scleredema	Rare	IgG-κ	Skin thickening (trunk/limbs)	Dermal mucin and fibrosis
Cutis laxa	Rare	IgG/A--κ/λ	Inelastic and wrinkled skin	Dermal loss of elastic fibers
Acquired angioneurotic edema	Rare	Unclear	Subcutaneous segmental edema (face/extremities)	Clinical/biological diagnosis
Xanthoderma/xanthotrichia	Constant	IgG-λ	Yellow skin/hairs	Clinical/biological diagnosis

MG monoclonal gammopathy, *HD* hematologic disease, *PAS* periodic acid-Schiff, *CR* Congo red, *EED* erythema elevatum diutinum, *PG* yoderma gangerenosum

Work-up of Patients with MG

Details of the work up are shown in Table 2.

Diagnosis of Monoclonal Gammopathy

The diagnosis of MG is done using serum and urine (on 24-hour urine collection) protein electrophoresis (SPE) and immunofixation. This examination allows the detection of MG in the form of a narrow band usually migrating in the region of

Table 2 Work-up of patients with MGUS

Investigations	Results and aims
Medical history and physical examination	Search for symptoms suggestive of an underlying hemopathy or complication (AL amyloidosis, infection, etc.)
Blood	
Blood cell count BUN, creatinine, total protein, CRP LDH, calcium, phosphate Beta-2-microglobulin, albumin	Cytopenias Phospho-calcic disturbance (bone lesion) Elevated LDH/beta-2-microglobulin (hemopathy) Elevated CRP (infection)
Bone marrow aspirate and biopsy	Medullary plasmacytoma
Imaging	
IgA and IgG: skeletal radiographies (skull, pelvis, vertebral column, and long bones)	Osteolytic defect (MM)
IgM: CT scan of chest, abdominal, and pelvis	Organomegaly, lymphadenopathy (WD)
Other pending on clinical evaluation	
Cryoglobulins, coombs tests	
Polyneuropathy: IgM anti-myelin-associated glycoprotein activity	
Total body MRI, 18FDG-PET/CT	Tumour (extramedullary plasmacytoma)

The proposed work-up does not include the tests which are necessary for the diagnosis of MG
BUN bun urea nitrogen, *CRP* C-reactive protein, *LDH* lactate dehydrogenase, *MRI* magnetic resonance imaging

gammaglobulins, sometimes in the region of beta-globulins or exceptionally in that of α2-globulins. Agarose gel electrophoresis is the gold standard.

Search for an Underlying Disease and Complications

The patient should be referred to a hematologist. The work-up aims at making a diagnosis of an underlying malignant hemopathy, in particular a MM or WD and severe complications. Various clinical, biological, or radiological manifestations should suggest MM or WD: weight loss, inflammatory bone pain, pathological fractures, anemia, hypercalcemia, renal failure, cookie-cutter deficiencies, compression, or an appearance of osteoporosis. Other manifestations immediately point to blood disease: lymphadenopathy, splenomegaly abnormalities of the blood cell count (anemia, thrombocytopenia, excessive lymphocytosis), or hyperviscosity syndrome.

Follow-Up

In the absence of symptoms, regular clinical monitoring (bone pain, palpation of the lymph nodes, liver, and spleen) and biological (blood cell count, urea, creatinine, calcemia, SPE for the dosage of the monoclonal pic) is necessary for life, at least once a year, to detect an underlying hemopathy.

The level of monoclonal Ig (e.g., IgG > 15 g/L) and the presence of symptoms and/or clinical, biological, and radiological signs should alert and strengthen clinical and paraclinical monitoring. However, assessing the individual risk of patients remains difficult.

Differential Diagnosis

Because skin manifestations of MG are numerous, the list of their differential diagnoses cannot be detailed here. MGUS is often diagnosed in the work-up of another disease: infections, autoimmune diseases, chronic liver disease, and immune deficiencies. They are however most often the cause of a polyclonal increase in Ig. All viral (EBV, CMV, HIV), bacterial (endocarditis, osteomyelitis, tuberculosis), or parasitic infections (leishmaniasis, malaria, toxoplasmosis) may be associated with a MG. Hepatitis C is often associated with a MG with cryoglobulinemia activity. All autoimmune diseases (rheumatoid polyarthritis, Sjögren, lupus, etc.) and all chronic liver diseases, regardless of the etiology (autoimmune, viral [HBV, HCV], toxic, etc.), can be accompanied by a MG. Paradoxically, immune deficiencies, the most common being common variable immune deficiency (CVID), may be responsible for the development of a MG.

Etiopathogenesis

The mechanisms driving skin invasion by clonal plasma cells in MM and WD are poorly understood, but may rely on the expression of various homing receptors by tumor cells [32] or endothelial cells [33]. The risk of infections in patients with MG, including MGUS, can be explained by underlying immunodeficiency due to reduced levels of uninvolved immunoglobulins. To note, patients with MGUS have lower CD4+ and CD8+ T cells as compared to healthy people.

The monoclonal Ig, itself (IgM-κ in Schnitzler's syndrome, IgG in xanthomas, IgG-κ in necrobiotic xanthogranuloma, IgG-λ in scleromyxedema, IgG-κ in scleredema), plays a role in the development of several skin disorders. The anti-C1 inhibitor properties of the monoclonal antibodies can explain acquired angioedema

[34]. Complement-consuming immune complexes made of monoclonal components of the Ig and lipoproteins, stored in extracellular tissues and/or macrophages, can explain the development of xanthomas and xanthogranulomas in the course of MG [35]. Although this has not been demonstrated, it is also conceivable that IgM bullous disease may be triggered by the biological activity of the monoclonal Ig, through complement activation, as in autoimmune junctional bullous diseases. Besides the biological activity of the monoclonal Ig, the overproduction of cytokines (VEGF and IL6 in POEMS and IL1 in SS) is involved in disease development. In SS, the deposition of the monoclonal Ig at the dermo-epidermal junction and in vessel's walls can explain chronic urticaria, but effectiveness of anti-IL1 treatments suggests that the IL1-L1R pathway is certainly involved. The link between the monoclonal Ig and cytokine production is however not known in these diseases.

Therapy

Treatment of skin manifestations of MG may rely on supportive care only in patients with mild symptoms and without underlying hemopathy. The therapeutic options are either directed toward the underlying plasma cell clone or to the skin manifestations themselves. In patients with MGUS, clone-directed therapies should only be used in patients with severe complications because of their potential side effects. IgM-related disease may be treated with rituximab, while non-IgM-related MGUS may benefit from anti-myeloma agents, such as melphalan, with auto-stem cell transplantation in younger patients, bortezomib, or lenalidomide. Other new therapeutic options may be used, and as an example, it has been recently shown that anti-CD38 humanized monoclonal antibodies (daratumuab) can improve the course of AL amyloidois [36].

A better understanding of pathophysiological mechanisms associated with skin manifestations of MG allowed the development of new efficient therapies. Coherently with the pathogenetic hypothesis, IL1 blockade is currently regarded as the most effective therapy in SS, and both anakinra and canakinumab were shown to be effective [37–39]. Plasma-derived C1-INH concentrate was shown to be effective in treating both C1 inhibitor deficiency and patients with anti-C1-INH autoantibodies. It is fast-acting and reduces attack duration [40]. Most patients with scleromyxedema can be successfully treated with intravenous immunoglobulin (IVIg) [41]. The suggested mechanism of action of IVIG is the neutralization of circulating autoantibodies by anti-idiotype antibodies. In a recent study, plasma cell-directed therapies using lenalidomide and/or bortezomib with dexamethasone in association with IVIg led to a significant improvement in severe cases [42]. IVIg has also been shown to be efficient in MG-associated capillary leak syndrome [43].

Prognosis and Course

The prognosis of MG associated with an underlying malignant hemopathy is tightly dependent on the course of the disease itself. The main complication of MGUS is evolution toward a malignant hemopathy (usually MM in IgG or IgA-MGUS and WD in IgM-MGUS), with an average risk of 1% per year [44]. Patients with MGUS also have an increased risk of developing bacterial and viral infections [45], as well as osteoporosis and fractures [46]. While most skin diseases associated with MG have an indolent course, some may be life-threatening, but mostly because of visceral involvement. There is no correlation between the intensity of the monoclonal peak and severity of skin manifestations or their subtypes. The prognosis of AL amyloidosis is heavily dependent on degree of organ involvement, in particular cardiac involvement, and median overall survival ranges from as short as 6 months to over 5 years [47]. Cardiac involvement predicts poor prognosis in light chain (AL) amyloidosis, and the current prognostic classification is based on cardiac biomarkers troponin-T (cTnT) and N-terminal pro-B-type natriuretic peptide (NT-ProBNP). However, long-term outcome is dependent on the underlying plasma cell clone, and incorporation of clonal characteristics may allow for better risk stratification. Acquired angioedema due to C1 inhibitor deficiency is a serious condition that may result in life-threatening asphyxiation due to laryngeal edema.

Scleromyxedema can develop organ complications that should be recognized, and both central nervous system and cardiac involvements can be life-threatening [26]. Patients typically respond well to therapy as highlighted in several larger series, but poor outcomes are reported in a few cases [48].

Conclusion

Although rare, many skin manifestations can be induced or associated with MG. These manifestations are very heterogeneous in terms of clinical-pathological presentation, severity, and pathophysiology. Some may be life-threatening, or can be the first manifestation of the disease, including MG with an underlying hemopathy. Thus, they are important to recognize through accurate clinical pathological confrontations and connections with hematologists.

References

1. Rongioletti F, Patterson JW, Rebora A. The histological and pathogenetic spectrum of cutaneous disease in monoclonal gammopathies. J Cutan Pathol. 2008;35:705–21.
2. Lacoste C, Ingen-Housz-Oro S, Ortonne N. [Dermatological manifestations of monoclonal gammopathies: contribution of cutaneous histopathology]. Ann Pathol 2015;35:281–93.

3. Lipsker D. Monoclonal gammopathy of cutaneous significance: review of a relevant concept. J Eur Acad Dermatol Venereol. 2017;31:45–52.
4. Requena L, Kutzner H, Palmedo G, Calonje E, Requena C, Pérez G, et al. Cutaneous involvement in multiple myeloma: a clinicopathologic, immunohistochemical, and cytogenetic study of 8 cases. Arch Dermatol. 2003;139:475–86.
5. Stien S, Durot E, Durlach A, Beylot-Barry M, Adamski H, Beltraminelli H, et al. Cutaneous involvement in Waldenström's macroglobulinaemia. Acta Derm Venereol. 2020;100:adv00225.
6. Daoud MS, Lust JA, Kyle RA, Pittelkow MR. Monoclonal gammopathies and associated skin disorders. J Am Acad Dermatol. 1999;40:507–35; quiz 536–8.
7. Wettle C, Springinsfeld G, Lipsker D. Cutaneous haemorrhage induced by minimal trauma as a sign of light chain-associated amyloidosis. Br J Haematol. 2012;159:383.
8. Gertz MA. Immunoglobulin light chain amyloidosis: 2014 update on diagnosis, prognosis, and treatment. Am J Hematol. 2014;89:1132–40.
9. Moon AO, Calamia KT, Walsh JS. Nodular amyloidosis: review and long-term follow-up of 16 cases. Arch Dermatol. 2003;139:1157–9.
10. Gressier L, Hotz C, Lelièvre J-D, Carlotti A, Buffet M, Wolkenstein P, et al. Cutaneous macroglobulinosis: a report of 2 cases. Arch Dermatol. 2010;146:165–9.
11. Bernstein LE, Shea CR, Baron JM. Erythematous papules on the legs. IgM storage papules in association with WM. Arch Dermatol. 2009;145:77–82.
12. Lowe L, Fitzpatrick JE, Huff JC, Shanley PF, Golitz LE. Cutaneous macroglobulinosis. A case report with unique ultrastructural findings. Arch Dermatol. 1992;128:377–80.
13. Tay LK, Lim FL, Ng HJ, Lee H-Y, Pang S-M, Thirumoorthy T. Cutaneous follicular hyperkeratotic spicules–the first clinical sign of multiple myeloma progression or relapse. Int J Dermatol. 2010;49:934–6.
14. Requena L, Sarasa JL, Ortiz Masllorens F, Martín L, Piqué E, Olivares M, et al. Follicular spicules of the nose: a peculiar cutaneous manifestation of multiple myeloma with cryoglobulinemia. J Am Acad Dermatol. 1995;32:834–9.
15. Bork K, Böckers M, Pfeifle J. Pathogenesis of paraneoplastic follicular hyperkeratotic spicules in multiple myeloma. Follicular and epidermal accumulation of IgG dysprotein and cryoglobulin. Arch Dermatol. 1990;126:509–13.
16. West NY, Fitzpatrick JE, David-Bajar KM, Bennion SD. Waldenström macroglobulinemia-induced bullous dermatosis. Arch Dermatol. 1998;134:1127–31.
17. Whittaker SJ, Bhogal BS, Black MM. Acquired immunobullous disease: a cutaneous manifestation of IgM macroglobulinaemia. Br J Dermatol. 1996;135:283–6.
18. Lipsker D, Rondeau M, Massard G, Grosshans E. The AESOP (adenopathy and extensive skin patch overlying a plasmacytoma) syndrome: report of 4 cases of a new syndrome revealing POEMS (polyneuropathy, organomegaly, endocrinopathy, monoclonal protein, and skin changes) syndrome at a curable stage. Medicine (Baltimore). 2003;82:51–9.
19. Gousseff M, Arnaud L, Lambert M, Hot A, Hamidou M, Duhaut P, et al. The systemic capillary leak syndrome: a case series of 28 patients from a European registry. Ann Intern Med. 2011;154:464–71.
20. Gusdorf L, Lipsker D. Neutrophilic urticarial dermatosis: an entity bridging monogenic and polygenic autoinflammatory disorders, and beyond. J Eur Acad Dermatol Venereol. 2020;34:685–90.
21. Akimoto R, Yoshida M, Matsuda R, Miyasaka K, Itoh M. Schnitzler's syndrome with IgG kappa gammopathy. J Dermatol. 2002;29:735–8.
22. Lipsker D. The Schnitzler syndrome. Orphanet J Rare Dis. 2010;5:38.
23. Cheng S, Edmonds E, Ben-Gashir M, Yu RC. Subcorneal pustular dermatosis: 50 years on. Clin Exp Dermatol. 2008;33:229–33.
24. Shoo BA, Shinkai K, McCalmont TH, Fox LP. Xanthogranulomas associated with hematologic malignancy in adulthood. J Am Acad Dermatol. 2008;59:488–93.

25. Wood AJ, Wagner MVU, Abbott JJ, Gibson LE. Necrobiotic xanthogranuloma: a review of 17 cases with emphasis on clinical and pathologic correlation. Arch Dermatol. 2009;145:279–84.
26. Rongioletti F, Merlo G, Cinotti E, Fausti V, Cozzani E, Cribier B, et al. Scleromyxedema: a multicenter study of characteristics, comorbidities, course, and therapy in 30 patients. J Am Acad Dermatol. 2013;69:66–72.
27. Rongioletti F, Cozzani E, Parodi A. Scleromyxedema with an interstitial granulomatous-like pattern: a rare histologic variant mimicking granuloma annulare. J Cutan Pathol. 2010;37:1084–7.
28. Stetsenko GY, Vary JC, Olerud JE, Argenyi ZB. Unusual granulomatous variant of scleromyxedema. J Am Acad Dermatol. 2008;59:346–9.
29. Berk DR, Bentley DD, Bayliss SJ, Lind A, Urban Z. Cutis laxa: a review. J Am Acad Dermatol. 2012;66:842.e1–17.
30. Castelli R, Deliliers DL, Zingale LC, Pogliani EM, Cicardi M. Lymphoproliferative disease and acquired C1 inhibitor deficiency. Haematologica. 2007;92:716–8.
31. Farhangi M, Osserman EF. Myeloma with xanthoderma due to an IgG lambda monoclonal anti-flavin antibody. N Engl J Med. 1976;294:177–83.
32. Marchica V, Accardi F, Storti P, Mancini C, Martella E, Dalla Palma B, et al. Cutaneous localization in multiple myeloma in the context of bortezomib-based treatment: how do myeloma cells escape from the bone marrow to the skin? Int J Hematol. 2017;105:104–8.
33. Tsutani H, Sugiyama T, Shimizu S, Iwasaki H, Ueda T, Ozaki K, et al. Discordant LFA-1/ICAM-1 expression in a case of secondary plasma cell leukemia associated with subcutaneous plasmacytoma. Am J Hematol. 1993;42:299–304.
34. Frémeaux-Bacchi V, Guinnepain M-T, Cacoub P, Dragon-Durey M-A, Mouthon L, Blouin J, et al. Prevalence of monoclonal gammopathy in patients presenting with acquired angioedema type 2. Am J Med. 2002;113:194–9.
35. Szalat R, Arnulf B, Karlin L, Rybojad M, Asli B, Malphettes M, et al. Pathogenesis and treatment of xanthomatosis associated with monoclonal gammopathy. Blood. 2011;118:3777–84.
36. Sidiqi MH, Gertz MA. Daratumumab for the treatment of AL amyloidosis. Leuk Lymphoma. 2019;60:295–301.
37. Néel A, Henry B, Barbarot S, Masseau A, Perrin F, Bernier C, et al. Long-term effectiveness and safety of interleukin-1 receptor antagonist (anakinra) in Schnitzler's syndrome: a French multicenter study. Autoimmun Rev. 2014;13:1035–41.
38. Krause K, Bonnekoh H, Ellrich A, Tsianakas A, Wagner N, Fischer J, et al. Long-term efficacy of canakinumab in the treatment of Schnitzler syndrome. J Allergy Clin Immunol. 2020;145:1681–1686.e5.
39. Bixio R, Rossini M, Giollo A. Efficacy of interleukin-1 blockade in Schnitzler's syndrome without detectable monoclonal gammopathy: a case-based review. Clin Rheumatol. 2020;
40. Bork K, Staubach-Renz P, Hardt J. Angioedema due to acquired C1-inhibitor deficiency: spectrum and treatment with C1-inhibitor concentrate. Orphanet J Rare Dis. 2019;14:65.
41. Guarneri A, Cioni M, Rongioletti F. High-dose intravenous immunoglobulin therapy for scleromyxoedema: a prospective open-label clinical trial using an objective score of clinical evaluation system. J Eur Acad Dermatol Venereol. 2017;31:1157–60.
42. Mahévas T, Arnulf B, Bouaziz J-D, Livideanu CB, Osio A, Servy A, et al. Plasma cell-directed therapies in monoclonal gammopathy-associated scleromyxedema. Blood. 2020;135:1101–10.
43. Pineton de Chambrun M, Gousseff M, Mauhin W, Lega J-C, Lambert M, Rivière S, et al. Intravenous immunoglobulins improve survival in monoclonal gammopathy-associated systemic capillary-leak syndrome. Am J Med. 2017;130:1219.e19–27.
44. Kyle RA, Therneau TM, Rajkumar SV, Remstein ED, Offord JR, Larson DR, et al. Long-term follow-up of IgM monoclonal gammopathy of undetermined significance. Blood. 2003;102:3759–64.

45. Kristinsson SY, Björkholm M, Andersson TM-L, Eloranta S, Dickman PW, Goldin LR, et al. Patterns of survival and causes of death following a diagnosis of monoclonal gammopathy of undetermined significance: a population-based study. Haematologica. 2009;94:1714–20.
46. Kristinsson SY, Tang M, Pfeiffer RM, Björkholm M, Blimark C, Mellqvist U-H, et al. Monoclonal gammopathy of undetermined significance and risk of skeletal fractures: a population-based study. Blood. 2010;116:2651–5.
47. Kumar S, Dispenzieri A, Lacy MQ, Hayman SR, Buadi FK, Colby C, et al. Revised prognostic staging system for light chain amyloidosis incorporating cardiac biomarkers and serum free light chain measurements. J Clin Oncol. 2012;30:989–95.
48. Hummers LK. Scleromyxedema. Curr Opin Rheumatol. 2014;26:658–62.

Lipophagic/Lipoatrophic Panniculitis: A TH1-Mediated Autoimmune Disorder of the Subcutaneous Fat

Cynthia M. Magro and Josh H. Mo

Introduction

The first reported series in the English literature can be traced to 1980 when Umbert and Winkelmann described three cases of lipophagic granulomatous lipoatrophy [1]. The authors emphasized that the lesions were dynamic in their morphology commencing as erythematous plaques which then progressed to atrophic lesions; constitutional symptoms were common.

Clinical Features

Lipophagic panniculitis is a unique form of panniculitis that has been described primarily in childhood [1–3]. One of the cardinal hallmarks is a clinically evolutionary pattern that commences with a nodular and infiltrative plaque-like phase (Fig. 1a, b) and ends in an atrophic one (Fig. 2) [1]. The extent of atrophy can at times be rather disfiguring and be a defining and dominant presentation. There are certain site predilections, most notably the ankles, whereby the progressive atrophy results in a characteristic bilateral annular lipodystrophic appearance, falling under the designation of annular lipoatrophic panniculitis of the ankles [4–6]. However proximal extremity involvement similar to that seen in other lymphocyte-mediated panniculitic syndromes is also seen. Since its initial description, the pathophysiology that underlies this distinctive panniculitis has remained somewhat elusive until recently [7]. When it was firstly described, the authors emphasized that the lesions were

C. M. Magro (✉) · J. H. Mo
Weill Cornell Medicine, Department of Laboratory Medicine, New York, NY, USA
e-mail: cym2003@med.cornell.edu

F. Rongioletti, B. R. Smoller (eds.), *New and Emerging Entities in Dermatology and Dermatopathology*, https://doi.org/10.1007/978-3-030-80027-7_21

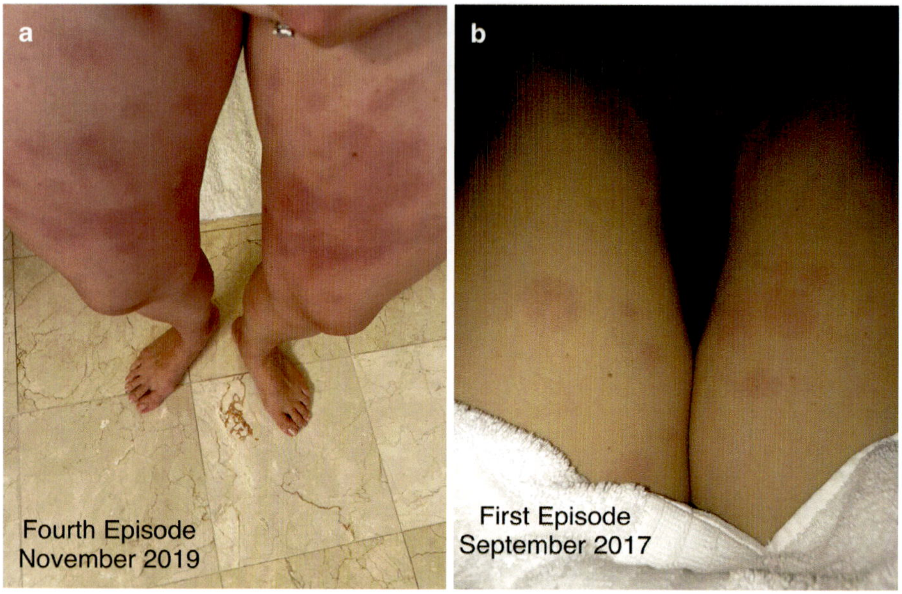

Fig. 1 (**a**, **b**) Lipophagic panniculitis is a unique form of panniculitis that has been described primarily in childhood. One of the cardinal hallmarks is a clinically evolutionary pattern that commences with a nodular and infiltrative plaque-like phase

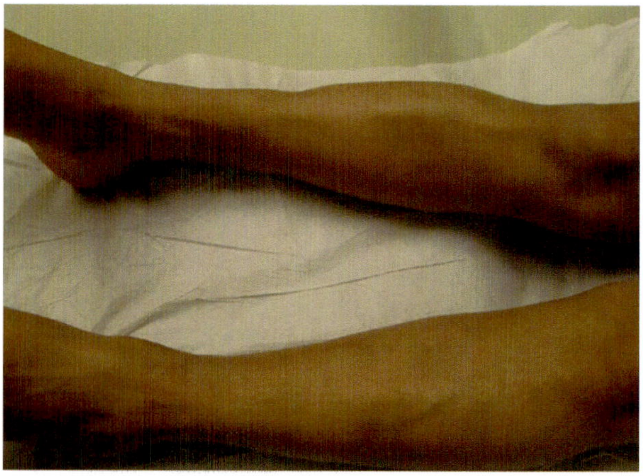

Fig. 2 Ultimately the inflammatory phase resolves and there is ensuing fibrosis and lipoatrophy eventuating in areas of cutaneous atrophy clinically

dynamic in their morphology commencing as erythematous plaques which then progressed to atrophic lesions with constitutional symptoms [8]. The cases we have seen in children also exhibited this metamorphosis beginning as erythematous painful nodules that eventuated into atrophic plaques. The patients typically had fevers, splenomegaly, and elevated liver function studies. Certain hematologic abnormalities, namely, a microcytic anemia and thrombocytosis, could be seen as well [9].

While much of the literature focuses on pediatric cases, this uncommon form of autoimmune panniculitis also affects adults; the clinical presentation and biopsy findings define a pattern most reminiscent of lipoatrophic panniculitis of childhood. As with the childhood cases, the patients were typically constitutionally unwell during flare-ups. While the episodes are associated with a state of constitutional unwellness, there are no cases of disease progression to subcutaneous panniculitis like T cell lymphoma (SPTCL) or a panniculitic variant of gamma delta T cell lymphoma. The occurrence of this panniculitis in adults indicates greater demographic heterogeneity that what had previously been reported.

The potential role of autoimmunity in the pathogenesis of lipophagic/lipoatrophic panniculitis lies in the association with certain autoimmune conditions, most notably insulin-dependent diabetes mellitus, juvenile rheumatoid arthritis, Graves' disease, Hashimoto's thyroiditis, alopecia areata, vitiligo, celiac disease, Crohn's disease, and partial IgA deficiency. Furthermore, even though the patient may not have a specific autoimmune condition, there can be serologies that point toward an autoimmune diathesis most typically a positive antinuclear antibody [7].

Histopathological Features

We have had the opportunity to study six cases of lipophagic panniculitis: two in the pediatric setting and four in the adult setting. The biopsies of all of these patients demonstrate a lobular panniculitis. One of the most striking features of this panniculitis is the degree of infiltration of the panniculus by lipid-laden macrophages (Fig. 3). The macrophages function as scavenger monocytes that imbibe lipid from damaged adipocytes. The extent of lipid-laden macrophage infiltration can be to a magnitude that it imparts an almost tumefactive quality to the histiocytic infiltrate

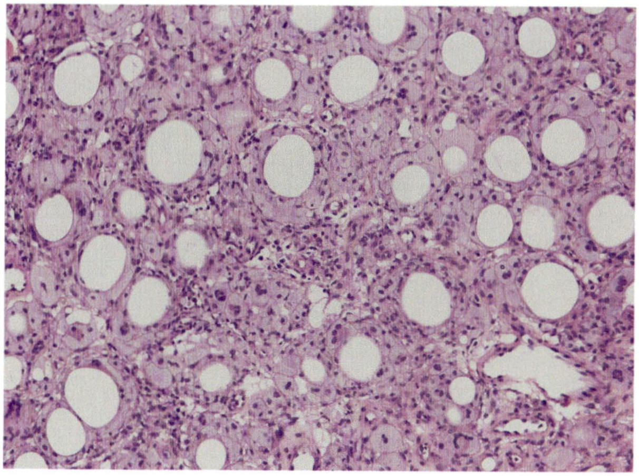

Fig. 3 The biopsies of all of these patients demonstrate a lobular panniculitis. One of the most striking features of this panniculitis is the degree of infiltration of the panniculus by lipid-laden macrophages. The macrophages function as scavenger monocytes that imbibe lipid from damaged adipocytes. The extent of lipid-laden macrophage infiltration can be to a magnitude that it imparts an almost tumefactive quality to the histiocytic infiltrate within the fat lobule

within the fat lobule. However, the incipient inflammatory milieu that presages the adipocyte injury is characterized by a relatively focal infiltrate of lymphocytes, neutrophils, and plasma cells intimately opposed to the adipocyte, resulting in a concentric ringlike pattern of infiltration around the adipocyte with focal disruption of the adipocyte membrane (Fig. 4a, b). Rarely there are germinal centers [10, 11]. While the macrophages engulf lipid, there is no significant phagocytosis of inflammatory cell debris nor is there red cell engulfment. As with any panniculitis, some degree of inflammation within the adventitial dermis of the eccrine coil is observed. Subcutaneous microcysts devoid of adipocytes and flanked by inflammation, including lipophages, are also noted. Vasculitic changes are not a significant morphologic feature. There are no significant differences between adult and pediatric cases from a pathology perspective. Once the adipocytes have been injured there is adipocyte dropout and ensuing fibrosis. The end-stage lesion is characterized by a relatively pauci-cellular appearing fat lobule exhibiting fibrosis, lipophage accumulation, and fibrosis (Fig. 5) [4, 12, 13].

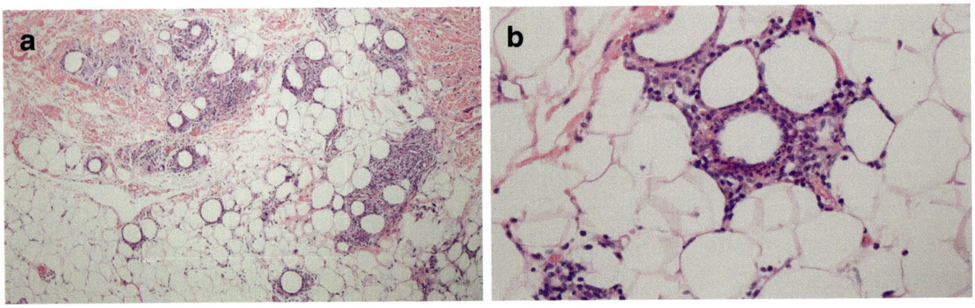

Fig. 4 (**a**, **b**) The incipient inflammatory milieu that presages the adipocyte injury is characterized by a relatively focal infiltrate of lymphocytes, neutrophils, and plasma cells intimately opposed to the adipocyte, resulting in a concentric ring-like pattern of infiltration around the adipocyte with focal disruption of the adipocyte membrane

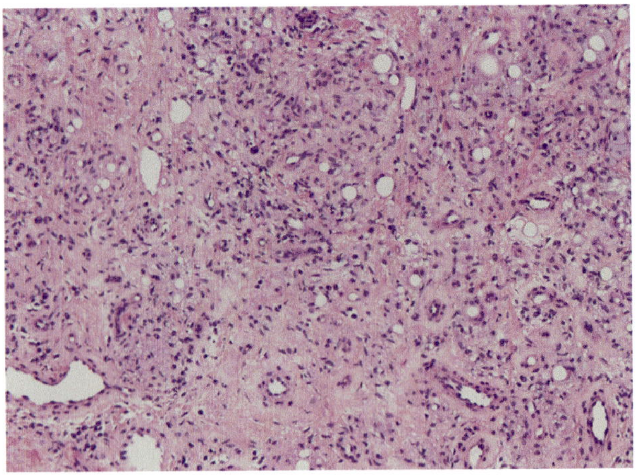

Fig. 5 Once the adipocytes have been injured, there is adipocyte dropout and ensuing fibrosis. The end-stage lesion is characterized by a relatively pauci-cellular appearing fat lobule exhibiting fibrosis, lipophage accumulation, and fibrosis

In examining the phenotypic profile, the lymphocytes are primarily of T-cell lineage; they are highlighted by T-cell receptor antibody beta F1 and various pan T-cell markers CD2, CD3, CD5, and CD7. The CD4 to CD8 ratio is variable, but there can be a predominance of CD8 T cells over those of the CD4 subset. ICOS and PD-1 positivity are frequently expressed by a subset of the reactive T cells although most of the lymphocytes do not show immunoreactivity with either ICOS or PD-1. This particular profile does not necessarily denote a follicular helper T-cell ontogeny but could simply indicate an activated T-cell phenotype. The CD8 T cells which can prevail also exhibit cytotoxic protein expression, likely contributing to the adipocyte injury (Fig. 6). Furthermore, the lymphocytes and monocytes stain positively for CCL5, a natural ligand for the CCR5 expressed on adipocytes accounting for the potential tropism of the infiltrate for the fat. CCL5 positivity amidst monocytes may also contribute to the ability of the monocyte to migrate into the fat [12].

A particularly intriguing finding that we have encountered is the rimming of adipocytes by CD83-positive and CD11c-positive histiocytes that would denote their categorization as a monocyte-derived dendritic cell; the histiocytes will express other monocyte markers such as CD68 and lysozyme (Fig. 7a, b). CD83 is the most

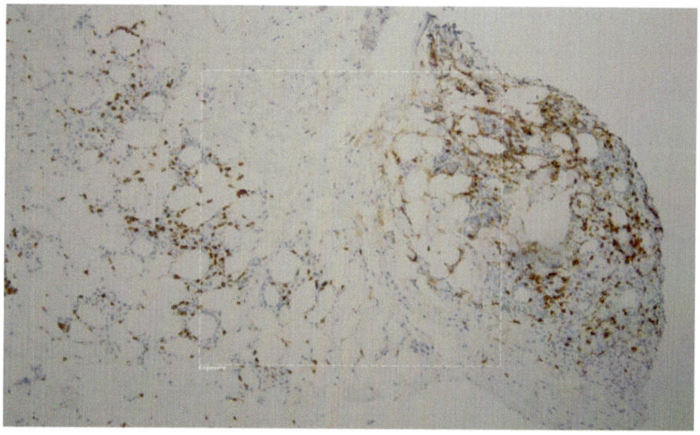

Fig. 6 The CD4 to CD8 ratio is variable, but there can be a predominance of CD8 T cells over those of the CD4 subset. The CD8 T cells which can prevail also exhibit cytotoxic protein expression, likely contributing to the adipocyte injury

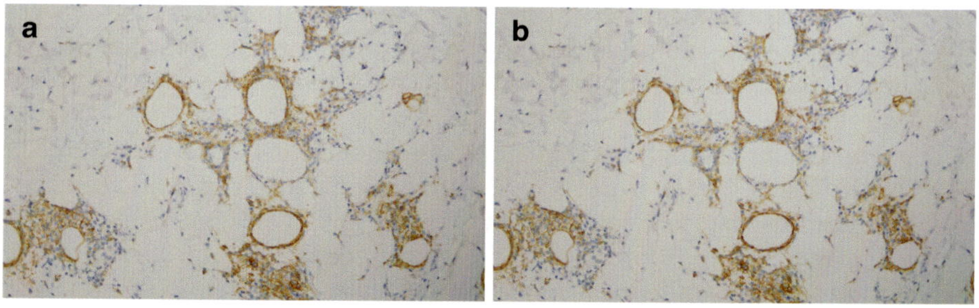

Fig. 7 (**a, b**) A particularly intriguing finding that we have encountered is the rimming of adipocytes by CD83-positive and CD11c-positive histiocytes that would denote their categorization as a monocyte-derived dendritic cell; the histiocytes will express other monocyte markers such as CD68 and lysozyme. CD83 is the most terminally differentiated dendritic cell marker involved in antigen presentation. The hallmark of a mature as opposed to an immature dendritic cell associated with antigen presentation is the expression of CD83 [14]

terminally differentiated dendritic cell marker involved in antigen presentation. The hallmark of a mature as opposed to an immature dendritic cell associated with antigen presentation is the expression of CD83 [14].

Differential Diagnosis

The differential diagnosis of lipophagic panniculitis would encompass SPTCL, gamma-delta T-cell lymphoma involving the fat, lupus profundus, the distinct prelymphomatous T-cell dyscrasia of atypical lymphocytic lobular panniculitis, and Weber-Christian disease [15]. In SPTCL, there is infiltration of the adventitial dermis of the eccrine coil and fat by atypical lymphocytes. A significant histiocytic component is identified, but instead of lipidization of the cytoplasm, the macrophages exhibit erythrocyte phagocytosis and phagocytosis of other inflammatory cells, a phenomenon observed in the dermis and subcutaneous fat. There is a distinctive pattern of adipocyte disruption resulting in the internalization of lymphocytes and histiocytes to reside within the adipocyte [16–18]. Over and above the eccrinotropic and subcutaneous infiltrate, infiltration of the dermal interstitium by histiocytes accompanied by dermal mucin is observed. The histiocytes have a plump polygonal appearance and demonstrate erythrocyte phagocytosis. There may be basilar vacuolar alteration with an accompanying low-density epitheliotropic lymphocytic infiltrate. From a cytomorphologic perspective, the lymphocytes are small to intermediate in size and appear hyperchomatic with nuclear contour irregularity although without a cerebriform appearance and without large cell transformation. Phenotypically the atypical lymphocytes are CD8 positive, exhibiting cytotoxic protein expression and demonstrating significant losses in the expression of the pan T-cell markers CD5 and CD7. Gamma delta T-cell lymphoma involving the fat has many overlapping features clinically and pathologically with SPTCL. However, there can be a greater tendency toward overlying dermal and epidermal involvement with many neoplastic cells infiltrating the epidermis and vessel walls leading to tissue compromise and ischemic-driven necrosis. The atypical cells are double negative for CD4 and CD8 and demonstrate cytotoxic protein expression with variable reductions in the expression of CD5 and CD7. The lymphocytes will not express beta F1.

Lupus profundus has a similar anatomic distribution as SPTCL and gamma delta T-cell lymphoma of the fat. Upper arm and proximal leg involvement is characteristic. There can also be facial involvement. The lesions can undergo regression and heal with significant lipoatrophy which is apparent clinically. The course can be episodic and the response to Plaquenil is usually very good. Microscopically there is a very distinctive morphology characterized by a striking lymphocytic lobular panniculitis and eccrine hidradenitis. One of the cardinal hallmarks in recognizing lupus profundus is in the context of overlying cutaneous changes of lupus erythematous revealed by the combination of an atrophying lymphocyte-mediated interface dermatitis, concomitant mesenchymal mucin deposition, and hyperkeratosis. Exceptionally we have seen cases of gamma delta T-cell lymphoma with overlapping features of lupus erythematosus in the overlying skin characterized by an atrophying interface dermatitis with follicular involvement marked hyperkeratosis and dermal mucin. Engulfment of cellular debris by macrophages is conspicuous, defining the in vivo equivalent of the so-called LE cell, while erythrocyte phagocytosis is distinctly uncommon. The pattern of diffuse infiltration of the interstitium by polygonal shaped macrophages containing red cells characteristic for SPTCL and gamma delta T-cell lymphoma is not observed. There can be germinal center formation. A hyalinizing alteration of the interstitial spaces of the fat is quite unique to lupus profundus. The lymphocytes are predominantly small to intermediate in size. It is not uncommon for lupus profundus to exhibit somewhat atypical lymphomatoid features as characterized by cytologic atypia and certain phenotypic abnormalities revealed by a loss in the expression of CD7 and even in some cases the identification of T cell clonality [16]. Focal colonization of the adipocyte by lymphocytes is observed. Injurious vascular alterations ranging from quiescent thickened microvessels reflective of vascular basement membrane zone reduplication to one of an active lymphocytic vasculitis with vascular thrombosis can be seen. The degree of lipophage accumulation that characterizes lipophagic panniculitis is not seen. There can be significant lipoatrophy hallmarked by diminutive appearing adipocytes. One of the cardinal phenotypic hallmarks phenotypically is the extent of myxovirus resistance protein A (MXA) staining. MXA is the surrogate type I interferon marker in paraffin-embedded formalin-fixed tissue and it is characteristically and significantly increased in the setting of lupus profundus. The positive staining is found in endothelium, inflammatory cells, and within epithelial structures.

Another important consideration would be atypical lymphocytic lobular panniculitis which is a unique form of panniculitic T-cell dyscrasia that can potentially presage SPTCL and gamma delta T-cell lymphoma of the fat [19]. The site distribution is similar to SPTCL, and hence involvement of the upper legs and upper arms is characteristic. The lesions following a course of spontaneous regression followed by recurrence oftentimes over years. If the lesions no longer regress and there are accompanying constitutional symptoms, then malignant transformation has likely occurred. One of the cardinal hallmarks histologically is a relatively modest pattern of lymphocytic infiltration without significant adipocyte injury and, therefore, lipophage accumulation is minimal. Acute and chronic vascular injury with or without vascular thrombosis is not usually observed. Cytologic atypia amidst the lymphocytes is observed but overall it is mild. As well, phenotypic abnormalities are observed characterized by some degree of loss in the expression of CD5 and CD7; there can be a predominance of CD8 T cells over those of the CD4 subset or the lymphocytes can be double negative for CD4 and CD8. T-cell clonality can be seen.

Weber-Christian disease encompasses a variety of lobular panniculitides which exhibit infiltration of the fat lobule by lymphocytes, histiocytes, and a variable number of neutrophils. The pattern of infiltration is very discrete and focal and can be associated with adipocyte injury and focal lipophage accumulation. In this regard the earliest phase of lipophagic panniculitis can resemble Weber-Christian disease. There is likely a subset of cases of Weber-Christian disease that in fact represent lipophagic panniculitis [20].

Etiopathogenesis

The composition of the infiltrate being one of T cells, CD83-positive mature antigen-presenting monocyte-derived dendritic cells, and neutrophils without significant tissue eosinophilia would suggest a TH1-dominant type IV immune response. Given the discrete rimming of adipocytes by CD83-positive monocytes and T cells, one would have to infer that the intended antigenic target is the adipocyte. The TH1 response is closely linked with tissue neutrophilia because among the TH1 cytokines are IL-17 and IL-23, potent neutrophil chemoattractants. The neutrophils likely damage the adipocyte, and then there is a secondary influx of scavenger macrophages which shows an even more exaggerated pattern of migration into the fat because of the expression of CCL5 by monocytes, the ligand for CCR5 expressed on adipocytes [12].

This panniculitic type IV autoimmune reaction could also tie in with the other underlying TH1-mediated autoimmune diseases that are associated with lipophagic panniculitis such as celiac disease, Crohn's disease, rheumatoid arthritis, and insulin-dependent diabetes mellitus.

Therapy and Prognosis

Lipoatrophic panniculitis is a rare disease, resulting in significant aesthetic atrophic sequelae which may be limited by early treatment initiation. Understanding the immunology that underlies lipophagic panniculitis could also have some important therapeutic implications; drugs that are successfully used to treat conditions like Crohn's disease such as a TNF-alpha inhibitor could have some efficacy in this condition. Due to the autoimmune nature of this form of panniculitis, a response to hydroxychloroquine has also been reported [10, 11]. Filling the secondary atrophy by fat grafting after the inflammatory period has ended could also be taken into consideration.

Conclusions

Lipophagic/lipoatrophic panniculitis is a rare condition notable clinically for an inflammatory panniculitis followed by the development of permanent lipoatrophy, mainly described in childhood. Additional designations include lipophagic panniculitis, lipoatrophic panniculitis, and annular lipoatrophic panniculitis of the ankles. Although lipophagic/lipoatrophic panniculitis has been associated with a number of autoimmune conditions, a paucity of reports and limited pathological analyses to date render this disease an elusive one whose pathogenesis is not yet understood. A cellular immunological reaction targeting the adipocyte at the crux seems to play a role in its pathogenesis. TNF-alpha inhibitors and antimalarials could have some efficacy in treating this condition.

References

1. Umbert IJ, Winkelmann RK. Adult lipophagic atrophic panniculitis. Br J Dermatol. 1991;124:291–5.
2. Weryńska-Kalemba M, et al. A case of lipoatrophic panniculitis in a 2-year-old boy. Adv Dermatol Allergol. 2016;2:155–6.
3. Ng SY, D'Arcy C, Orchard D. Acquired idiopathic lipoatrophic panniculitis in a 12-month-old infant: lipoatrophic panniculitis. Australas J Dermatol. 2015;56:e102–4.
4. Fernandez-Flores A, Barja-Lopez J-M. Immunohistochemical study of another case of lipoatrophic panniculitis of the ankles in childhood. Am J Dermatopathol. 2013;35:524–6.
5. Corredera C, et al. Annular lipoatrophic panniculitis of the ankles: panniculitis of the ankles. Pediatr Dermatol. 2011;28:146–8.
6. Dimson OG, Esterly NB. Annular lipoatrophy of the ankles. J Am Acad Dermatol. 2006;54:S40–2.
7. Billings JK. Lipoatrophic panniculitis: a possible autoimmune inflammatory disease of fat. Report of three cases. Arch Dermatol. 1987;123:1662–6.
8. Peters MS, Winkelmann RK. Localized lipoatrophy (atrophic connective tissue disease panniculitis). Arch Dermatol. 1980;116:1363–8.
9. Winkelmann RK. Lipophagic panniculitis of childhood. 1989;21:8.
10. Moulonguet I, Braun-Arduz P, Plantier F, Lerolle N, Petit A. Panniculite lipoatrophiante de l'adulte : traitement par hydroxychloroquine. Ann Dermatol Venereol. 2011;138:681–5.
11. Cornille H, Adelmand L, Garmi R, Comoz F, Verneuil L. Panniculite lipoatrophiante idiopathique de l'adulte traitée par hydroxychloroquine et autogreffe de cellules graisseuses. Ann Dermatol Venereol. 2018;145:694–701.
12. Levy J, Burnett ME, Magro CM. Lipophagic panniculitis of childhood: a case report and comprehensive review of the literature. Am J Dermatopathol. 2017;39:8.
13. Torrelo A, et al. Recurrent lipoatrophic panniculitis of children. J Eur Acad Dermatol Venereol. 2017;31:536–43.
14. Twist CJ, Beier DR, Disteche CM, Edelhoff S, Tedder TF. The mouse Cd83 gene: structure, domain organization, and chromosome localization. Immunogenetics. 1998;48:383–93.
15. Santonja C, Gonzalo I, Feito M, Beato-Merino MJ, Requena L. Lipoatrophic panniculitis of the ankles in childhood: differential diagnosis with subcutaneous panniculitis-like T-cell lymphoma. Am J Dermatopathol. 2012;34:6.
16. Magro CM, Crowson AN, Kovatich AJ, Burns F. Lupus profundus, indeterminate lymphocytic lobular panniculitis and subcutaneous T-cell lymphoma: a spectrum of subcuticular T-cell lymphoid dyscrasia. J Cutan Pathol. 2001;28:235–47.
17. Magro CM, Wang X. CCL5 expression in panniculitic T-cell dyscrasias and its potential role in adipocyte tropism. Am J Dermatopathol. 2013;35:332–7.
18. Magro CM, Wang X. Indolent primary cutaneous γ/δ T-cell lymphoma localized to the subcutaneous panniculus and its association with atypical lymphocytic lobular panniculitis. Am J Clin Pathol. 2012;138:50–6.

19. Magro CM, Neil Crowson A, Byrd JC, David Soleymani A, Shendrik I. Atypical lymphocytic lobular panniculitis. J Cutan Pathol. 2004;31:300–6.
20. Al-Niaimi F, Clark C, Thorrat A, Burden AD. Idiopathic lobular panniculitis: remission induced and maintained with infliximab. Br J Dermatol. 2009;161:691–2.

COVID-19-Related Cutaneous Manifestations

Franco Rongioletti and Valentina Caputo

Introduction

In December 2019, the first cases of coronavirus disease 2019 (COVID-19), an infectious interstitial pneumonitis caused by a novel, RNA betacoronavirus named severe acute respiratory syndrome coronavirus 2 (SARS-CoV-2), were detected in Wuhan, China [1]. On March 11, 2020, the World Health Organization officially designated the Coronavirus Disease 2019 (COVID-19) as a global pandemic [2]. After more information has been gathered on the characteristics of COVID-19, it became clear that skin symptoms are not rare and many cutaneous manifestations have been increasingly described in association with SARS-CoV-2 infection. A recent systematic review indicates a worldwide incidence of skin involvement around 1–2%, while the prevalence ranges from 0.2% in a cohort of Chinese patients to 20.4% in an Italian study [3–5]. Covid-19-related skin manifestations can be classified into five groups: (1) chilblain-like lesions (pernio-like); (2) acro-ischemic-necrotic lesions; (3) exanthematous eruptions including (a) varicelliform-like/vesicular, (b) confluent erythematous/maculopapular/morbilliform, (c) urticarial, (d) erythema multiforme-like, and (e) purpuric/petechial; (4) skin manifestations of multisystem inflammatory syndrome in children (MIS-C)/pediatric inflammatory multisystem syndrome (PIMS) (atypical Kawasaki disease); (5) miscellanea (pityriasis rosea-like eruption, digitate papulosquamous, transient livedo reticularis, erythema nodosum/Sweet's-like, SDRIFE-like lesions. Erythema annulare centrifugum with ageusia and anosmia), erythema (Table 1).

F. Rongioletti (✉)
Unit of Dermatology, IRCCS San Raffaele Hospital Vita Salute San Raffaele University, Milan, Italy

Unit of Dermatology, Department of Medical Sciences and Public Health, University of Cagliari, Cagliari, Italy

V. Caputo
Unit of Surgical Pathology, ASST Grande Ospedale Metropolitano Niguarda, Milan, Italy

F. Rongioletti, B. R. Smoller (eds.), *New and Emerging Entities in Dermatology and Dermatopathology*, https://doi.org/10.1007/978-3-030-80027-7_22

Table 1 Clinico-pathologic characterization of current COVID-19 associated skin manifestations

Skin manifestation	Clinical features	Histopathology	COVID-19 course
Chilblain-like eruption (pernio-like)	Acral: dorsal aspect of the toes (Covid-19 toe), lateral sides of the feet, soles and less frequently fingers Variable symptoms: asymptomatic, itching, painful	Superficial and deep perivascular lymphocytic infiltrate, perieccrine extension and intramural lymphocytes with thickening and enlargement of endothelium ("lymphocytic vasculitis") Vacuolar interface dermatitis with scattered necrotic (apoptotic) keratinocytes. Sometimes, microthrombi in superficial capillaries and epidermal necrosis in acral lesions overlapping with livedoid/Ischemic/necrotic lesions Direct immunofluorescence negative	Children/young person: asymptomatic or mild disease often with negative Covid-19 tests and serology
Ischemic/livedoid/necrotic lesions	Acral acute painful lesions; often bullae; possible progression to dry gangrene	Epidermal necrosis Thrombotic vasculopathy of small and medium vessels in superficial and deep dermis Sweat gland necrosis Slight perivascular lymphocytic infiltrate No sign of leucocytoclastic vasculitis Complement deposition in vessel walls	Severe disease; 10% mortality in a Spanish survey
Varicella-like/vesicular eruption	Diffuse, constant trunk involvement Itching	Earlier lesions: Vacuolar degeneration of basal layer Multinucleate, hyperchromatic keratinocytes with many dyskeratotic (apoptotic) cells Pauci to absent inflammatory infiltrate Well-established lesion: Intraepidermal vesicle containing multinucleated and ballooned keratinocytes, with acantholytic and dyskeratotic cells (similar to herpetic lesions or pseudo-herpetic Grover's disease)	Unpredictable Severe pulmonary disease in 42% of Spanish patients; 13.6% fatal outcome in an Italian survey

Table 1 (continued)

Skin manifestation	Clinical features	Histopathology	COVID-19 course
Confluent erythematous/ maculo-papular/ morbilliform eruptions	Widespread sparing palmo-plantar surfaces and mucosae	Variable features consistent with viral exanthem: Spongiosis, basal cell vacuolization, perivascular lymphocytic infiltrate with some neutrophils and eosinophils in early lesions. Interstitial histiocytes in late lesions Lymphocytic vasculitis Grover's like feature Microthrombi (rarely)	Early symptomatic disease, variable course Adults
Urticarial eruptions	Widespread small or larger wheals (giant)	From normal epidermis to spongiosis with perivascular infiltrate to interface dermatitis (two cases) to small vessels vasculitis (urticarial vasculitis) Variable tissue eosinophilia	Variable prognosis. Presence of eosinophils suggested as sign of a better prognosis.
Erythema multiforme-like eruptions	Variable: Acral in young persons and children Generalized in older adults	Acral type in youngsters: Reminiscent of chilblain-like lesions with a superficial and deep perivascular CD3+ lymphocytic infiltrate with perieccrine involvement and some vasculopatic changes. Positivity of SARS-CoV/ SARS-CoV-2 spike protein in endothelial cells and epithelial cells of eccrine glands with immunohistochemistry. Diffuse type in adults: Consistent with EM, although not typical Normal epidermis or spongiosis, exocytosis, variable degrees of interface dermatitis, absent or a few necrotic keratinocytes. Absence of fibrinoid necrosis, thrombosis, eosinophils.	Mild disease in youngsters Symptomatic disease with variable outcome in adults

(continued)

Table 1 (continued)

Skin manifestation	Clinical features	Histopathology	COVID-19 course
Petechial/purpuric rash	Variable: Periflexural onset Limited to lower limb Generalized	Two different patterns from few biopsies: Superficial perivascular lymphocytic infiltrate with hemorrhages, papillary edema and some dyskeratotic cells in the absence of vasculopathy Leucocytoclastic vasculitis	Symptomatic disease with variable outcome
Multisystem inflammatory syndrome – Atypical Kawasaki Disease	Generalized, variable morphology	Two different patterns from few biopsies: Leukocytoclastic vasculitis Erythema multiforme-like	Multiorgan symptoms in children Nasopharingeal swab often negative 1 case in adult
Miscellanea Pityriasis rosea like Digitate papulosquamous Livedo reticularis Skin mottling (neonate) Intertriginous and flexural exanthema Erythema annulare centrifugum	Anecdotal reports with various morphology	Usually not biopsy. In the digitate papulosquamous: Spongiosis, with vesicles containing lymphocytes, and Langerhans cells Mild papillary edema, and a superficial lympho-histiocytic infiltrate	Associated with symptomatic disease, but benign course Only one fatal outcome (digitate papulosquamous eruption)

Chilblain-Like Lesions

Clinical Features

Chilblain-like lesions have been reported to occur in younger patients (median age of presentation of 14 years) with less severe systemic involvement and manifested late during the course of the disease. The lesions are considered one of the most specific manifestations of COVID-19, occurring in 19% of a Spanish series [6] and 18% of the American Academy of Dermatology and International League of Dermatological Societies registry [7]. The clinical presentation is characterized by dusky erythematous and edematous macules or plaques, sometimes with a purpuric hue (Fig. 1a) and the development of blisters involving the dorsal aspect of the toes (Covid-19 toe), the lateral sides of the feet, soles, and less frequently the hands. Distribution is usually asymmetrical and lesions may be asymptomatic, itching, or painful [8, 9]. In children, a pattern resembling erythema multiforme has also been

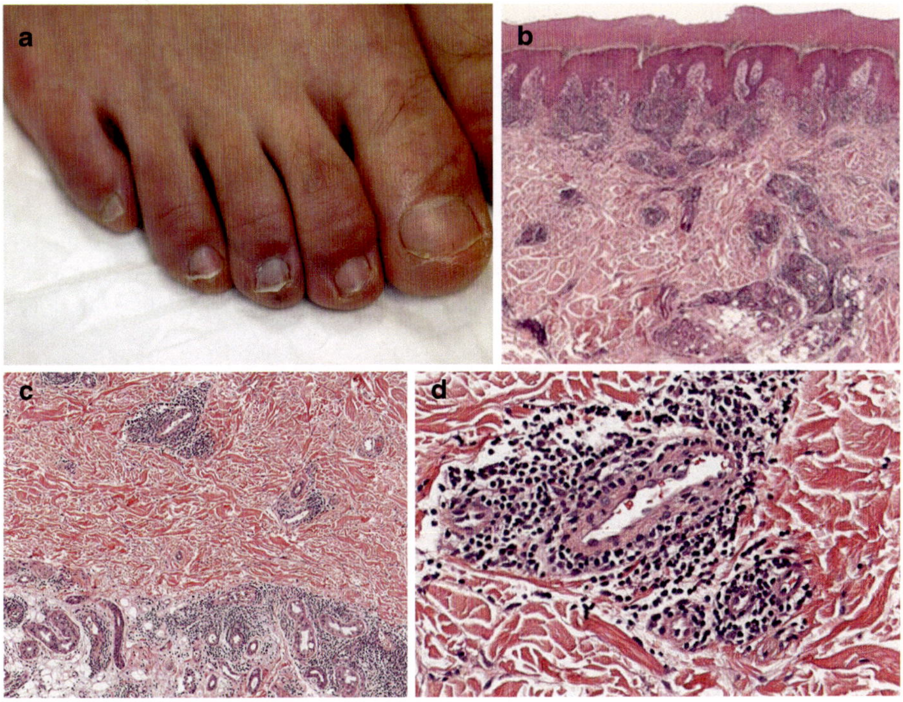

Fig. 1 (**a**) Chilblain-like lesions of the dorsal aspect of the toes (COVID-19 toe), with dusky erythematous edematous macules and plaques, with a purpuric hue. (**b**) Papillary edema with a superficial and deep perivascular lymphocytic infiltrate with perieccrine accentuation. (**c**) Perivascular and perieccrine inflammatory infiltrate. (**d**) The dermal infiltrate tightly cuffs the vessel walls ("lymphocytic vasculitis") with endothelium thickening, without true thrombosis

described, although histopathology was consistent with chilblains [10]. Although highly suspect, several patients with acral chilblain-like lesions demonstrated negative tests for SARS-CoV-2 polymerase chain reaction and serology [11–14]. A prospective study in Spain found only 14.8% positive patients [15]. Dermatoscopy revealed a red, purple, brown, or gray background area with red to purple globules and a gray-brown reticular network located peripherally within the background area [16].

Histopathologic Features

Microscopic features are reproducible and are similar to idiopathic chilblains or chilblain lupus erythematosus [17, 18], showing a superficial and deep perivascular lymphocytic infiltrate with peri-eccrine accentuation (Fig. 1b, c). The lymphocytic dermal infiltrate tightly cuffs the vessel walls ("lymphocytic vasculitis") whose endothelium is thickened without occlusive features (Fig. 1c, d), although small thrombi may occasionally be present in the superficial dermis. Scattered necrotic (apoptotic) keratinocytes and smudging of the basement membrane may be associated findings, but epidermal necrosis is usually absent [19]. Dermal and perieccrine mucin deposition is also seen [20]. Direct immunofluorescence is negative [21, 22]. A recent study on seven children with chilblains found the SARS-CoV-2 immunohistochemistry positive in endothelial cells and epithelial cells of eccrine glands [23]. Moreover, electron microscopy depicted Coronavirus particles in the cytoplasm of endothelial cells. In the same patients, SARS-CoV-2 PCR from nasopharyngeal and oropharyngeal swabs was negative [23].

Work-up

Chilblain-like skin changes of the feet and hands, without another explanation, may suggest COVID-19 infection and should prompt consideration of testing for both PCR and IgM and IgG antibodies.

Differential Diagnosis

Although the clinical appearance of the chilblain-like lesions is similar, if not identical, to that of both idiopathic and autoimmune-related chilblains, these lesions are distinct because they appeared in a relatively warm setting in the absence of a previous history of chilblains, Raynaud's syndrome, or collagen vascular disease.

Etiopathogenesis

An upregulation of interferon and other cytokine signaling pathways is associated with a peripheral microangiopathy, clinically visible as chilblain-like lesions. Early type 1 interferon upregulation can effectively limit SARS-CoV-2 infection, without intervention of the adaptive immune system, explaining the lack of specific antibodies in most of the patients [18]. Effective host innate response also explains the otherwise indolent course of the infection in the majority of young patients, mostly asymptomatic or negative for COVID-19 at nasopharyngeal swabs. A delayed immune-mediated reaction to the virus in genetically predisposed patients has also been proposed [24]. However, some authors have suggested that chilblains are related to a series of environmental conditions due to lockdown such as little physical activity, considerable sedentary position, barefoot, or only wearing socks [14].

Therapy

No treatment is usually recommended [20, 24]. High-potency topical corticosteroids may be helpful if the lesions are causing discomfort [25].

Prognosis and Course

Chilblain-like lesions in the setting of SARS-CoV-2 infection have primarily been described in relatively younger patients who tend to have a milder disease course of COVID-19. Prognosis is excellent, with recovery in all cases after 4–8 weeks. Although some patients experienced new lesions during this time, the outcome has not been affected [22].

Acro-Ischemic-Necrotic Lesions (Retiform Purpura, Acral Livedo Racemosa)

Clinical Features

Acro-ischemia is a vasomotor disorder of the extremities involving severely ill patients in a more or less advanced age which is characterized by different clinical patterns including purplish retiform and roundish dusky patches, some with angled edges or persistent broken, sometimes ulcerated rings (livedo racemosa), livedo

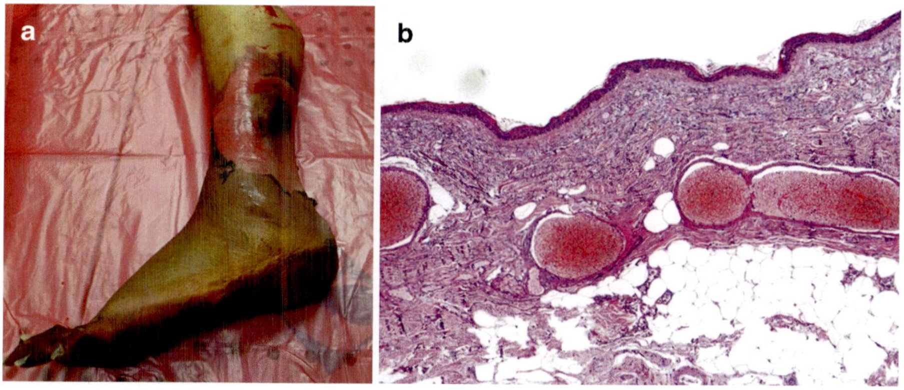

Fig. 2 (**a**) (Acro)ischemic/livedoid/necrotic lesions of the leg with erosion and dry gangrene. (**b**) Thrombotic vasculopathy of dermal vessels with pauci-perivascular inflammatory infiltrate in the absence of leukocytoclastic vasculitis

reticularis, purpura to ecchymoses, bullae formation, necrosis, and dry gangrene [26] (Fig. 2a). A continuum spectrum has been also postulated, ranging from mild chilblain-like manifestations to dry gangrene [27]. The first cases have been reported in severely ill Chinese patients (median age of 59 years) [28], then in 6% of the Spanish COVID-19 patients [6], and in three US patients, presenting with a diffuse purpuric, livedo racemosa-like eruption involving the chest, buttocks, and extremities [29].

Histopathological Features

Acro-ischemic-livedoid-necrotic lesions in severely ill patients are characterized by epidermal necrosis with features of thrombotic vasculopathy, involving the superficial and deep vessels, most of them filled with hyaline thrombi [30] (Fig. 2b). A slight perivascular lymphocytic or neutrophilic infiltrate is seen. Sweat gland necrosis, more evident in the secretory portion of the eccrine sweat coil, with preserved eccrine ducts is a peculiar finding. In some areas, arterioles at the dermo-hypodermal junction showed focal fibrinoid necrosis surrounded by a scarce neutrophilic infiltrate, but no findings of leukocytoclastic vasculitis have been observed. Magro et al. described a pauci-inflammatory thrombogenic vasculopathy [29], with deposition of C5b-9 and C4d in both grossly involved and normally appearing skin, whose microscopic features were similar to those observed in the lungs of three patients who died for severe pneumonitis due to SARS-Cov2.

Etiopathogenesis

SARS-CoV-2 predispose patients to thrombotic disease, both in the venous and arterial circulations for several mechanisms including (i) disseminated intravascular coagulation, (ii) properties of the virus itself, (iii) antiphospholipid syndrome, (iv) activation of complement cascade, (v) endothelial dysfunction, and (vi) drug interactions [26].

Work-up

Elevated levels of D-dimer, fibrinogen, and fibrinogen degradation products are usually found, as well as a prolonged prothrombin time in the setting of disseminated intravascular coagulation [30].

Therapy

Topical corticosteroids, alone or in combination with topical antibiotics, are the most widely reported therapy for acro-ischemic lesions [6, 7]. As these manifestations occur in severely ill patients, as part of the pro-thrombotic setting, treatment with low molecular weight heparin can be beneficial and it is currently included in standard COVID-19 protocols [2].

Prognosis and Course

The prognosis of acro-ischemic-necrotic lesions is serious, being associated with a hypercoagulation state [29, 31]. In the Spanish survey, the mortality rate was approximately 10% [6], while median time from acro-ischemia onset to death in the Chinese study was 12 days [28]. However, an anecdotal COVID-19-positive 74-year-old woman with acral necrotic lesions recovered completely, without systemic implications [31].

Exanthematous Eruptions

Morphology of skin eruptions associated with COVID-19 outbreak is very polymorphic, and classification is limited by the subjectivity of the description in different reports [32]. At least five patterns can be recognized: (a) varicella-like/vesicular, (b) erythematous/maculopapular/morbilliform, (c) urticarial, (d) erythema multiforme-like, and (e) petechial/purpuric [33].

Varicella-Like/Vesicular Eruption

Clinical Features

Among the COVID-19-related diffuse cutaneous eruptions, the varicella-like/vesicular rash is considered the most specific one. It has been described for the first time in a case series of 22 Italian COVID-19-positive patients [34] and in up to 9% of middle-aged Spanish patients [6]. A systematic review confirmed a prevalence ranging from 11% to 18% among COVID-19 patients [3]. The rash is characterized by small, scattered monomorphic vesicles, very similar to chicken pox, with constant trunk involvement and mild/absent pruritus (Fig. 3a), occurring 3 days after systemic

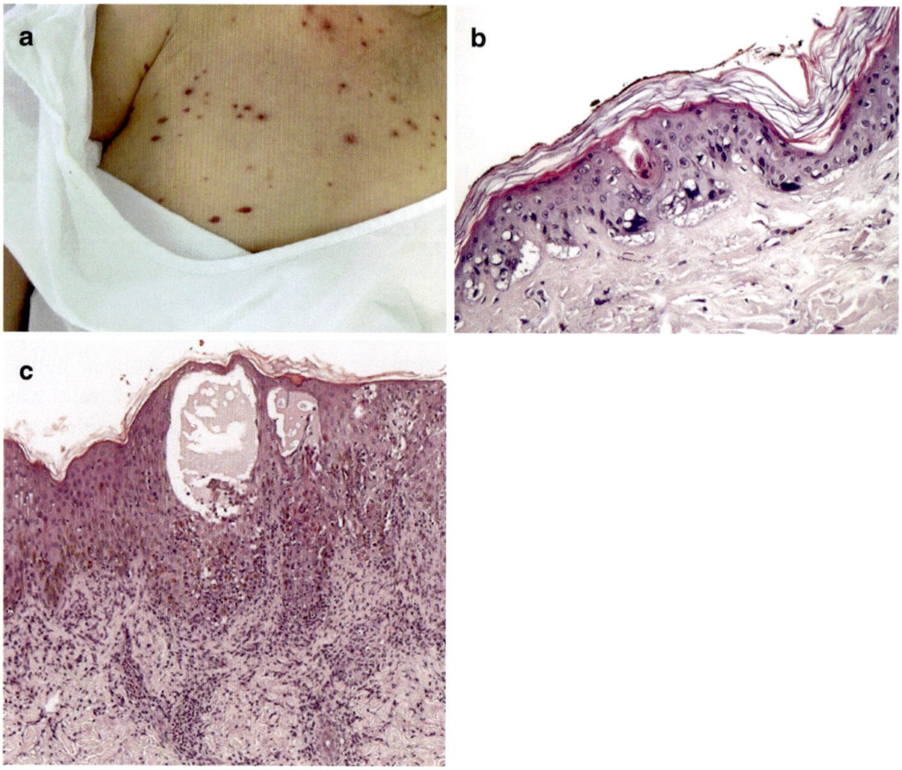

Fig. 3 (**a**) Varicella-like/vesicular eruption with small, scattered vesicles and crusted papules on the trunk. (**b**) Slightly atrophic epidermis, vacuolar degeneration of the basal cell layer, and multinucleate, hyperchromatic keratinocytes with dyskeratotic (apoptotic) cells associated with minimal to absent inflammatory infiltrate in early lesions. (**c**) Later findings include intraepidermal unilocular vesicles, exocytosis, reticular degeneration of the epidermis, acantholytic cells, and scattered dyskeratotic keratinocytes similar to herpetic lesions

symptoms [34]. Alongside this typical vesicular rash, a more polymorphic pattern with addition of papules and pustules has been recently outlined [35]. In some patients the rash was reminiscent of Grover's diseases or herpes-like lesions [36].

Histopathological Features

Histopathology shows cytopathic changes consistent with a viral exanthem. In early lesions [34], a slightly atrophic epidermis with vacuolar degeneration of the basal layer and multinucleate, hyperchromatic keratinocytes with dyskeratotic (apoptotic) cells associated with minimal to absent inflammatory infiltrate has been observed (Fig. 3b). Later findings include intraepidermal unilocular vesicle, reticular degeneration of the epidermis, multinucleated and ballooned keratinocytes, and acantholytic cells, some of them with dyskeratotic features similar to herpetic lesions (Fig. 3c) or pseudo-herpetic Grover's disease [36]. Prominent dyskeratosis, with "pomegranate-like" aspect due to suspected nuclear viral inclusions in multinucleated cells, has also been described [37]. The direct immunofluorescence and SARS-CoV-2 PCR tests performed on vesicles were negative [37].

Differential Diagnosis

The differential diagnosis with true chicken pox is difficult, but typical microscopic findings such as nuclear atypia, large multinucleated cells, acantholysis secondary to ballooning degeneration, and vasculitis which are prominent in varicella have never been outlined in COVID-19 cases with vesicular eruptions. Grover's disease presents with a distinct clinical context, but prevalence of dyskeratosis and acantholytic changes has induced the proposal to name this entity as "COVID-19-associated acantholytic rash" [37].

Etiopathogenesis

Histopathologic findings and reproducible timing from COVID-19 symptom onset support a direct viral effect. Identification of angiotensin-converting enzyme 2 [38], the receptor for SARS-CoV-2 spike protein, expressed in the basal cell layer keratinocytes, supports this hypothesis. Viral interaction with the ACE-2 seems able to induce acantholysis and dyskeratosis.

Therapy

No specific therapy exists. The skin lesions are self-healing and a wait-and-see approach is recommended [34].

Prognosis and Course

The varicella-like/vesicular rash tends to disappear upon 8 days, without leaving scarring [12]. Prognostic significance is variable, as 42% of the Spanish patients developed pneumonia and 13.6% of the Italian patients died of COVID-19 [34].

Erythematous/Maculopapular/Morbilliform Eruption

Clinical Features

A slightly itching widespread erythematous rash is the most frequent cutaneous manifestation associated with COVID-19, although less specific. The Italian first study reported its occurrence in 16% of patients [21], while two Spanish studies reported a prevalence ranging from 30% [39] to 47% [6]. A systematic review assessed a prevalence of 44% [9]. However, in most of the reports, the terms that have been used are variable [32], going from erythema to erythematous eruption to maculopapular (Fig. 4a) or morbilliform rash (Fig. 4a). The palmar and plantar skin and mucosae are spared. Characteristically, it appears at a late stage of the disease [3] and is uncommon among COVID-19-positive children [40].

Histopathologic Features

Morbilliform rash concomitant to SARS-CoV-2 infection is characterized by mild and unspecific histopathological features with no detectable viral RNA and protein and does not seem to be directly caused by the virus [41]. In fact, although infrequently performed, histopathology shows variable features of spongiotic dermatitis, slight vacuolar degeneration with a superficial perivascular and mixed inflammatory infiltrate with lymphocytes, histiocytes, eosinophils, and sometimes neutrophils (Fig. 4b) [39, 42]. Nests of Langerhans cells within the epidermis were also observed. A lymphocytic vasculitis with rare microthrombi and extravasated red blood cells or overlapping features with those of the varicelliform eruption (see above) showing dyskeratotic, ballooning, and necrotic keratinocytes with lymphocytic exocytosis and Grover-like features has also been described. No virally induced cytopathic alterations or intranuclear inclusions have been identified [43].

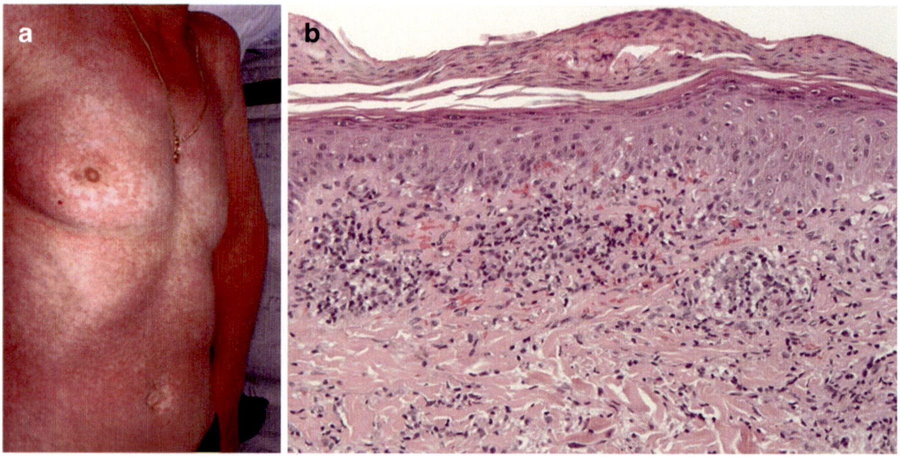

Fig. 4 (**a**) Maculopapular eruption of the trunk in a COVID-19 symptomatic patient. (**b**) Parakeratosis, slight spongiosis, vacuolar degeneration of basal cell layer, and perivascular and interstitial infiltrate made by lymphocytes, histiocytes, and some neutrophils with red blood cell extravasation

Etiopathogenesis

From the few information recovered, it can be postulated that viral particles circulating in the blood of patients with COVID-19 infection reach the skin vessels, where they set off a lymphocytic vasculitis [42]. Immune complex deposition and activated cytokines might produce alterations similar to what happens in thrombophylic arteritis. Keratinocytes may be a secondary target, after Langerhans cells activation, thus inducing a spectrum of different clinical and pathological manifestations, going from simple vasodilation and spongiosis to lymphocytic vasculitis and microthrombi formation. Actually, it is well reported that SARS-CoV-2 infection can cause overactive immune responses that may induce immunopathological conditions, named as *cytokine storm*. Cytokines could reach not only the lung but all other organs, including the skin. By stimulating inflammatory cells, cytokines could promote eruptions such as erythema, urticarial lesions, vesicles, and others. In this view, rashes may be paraviral due to cytokine release [44].

Differential Diagnosis

Drug hypersensitivity reaction and viral infections are the most common cause of morbilliform eruptions, with significant and often problematic clinical overlap. Drug-induced rashes usually develop within 3 days to 3 weeks after initiation of a novel drug and may last up to 2 weeks after cessation of attributable treatment. Blood hypereosinophilia can be an argument, although weak, in favor of drug-induced rash. Histopathological features of these two types of eruptions are also overlapping. Subtle microscopic clues in favor of drug hypersensitivity reaction are eosinophilic infiltrate in the dermis, lymphocytic exocytosis, basal cell damage with apoptotic keratinocytes, and usually more marked lymphocytic dermal infiltrate than in viral exanthem [45].

Therapy

The erythematous/maculopapular/morbilliform eruptions have a self-limiting course and resolve without specific therapy [46]. However, several authors suggest treatment with topical corticosteroids, oral antihistamines, and oral corticosteroids [6, 47]. Vitamin C and topical steroid have also been used [47].

Prognosis and Course

The erythematous/maculopapular/morbilliform rash lasts for about 9 days and seems to be sometimes associated with a variable course, including also a severe outcome [6, 33].

Urticarial Eruption

Clinical Presentation

Acute urticaria, albeit nonspecific, has been reported as a prodromal clinical finding among adult COVID-19 patients, with a variable timing: some lesions appeared before onset of fever, while others in combination with pyrexia and cough [48–50]. Presentation is not different from idiopathic urticaria (Fig. 5a), with small or larger itching wheals. In the Spanish cohort of COVID-19-positive patients, 19% of them presented an urticarial eruption lasting a mean time of 6.8 days [6].

Histopathological Features

The prevalent pattern is reminiscent of idiopathic urticaria, with a perivascular lymphocytic infiltrate, upper dermal edema, and some eosinophils, without virally-induced cytopathic alterations or intranuclear inclusions [51]. Urticarial vasculitis has also been documented in two patients with persistent urticarial plaques and residual purpura, showing a small vessel leukocytoclastic vasculitis, with red blood cell extravasation, perivascular infiltrate of neutrophils and karyorrhexis, endothelial swelling and fibrinoid necrosis [52]. Finally, a superficial perivascular lymphocytic infiltrate without eosinophils, accompanied by a lichenoid and vacuolar interface dermatitis with occasional dyskeratotic keratinocytes in the basal layer, has been described in a 39-year-old man with a widespread erythematous and edematous, non-pruritic urticarial-like eruption [53].

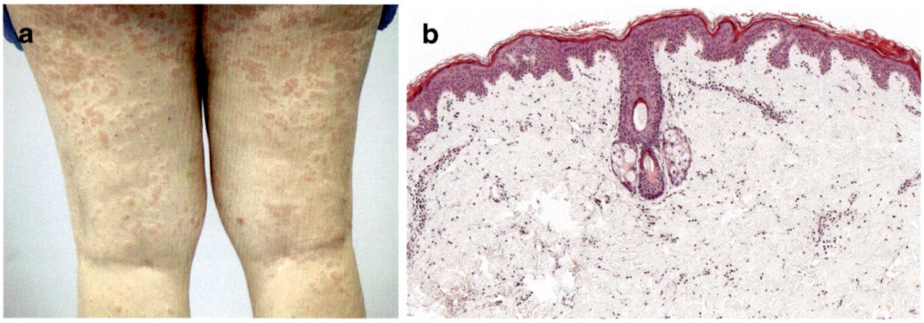

Fig. 5 (**a**) Figurate urticarial eruption of the limbs in a COVID-19 symptomatic woman. (**b**) Normal epidermis and a superficial perivascular mixed infiltrate with lymphocytes, some eosinophils and neutrophils with slight edema

Etiopathogenesis

Sars-Cov-2 might directly and/or indirectly induce mast cell and basophil activation, although not yet demonstrated [54] Late-onset persistent lesions are probably related to the general immune system activation, confirmed by the association with vasculitis and absence of eosinophils in the infiltrate, with spongiotic or lichenoid interface dermatitis [52, 53].

Therapy

A systematic review and case series of acute urticaria in COVID-19 patients recommend treatment with antihistamines [55–58] with additional low-dose prednisone to be considered on an individualized basis [59]. Skin lesions resolved from less than 24 hours to up to 2 weeks, without recurrence at steroidal dismission.

Prognosis and Course

In a Spanish study, urticarial eruption seems to carry rarely a severe prognosis with a mortality rate of 2% [6]. Concomitant systemic eosinophilia has been suggested to be predictor of a better outcome [60].

Erythema Multiforme-Like Eruption

Clinical Presentation

The occurrence of erythema multiforme (EM) lesions is reported both in young patients, with good prognosis [6, 21], and in older persons, associated with severe COVID-19 symptoms [61]. In youngsters, the lesions vary from target (three rings) to targetoid (two rings) confluent macules, papules, and plaques, some with hemorrhages and central crusts and are associated with chilblain-like lesions on acral sites such as the palms, elbows, and knees. Lesions recover spontaneously within 1–3 weeks. By converse, in older patients (mean age 67 years), the eruption is widespread, with palatal macules and petechiae and sparing palms and soles, and is associated with mild alterations of the coagulation system [61]. In one patient the skin rash had occurred concomitantly to COVID-19 symptoms, while three additional patients presented with EM-like eruption after the discharge for disease recovery, thus causing a new hospitalization.

Histopathological Features

Histopathology confirms different patterns: acral lesions in adolescents with chilblain-like showed a superficial and deep perivascular lymphocytic infiltrate with perieccrine involvement and some vasculopathic changes, reminiscent of what is observed in chilblain-like lesions [12]. The infiltrate was made of CD3+ T cells, with a mix of CD4+ and CD8+ lymphocytes. Immunohistochemical stain with the antibody against SARS-CoV/SARS-CoV-2 spike protein in two cases showed granular positivity in the endothelial cells and epithelial cells of eccrine glands. In the diffuse form involving adults [61], histopathology was consistent with true EM, showing spongiosis, lymphocytic exocytosis, variable degrees of interface dermatitis, and focal necrotic keratinocytes.

Etiopathogenesis

It is likely that the acral EM-like lesions in young persons are a clinical variant of chilblain-like lesions [12], while the more generalized adult EM-like eruption, with enanthem, corresponds to EM related to a late response to SARS-Cov2, as the majority of patients recovered from COVID-19 at the onset of skin lesions. An adverse drug reaction could not be ruled out, because of the relative multidrug intake, as well as other possible triggers [61].

Therapy

More severe erythema multiforme-like eruptions can be treated with systemic steroids [62].

Prognosis and Course

Erythema multiforme (EM) lesions in young patients recover spontaneously within 1–3 weeks and are associated with a good prognosis [6, 21] while lesions in older people are associated with more severe COVID-19 symptoms [61].

Petechial/Purpuric Eruption

A petechial/purpuric rash should be considered herald of symptomatic COVID-19 in aged patients, carrying a benign course with complete recovery. Lesions distribution was variable, from symmetric periflexural confluent erythematous macules, papules, and petechiae in a 48-year-old patient [63] to a more generalized petechial eruption in a 59-year-old man (Fig. 6a) [64], as well as limited to the lower limbs in 61-year-old woman [65].

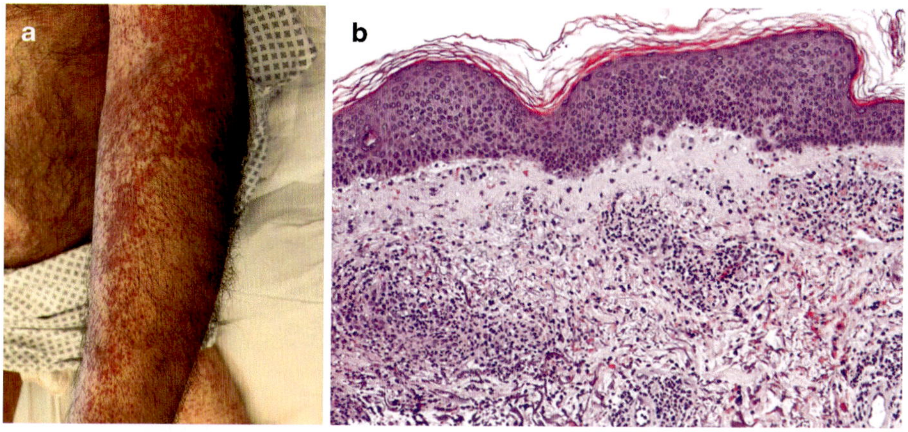

Fig. 6 (**a**) Petechial/purpuric eruption in asymptomatic COVID-19 man. (**b**) Histopathologic findings showing a typical leukocytoclastic vasculitis of small vessels with red blood cell extravasation

Histopathological Features

Results from the few histopathological studies are again variable. One survey shows a superficial perivascular lymphocytic infiltrate with hemorrhages and papillary edema with some dyskeratotic epidermal cells in the absence of vasculopathy [63]. The two other reports found a typical leukocytoclastic vasculitis of small vessels (Fig. 6b) [64, 65]. No viral cytopathic changes were observed.

Etiopathogenesis

Purpuric lesions with features of leukocytoclastic vasculitis may represent an immune complex hypersensitivity reaction to antigens of SARS-CoV2 [64, 65]; however, an immune-mediated reaction to drugs cannot be ruled out.

Differential Diagnosis

The petechial rash related to COVID-19 can be a misleading feature in tropical countries, where dengue fever is endemic, and overlapping signs and symptoms would make diagnosis and treatment difficult [68]. From the first case reported in Thailand [66], a general alert has been diffused, and presence of high dengue antibodies can give false-negative testing for SARS-CoV-2. In this setting, only reverse transcription polymerase chain reaction (RT-PCR) testing is resolutive [67].

Therapy

Topical corticosteroids have been successfully used for treating mild cases of purpuric rash. Leukocytoclastic vasculitis associated with COVID-19 can be treated with a dose of 0.5 mg/Kg/daily of prednisone [68, 69], although a patient already under steroids developed a purpuric leukocytoclastic vasculitis [64].

Prognosis and Course

Purpuric lesions seem to occur more frequently in elderly patients with severe COVID-19, representing a skin manifestation associated with a guarded prognosis [6, 64].

Skin Manifestations of Multisystem Inflammatory Syndrome in Children (MIS-C) and Pediatric Inflammatory Multisystem Syndrome (PIMS) (Atypical Kawasaki Disease)

During the pandemic course, European and US pediatricians started to notice cases of a severe hyperinflammatory condition, sharing some features with toxic shock syndrome, Kawasaki disease, and macrophage activation syndrome in otherwise healthy patients. Multisystem inflammatory syndrome in children (MIS-C) and pediatric inflammatory multisystem syndrome (PIMS) have designated this new entity in the USA and Europe, respectively. The mean age of patients with MIS-C/PIMS is higher than that usually seen with classic Kawasaki disease ranging from 3.7 to 16.6 years (median 7.9 years). Generally, in comparison with Kawasaki disease, children with MIS-C/PIMS display an overrepresentation of gastrointestinal symptoms, cardiac involvement, and shock syndrome [70].

Clinical Features

This syndrome was described initially by Riphagen, presenting with unrelenting fever, conjunctivitis, and abdominal pain, progressing to hemodynamic shock and severe myocardial involvement [71]. An Italian survey reported a 30-time increase in the rate of Kawasaki-like presentation during the COVID-19 pandemic among children [72] The nasopharyngeal swabs taken from these children were mostly negative, once again putting into discussion a direct responsibility of SARS-CoV-2 infection. However, further reports highlighted that most patients had a clinical history of exposure to COVID-19 patients and/or SARS-COV2 biological diagnosis. The spectrum of severity ranged from standard hospitalization to pediatric intensive care unit management. In addition to general symptoms such as fever for >5 days, cardiac involvement (hypotension, myocarditis), gastrointestinal symptoms (diarrhea), hematological features, or other organ dysfunctions, patients may present with mucocutaneous manifestations. Skin morphology, however, has been poorly characterized, mostly suggestive of erythema multiforme, but also maculopapular, morbilliform rashes and vasculitis [73–75]. Transient and protean mucocutaneous changes, including conjunctival injection, palmoplantar erythema, lip hyperemia, periorbital erythema and edema, strawberry tongue, and malar erythema, have also been described [76].

Recently, MIS occurrence in an adult with SARS-CoV-2 infection has been reported, and dermatological findings were also described as erythema multiforme-like lesions [77].

Histopathological Features

Two different microscopic patterns from few biopsies have been at least identified: the former is consistent with leukocytoclastic vasculitis [11], while the latter is characterized by erythema multiforme-like changes, showing a nonspecific sparse inflammatory infiltrate with few intraepidermal neutrophils and necrotic keratinocytes. Direct immunofluorescence has outlined the presence of IgA and complement in the vessel walls, which might be a key factor of the vasculitis [76].

Work-up

Markers of inflammation, including erythrocyte sedimentation rate, CRP, neutrophil count, and ferritin, are elevated in almost all cases. Leukopenia may be a finding. Interleukin-6 level was shown to be elevated in the setting of a cytokine storm.

Etiopathogenesis

Exaggerated innate immunologic activation causing multisystem vasculitis involving medium-sized arteries is implicated in MIS-C/PIMS, with similar pathological abnormalities in affected internal organs and the skin, rather than direct viral injury.

Therapy

Most children will need to be treated in a hospital. Treatments include corticosteroids, intravenous immunoglobulin, ASA, and anticoagulation therapy. However, additional immunomodulator agents such as antitumor necrosis factor alpha, anti-IL-6, and interleukin-1 receptor antagonist could play a role in difficult cases [78].

Prognosis and Course

The prognosis of MIS-C seemed favorable without sequelae in most patients despite a reported mortality rate of approximately 1.5%. Cutaneous findings are responsive to the main treatment [78].

Miscellanea

A widespread *pityriasis rosea-like rash* in a 27-year-old COVID-19-positive patient occurred 3 days after mild systemic symptoms including low-grade fever, fatigue, anorexia, and gastroenteritis [79]. No biopsy was taken. The patient recovered completely.

A *papulosquamous eruption* with a peculiar *digitate* morphology presented in a hospitalized elderly diabetic man [80]. The patient died from COVID-19-related complications, although the eruption had spontaneously resolved in 1 week. A skin biopsy revealed diffuse spongiosis with vesicles containing lymphocytes and Langerhans cells. The dermis showed mild papillary edema and a superficial lympho-histiocytic infiltrate. The real-time PCR for SARS-CoV-2 in the fresh tissue resulted negative.

Manifestations suggestive of *livedo reticularis* in COVID-19-positive adults have been reported [81, 82]. The dusky not blanching lacelike network, forming annular patches around a pale center, may be unilateral and transitory or symmetrical and more generalized without signs of vasculitis. Biopsy was not performed.

Similar to transient livedo, *skin mottling* developed in an Iranian neonate [83] with positive history of COVID-19 in the mother. Fever, sepsis signs, and positive SARS-CoV-2 testing confirmed disease in the child, but the course was benign, with dismission 2 days after referral. No skin biopsies were performed.

An *intertriginous and flexural exanthema*, similar to the symmetrical drug-related intertriginous and flexural exanthema (SDRIFE), developed in a diabetic 64-year-old woman 4 days after the onset of COVID-19 symptoms [84]. Biopsy was not performed.

An *erythema annulare centrifugum* with anosmia and ageusia in a SARS-CoV-2-exposed patient successfully treated with doxycycline has been signaled [85].

Conclusions

A great heterogeneity of cutaneous manifestations is increasingly associated with SARS-CoV2 infection. Actually, only three patterns are considered specifically related to COVID-19 with a consistent degree of reliability, because they have occurred in many patients in the course of the pandemic, and they have been described by independent investigators. They include chilblain-like lesions, acro-ischemic-necrotic-livedoid lesions, and varicelliform-like/vesicular eruptions [2, 12, 22–48]. Histopathologic correlation has provided more insights not only on the diagnosis but also on the possible mechanisms and course of these diseases. Chilblain-like lesions are associated with a pauci or asymptomatic course, while acro-ischemic-necrotic-livedoid manifestations alert about the severe thrombotic vasculopathy in progress. Although the varicelliform-like/vesicular eruptions are associated with variable outcome, they represent the most specific manifestation of the viral direct cytopathic interaction with the skin. As regards the plea of other skin patterns, the association with COVID-19 remains presumptive. Clinical-pathologic correlation confirms its crucial role in the differential diagnosis with skin lesions related to different viral conditions and skin adverse drug reactions, but more skin biopsies are warranted. Improvement of accessibility to immunohistochemical staining with antibodies to SARS-CoV/SARS-CoV-2 spike protein on paraffin-embedded specimens, RNA detection of SARS-CoV-2 strain by real-time PCR-based assay, and electron microscopy studies would make the final difference, especially in patients with negative nasopharyngeal swab and serology. Dermatologists and dermatopathologists should stay up-to-date on the rapidly changing literature to continue playing a vital role in aiding in the diagnosis and understanding of COVID-19 infection.

References

1. Zhu N, Zhang D, Wang W, et al. A novel coronavirus from patients with pneumonia in China, 2019. N Engl J Med. 2020;382:727–33.
2. Kakodkar P, Kaka N, Baig M. A comprehensive literature review on the clinical presentation, and management of the pandemic coronavirus disease 2019 (COVID-19). Cureus. 2020;12(4):e7560.
3. Matar S, Oulès B, Sohier P, et al. Cutaneous manifestations in SARS-CoV-2 infection (COVID-19): a French experience and a systematic review of the literature [published online ahead of print, 2020 Jun 26]. J Eur Acad Dermatol Venereol. 2020.
4. Guan WJ, Ni ZY, Hu Y, et al. Clinical characteristics of coronavirus disease 2019 in China. N Engl J Med. 2020;382:1708–20.
5. Recalcati S. Cutaneous manifestations in COVID-19: a first perspective [published online ahead of print, 2020 Mar 26]. J Eur Acad Dermatol Venereol . 2020.
6. Galván Casas C, Català A, Carretero Hernández G, et al. Classification of the cutaneous manifestations of COVID-19: a rapid prospective nationwide consensus study in Spain with 375 cases Br J Dermatol 2020;183:71–7.
7. Freeman EE, McMahon DE, Lipoff JB, et al. The spectrum of COVID-19-associated dermatologic manifestations: an international registry of 716 patients from 31 countries [published online ahead of print, 2020]. J Am Acad Dermatol. 2020;S0190-9622(20):32126–5.
8. Wollina U, Karadağ AS, Rowland-Payne C, Chiriac A, Lotti T. Cutaneous signs in COVID-19 patients: a review Dermatol Ther. 2020;33(5):e13549.
9. Zhao Q, Fang X, Pang Z, Zhang B, Liu H, Zhang F. COVID-19 and cutaneous manifestations: a systematic review J Eur Acad Dermatol Venereol. 2020;34:2505–10.
10. Roca-Ginés J, Torres-Navarro I, Sánchez-Arráez J, et al. Assessment of acute acral lesions in a case series of children and adolescents during the COVID-19 pandemic. JAMA Dermatol. 2020;156:992–7.

11. Schnapp A, Abulhija H, Maly A, et al. Introductory histopathological findings may shed light on COVID-19 paediatric hyperinflammatory shock syndrome J Eur Acad Dermatol Venereol. 2020;34:e665–7.
12. Torrelo A, Andina D, Santonja C, et al. Erythema multiforme-like lesions in children and COVID-19 [published online ahead of print, 2020]. Pediatr Dermatol . 2020;37:442–6.
13. Caselli D, Chironna M, Loconsole D, et al. No evidence of SARS-CoV-2 infection by polymerase chain reaction or serology in children with pseudo-chilblain Br J Dermatol. 2020; 183:784–5.
14. Herman A, Peeters C, Verroken A, et al. Evaluation of chilblains as a manifestation of the COVID-19 pandemic . JAMA Dermatol . 2020:156:998–1003.
15. Docampo-Simón A, Sánchez-Pujol MJ, Juan-Carpena G, et al. Are chilblain-like acral skin lesions really indicative of COVID-19? A prospective study and literature review J Eur Acad Dermatol Venereol. 2020;34:e445–7.
16. Navarro L, Andina D, Noguera-Morel L et al. Dermoscopy features of COVID-19-related chilblains in children and adolescents. J Eur Acad Dermatol Venereol . 2020;34:e762–4.
17. Locatelli AG, Robustelli Test E, Vezzoli P, et al. Histologic features of long-lasting chilblain-like lesions in a pediatric COVID-19 patient. J Eur Acad Dermatol Venereol. 2020;34:e365–8.
18. Kolivras A, Dehavay F, Delplace D, et al. Coronavirus (COVID-19) infection-induced chilblains: a case report with histopathologic findings. JAAD Case Rep. 2020;18:489–92.
19. de Masson A, Bouaziz JD, Sulimovic L, et al. Chilblains is a common cutaneous finding during the COVID-19 pandemic: a retrospective nationwide study from France. J Am Acad Dermatol. 2020;83:667–70.
20. El Hachem M, Diociaiuti A, Concato C, et al. A clinical, histopathological and laboratory study of 19 consecutive Italian paediatric patients with chilblain-like lesions: lights and shadows on the relationship with COVID-19 infection [published online ahead of print, 2020]. J Eur Acad Dermatol Venereol. 2020;34:2620–9.
21. Recalcati S, Barbagallo T, Frasin LA, et al. Acral cutaneous lesions in the time of COVID-19 [published online ahead of print, 2020]. J Eur Acad Dermatol Venereol. 2020;34:e346–7.
22. Andina D, Noguera-Morel L, Bascuas-Arribas M, et al. Chilblains in children in the setting of COVID-19 pandemic. Pediatr Dermatol. 2020;37:406–11.
23. Colmenero, I., Santonja, C., Alonso-Riaño, M., et al. SARS-CoV-2 endothelial infection causes COVID-19 chilblains: histopathological, immunohistochemical and ultrastructural study of seven paediatric cases. Br J Dermatol. 2020;183:729–37.
24. Piccolo V, Neri I, Filippeschi C, et al. Chilblain-like lesions during COVID-19 epidemic: a preliminary study on 63 patients [published online ahead of print, 2020]. J Eur Acad Dermatol Venereol. 2020;34:e291–3.
25. Ladha MA, Luca N, Constantinescu C, Naert K, Ramien ML. Approach to chilblains during the COVID-19 pandemic [Formula: see text]. J Cutan Med Surg. 2020;24(5):504–17.
26. Alonso MN, Mata-Forte T, García-León N, Vullo PA, Ramirez-Olivencia G, Estébanez M, Álvarez-Marcos F. Incidence, characteristics, laboratory findings and outcomes in acroischemia in COVID-19 patients. Vasc Health Risk Manag. 2020;16:467–78.
27. Suarez-Valle A, Fernandez-Nieto D, Diaz-Guimaraens B, Dominguez-Santas M, Carretero I, Perez-Garcia B. Acro-ischemia in hospitalized COVID-19 patients J Eur Acad Dermatol Venereol. 2020;34:e455–7.
28. Zhang Y, Cao W, Jiang W, et al. Profile of natural anticoagulant, coagulant factor and anti-phospholipid antibody in critically ill COVID-19 patients [published online ahead of print, 2020]. J Thromb Thrombolysis. 2020:1–7.
29. Magro C, Mulvey JJ, Berlin D, et al. Complement associated microvascular injury and thrombosis in the pathogenesis of severe COVID-19 infection: a report of five cases [published online ahead of print, 2020]. Transl Res. 2020;S1931–5244(20)30070-0.
30. Llamas-Velasco M, Muñoz-Hernández P, Lázaro-González J, et al. Thrombotic occlusive vasculopathy in skin biopsy from a livedoid lesion of a COVID-19 patient Br J Dermatol. 2020;183:591–3.

31. Balestri R, Termine S, Rech G, Girardelli CR. Late onset of acral necrosis after SARS-CoV-2 infection resolution J Eur Acad Dermatol Venereol. 2020;34:e448–9.
32. Guarneri C, Venanzi Rullo E, Gallizzi R, Ceccarelli M, Cannavò SP, Nunnari G. Diversity of clinical appearance of cutaneous manifestations in the course of COVID-19. J Eur Acad Dermatol Venereol. 2020;34:e449–50.
33. Català A, Galván-Casas C, Carretero-Hernández G, et al. Maculopapular eruptions associated to COVID-19: a subanalysis of the COVID-Piel study. Dermatol Ther. 2020;33:e14170.
34. Marzano AV, Genovese G, Fabbrocini G, et al. Varicella- like exanthem as a specific COVID-19-associated skin manifestation: multicenter case series of 22 patients. J Am Acad Dermatol. 2020;83:280–5.
35. Fernandez-Nieto D, Ortega-Quijano D, Jimenez-Cauhe J, et al. Clinical and histological characterization of vesicular COVID-19 rashes: a prospective study in a tertiary care hospital. Clin Exp Dermatol. 2020;45:872–5.
36. Llamas-Velasco M, Chicharro P, Rodríguez-Jiménez P, et al. Reply to "Clinical and histological characterization of vesicular COVID-19 rashes: a prospective study in a tertiary care hospital": pseudo herpetic Grover disease seems to appear in patients with COVID-19 infection. Clin Exp Dermatol. 2020;45:896–8.
37. Mahé A, Birckel E, Merklen C, et al. Histology of skin lesions establishes that the vesicular rash associated with COVID-19 is not 'varicella-like'. J Eur Acad Dermatol Venereol. 2020;34:e559–61.
38. Hamming I, Timens W, Bulthuis ML, Lely AT, Navis G, van Goor H. Tissue distribution of ACE2 protein, the functional receptor for SARS coronavirus. J Pathol. 2004;203:631–7.
39. Ahouach B, Harent S, Ullmer A, et al. Cutaneous lesions in a patient with COVID-19: are they related? Br J Dermatol. 2020;183(2):e31.
40. Morey-Olivé M, Espiau M, Mercadal-Hally M, Lera-Carballo E, García-Patos V. Cutaneous manifestations in the current pandemic of coronavirus infection disease (COVID 2019). An Pediatr (Engl Ed). 2020;92:374–5.
41. Fattori A, Cribier B, Chenard MP, Mitcov M, Mayeur S, Weingertner N. Cutaneous manifestations in patients with coronavirus disease 2019: clinical and histological findings. Hum Pathol. 2020;107:39–45.
42. Vesely MD, Perkins SH. Caution in the time of rashes and COVID-19 [published online ahead of print, 2020 Jul 15]. J Am Acad Dermatol. 2020;S0190-9622(20)32190–3.
43. Rongioletti F, Ferreli C, Sena P, Caputo V, Atzori L. Clinicopathologic correlations of COVID-19–related cutaneous manifestations with special emphasis on histopathologic patterns. Clin Dermatol. 2021;39:149–62.
44. Lipsker D. Paraviral eruptions in the era of COVID-19: do some skin manifestations point to a natural resistance to SARS-CoV-2? Clin Dermatol. 2020;38(6):757–61.
45. Atzori L, Perla S, Atzori MG, Ferreli C, Rongioletti F. Cutaneous drug eruptions associated with COVID-19 therapy. JAAD Int. 2020;1(1):73–6.
46. De Giorgi V, Recalcati S, Jia Z, et al. Cutaneous manifestations related to coronavirus disease 2019 (COVID-19): a prospective study from China and Italy. J Am Acad Dermatol. 2020;83:674–5.
47. Iancu GM, Solomon A, Birlutiu V. Viral exanthema as manifestation of SARS-CoV-2 infection: a case report. Medicine (Baltimore). 2020;99:e21810.
48. Henry D, Ackerman M, Sancelme E, Finon A, Esteve E. Urticarial eruption in COVID-19 infection J Eur Acad Dermatol Venereol. 2020;34:e244–5.
49. van Damme C, Berlingin E, Saussez S, Accaputo O. Acute urticaria with pyrexia as the first manifestations of a COVID-19 infection. J Eur Acad Dermatol Venereol . 2020;34:e300–1.
50. Fernandez-Nieto D, Ortega-Quijano D, Segurado-Miravalles G, Pindado-Ortega C, Prieto-Barrios M, Jimenez-Cauhe J. Comment on: cutaneous manifestations in COVID-19: a first perspective. Safety concerns of clinical images and skin biopsies J Eur Acad Dermatol Venereol. 2020;34:e252–4.

51. Rodríguez-Jiménez P, Chicharro P, De Argila D, Muñoz-Hernández P, Llamas-Velasco M. Urticaria-like lesions in COVID-19 patients are not really urticaria – a case with clinico-pathological correlation. J Eur Acad Dermatol Venereol. 2020;34:e459–60.
52. de Perosanz-Lobo D, Fernandez-Nieto D, Burgos-Blasco P, et al. Urticarial vasculitis in COVID-19 infection: a vasculopathy-related symptom? J Eur Acad Dermatol Venereol. 2020;34:e566–8.
53. Amatore F, Macagno N, Mailhe M, et al. SARS-CoV-2 infection presenting as a febrile rash. J Eur Acad Dermatol Venereol. 2020;34(7):e304–6.
54. Criado PR, Abdalla BMZ, de Assis IC, van Blarcum de Graaff MC, Caputo GC, Vieira IC. Are the cutaneous manifestations during or due to SARS-CoV-2 infection/COVID-19 frequent or not? Revision of possible pathophysiologic mechanisms. Inflamm Res. 2020;69(8):745–56.
55. Abuelgasim E, Dona ACM, Sondh RS, Harky A. Management of urticaria in COVID-19 patients: a systematic review. Dermatol Ther. 2020:e14328.
56. Henry D, Ackerman M, Sancelme E, Finon A, Esteve E. Urticarial eruption in COVID-19 infection. J Eur Acad Dermatol Venereol. 2020;34:e244–5.
57. Van Damme C, Berlingin E, Saussez S, Accaputo O. Acute urticaria with pyrexia as the first manifestations of a COVID-19 infection. J Eur Acad Dermatol Venereol. 2020;34:e300–1.
58. Quintana-Castanedo L, Feito-Rodriguez M, Valero-Lopez I, Chiloeches-Fernandez C, Sendagorta-Cudos E, Herranz-Pinto P. Urticarial exanthem as early diagnostic clue for COVID-19 infec-tion. JAAD Case Rep. 2020;6:498–9.
59. Shansai M. Low-dose systemic steroids, an emerging therapeutic option for COVID-19 related urticaria. J Dermatol Treat. 2020;16:1–2.
60. Dastoli S, Bennardo L, Patruno C, Nisticò SP. Are erythema multiforme and urticaria related to a better outcome of COVID-19?. Dermatol Ther. 2020:e13681.
61. Jimenez-Cauhe J, Ortega-Quijano D, Carretero-Barrio I, et al. Erythema multiforme-like eruption in patients with COVID-19 infection: clinical and histological findings. Clin Exp Dermatol. 2020;45:892–5.
62. Demirbaş A, Elmas OF, Atasoy M, Türsen U, Lotti T. A case of erythema multiforme major in a patient with COVID 19: the role of corticosteroid treatment. Dermatol Ther. 2020:e13899.
63. Diaz-Guimaraens B, Dominguez-Santas M, Suarez-Valle A, et al. Petechial skin rash associated with severe acute respiratory syndrome coronavirus 2 infection. JAMA Dermatol. 2020;156:820–22.
64. Caputo V, Schroeder J, Rongioletti F. A generalized purpuric eruption with histopathologic features of leucocytoclastic vasculitis in a patient severely ill with COVID-19. J Eur Acad Dermatol Venereol. 2020;34:e579–81.
65. Dominguez-Santas M, Diaz-Guimaraens B, Garcia Abellas P, Moreno-Garcia Del Real C, Burgos-Blasco P, Suarez-Valle A. Cutaneous small-vessel vasculitis associated with novel 2019 coronavirus SARS-CoV-2 infection (COVID-19). J Eur Acad Dermatol Venereol. 2020;34:e536–7.
66. Joob B, Wiwanitkit V. COVID-19 can present with a rash and be mistaken for dengue. J Am Acad Dermatol. 2020;82(5):e177.
67. Lokida D, Lukman N, Salim G, et al. Diagnosis of COVID-19 in a dengue-endemic area. Am J Trop Med Hyg. 2020;103:1220–2.
68. Mayor-Ibarguren A, Feito-Rodriguez M, Quintana Castanedo L, Ruiz-Bravo E, Montero Vega D, Herranz-Pinto P. Cutaneous small vessel vasculitis secondary to COVID-19 infection: a case report. J Eur Acad Dermatol Venereol. 2020;34:e541–2.
69. Camprodon Gómez M, González-Cruz C, Ferrer B, Barberá MJ. Leucocytoclastic vasculitis in a patient with COVID-19 with positive SARS-CoV-2 PCR in skin biopsy. BMJ Case Rep. 2020;13:e238039.
70. Andina D, Belloni-Fortina A, Bodemer C, et al. Skin manifestations of COVID-19 in children: part 2. Clin Exp Dermatol. 2021;46:451–61.
71. Riphagen S, Gomez X, Gonzalez-Martinez C, et al. Hyperinflammatory shock in children during COVID-19 pandemic. Lancet. 2020;395:1607–8.

72. Verdoni L, Mazza A, Gervasoni A, et al. An outbreak of severe Kawasaki-like disease at the Italian epicentre of the SARS-CoV-2 epidemic: an observational cohort study. Lancet. 2020;6736:1.
73. Bapst T, Romano F, Müller M, Rohr M. Special dermatological presentation of paediatric multisystem inflammatory syndrome related to COVID-19: erythema multiforme. BMJ Case Rep. 2020;13:e236986.
74. Moghadam P, Blum L, Ahouach B, et al. Multisystem inflammatory syndrome with particular cutaneous lesions related to COVID 19 in a young adult [published online ahead of print, 2020]. Am J Med. 2020;S0002-9343(20):30608–2.
75. Yozgat CY, Uzuner S, Bursal Duramaz B, et al. Dermatological manifestation of pediatrics multisystem inflammatory syndrome associated with COVID-19 in a 3-year-old girl. Dermatol Ther. 2020:e13770.
76. Young TK, Shaw KS, Shah JK, Noor A, Alperin RA, Ratner AJ, Orlow SJ, Betensky RA, Shust GF, Kahn PJ, Oza VS. Mucocutaneous manifestations of multisystem inflammatory syndrome in children during the COVID-19 pandemic. JAMA Dermatol. 2020:e204779.
77. Shaigany S, Gnirke M, Guttmann A, et al. An adult with Kawasaki-like multisystem inflammatory syndrome associated with COVID-19. Lancet. 2020;396:e8–e10.
78. Kwak JH, Lee SY, Choi JW, Korean Society of Kawasaki Disease. Clinical features, diagnosis, and outcomes of multisystem inflammatory syndrome in children associated with coronavirus disease 2019. Clin Exp Pediatr. 2021;64:68–75.
79. Ehsani Ehsani AH, Nasimi M, Bigdelo Z. Pityriasis rosea as a cutaneous manifestation of COVID-19 infection. J Eur Acad Dermatol Venereol. 2020;34:e436–7.
80. Sanchez A, Sohier P, Benghanem S, et al. Digitate papulosquamous eruption associated with severe acute respiratory syndrome coronavirus 2 infection. JAMA Dermatol. 2020;156:819–20.
81. Manalo IF, Smith MK, Cheeley J, Jacobs R. A dermatologic manifestation of COVID-19: transient livedo reticularis. J Am Acad Dermatol. 2020;83(2):700.
82. Verheyden M, Grosber M, Gutermuth J, Velkeniers B. Relapsing symmetric livedo reticularis in a patient with COVID-19 infection. J Eur Acad Dermatol Venereol. 2020;34:e684–6.
83. Kamali Aghdam M, Jafari N, Eftekhari K. Novel coronavirus in a 15-day-old neonate with clinical signs of sepsis, a case report. Infect Dis (Lond). 2020;52(6):427–9.
84. Mahé A, Birckel E, Krieger S, Merklen C, Bottlaender L. A distinctive skin rash associated with Coronavirus Disease 2019? J Eur Acad Dermatol Venereol. 2020;34:e246–7.
85. Montinari M, Atzori L, Valdevit S, Rongioletti F. Erythema annulare centrifugum with anosmia and ageusia in a SARS-CoV-2 exposed patient successfully treated with doxycycline. Int J Dermatol 2021;60:384–6.

PAPA, PASH, PAPASH, PsAPASH, and PASS: Autoinflammatory Syndromes of Hidradenitis Suppurativa

Giovanni Genovese, Chiara Moltrasio, and Angelo Valerio Marzano

Introduction

Hidradenitis suppurativa (HS) is a chronic inflammatory dermatosis involving the epithelium of the pilosebaceous units localized in the apocrine gland-rich intertriginous areas. It is characterized by recurrent suppurative painful lesions leading to tissue destruction and scarring [1].

HS pathogenesis is multifaceted, resulting from the interplay between genetic factors, host-specific aspects, and environmental influences [2]. A family history of HS is observed in almost 30% of cases, and some familial variants of HS have been proposed to be diseases with autosomal dominant inheritance [3, 4]. Genetic factors underlying familial HS have been reported only in few patients, with mutations of the genes encoding for the gamma-secretase complex being related to some familial pedigrees and specific disease subsets [5].

Rarely, HS can be associated with other autoinflammatory disorders (a heterogeneous group of systemic/organ-specific diseases) which share a dysregulation of the innate immune system with exaggerated interleukin (IL)-1 signaling, in the absence of infectious causes or typical features of autoimmunity such as high titers of circulating autoantibodies/autoreactive T cells [6]) or inherited conditions, presenting as "syndromic HS" [7].

Syndromic HS may present with a wide spectrum of clinical manifestations. Gasparic et al. proposed a provisional classification of syndromic HS that distinguished three main categories based on the main pathomechanisms involved and availability of specific diagnostic tests [7] (Table 1):

G. Genovese · C. Moltrasio · A. V. Marzano (✉)
Dermatology Unit, Department of Pathophysiology and Transplantation, Università degli Studi di Milano, Milan, Italy
e-mail: chiara.moltrasio@policlinico.mi.it; angelo.marzano@unimi.it

F. Rongioletti, B. R. Smoller (eds.), *New and Emerging Entities in Dermatology and Dermatopathology*, https://doi.org/10.1007/978-3-030-80027-7_23

Table 1 Spectrum of conditions associated with syndromic HS

Classification	Syndromes	Involved genes or chromosomal alterations
Group 1	Keratitis-ichthyosis-deafness syndrome (KIDS)	GJB2
	Down syndrome	Trisomy chromosome 21
	Dowling-Degos disease	KRT5 POFUT1, POGLUT1, and PSENEN
Group 2	Follicular occlusion syndrome	//
Group 3	Pyoderma gangrenosum, acne, suppurative hidradenitis (PASH)	MEFV, NOD2, NLRP3, IL1RN, PSTPIP1, PSMB8, NCSTN
	Pyogenic arthritis, pyoderma gangrenosum, acne, suppurative hidradenitis (PAPASH)	PSTPIP1, IL1RN, MEFV
	Psoriatic arthritis, pyoderma gangrenosum, acne, suppurative hidradenitis (PsaPASH)	//
	Pyoderma gangrenosum, acne, suppurative hidradenitis, ankylosing spondylitis (PASS)	//
	Familial Mediterranean fever (FMF)	MEFV
	Synovitis, acne, pustulosis, hyperostosis, osteitis (SAPHO)	LPIN2, NOD2, PSTPIP2, IL1RN

Abbreviations: *GJB2* Gap junction beta-2 protein, *IL1RN* interleukin-1 receptor antagonist, *KRT5* keratin 5, *LPIN2* lipin 2, *MEFV* Mediterranean fever, *NCSTN* nicastrin, *NOD2* nucleotide-binding oligomerization domain-containing protein 2, *NLRP3* NOD-, LRR-, and pyrin domain-containing protein 3, *POFUT1* protein O-fucosyltransferase 1, *POGLUT1* protein O-glucosyltransferase 1, *PSENEN* presenilin enhancer, *PSMB8* proteasome subunit beta type 8, *PSTPIP1* proline-serine-threonine phosphatase interacting protein 1, *PSTPIP2* proline-serine-threonine phosphatase interacting protein 2

- Group 1: syndromic HS associated with a genetic condition and related diagnostic testing – Dowling-Degos disease (DDD), Down syndrome (DS), keratitis-ichthyosis-deafness syndrome (KIDS), and PAPASH
- Group 2: syndromic HS associated with follicular keratinization disorders or structural disorders – follicular occlusion syndrome (FOS), DDD, DS, and KIDS
- Group 3: syndromic HS associated with autoinflammatory disease (monogenic, polygenic, other) – familial Mediterranean fever (FMF), PASH, PAPASH, PsaPASH, PASS, and SAPHO

In syndromic HS, a prevalent pathogenetic factor induces the follicular occlusion or a hyperactivation of the innate immune response, leading to the suppurative inflammation of the hair follicle. The diagnosis of syndromic HS is complex and should result from the combination of clinical evaluation (including HS-specific diagnostic criteria) (Fig. 1), histology of skin lesions (Fig. 2), laboratory findings, and genetic testing.

In the present chapter, we aimed at providing a comprehensive description of the main pathophysiological and clinical features of the following entities associated with HS belonging to the Group 3 of the classification by Gasparic et al., which are regarded as a paradigm of autoinflammatory syndromes: (i) PASH (pyoderma

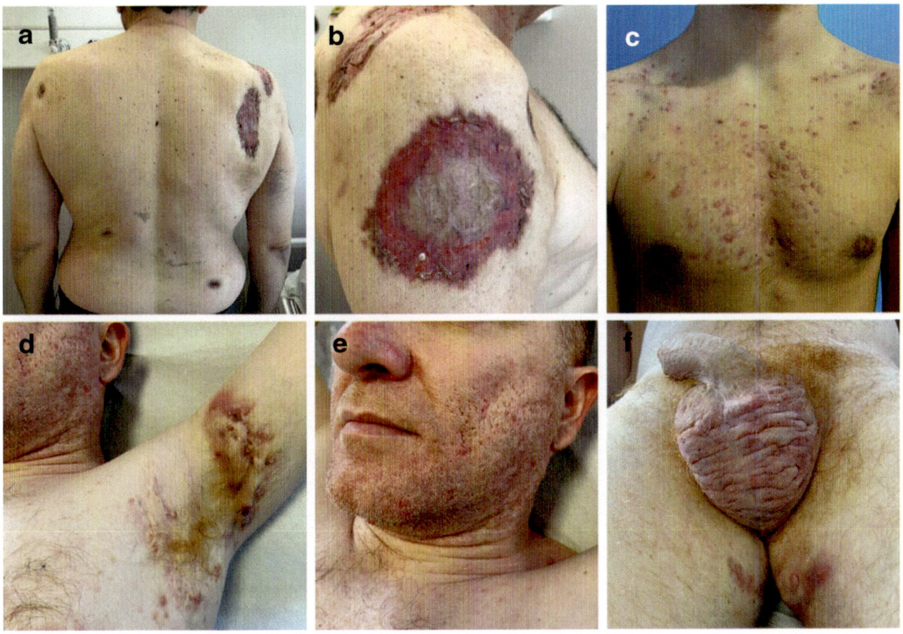

Fig. 1 Clinical features of syndromic hidradenitis suppurativa (HS) in the context of PASH syndrome: (**a**) multiple pyoderma gangrenosum ulcerative lesions on the back; (**b**) a close-up view of a pyoderma gangrenosum lesion on the right arm; (**c**) acne lesions on the chest; (**d**) nodules, abscesses, and draining fistulas in the axillary cavity of a patient with severe HS in the context of PASH syndrome; (**e**) ice-pick acne scars on the face; (**f**) HS involvement of the scrotum manifesting as confluent fistulous tracts and abscesses. Pictures **a** and **b** and pictures **d**, **e**, and **f** show the same patient

gangrenosum, acne, and suppurative hidradenitis), (ii) PAPASH (all features of PASH combined with pyogenic sterile arthritis), (iii) PsAPASH (PASH associated with psoriatic arthritis [PsA]), and (iv) PASS (PG, acne, ankylosing spondylitis, with or without HS).

Syndromic HS Associated with Autoinflammatory Diseases

The presence of HS is characteristic of PASH, PAPASH, PsAPASH, and PASS syndromes, which can be regarded as a clinical spectrum of autoinflammatory disorders with prevalent cutaneous/articular involvement [8]. In contrast to other autoinflammatory conditions, caused by mutations in known inflammatory genes, the genetic background of these conditions is still poorly understood and actively explored with new molecular approaches, such as whole exome sequencing (WES), also by our group [9].

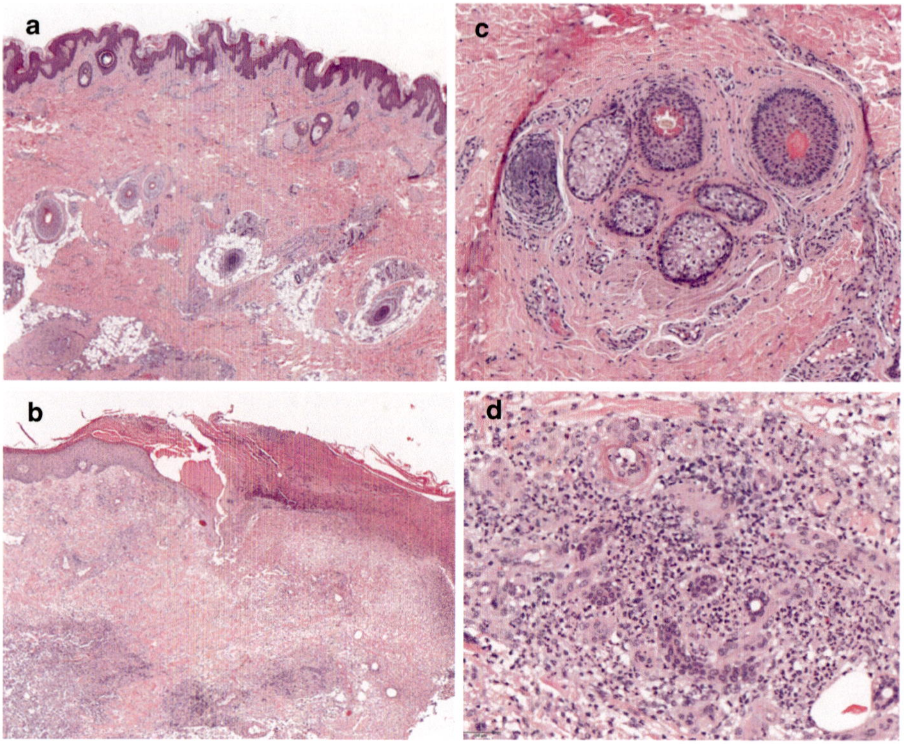

Fig. 2 Histopathological features of hidradenitis suppurativa: (**a**) inflammatory infiltrates surrounding pilosebaceous units; (**c**) close-up view of perifollicular infiltrates mainly consisting of lympho-histiocytic cells. Histopathological features of pyoderma gangrenosum: (**b**) epidermal ulceration with mild pseudo-epitheliomatous hyperplasia and dermal inflammatory infiltrate associated with necrosis; (**d**) close-up view of the dermal infiltrate mainly consisting of neutrophils with several lympho-histiocytic cells and scattered giant cells

PASH

PASH is an autoinflammatory syndrome clinically characterized by the triad of PG, acne, and HS [10–12]. It was first described by Braun-Falco et al. in 2012 [13], and it was originally considered as a monogenic disease.

Clinical Features

Inception of PASH occurs usually in the third or fourth decade of life, with acne being generally the first sign of this syndrome [12, 14–16]. Cutaneous manifestations include (i) ulcers, which may have also vegetating features, ascribable to PG; (ii) nodules, abscesses, fistulae, and scarring lesions consistent with HS; and (iii) mild-moderate to severe acne, including acne fulminans. Leukocytoclastic vasculitis [17] and focal segmental glomerulosclerosis resulting in end-stage renal disease [18] as well as inflammatory bowel diseases and obesity [11, 12] may be associated with PASH. In a patient, coccyx destruction by direct extension of HS has been reported [19].

Histopathology

The histopathologic findings of PG in the setting of PASH are not specific. Cutaneous biopsy specimens taken from the ulcer border typically show mixed cellular inflammation with predominance of neutrophils. Necrosis of dermal or pannicular blood vessels (mainly characterized by lymphocytic infiltrates) may be observed in skin biopsy specimens of perilesional areas. In some cases, vegetating aspects and pseudoepitheliomatous hyperplasia may be found [13].

Also HS show nonspecific histopathological findings, such as neutrophilic or mixed inflammatory infiltrates around apocrin gland. Hyperkeratosis of the terminal follicles and follicle ruptures with perifolliculitis along with suppurative changes of connective tissue and foreign body-type reaction are other remarkable histopathological findings of HS in the context of PASH [13].

Etiopathogenesis

However, new scientific findings are proving its polygenic autoinflammatory nature [14]. In the first two reported PASH patients, a heterozygous increased number of CCTG microsatellite repeats was identified in the promoter region of the *PSTPIP1* (proline-serine-threonine phosphatase interacting protein 1) gene, previously associated with aseptic abscesses and Crohn's disease [10]. Nevertheless, the biological relevance of this microsatellite amplification is controversial. Indeed, there is no direct evidence for a functional effect of this motif on *PSTPIP1* expression and consequently the influence on the disease phenotype [14].

In 2015, Duchatelet and colleagues described a PASH pedigree where one proband showed a mutation in the exon 4 of the *NCSTN* (nicastrin) gene (c.344_351del), causing a loss of the normal protein function [14]. Nicastrin is a component of the gamma-secretase complex, a group of intramembrane-cleaving proteases involved in several biological pathways. Mutations in this gene as well as in *PSENEN* (presenilin enhancer-2) gene are often associated with familial forms of HS leading to an impairment of Notch signaling, a conserved pathway that regulates cell fate determination, and it is involved in the growth and differentiation of many cellular types [20]. In animal models, both deficiency of gamma secretase proteins and alterations in Notch signaling pathway lead to a phenotype like HS in humans [21]. Targeted sequencing approach has been performed in four PASH subjects [12] in order to unravel causative mutations in ten candidate inflammatory genes. In three of these four PASH patients, the authors described pathogenic mutations in three target genes: A>G p.I591T in the *MEFV* (Mediterranean fever) gene, C>T p.R702W and G>C p.G908R in the *NOD2* (nucleotide-binding oligomerization domain-containing protein 2) gene, and finally C>T p.G8R in the *PSMB8* (proteasome 20S subunit beta 8) gene. In addition, genetic analyses showed, in one proband, a mutation in *NLRP3* (NOD-like receptor family, pyrin domain-containing 3) gene, already described as variant of uncertain significance. The lack of functional and clinical effect of this point mutation, p.Q703K, was later confirmed by other studies, with the indication not to report it [22].

The same authors also analyzed the expression of cytokines, chemokines, and other effector molecules either in lesional skin and serum of these patients [12].

The key finding was the increased expression of IL-1β (interleukin-1β) and its receptors in the skin, probably due to the dysregulation of inflammasome. Skin biopsies from PG ulcers also showed overexpression of TNF-α (tumor necrosis factor- α), IL-17 (interleukin-17), and their receptor.

On the other hand, serum levels of these cytokines were within the normal range, suggesting that PASH is characterized by an inflammatory status confined to the skin. Finally, several chemokines involved in neutrophilic activation and transendothelial migration such as IL-8 (interleukin-8), CXCL (C-X-C motif ligand) 1/2/3 e 16, and RANTES (regulated upon activation, normal T cell expressed and presumably secreted) were also overexpressed.

In 2018, novel *PSTPIP1* gene mutation has been described in a 37-year-old Japanese woman. Sanger sequencing revealed a heterozygous mutation, c.1034A>G (p.Y345C) in exon 15 of this gene both in proband and in their relatives. Of note, her mother suffered from HS/acne while one sister presented with only manifestations of acne [23]. This finding highlighted the incomplete penetrance and variable expression of this condition as well as the need to shed more light on the pathogenesis of this disease. Zhang et al. [19] reported, for the first time, a *PSENEN* mutation (c.228_229insCACC; p.Ile77Hisfs*45) in a PASH syndrome Chinese family. The imbalance discovered refers to 4bp of insertion leading to a premature stop codon in the nucleotide sequence with the loss of normal function of its protein product [24].

In conclusion, our group, through a novel genetic strategy retrieved four altered pathways shared by four PASH patients: (i) vitamin D metabolism, (ii) keratinization, (iii) formation of the cornified envelope, and (iv) steroid metabolism. In particular, the mainly affected pathway was vitamin D metabolism, followed by the one involved in keratinization [9].

PAPASH

The term PAPASH was coined by two independent groups to describe two distinct autoinflammatory syndromes [25, 26].

Marzano and colleagues first described PAPASH syndrome, reporting the case of a 16-year-old girl with pyogenic arthritis, PG, acne, and HS, in whom genetic analyses evaluating exons 10 and 11 of the *PSTPIP1* gene detected a new missense mutation (p.E277D) [25]. Moreover, mutations in *IL1RN* (interleukin 1 receptor antagonist) gene (G>A p.A106T) and in *MEFV* gene T>C p.M694V; A>G p.V726A) were revealed [12].

Soon after, Garzorz and coworkers [26] suggested utilizing the same acronym to define the combination of PG, acne, psoriasis, arthritis, and HS that they described in a 39-year-old woman. They hypothesized that the main molecular feature in this patient was neutrophil activation by the Th17/TNF-α axis, a pathogenic immunological basis shared by all four conditions included in this syndrome. Finally, Gottlieb et al. reported two further cases of PAPASH, one of whom was effectively treated with an association of infliximab and methotrexate [27].

PsAPASH

PsAPASH represents another clinical variant of PASH, characterized by the combination of PsA, PG, acne, and HS. To date, genotype-phenotype correlations have not yet been found [28]. It was first described in 2015 by Saraceno et al. in a 50-year-old man [29]. To our knowledge, only two other patients with PsAPASH syndrome in addition to the first one have been described in the literature up to now [27, 30]. Adalimumab at the recommended dose for PsA was successfully used in all of three cases [27, 29, 30].

PASS

PASS is a rare condition included within the spectrum of syndromic HS that was first reported in 2012 by Bruzzese [31], who described a patient with concomitant PG, acne conglobata, HS, and axial non-pyogenic, seronegative spondyloarthritis. The author proposed that the synchronous development of these four entities may represent a distinct condition, termed the PASS syndrome.

Five further patients with PASS disease have been subsequently reported by Gottlieb et al., who observed a good response to TNF-α inhibitors in four out of five cases [27].

Laboratory investigations show elevated IL-1β and IL-1Ra serum levels, supporting a causative role of this interleukin in PASS syndrome. However, no pathogenic mutations in autoinflammatory genes have been yet reported. Further biomolecular studies are needed to clarify the pathogenesis of this condition.

Treatment Strategies for Syndromic HS

Since HS may be a difficult-to-treat condition, therapeutic strategies include conservative, medical, and surgical treatments based on clinical stage, disease severity, and impact of patient-reported outcome measures [32]. Adalimumab, a humanized monoclonal antibody targeting TNF-α, is currently the only approved biologic drug for the treatment of moderate-to-severe HS. Most of the other treatments, including systemic antibiotics, are supported only by limited evidence. The complexity of clinical presentation and increased severity of HS-related manifestations make syndromic HS generally challenging to treat. Indeed, autoinflammatory syndromes commonly present with moderate-severe (Hurley II–III) disease, systemic inflammatory symptoms (fever, fatigue, increased inflammatory markers), and refractoriness to traditional first-line topical and/or systemic treatments [7].

The treatment of syndromic HS associated with autoinflammatory diseases (Group 3), which is clinically characterized by severe cutaneous and/or joint manifestations and by aberrant expression of IL-1β, may be pathogenesis-driven. Biological immune response modifiers, targeting specific cytokines of the autoinflammatory cascade, such as IL-1 and the downstream mediators TNF-α, IL-23 (interleukin-23), and IL-36 (interleukin-36), are invoked as relevant treatments in this subset of patients [33].

Gottlieb et al. reported the efficacy of TNF-α inhibitors such as adalimumab and infliximab either as monotherapy or in combination with traditional immunosuppressants (methotrexate, systemic corticosteroids, calcineurin inhibitors) in treating patients with severe HS in the context of PAPASH, PsAPASH, or PASS syndromes [27].

Infliximab induced partial control of the skin manifestations in two PASH patients [12], while adalimumab induced complete remission of both PG and HS in a PASH patient with end-stage renal disease [19].

A combination of intravenous infliximab, cyclosporine, and dapsone was also described to lead to rapid and sustained improvement of the clinical symptoms in a patient with PASH [34].

The effectiveness of IL-1 blockade with anakinra or canakinumab has been reported in many reports of autoinflammatory syndromes, such as PASH and PAPASH, corroborating the role of dysregulated IL-1 signaling pathway in these diseases. IL-1 blockade has also been successfully applied to sporadic HS, as recently described in a randomized clinical trial with anakinra, in cases series with canakinumab and in a recent open label study with bermekimab, an IL-1α inhibitor [35–38].

Systemic antibiotics have also been recommended as an alternative treatment option for autoinflammatory syndromic HS. The efficacy of systemic antibiotics could be conceivably associated with their indirect anti-inflammatory effect (see rifampicin and tetracyclines) and to a reduced bacterial load, which constitutes a possible trigger factor for the autoinflammatory process [39].

Systemic antibiotics failed to control disease activity in some cases [12]. Conversely, intravenous meropenem allowed to control extremely severe HS and to start adalimumab in a patient with PASH [24]. Furthermore, in patients intolerant to anakinra and with PG refractory to etanercept, a combination of rifampicin and clindamycin induced remission of both PG and HS [40]. Finally, Join-Lambert *and colleagues* showed that in four PASH patients protracted remission was achieved with prolonged broad-spectrum antibiotics (variable schemes including ceftriaxone, metronidazole, ertapenem, rifampicin, moxifloxacin, metronidazole, amoxicillin, linezolid, pristinamycin, or cotrimoxazole) [39].

Unlike monogenic autoinflammatory disorders, diseases included in the PASH spectrum disorders show a partial response to IL-1 blockade in the long term; thus, combination treatment regimens with targeted biologic agents and conventional immunomodulating agents such as colchicine, cyclosporine, and dapsone need to be used for controlling recurrences and relapses [27].

Systemic corticosteroids, variably combined with azathioprine, cyclosporine, or mycophenolate, demonstrated to be effective in different cases of PASH [27]. Dapsone in combination with systemic corticosteroids allowed to control disease activity in two PASH patients [34]. Intravenous immunoglobulin therapy induced partial response in a case of PASH [16].

Follicular keratinization observed in syndromic HS may benefit from retinoids (such as isotretinoin and acitretin) combined with anti-inflammatory agents, in order to reduce the exaggerated epidermal proliferation. The role of isotretinoin in the management of sporadic HS is controversial, but it can be a useful add-on treatment for syndromic HS with prominent features of truncal acne and follicular occlusion. Acitretin is an established second- and third-line agent for the treatment of moderate-to-severe HS, albeit with a limited tolerability profile at the high doses required (0.25–0.88 mg/kg daily) [41].

References

1. Saunte DML, Jemec GBE. Hidradenitis suppurativa: advances in diagnosis and treatment. JAMA. 2017;318(20):2019–32.
2. Kurayev A, Ashkar H, Saraiya A, Gottlieb AB. Hidradenitis suppurativa: review of the pathogenesis and treatment. J Drugs Dermatol. 2016;15(8):1017–22.
3. Fitzsimmons JS, Fitzsimmons EM, Gilbert G. Familial hidradenitis suppurativa: evidence in favour of single gene transmission. J Med Genet. 1984;21(4):281–5.
4. Von Der Werth JM, Williams HC, Raeburn JA. The clinical genetics of hidradenitis suppurativa revisited. Br J Dermatol. 2000;142(5):947–53.
5. Wang B, Yang W, Wen W, Sun J, Su B, Liu B, Ma D, Lv D, Wen Y, Qu T, Chen M, Miao S, Shen Y, Zhan X. Gamma-secretase gene mutations in familial acne inversa. Science. 2010;330(6007):1065.
6. Kastner DL, Aksentijevich I, Goldbach-Mansky R. Autoinflammatory disease reloaded: a clinical perspective. Cell. 2010;140(6):784–90.
7. Gasparic J, Theut Riis P, Jemec GB. Recognizing syndromic hidradenitis suppurativa: a review of the literature. J Eur Acad Dermatol Venereol. 2017.

8. Cugno M, Borghi A, Marzano AV. PAPA, PASH and PAPASH syndromes: pathophysiology, presentation and treatment. Am J Clin Dermatol. 2017;18(4):555–62.
9. Brandao L, Moura R, Tricarico PM, Gratton R, Genovese G, Moltrasio C, Garcovich S, Boniotto M, Crovella S, Marzano AV. Altered keratinization and vitamin D metabolism may be key pathogenetic pathways in syndromic hidradenitis suppurativa: a novel whole exome sequencing approach. J Dermatol Sci. 2020;99(1):17–22.
10. Braun-Falco M, Kovnerystyy O, Lohse P, Ruzicka T. Pyoderma gangrenosum, acne, and suppurative hidradenitis (PASH)—a new autoinflammatory syndrome distinct from PAPA syndrome. J Am Acad Dermatol. 2012;66(3):409–15.
11. Marzano AV, Ishak RS, Colombo A, Caroli F, Crosti C. Pyoderma gangrenosum, acne and suppurative hidradenitis syndrome following bowel bypass surgery. Dermatology. 2012;225(3):215–9.
12. Marzano AV, Ceccherini I, Gattorno M, Fanoni D, Caroli F, Rusmini M, Grossi A, De Simone C, Borghi O, Meroni PL, Crosti C, Cugno M. Association of pyoderma gangrenosum, acne, and suppurative hidradenitis (PASH) shares genetic and cytokine profiles with other autoinflammatory diseases. Medicine (Baltimore). 2014;93:e187.
13. Szymanski AM, Ombrello MJ. Using genes to triangulate the pathophysiology of granulomatous autoinflammatory disease: NOD2, PLCG2 and LACC1. Int Immunol. 2018;30(5):205–13.
14. Duchatelet S, Miskinyte S, Join-Lambert O, Ungeheuer MN, Frances C, Nassif A, Hovnanian A. First nicastrin mutation in PASH (pyoderma gangrenosum, acne and suppurative hidradenitis) syndrome. Br J Dermatol. 2015;173:610–2.
15. Jorissen E, De Strooper B. Chapter six-γ-secretase and the intramembrane proteolysis of notch. Current topics in developmental biology. Academic Press. 2010;92:201–30.
16. Jfri AH, O'Brien EA, Litvinov IV, Alavi A, Netchiporouk E. Hidradenitis suppurativa: comprehensive review of predisposing genetic mutations and changes. J Cutan Med Surg. 2019;23(5):519–27.
17. Naselli A, Penco F, Cantarini L, Insalaco A, Alessio M, Tommasini A, Maggio C, Obici L, Gallizzi R, Cimmino M, Signa S, Lucherini OM, Carta S, Caroli F, Martini A, Rubartelli A, Ceccherini I, Gattorno M. Clinical characteristics of patients carrying the Q703K variant of the NLRP3 gene: a 10-year multicentric national study. J Rheumatol. 2016;43(6):1093–100.
18. Saito N, Minami-Hori M, Nagahata H, Nozaki H, Iinuma S, Igawa S, Kanno K, Kishibe M, Kanazawa N, Ishida-Yamamoto A. Novel PSTPIP1 gene mutation in pyoderma gangrenosum, acne and suppurative hidradenitis syndrome. J Dermatol. 2018;45(8):e213–4.
19. Zhang X, He Y, Xu H, Wang B. First PSENEN mutation in PASH syndrome. J Dermatol. 2020;47(11):1335–7.
20. Ead JK, Snyder RJ, Wise J, Cuffy C, Jafary H, Fischborn K. Is PASH syndrome a biofilm disease?: a case series and review of the literature. Wounds. 2018;30:216–23.
21. Sonbol H, Duchatelet S, Miskinyte S, Bonsang B, Hovnanian A, Misery L. PASH syndrome (pyoderma gangrenosum, acne and hidradenitis suppurativa): a disease with genetic heterogeneity. Br J Dermatol. 2018;178:e17–8.
22. Niv D, Ramirez JA, Fivenson DP. Pyoderma gangrenosum, acne, and hidradenitis suppurativa (PASH) syndrome with recurrent vasculitis. JAAD Case Rep. 2017;3(1):70–3.
23. De Wet J, Jordaan HF, Kannenberg SM, Tod B, Glanzmann B, Visser WI. Pyoderma gangrenosum, acne, and suppurative hidradenitis syndrome in end-stage renal disease successfully treated with adalimumab. Dermatol Online J. 2017;23(12):13030/qt82d4m2zw.
24. McCarthy S, Foley CC, Dvorakova V, Quinlan C, Murphy M, Maher M. PASH syndrome with bony destruction. Clin Exp Dermatol. 2019;44(8):918–20.
25. Marzano AV, Trevisan V, Gattorno M, Ceccherini I, De Simone C, Crosti C. Pyogenic arthritis, pyoderma gangrenosum, acne, and hidradenitis suppurativa (PAPASH): a new autoinflammatory syndrome associated with a novel mutation of the PSTPIP1 gene. JAMA Dermatol. 2013;149(6):762–4.
26. Garzorz N, Papanagiotou V, Atenhan A, Andres C, Eyerich S, Eyerich K, Ring J, Brockow K. Pyoderma gangrenosum, acne, psoriasis, arthritis and suppurative hidradenitis (PAPASH)-

syndrome: a new entity within the spectrum of autoinflammatory syndromes? J Eur Acad Dermatol Venereol. 2016;30(1):141–3.
27. Gottlieb J, Madrange M, Gardair C, Sbidian E, Frazier A, Wolkenstein P, Hickman G, Schneider P, Baudry C, Claudepierre P, Bertheau P, Richette P, Smahi A, Bachelez H. PAPASH, PsAPASH and PASS autoinflammatory syndromes: phenotypic heterogeneity, common biological signature and response to immunosuppressive regimens. Br J Dermatol. 2019;181(4):866–9.
28. Brenner M, Ruzicka T, Plewig G, Thomas P, Herzer P. Targeted treatment of pyoderma gangrenosum in PAPA (pyogenic arthritis, pyoderma gangrenosum and acne) syndrome with the recombinant human interleukin-1 receptor antagonist anakinra. Br J Dermatol. 2009;161:1199–201.
29. Saraceno R, Babino G, Chiricozzi A, Zangrilli A, Chimenti S. PsAPASH: a new syndrome associated with hidradenitis suppurativa with response to tumor necrosis factor inhibition. J Am Acad Dermatol. 2015;72:e42–4.
30. Gadelha RL, Paiva RDSR, Palitot EB, Costa JEFD. PsAPASH: a rare and recent autoinflammatory syndrome associated with hidradenitis suppurativa. An Bras Dermatol. 2020;95(2):203–6.
31. Bruzzese V. Pyoderma gangrenosum, acne conglobata, suppurative hidradenitis, and axial spondyloarthritis: efficacy of anti-tumor necrosis factor α therapy. J Clin Rheumatol. 2012;18:413–5.
32. Gulliver W, Zouboulis CC, Prens E, Jemec GBE, Tzellos T. Evidence-based approach to the treatment of hidradenitis suppurativa/acne inversa, based on the European guidelines for hidradenitis suppurativa. Rev Endocr Metab Disord. 2016;17(3):343–51.
33. Garcovich S, De Simone C, Berti E, Marzano AV. Drug management of neutrophilic dermatoses. Expert Rev Clin Pharmacol. 2017;10(10):1119–28.
34. Staub J, Pfannschmidt N, Strohal R, Braun-Falco M, Lohse P, Goerdt S, Leverkus M. Successful treatment of PASH syndrome with infliximab, cyclosporine and dapsone. J Eur Acad Dermatol Venereol. 2015;29:2243–7.
35. Houriet C, Seyed Jafari SM, Thomi R, Schlapbach C, Borradori L, Yawalkar N, Hunger RE. Canakinumab for severe hidradenitis suppurativa: preliminary experience in 2 cases. JAMA Dermatol. 2017;153(11):1195–7.
36. Tzanetakou V, Kanni T, Giatrakou S, Katoulis A, Papadavid E, Netea MG, Dinarello CA, van der Meer JWM, Rigopoulos D, Giamarellos-Bourboulis EJ. Safety and efficacy of anakinra in severe hidradenitis suppurativa: a randomized clinical trial. JAMA Dermatol. 2016;152(1):52–9.
37. Andre R, Marescassier H, Gabay C, Pittet B, Laffitte E. Long-term therapy with anakinra in hidradenitis suppurativa in three patients. Int J Dermatol. 2019;58(11):e208–9.
38. Gottlieb A, Natsis NE, Kerdel F, Forman S, Gonzalez E, Jimenez G, Hernandez L, Kaffenberger J, Guido G, Lucas K, Montes D, Gold M, Babcock C, Simard J. A phase II openlabel study of bermekimab in patients with hidradenitis suppurativa shows resolution of inflammatory lesions and pain. J Invest Dermatol. 2020;140(8):1538–1545.e2.
39. Join-Lambert O, Duchatelet S, Delage M, Miskinyte S, Coignard H, Lemarchand N, Alemy-Carreau M, Lortholary O, Nassif X, Hovnanian A, Nassif A. Remission of refractory pyoderma gangrenosum, severe acne, and hidradenitis suppurativa (PASH) syndrome using targeted antibiotic therapy in 4 patients. J Am Acad Dermatol. 2015;73:S66–9.
40. Lamiaux M, Dabouz F, Wantz M, Lebas D, Lasek A, Courivaud D, Modiano P. Successful combined antibiotic therapy with oral clindamycin and oral rifampicin for pyoderma gangrenosum in patient with PASH syndrome. JAAD Case Rep. 2017;4:17–21.
41. Matusiak Ł, Bieniek A, Szepietowski JC. Acitretin treatment for hidradenitis suppurativa: a prospective series of 17 patients. Br J Dermatol. 2014;171(1):170–4.

Re-emerging and New Skin Infections

Francisco G. Bravo and Patricia J. Alvarez

Buruli Ulcer

Introduction

Buruli ulcer (BU), also known as Bairnsdale ulcer and Kumusi ulcer, is an infection caused by a particularly distinct microbia, *Mycobacterium ulcerans*. The disease is the third most common mycobacteriosis in the world (after tuberculosis and leprosy) and is one of the 17 neglected tropical diseases worldwide [1]. The disease was initially described in Australia in 1948, although the same clinical picture was already described by Cook in 1897. The name Buruli comes from the old denomination of the Uganda province (currently Nakasongola) where the disease was best described [2]. It has been reported in 33 countries in Africa, Australia, Southeast Asia, South America, and the Western Pacific, with the highest incidence in impoverished communities of West and Central Africa. Between 5000 and 6000 cases are reported annually by 15 of the 33 countries. The reported incidence in Africa seems to be decreasing since 2010, with no clear explanation for that. The decline may be the result of specific control programs or a collateral effect from other health programs. The disease is most likely acquired in low-lying wetlands and slow-moving rivers, and the environmental reservoirs are natural biofilms, soil, and aquatic insects. The disease is one of low mortality but high morbidity, causing incapacity with physical and socioeconomic impacts on the affected population. The exposure to insect bites near rivers, swimming, wading, bathing, and farming near lacustrine systems are all considered risk factors to contract the disease. Poor socioeconomic

F. G. Bravo (✉)
Universidad Peruana Cayetano Heredia, Peru

P. J. Alvarez
Universidad de Piura, Peru

F. Rongioletti, B. R. Smoller (eds.), *New and Emerging Entities in Dermatology and Dermatopathology*, https://doi.org/10.1007/978-3-030-80027-7_24

conditions, young people less than 15 years of age, poor wound care, and failure to wear appropriate clothing seem to increase the risk as well.

Clinical Features

The earliest clinical lesion consists of a papule that evolves into a nodule, progressing later to a plaque that eventually becomes an ulcer. The ulcer classically will have undermined borders (Fig. 1). The ulcer becomes deeper and tends to involve the subcutaneous tissue, with marked necrosis at the base. A remarkable lack of symptoms such as pain, high fever, or malaise is quite characteristic of the disease, unless it becomes superinfected. Most lesions tend to be in exposed areas, such as the extremities and the face. A purely edematous form is also described affecting a limb, and the disease may progress to involve the bone, causing osteomyelitis. If the diagnosis is not established in an initial state, the resulting incapacity will be so severe that it will result in deformities affecting the life of the affected individual. The clinical evolution may take from 3 weeks through a year. Most patients do have a single lesion, but satellite lesions are not unusual.

The World Health Organization has established three different categories. In category I, the lesion has a diameter of less than 5 cm. Category II include nodules, plaques, and ulcers from 5 to 15 cm in diameter. Category III includes lesions larger than 15 cm or those that compromise critical sites, such as the eye, breast, genitalia, joint, or bone, or those who have disseminated disease. African patients will present with equal numbers in each category, whereas most Australian patients will be diagnosed in Category I [3].

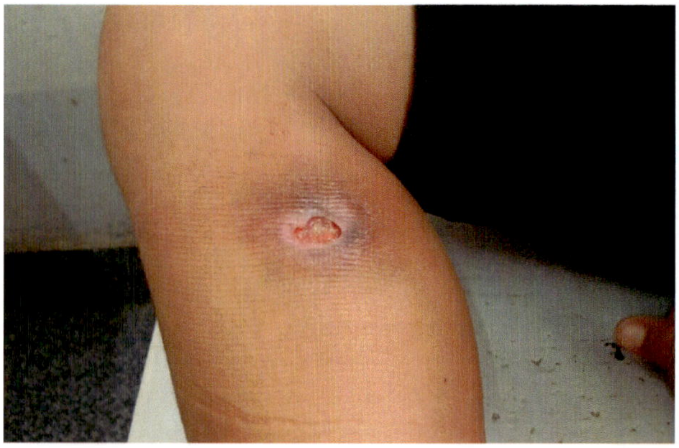

Fig. 1 Buruli ulcer: large ulceration on the leg; notice clear undermined borders

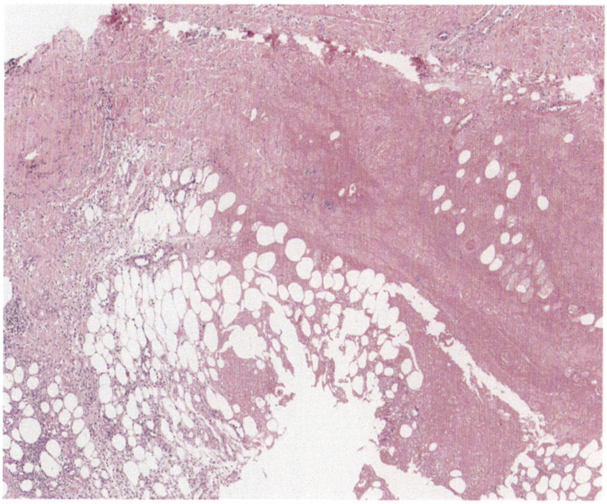

Fig. 2 Buruli ulcer: massive necrosis of the deep dermis and panniculus in the absence of significant inflammatory infiltrate. H/E, 100×

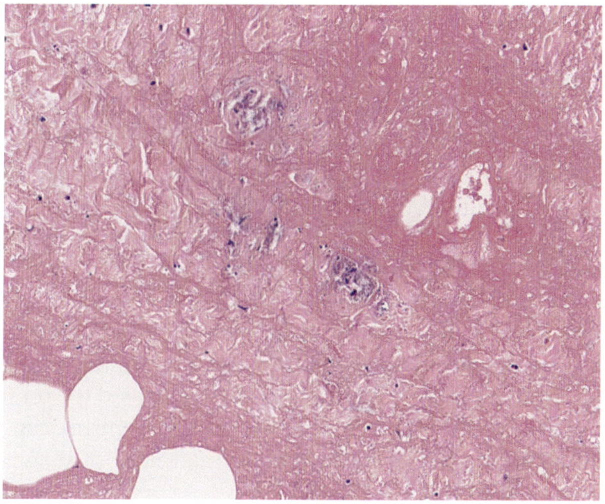

Fig. 3 Buruli ulcer: bluish material in the necrosis representing cumuli of bacilli. H/E, 400×

Histopathologic Features

The main histological findings consist of extensive areas of necrosis involving deep dermis and subcutaneous tissue (Fig. 2), lacking any significant inflammatory infiltrate. The epidermis is most likely ulcerated but may also show epidermal hyperplasia at the edges. Sometimes, a bluish material may be seen in the areas of necrosis (Fig. 3). With appropriate mycobacterial staining such as Ziehl-Neelsen or Fite-Faraco, a remarkable number of mycobacteria can be identified in those areas (Fig. 4), comparable to what can be seen in lepromatous leprosy or *Mycobacterium avium-intracellulare* infections. Interestingly, the mycobacteria may show different

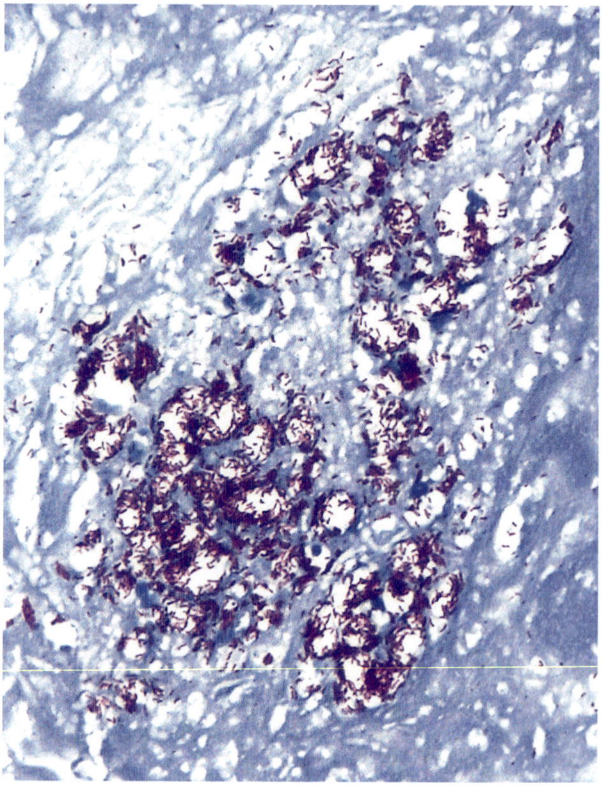

Fig. 4 Buruli ulcer: the same area of Fig. 3 stained with Ziehl-Neelsen demonstrating large number of bacilli. Z-N,1000×

degrees of staining in a single slide. Non-ulcerated lesions may have less amount of detectable microorganism even with the appropriate staining. Granulomas may be seen at the advancing edge. Perivascular infiltrates and thrombosis may be seen in affected tissue. A PCR study has demonstrated the presence of mycobacterial DNA even beyond the areas where the microorganisms can be seen with special stains. Histopathology can confirm more than 90% of diagnosed cases and 70% of suspected cases [2].

Etiopathogenesis

Mycobacterium ulcerans has been postulated to be dated back to the Jurassic period. It is closely related genetically to *M. marinum* and probably represents an evolutionary state of the same organisms that acquired the ability to make specific toxins by the way of a plasmid. The toxin, known as mycolactone, is a polyketide, of the family of macrolides; it has a lactone core and a fatty acid chain. Six variants of mycolactone have been studied: A/B, C, D, E, F, and G. Each variant of mycolactone is associated with a geographic region; A/B mycolactones are classically associated with isolates from Africa and Malaysia. The variability of mycolactone may also explain the variability in clinical pictures; the African variant seems to cause more damage than the isolates from Asia, Australia, Central America, and Mexico. Mycolactone is capable of inducing cytotoxicity that translates clinically into necrosis and ulceration; the toxin also has anesthetic capabilities and has an immunosuppressive, anti-inflammatory effect. These capabilities explain the existence of clinically large ulcerations in the absence of pain and paucity of local inflammation [4].

Differential Diagnosis

The diagnosis of Buruli ulcer should be considered in the presence of a large ulceration with an undermined border in a patient living in an endemic area or with a history of visiting an endemic area. Confirmatory tests include direct microscopy, either swab or touch prep, and staining with Ziehl-Neelsen. The number of bacilli detectable on direct examination varies, being more abundant in nodules than in ulcers. Culture is a gold standard technique but requires specialized laboratories. The microbe takes 9–12 weeks to grow even under optimal conditions (temp, 29–33 °C; oxygen concentration of 2.5–5%). If the mycobacterium is isolated, it still must be identified by PCR or by MALDI-TOF mass spectrometry. PCR techniques are quite sensitive, detecting the microorganism in 50–80% of cases; it is quite specific when the target is the IS2404 gene. The sample can be taken in the field, but it requires sophisticated equipment and expert laboratory technicians to process it. Another technique requiring less cold chain transportation for the reagents is the loop-mediated isothermal amplification (LAMP) technique; it has also proven to be useful for the early diagnosis of Buruli ulcer (2).

Differential diagnosis of Buruli ulcer depends on the clinical form: nodules must be differentiated from tumoral and cystic lesions of the skin, insect bites, and other mycobacterial disease. For plaque lesions the differential diagnosis will include cutaneous tuberculosis, leishmaniasis, and subcutaneous mycosis. The differential diagnosis for the ulcers includes vascular ulcers (arterial or venous), diabetic ulcers, leishmaniasis, ulcerative yaws, tropical ulcer, and squamous cell carcinomas.

Prognosis

Early intervention after a prompt diagnosis results in less morbidity and reduces disfiguring and tissue damage. Again, the disease carries low mortality, but when the therapeutic intervention is too late, the sequelae may incapacitate the patient for the rest of his life.

Therapy

Before 2004, the only therapeutic option was surgical cleaning of injured and damaged tissues. Since then, the World Health Organization started proposing medical management with systemic antibiotics, either alone or in conjunction with surgery. The first recommended regimen included an 8-week period of administration of intramuscular streptomycin (15 mg/kg) plus oral administration of rifampin (10 mg/kg). This scheme resulted in a marked decrease in the recurrence rate of the infection and less patients requiring surgery. However, the IM streptomycin was difficult to provide in rural, distant settings and became overly complicated if it had to be administered daily for 8 weeks. During treatment, patients may present a paradoxical reaction, that is, worsening of their symptoms in the first weeks of therapy, as the result of restoring local and systemic immune responses.

The current trend is toward the use of an all oral regimen including rifampin, levofloxacin, and clarithromycin. Since 2017, the therapy recommended by WHO has been reduced to an oral regimen that includes rifampin (10 mg/kg once daily) and clarithromycin (7.5 mg/kg twice daily). Surgery is still recommended for debridement and cleaning of large lesions.

Infection by the Free-Living Amoeba *Balamuthia Mandrillaris*

Introduction

Infections by free-living amoebas that involve the skin are relatively rare but associated with delayed diagnosis and extremely high mortality. There are four genus of free-living amoebas causing disease in humans: *Naegleria*, *Acanthamoeba*, *Balamuthia*, and *Sappinia*. *Naegleria* causes acute encephalitis, whereas *Acanthamoeba*, *Sappinia*, and *Balamuthia* cause subacute granulomatous meningoencephalitis. Relevant to dermatologists is the fact that, occasionally in the case of *Acanthamoeba*, and quite frequently in the case of *Balamuthia*, the disease may have cutaneous manifestations that precede the CNS involvement. The identification and early diagnosis of such infection may be lifesaving, especially when considering the current developments in the therapy of an otherwise fatal disease.

Balamuthia mandrillaris belongs to the kingdom Protista, subkingdom Protozoa, superclass Rhizopodia. The first description of the microorganism causing disease in mammals goes back to 1986, when the amoeba was identified as the cause of meningoencephalitis in a pregnant baboon at the San Diego Zoo. The amoeba was initially classified as belonging to the Leptomyxid family, and a series of cases in humans was reported along with the original animal case [5]. Following further publications, the microorganism was found to have unique microbiologic characteristics, and by 1993, it was reclassified as belonging to a new genus and was given its final name *Balamuthia mandrillaris* (after William Balamuth, a prominent Californian parasitologist) [6]. Since then, multiple human cases have been described, mainly from the USA [7], Peru [8], and recently China [9]. Other countries where the disease has been reported include Japan [10], Australia [11, 12], Thailand [13], Czech Republic [14], Portugal [15], and Turkey [16]. In the American continent, besides the USA and Peru, *Balamuthia* infections have been reported in Mexico [17, 18], Chile [19], Argentina [20], Venezuela [21], Brazil [22], and Bolivia [23] during the last 15 years.

In Peru, most patients come from the country's coastal region that is topographically characterized by a succession of alternating valleys with desertic areas. In the USA, most patients concentrate in California (which geographically has some similarities with the Peruvian coast) and the Southwestern States. In the case of China, the cases come from many provinces, affecting people living in rural environments. For the most part, *Balamuthia* infections affect the immunocompetent patient, as opposed to what is seen in the case of *Acanthamoeba* infections, where the patients are usually immunocompromised. Whereas in most cases *Balamuthia* is acquired directly from the environment, most likely through trauma, there is currently evidence that the infection can also be transmitted through solid organ transplantation [24].

Clinical Features

Patients presenting with *Balamuthia* infection are usually young, but the disease has been described affecting children as young as 3 years old to seniors above 70 year of age. Half of the patients are 15 years old or younger. Males are affected twice as common as females. Generally, they are involved in agricultural work, are gardeners, or are exposed to dirt or soil. As opposed to *Naegleria* infections, patients do not

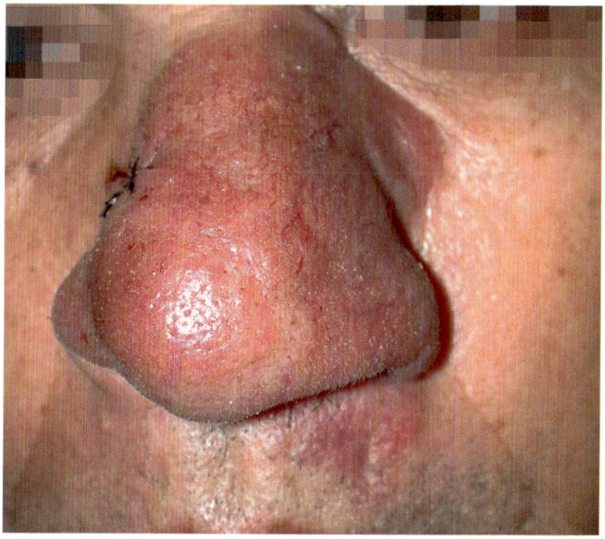

Fig. 5 Large smooth-surface plaque on the central face: this is the typical clinical presentation of *Balamuthia* infection on the skin

need to have a history of being exposed to stagnant water or swimming in ponds or lakes. History of trauma as the site of infection is a common event in Chinese patients [9]. Most patients are immunocompetent.

The presence of the cutaneous lesion preceding the development of neurological symptoms seems to be the rule in Peruvian and Chinese cases, but a cutaneous lesion has been described only in 10% of cases of *Balamuthia* infection in the USA.

The classical cutaneous lesion at the time of presentation is a non-tender, painless plaque on the central face, either exactly on the nose (Fig. 5) or cheeks, but also on the forehead or the chin, measuring from one to several centimeters in diameter. It usually has a smooth surface, and ulceration is exceptional (as opposite to *Acanthamoeba* infection). Lesions are more commonly single, but occasionally one may see small satellite lesions at the periphery of the initial plaque. If the lesion progresses naturally, it will become more infiltrating and the border will become blunted. Second to the face, the most common locations are the knee, the arm, or the chest. Again, the surface of the plaque tends to be smooth in extra facial locations, although it may adopt a multinodular aspect on the surface, but not verrucous.

The time between the development of the skin lesion and the development of neurological symptoms may vary, from months to years. In fact, recognizing the cutaneous lesion early may precede the neurological involvement; at that point, no affectation of the central nervous system would be detectable by imaging techniques such as computer tomography or magnetic resonance. Thus, an early diagnosis when the disease is limited to the skin will be critical to initiate therapy and to prevent CNS disease and a fatal outcome.

Histopathologic Features

The best way to diagnose cutaneous *Balamuthia* infection is to recognize the disease on the skin biopsy. As a rule, the process does not affect the epidermis, except for mild hyperplasia. Most of the pathological process is in the reticular dermis (Fig. 6). The classical picture is of a granulomatous reaction, with formation of ill-defined granulomas; multinucleated giant cells are present inside and outside the granulomas, accompanied by a mixed inflammatory infiltrate containing lymphocytes and plasma cells (Fig. 7). Occasionally neutrophils and eosinophils are present in focal areas. Involvement of the subcutaneous fat has been associated secondary to traumatic penetration of foreign material.

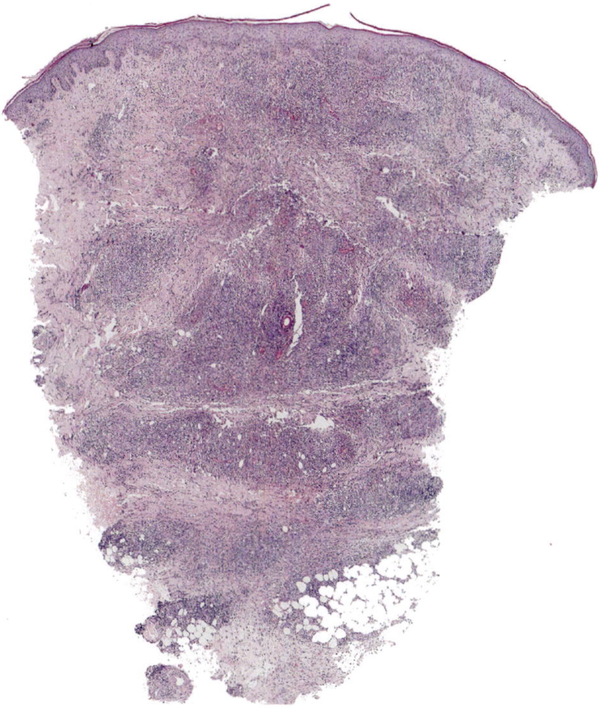

Fig. 6 Cutaneous involvement of *Balamuthia* infection: diffuse infiltration of the whole dermis by a granulomatous infiltrate with ill-defined granulomas. H/E, 40×

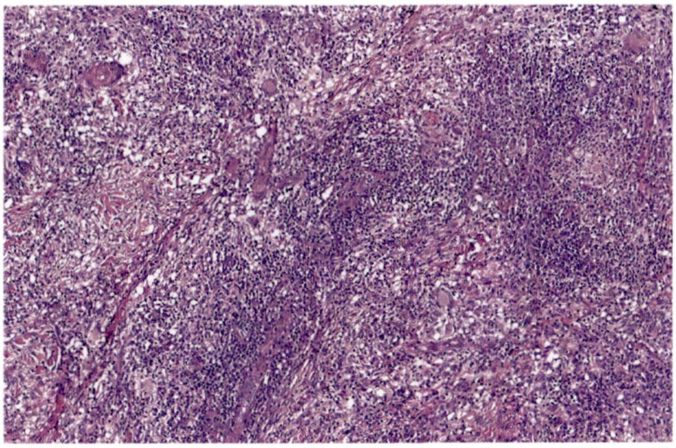

Fig. 7 *Balamuthia* infection: ill-defined granulomas with giant cells surrounded by lymphocytes and plasma cells. H/E 100×

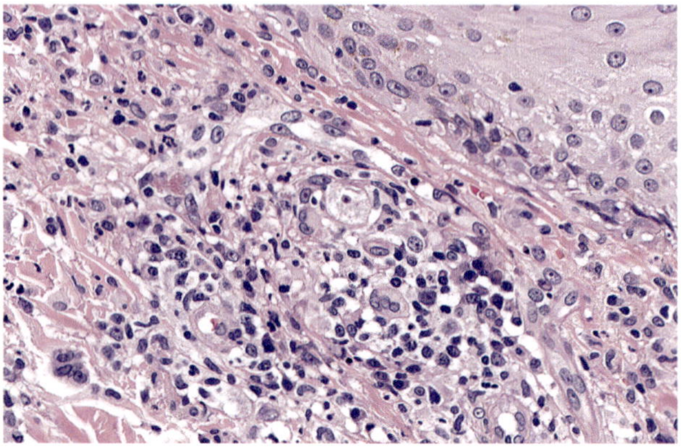

Fig. 8 *Balamuthia* infection: a distinct trophozoite of ameba showing a visible cytoplasm, nucleus, and nucleolus. H/E 800×

The most important clue for the diagnosis is to find the trophozoites in the tissue. They measure from 10 to 30 μm in diameter. As a rule, they are very scarce in number, and when they are abundant, they have a special predilection for areas around vessels. To recognize a trophozoite as such, one must see the distinct nucleus and nucleolus (Fig. 8); otherwise, the amebic cytoplasm may be easily confused with a histiocyte. Sometimes the shape is not ameboid, but more oval, with a "bubbly" cytoplasm. It is not uncommon to see the trophozoite inside a tissue retraction artifact. Cysts are rarely seen in the skin.

Perineural invasion can be seen in some cases; when the trophozoites are abundant, vasculitis with fibrin deposits may be recognized.

No particular stain represents some advantage in looking for the amoeba besides H/E; however, direct immunofluorescence and specific immunohistochemistry techniques are already available to demonstrate the presence of the microbe in skin and brain tissue [25]. The most recent advances in the diagnosis of *Balamuthia* infection include real-time polymerase chain reaction (PCR) aiming for the *16s* rRNA and *18s* rRNA gene [26]. Also, next-generation sequencing is a promising method that already has demonstrated its usefulness in diagnosing this infection, using cerebrospinal fluid, brain tissue, and even plasma as a substrate [27].

Etiopathogenesis

Whereas in *Naegleria* infections the risk factors are clearly associated with contact with stagnant water, *Balamuthia* is a microbe of water and soil [28–30]. The patient may report a history of trauma as the port of entry into the skin. In cases with cutaneous involvement, there seems to be a containment process at the dermal level and then an hematogenous spreading to CNS. There is some autopsy evidence that the infection may involve other organs as well, such as the kidneys [31], which may explain the reported cases of transmission of the infection by solid organ transplant [24].

It has been shown that there is alteration of the hemato-cephalic barrier associated with an increment of IL6 [32] induced by *Balamuthia,* thus the importance of selecting antimicrobials that can penetrate the brain tissue to reach good therapeutic levels.

Differential Diagnosis

The differential diagnosis for the disease affecting the central face includes infectious processes such as tuberculosis, leishmaniasis, subcutaneous and systemic mycosis such as mucormycosis and rhinoentomophthoromycosis, leprosy, endemic syphilis, granulomatous non-infectious processes such as sarcoidosis and granulomatosis with angiitis, and neoplastic processes such as skin carcinomas and NK/T--cell lymphomas. For lesions outside the face the diagnosis is even wider; the absence of verrucous hyperplasia of the epidermis may allow the distinction from verrucous tuberculosis, verrucous leishmaniasis, and chromoblastomycosis.

Prognosis

If the disease progresses to involve the CNS, the prognosis is dismal, and the fatal outcome may be inevitable. Thus, there is great importance for dermatologists being able to recognize the cutaneous involvement early in the course of the disease.

Therapy

There is no therapeutic scheme that has been proved to be effective in all cases. The selection of antimicrobial agents should be reached through a consensus with other specialists, such as neurologists and infection disease specialists. A basic concept is that therapy should be based on a multiple drug approach, including the use of the antiparasitic drug miltefosine [33]. Also, the period of treatment should be prolonged up to a year. An excellent clinical response of the skin lesion to therapy does not mean that the CNS is free of disease, and neuroimaging and neurological assessment are required for the follow-up of the patient for potential neurological involvement.

Infective Dermatitis as a Cutaneous Manifestation of HTLV-1 Infection

Introduction

The human T-cell lymphotropic virus 1 (HTLV-1) is a delta retrovirus known to cause lifelong infections in human beings. In 1979, Robert Gallo isolated the virus from a man suffering from a lymphoid malignancy [34]. Interestingly, some skin manifestations of this viral infection had already been described, even when an infectious etiology was not even suspected. That is the case for what was called an infectious dermatitis by Robert Sweet in Jamaican children [35]. The connection between the virus and what was described in those Jamaican children was made several years later, in 1990, by Lois La Grenade [36].

Between 10 and 20 million people around the world are infected by the virus; the microorganism, the first human retrovirus described, causes asymptomatic infections in a great majority of patients, where less than 10% of patients will develop some sort of clinical manifestations. This is just the opposite of what is seen in the infection by the most relevant retrovirus known nowadays, the human immunodeficiency virus (HIV). The HTLV-1 has been link to neurological manifestations, such as tropical spastic paraparesis (TSP), to hematological malignancies, such as the adult T-cell leukemia lymphoma (ATL), to ocular manifestations such as uveitis, and to a myriad of cutaneous manifestations including crusted scabies, extensive dermatophytosis, and xerosis. The following discussion will put emphasis on discussing the clinical and histological manifestations of infective dermatitis and its relevance regarding the risk of developing the T-cell malignancies associated with the retrovirus.

Countries in the world known to have significant prevalence of HTLV-1 infection include Jamaica, Barbados, Martinique, Guadalupe, Dominican Republic, Trinidad and Tobago, and Haiti, in the Caribbean. French Guyana, Colombia, Chile, Peru, Argentina, and Brazil are South American countries with well-documented studies of prevalence [37]. In Europe, countries such as the UK and metropolitan areas of France are known to have significant prevalence in populations of Caribbean and African ancestors. In Spain, Italy, and Ireland, intravenous drug users represent an endemic population for HTLV-1. Africa is probably the largest endemic area for HTLV-1, but the actual status of each country is not well known. Several countries of West Africa including Senegal, Mauritania, Mali, Cote d'Ivoire, and Nigeria have reported cases of ATL as well as TSP. In Central Africa, serological prevalence has been reported in Cameroon, Gabon, the Central African Republic, and the Democratic Republic of the Congo. Studies in East Africa are few, but it seems that this area is less endemic for the infection than West and Central Africa. In the South African region, the country with more serological surveys and known described cases of ATL, TSP, or infective dermatitis is South Africa. In Australia, the most affected population are the aborigines, and, in Asia, significant number of cases are reported in Iran, Japan, and Taiwan. One remarkable fact is that, in Japan, where the

HTLV-1 infection and its clinical manifestations have been extensively studied, infective dermatitis is extremely rare, pointing to the fact that not only prevalence of the infection but other factors, such as a genetic predisposition, malnutrition, and poor sanitary conditions, may play a role in the etiopathogenesis of the dermatitis. Not only dermatologists working in endemic areas but those who practice in non-endemic countries should be aware of this entity, especially while working in metropolitan areas with large migratory populations from endemic countries [38].

In children, the main route of acquiring the infection is by breastfeeding, whereas in adults, there are other possibilities such as sexual transmission and transfusion.

Clinical Features

The most common age of presentation of infective dermatitis is during childhood, although observations made in Peru [39], Paraguay [40], and Brazil [41, 42] have widened the spectrum of the age of onset of the disease into adulthood, up to the seven decade. Male and females are similarly affected. For a dermatologist, at a

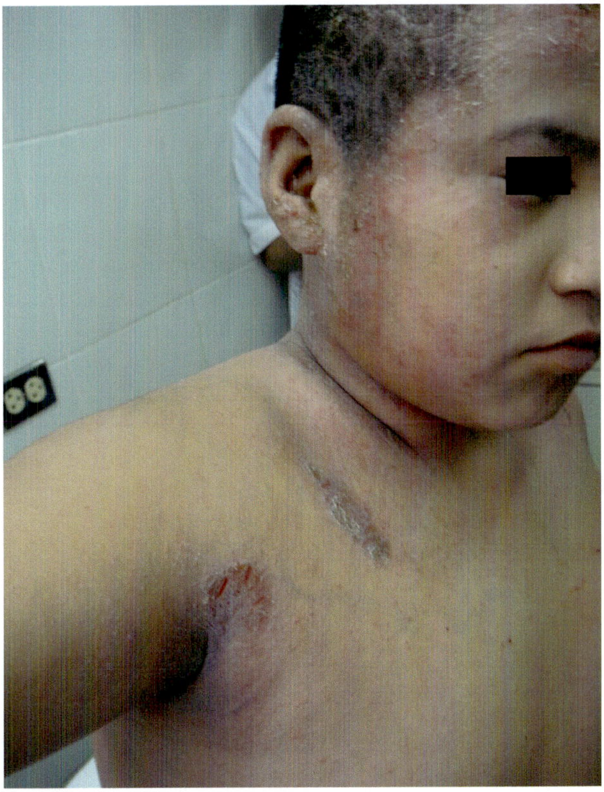

Fig. 9 Infective dermatitis: eczematous process involving the scalp, face, periauricular area, neck, and axillae: this is the classical picture of affected children

first impression, infective dermatitis may look like a nonspecific form of eczematous process, but after seeing several cases, the clinician may observe the repetitive anatomic pattern of involvement of the eczema. Characteristically, the process is localized on the scalp, the retro-auricular areas, the nape, the face, especially along the hairline, the seborrheic areas of the face, and a special preference for involving the axillary (Fig. 9) and groin areas. Very commonly, the lesions are exudative, with honey-crusting, but occasionally scalier and drier. There is classically certain degree of impetiginization that makes the clinician to presume superinfection by pyogenic microorganisms such as *Staphylococcus* or *Streptococcus*. Reading the description of Robert Sweet, one realizes that infectious was the first word that came to his mind when he described his experience when seeing such patients in Jamaica [35].

The criteria used for diagnosing the disease include the presence of erythematous, scaly, exudative, and crusted lesions in the body regions previously described and other areas such as the chest or the back. Although crusting of nostrils was described as one of the main criteria, it is not always present. Another useful criterion is the chronic course of the disease. The lesions will subside rapidly with the administration of oral antibiotics, but eventually the lesions will relapse after a few weeks with the discontinuation of therapy. In children, such a course may persist up to the adolescence, around the 15 years of age; then, the dermatitis will spontaneously disappear, mimicking the course seen in pediatric atopic dermatitis. Adult infective dermatitis tends to have a more chronic course, without spontaneous remission. One important diagnostic criterion is a positive test for HTLV-1, either by serology or molecular biology testing.

The disease in children usually starts at 1 and a half years of age, but exceptionally, it can be seen in younger patients. The patients for the most part will be superinfected by either *Staphylococcus aureus* or beta hemolytic *Streptococcus*; those microorganisms can be isolated from the skin or the nostrils. It is not uncommon that the infected *Staphylococcus* may include methicillin-resistant strains, which will increase the difficulty in managing the cases. Because of the underlying immune dysfunction, the patients may simultaneously develop scabies, corneal opacities, acquired ichthyosis, chronic bronchiectasis, glomerulonephritis, and lymphocytic interstitial pneumonitis [43].

Other clinical features include lymphocytosis, anemia, lymphadenopathy, elevated erythrocyte sedimentation rate (ESR), hypergammaglobulinemia, increased CD4 and CD8 counts, and elevated CD4/CD8 ratios [44]. Although TSP seems to occur later in life, the two diseases may coexist. The role of ID as precursor or as a risk factor for the ulterior development of ATL has yet to be elucidated.

Histological Features

The histological findings of infective dermatitis can be quite unspecific and there are no diagnostic criteria to make a diagnosis without clinic-pathologic correlation. Histologically it can be either a superficial perivascular or a lichenoid infiltrate. The

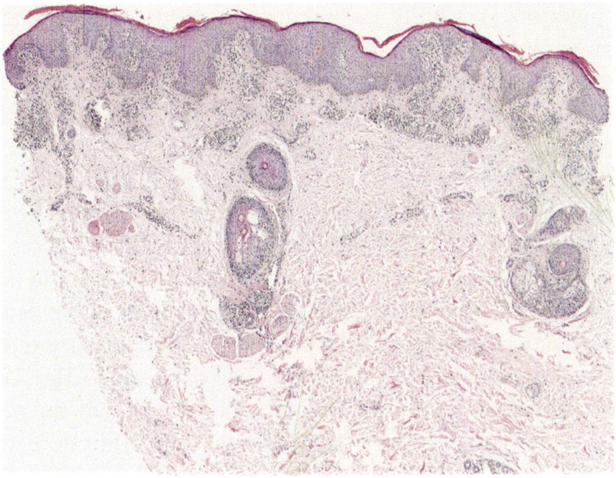

Fig. 10 Infective dermatitis, spongiotic dermatitis: acanthosis, parakeratosis, spongiosis; this pattern may be misinterpreted as any other type of eczema. H/E, 40 ×

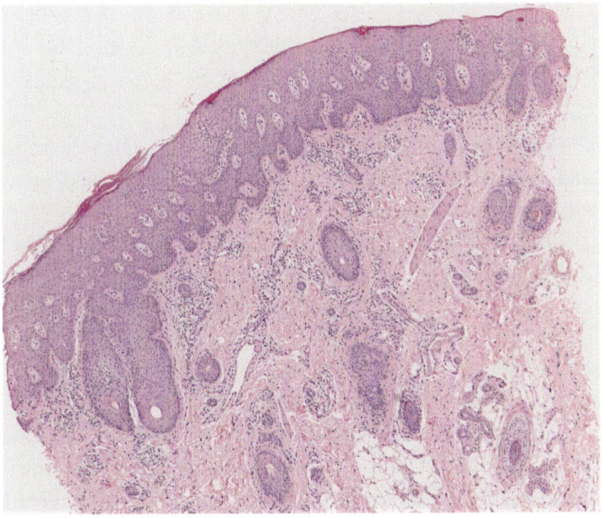

Fig. 11 Infective dermatitis, spongiotic, psoriasiform pattern: this pattern may be misinterpreted as psoriasis

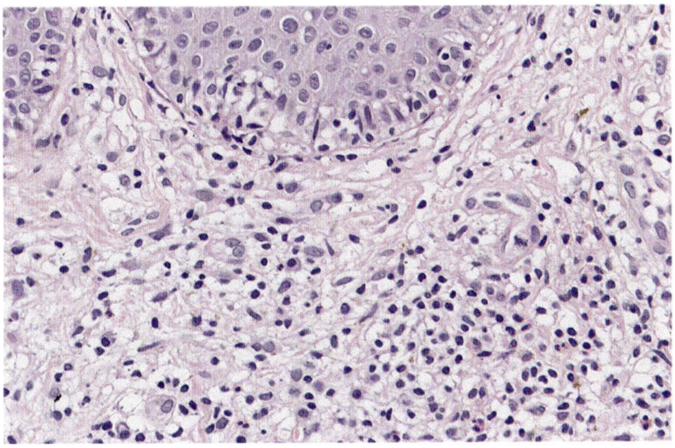

Fig. 12 Some exocytosis plus a mixed infiltrate of lymphocytes, eosinophils, and plasma cells are seen at high power in this case of infective dermatitis. The plasma cells and the exocytosis, in the clinical context, should raise the possibility of ID. H/E, 400×

epidermis is usually involved, from mild acanthosis and spongiosis (Fig. 10) to a more psoriasiform pattern (Fig. 11); signs of lichenification are rare because pruritus itself is rare. Spongiosis and exocytosis can be seen. Neutrophils may be present in the stratum corneum, and in cases with psoriasiform hyperplasia, psoriasis becomes an important differential diagnosis. Parakeratosis around the follicular infundibulum may be reminiscent of seborrheic dermatitis. The lymphocytes may be aligned along the dermal epidermal junction and added to the exocytosis as well as some wiring of the dermal collagen, so the whole constellation of findings may mimic mycosis fungoides. The observer may use the lack of lymphocytic atypia as the one criterion to be used to distinguish infective dermatitis from the patch stage of mycosis fungoides. Plasma cells in the papillary dermis in a psoriasiform spongiotic dermatitis will favor infective dermatitis (Fig. 12) instead of regular eczema or psoriasis. Eosinophils may also be present as part of the dermal infiltrate. Immunohistochemistry will show that the infiltrate is usually predominantly CD8-positive lymphocytes. There is scarcity of T-reg cells in the infiltrate [45].

Etiopathogenesis

The proposed etiopathogenesis of ID includes a dysregulation produced by the virus leading to immunosuppression and an increased susceptibility to staphylococcal and streptococcal infections.

The virus has special predilection for infecting CD4 lymphocytes but also infects CD8 lymphocytes, dendritic cells, B cells, monocyte natural killer cells, and microglial cells [44]. Once the cell is infected, there is an integration of the viral DNA inside the cellular DNA. From there on, the HTLV-1 becomes a pro-virus, and, as a result, there is no viral load detectable in blood, a mechanism that favors its avoidance of the host immune system.

The HTLV-1 uses the machinery of the cell to produce viral proteins, such as tax, rex, p12, p13, p21, and basic leucine zipper protein/factor. Among them, the tax protein is the most pathogenic, causing cell proliferation and exuberant inflammatory reaction. The cell proliferation results in immortal CD4+ and CD8+ clones.

ID is associated with increased viral loads and the presence of HTLV-1 antibodies. The profile of ID is more of a Th1 response, similar in a way to what is seen in TSP; however, in the last one, the CD8+ cells produce perforin and granzyme B, which is either absent or only present in small amounts in ID.

Genetics seems to play a role in the etiopathogenesis of ID. Among evidence in favor, carrying some human leukocyte antigen (HLA) increases the transmission from mother to child. Also, major histocompatibility complex (MHC) HLA class II haplotype DRB1* has been found in patients with ID and TSP and is associated with increased immune response.

Genetic factors seem to make some patients fewer immune responders to the virus and major risk to develop ATL, whereas other patients will have exuberant immune reactions and a higher risk of developing TSP.

Also, patients with malnutrition and poor economic status tend to develop ID, which may also explain the lack of DI cases in Japan, despite a high prevalence of the virus in the general population.

In ID biopsies, compared to asymptomatic carriers and normal population, there is an increased expression of Fox-p3 cells in the dermis and epidermis, as well as downregulation of filaggrin expression in lesional skin. The increased Fox-p3 expression results in immunosuppression and tumorigenesis, with an increment in T-reg cells. Filaggrin deficiency may also explain the similarities found between ID and atopic dermatitis.

The role of pyogenic bacteria such as *Staphylococcus* and *Streptococcus* is indubitable, considering the excellent clinical response of the dermatosis to oral antibiotics. ID is a disease easy to control by controlling the infection, compared to atopic dermatitis, where the emphasis is put in controlling the inflammation.

Differential Diagnosis

The most important differential diagnosis of ID is with atopic dermatitis, seborrheic dermatitis, contact eczema, and even psoriasis and mycosis fungoides in adults.

Criteria for the diagnosis have been established and revised (see Table 1). A small number of pediatric patients may have simultaneous findings of ID and atopic dermatitis. The dermatologist should raise the possibility of ID whenever he/she sees "atopic dermatitis" with marked scalp involvement, "impetiginized seborrheic dermatitis," or what it looks like heavily infected scalp psoriasis that responds too quickly to the administration of antibiotics. Also, the diagnosis should be considered in any case of recalcitrant intertrigo of axillary and groin areas with an exudative, honey-crusting component. In children, retro-auricular eczematous

Table 1 Diagnostic criteria for the diagnosis of HTLV-1-related infective dermatitis

1. Presence of erythematous, scaly, exudative, and crusted lesions of the scalp, retro-auricular areas, neck, axillae, groin, paranasal and perioral skin, ears, thorax, abdomen, and other sites
2. Crusting of nostrils
3. Chronic relapsing course with prompt response to appropriate therapy followed by prompt recurrence after discontinuation of therapy.
4. Diagnosis of HTLV-1 infection (by serology or molecular biologic testing)

Modified from Hlela and Bittencourt [43]
Of the four major criteria, three are required for diagnosis with mandatory inclusion of number 1, 2, and 4
To fulfill criterion 1, at least three sites should be involved, including scalp and retro-auricular areas

involvement should be distinguished from what is seen in hyperimmunoglobulin E syndrome.

Prognosis

ID in the pediatric age tends to resolve during adolescence, in an analogous fashion to atopic dermatitis. In adulthood, the disease follows a more chronic course, with the disease lasting for a long time. The risk of ID children to develop ATL in adulthood has not been established with certainty but seems to be the case in retrospective studies. In a group of patients with ATL and cutaneous involvement, 37.5% of those had a history compatible with ID in their childhood [46].

Therapy

Most patients with ID, including children and adults, will respond rapidly to administration of oral antibiotics directed to clear the staphylococcal and streptococcal infection. The risk of developing resistance by the prolonged administration of antibiotic therapy is reduced by using trimethoprim/sulfamethoxazole combinations. Rarely, the patient may require the addition of topical or systemic steroid for the complete resolution of the dermatitis.

Gnathostomiasis

Introduction

Gnathostomiasis is a disease produced by the migration in tissue (mostly cutaneous) of the third larval state (L3) of nematodes of the genus *Gnathostoma*. The disease is acquired by ingestion of raw freshwater fish contaminated with the larva. It is commonly seen in Asia and in endemic countries such as Japan, Thailand, Cambodia, Laos, Myanmar, Indonesia, the Philippines, Malaysia, and Vietnam. Additional cases also have been reported in India, China, Taiwan, and Sri Lanka [47].

In the Americas, the largest number of cases is reported from Mexico, Ecuador, and Peru, with additional cases in Guatemala and Colombia. Most recently, autochthonous cases of gnathostomiasis have been described in Brazil [48, 49] and the USA [50].

The disease has also been described in Europe, especially in international travelers coming back home after visiting endemic countries [51–53].

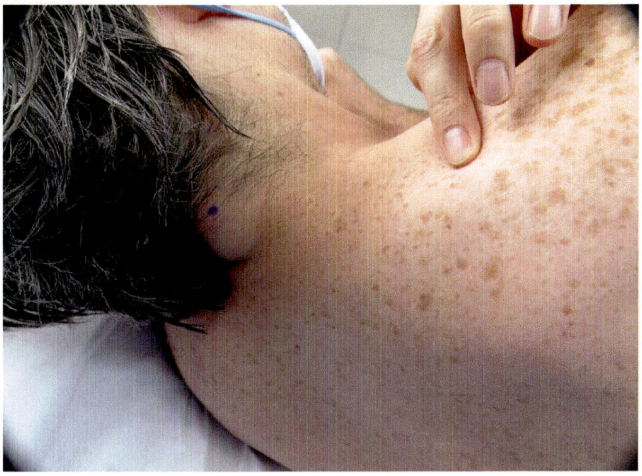

Fig. 13 Gnathostomiasis: the patient is pointing toward the original area where he noticed the first swelling, 2 weeks ago. The blue dot is marking the nodule he just developed 24 hours ago on the posterior neck

The disease is associated with the consumption of raw freshwater fish, in the form of ceviche, sushi, or sashimi. However, the disease may also occur after the consumption of brackish water fish. It is likely that, for every country and every location where the disease is seen, a specific species of fish may be responsible for carrying the larva.

Clinical Features

In the acute phase of infection, the patient may complain of abdominal symptoms, such as abdominal pain and discomfort, produced by the perforation of the gastric wall by the invasive larva into the peritoneal space.

Most commonly, the main complaint is the development of a single, indurated nodule or plaque, located on the abdominal wall, the chest, or extremities, but potentially in anywhere of the body, including the head, neck, vulvar area [54], or eye. The lesion usually measures a few centimeters in diameter, is red and hot, and may have a "peau d'orange" appearance on its surface. The lesion may be itchy or painful. The patient may be misdiagnosed as suffering some form of bacterial infection, and the nodule may disappear after the administration of antibiotics, to later recur a few centimeters beyond the original location, giving the idea of a migratory panniculitis. It would be extremely unusual to have two similarly active sites simultaneously, but it has been reported [55]. The lesions may appear and disappear cyclically, giving the idea of a wandering swelling (Fig. 13). This migratory quality is one of the main clues for the diagnosis, even more with a previous recent history of consuming raw fish. The lesion tends to appear within 3–4 weeks after the ingestion of the larva, and each episode of swelling may last up to 2 weeks. In the untreated patient, the migration may continue for prolonged periods for up to 12 years [55].

On occasion, the clinical picture is almost identical to larva migrans, especially after the administration of antiparasitic medication, except for the location. Whereas cutaneous larva migrans seems to prefer acral locations, such as the feet, or gluteal location as in children, the superficial migratory lesion of gnathostomiasis will be seen in the abdomen, anterior chest, back, or proximal limbs. It is possible to see a mixed lesion, where a nodular lesion is almost in continuity with the superficial "larva migrans" pattern.

The so-called furuncular form of gnathostomiasis represents the most extreme case of superficialization of the larva. It is classically seen after the patient receives treatment. Instead of traveling through the panniculus or the reticular dermis, the larva adopts a position perpendicular to the epidermis, and rarely, the larva emerges through the skin surface. When the whole nodule or plaque has been reduced to a single papule, the chances of catching the parasite in a punch biopsy are the highest, as has been demonstrated in the literature [56].

Even when the classical migration does occur at the skin level, the larva may migrate inside the body, producing pulmonary, gastrointestinal, and genitourinary involvement. The most dangerous migrations are those that affect the central nervous system and the ocular globe. In the central nervous system, it may produce radiculomyelitis, radiculomyeloencephalitis, eosinophilic meningitis, and subarachnoid hemorrhage. Classically, it will manifest as excruciating radicular pain or headache, with subsequent paralysis of extremities or focal palsy. Ocular involvement implies the penetration of the larvae inside the ocular globe; it is the only situation where the larva can be visualized in vivo, most commonly in the anterior chamber. Ocular involvement is characterized by the absence of peripheral eosinophilia.

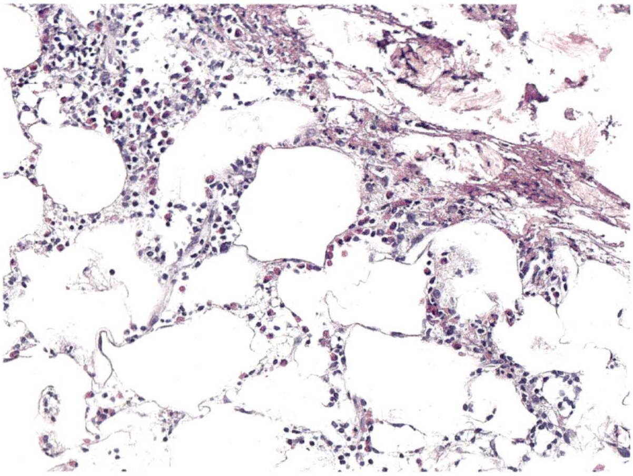

Fig. 14 Gnathostomiasis: lobular panniculitis with heavy infiltrate mostly of eosinophils. H/E, 40×

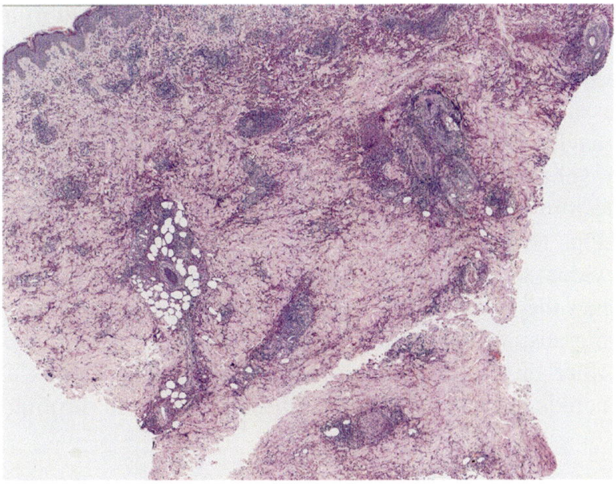

Fig. 15 Gnathostomiasis: superficial and deep, perivascular and periadnexal infiltrate of lymphocytes and several eosinophils. H/E, 100×

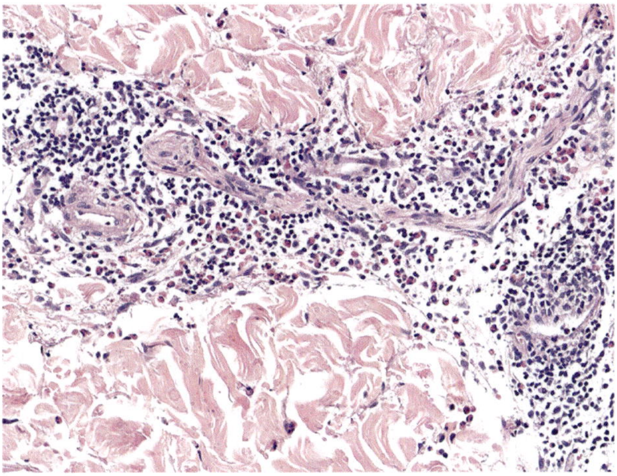

Fig. 16 Gnathostomiasis: perivascular infiltrate of eosinophils. H/E, 40×

Histological Features

The clue for the diagnosis of gnathostomiasis from the histopathological point of view is the presence of eosinophils in the skin. When dealing with nodules clinically, one should expect a dense inflammatory infiltrate at the subcutaneous level, as in a lobular panniculitis (Fig. 14), although sometimes eosinophils are scarce. In cases where the clinical lesion is most of a plaque or a papule, the infiltrate may be in the reticular dermis with an important interstitial component of mainly eosinophils (Figs. 15 and 16). Occasionally, edema of the papillary dermis is present, as well as some spongiosis at the epidermal level. Dense infiltration of eosinophils in the dermis may result in the formation of flame figures, with eosinophilic degeneration of the collagen fibers accompanying the cellular infiltrate.

As a rule, the possibilities of finding the worm in histological cuts are low, but the chances increase if the biopsy is taken from a new developing papule after therapy. The larva is large, located either in the reticular dermis or in the subcutaneous tissue. Sections of the larva may show either a thick esophagus or an intestine with heavily pigmented epithelial cells surrounded by lateral cavernous cords. Nematodes are characteristically roundworms, with internal organs, as opposed to flatworms as seen in sparganosis, where there is no distinct intestine. Another characteristic that helps to identify the *Gnathostoma* larva is the presence of cuticular spines, more evident toward the cephalic pole. Considering the size of the larva, it is quite larger than the larva of *Strongyloides* and all the larva associated with cutaneous larva migrans; this last microorganism does its traveling only at the epidermal level. Other migratory larvae that can be seen in dermis and have a comparable size include the larva of onchocerciasis and animal dirofilariasis.

Etiopathogenesis

There are at least 13 species of *Gnathostoma*, but only five have been known to cause disease in humans: *G. spinigerum*, which is the most commonly reported in Asia, *G. hispidum*, *G. doloresi*, *G. nipponicum*, and, more recently, *G. binucleatum*, which seem to be the predominant species in cases reported in Mexico and Ecuador [57].

The final natural hosts are cats and dogs. The cycle starts in the gastric mucosae of the domestic animals. In such a nest, a fertilized female liberates eggs that come outside with the animal feces. The unembryonated eggs get into the nearby current water of creeks and rivers and mature into embryonated eggs that after hatching give origin to the first larvarial stage or L1. The L1 is then ingested by copepods and evolve into a second larvarial stage or L2 and then into a third larvarial stage or L3. The L3, following the aquatic alimentary chain, is again ingested by larger fishes or frogs. The L3 mature in the tissue of the secondary host. The second host may directly be ingested by the final host or end up being ingested by paratenic hosts. As described by W. Ollague in the Guayas region of Ecuador, local fishermen feed their domestic animals with rotten fish, so the vital cycle is completed [58].

Humans get the infection by ingesting the flesh contaminated with L3, either from fish or other intermediate hosts such as frogs, snakes, and chicken. Two alternative modes of infection are also described: human beings getting the infection from drinking water contaminated with viable L2 and human beings functioning as intermediate hosts or fish handlers that get in contact with L3 from contaminated meat and get the infection directly through the skin [55].

The larvae usually measure up to 12.5 mm long and 1.2 mm wide and are reddish white in color.

The cephalic bulb of the invasive larva has anatomic structures that allow it to penetrate human tissue including burrowing hooks while releasing secretory proteins including hyaluronidases, hemolysins, and metalloproteinases [59].

Differential Diagnosis

The diagnosis of gnathostomiasis requires the history of ingesting contaminated fish in the form of ceviche, sushi, or sashimi, as well as the alternatives ways to acquire the disease (drinking contaminated water or manipulating contaminated fish flesh). The clinical lesion should be characterized as a migratory swelling accompanied by the presence of tissue or peripheral eosinophilia (present in 50% of cases). The history of living or traveling into an endemic area also is quite important, although the recent description of autochthonous cases in countries where the disease has not been previously recognized should make the clinician more suspicious even when the epidemiological data is absent.

The best recognized serological test for gnathostomiasis is the *G. spinigerum*-antigen-based immunoblot; however, it is only available in research centers, such as the Mahidol University in Thailand and the Swiss Tropical and Public Health Institute, in Basil.

The diagnosis of gnathostomiasis should be based on clinical and histological grounds, and considering the low rate of complications from therapy, the treatment should be given just based on those clinical criteria.

Other infections and infestations that may behave similarly include dracunculiasis, toxocariasis, cutaneous larva migrans, strongyloidiasis, dirofilariasis, sparganosis, and migratory myiasis.

Prognosis

Most cases of gnathostomiasis respond to antiparasitic medication. The benign prognosis in cases of cutaneous gnathostomiasis should be compared with the prognosis in visceral disease and especially in cases with ocular and central nervous system involvement; the last involvement may carry mortality rates of 8–25%, with 30% of patients reported to have long-term sequelae [55].

Therapy

The best medications in gnathostomiasis include oral albendazole and oral ivermectin. Albendazole should be given in doses of 400–800 mg daily for 21 days. Ivermectin can function as an alternative drug, using 200 mcg/kg as a single dose, every 7 days for two to three doses. Some patients will be required more than one cycle of treatment. Consideration to the simultaneous use of both medications should be given in special cases such as patients with disease in the head and neck region or near the eyes or in cases associated with neurological involvement.

Rational use of oral steroids is recommended in patients with involvement of the central nervous system.

Surgery as the extirpation of small lesions following oral therapy may increase the chances of successfully extracting the larvae.

Paederus Dermatitis

Introduction

Paederus dermatitis, also known as dermatitis linearis, whiplash dermatosis, "latigazo," or "potó" is a vesicating irritant dermatosis following the contact of the skin with beetles of the genus *Paederus*, of the Staphylinidae family, Paederinae subfamily. There are 622 species of the genus, about 30 described as causing the dermatosis [60]. The disease is seen around the world, although it is more frequent in places with hot, humid, and a rainy climate.

Countries with high incidence and reporting include India, Pakistan, China, and countries of Southeast Asia. The disease is increasingly reported in travelers [61], military personnel stationed in endemic areas [62], and factory workers [63]. The disease has been reported affecting rural workers as well as in urban settings. Rice fields seem to be ideal for breeding [64]. The disease is reported as isolated cases as well as in epidemic fashion. The epidemics are associated with overgrowing of a specific *Paederus* species because of climate changes, especially with heavy rainfall. The epidemics have been associated with "El Niño" climate phenomenon in Peru [65], and a similar occurrence was reported in Africa as increased incidence of the Nairobi "fly" (*P. sabaeus*) [66].

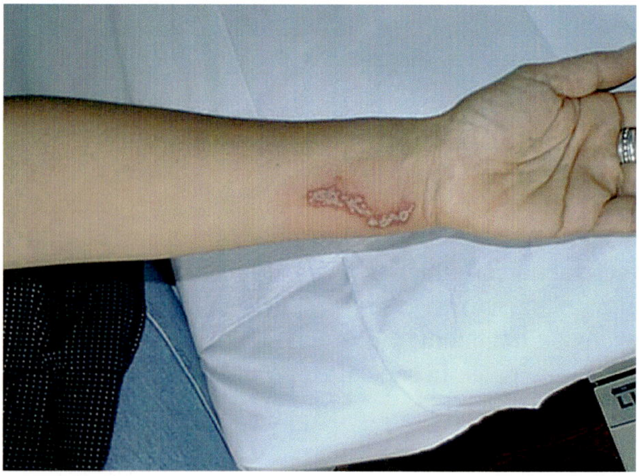

Fig. 17 A linear pustular dermatosis typical of Paederus dermatitis

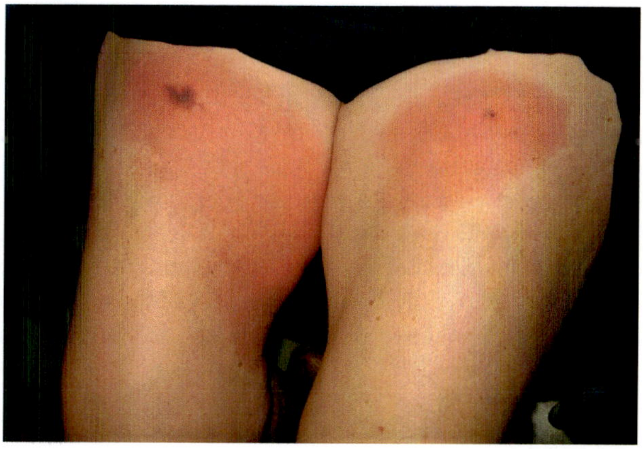

Fig. 18 "Kissing" lesions commonly described in Paederus dermatitis

Clinical Features

The disease is induced by the crushing and smearing of the beetle body against the skin, following a natural reflex movement after the crawling sensation. This is the origin of the linear fashion of the dermatosis. The symptoms start 24–48 hours after the contact with the insect, as itching and burning at the site, followed by appearance of erythema, edema, vesiculation, and blistering. Vesicles start to appear at the center of the lesion, and, then, they may evolve into pustules (Fig. 17). The presence of inflammatory signs as erythema allows the distinction from cantharidin contact, where the vesicles and bullae are not associated with erythema. Clinical symptoms can be classified as mild, moderate, or severe. Mild cases consist mainly of erythema; moderate cases are characterized by vesicle and bullae formation; the erythema is seen in the first 24 hours, whereas the blister formation is seen at 48 hours. Severe cases are characterized by extensive lesions, accompanied by systemic involvement, including, fever, neuralgia, arthralgia, and vomiting. Lesions evolve into crusting and hyperpigmentation that may last for weeks. A persistent erythema has also been described. Other complications include secondary infections, rhinitis, tympanitis, and ocular injury. The common areas of involvement are the face, neck, and arms; palms and soles are usually spared. The dermatosis is classically linear, but it is not uncommon to see "kissing lesions," where there is anatomical contact between two corporal surfaces such as in the flexure of the elbows or the anterolateral aspect of the inner thighs (Fig. 18). By transferring of the toxin by fingers, eye or genital involvement can occur. Eye involvement may progress to conjunctivitis, keratitis, and temporal eye loss.

Histological Features

Histology is not required to make the diagnosis. However, in documented cases where biopsy has been performed, remarkable findings include intra- and subepidermal vesiculation, spongiosis, ballooning, necrotic keratinocytes, and reticular necrosis of the epidermis, marked edema of the papillary dermis, and acantholysis. The dermal infiltrate is superficial and deep, wedge-shaped, composed by lymphocytes and abundant eosinophils; other findings include exocytosis into the epidermis and nuclear dust. Subacute changes include persistence of the lymphocytic infiltrate around vessels and even perineural, associated with clinical dysesthesias [64].

Etiopathogenesis

Several species have been associated with dermatitis linearis, including *Paederus fuscipes* in Asia and Europe, *P. sabaeus* in Africa, and *P. columbinus* and *P. brasiliensis* in South America. The adult measures 7–8 mm in length, 0.5–1 mm in width, and 4 mg in weight [67]. The adult has a distinct color pattern: black head, orange prothorax, iridescent blue elytra, and orange abdomen with black apex; it can be mistaken for ants [64] . The insect is active in broad light and resides on vegetation, especially in moist habitats. The *Paederus* is attracted to incandescent and fluorescent lights; some adults can fly, but others are flightless. In cases of epidemics, the insects are abundant, but isolated cases can be caused by occasional encounters with the normal population of beetles.

The cause of the dermatitis is the action of one or the mix of vesicating toxins called pederin, pseudopaederin, and pederone. The toxins are produced by endosymbiotic bacteria of the genus *Pseudomonas* that is present in the endolymph of females. Pederin ($C_{25}H_{45}O_9N$) is an amide with two tetrahydropyran rings. The toxins are liberated when the insect body is crushed and smashed on the patient skin. The effect of the toxin is by blocking mitosis even with levels as low as 1 ng/mL, inhibiting protein and DNA synthesis without affecting RNA synthesis.

Differential Diagnosis

The differential diagnosis includes any cause of irritant and contact dermatitis, thermal and chemical burns, herpetic infections, phytophotodermatitis, cutaneous larva migrans, autoimmune blistering diseases, and injuries caused by caterpillars and moths. Capturing the provoking insect, the linear array of the lesion, the involvement of exposed areas, the presence of kissing lesions, and the epidemiologic data all contribute to make a clinical diagnosis.

Prognosis

Although the clinical course may vary, most patients evolve favorably, toward the complete resolution of symptoms. Pigmentary alterations and local erythema may persist for a while. Dysesthesia, acute as well as chronic, may complicate some cases, but the use of low-dose anticonvulsants such as gabapentin or pregabalin may help in most refractory cases.

Therapy

Recommended therapy by most authors consists of measures normally used in irritant and allergic contact dermatitis, from soothing compresses to emollients, oral antihistamines, and rarely the use of systemic steroids.

References

1. Yotsu RR, Murase C, Sugawara M, et al. Revisiting Buruli ulcer. J Dermatol. 2015;42(11):1033–41.
2. Zingue D, Bouam A, Tian RBD, Drancourt M. Buruli ulcer, a prototype for ecosystem-related infection, caused by Mycobacterium ulcerans. Clin Microbiol Rev. 2017;31(1):e00045–17.
3. Guarner J. Buruli ulcer: review of a neglected skin mycobacterial disease. J Clin Microbiol. 2018;56(4):e01507–17.
4. Yotsu RR, Suzuki K, Simmonds RE, Bedimo R, Ablordey A, Yeboah-Manu D, Phillips R, Asiedu K. Buruli ulcer: a review of the current knowledge. Curr Trop Med Rep. 2018;5(4):247–56.
5. Visvesvara GS, Martinez AJ, Schuster FL, Leitch GJ, Wallace SV, Sawyer TK, Anderson M. Leptomyxid ameba, a new agent of amebic meningoencephalitis in humans and animals. J Clin Microbiol. 1990;28(12):2750–6.
6. Visvesvara GS, Schuster FL, Martinez AJ. Balamuthia mandrillaris, N. G., N. Sp., agent of amebic meningoencephalitis in humans and other animals. J Eukaryot Microbiol. 1993;40(4):504–14.
7. Cope JR, Landa J, Nethercut H, et al. The epidemiology and clinical features of Balamuthia mandrillaris disease in the United States, 1974–2016. Clin Infect Dis. 2019;68(11):1815–22.
8. Bravo FG, Seas C. Balamuthia mandrillaris amoebic encephalitis: an emerging parasitic infection. Curr Infect Dis Rep. 2012;14(4):391–6.
9. Wang L, Cheng W, Li B, et al. *Balamuthia mandrillaris* infection in China: a retrospective report of 28 cases. Emerg Microbes Infect. 2020;9(1):2348–57.
10. Itoh K, Yagita K, Nozaki T, et al. An autopsy case of Balamuthia mandrillaris amoebic encephalitis, a rare emerging infectious disease, with a brief review of the cases reported in Japan. Neuropathology. 2015;35(1):64–9.
11. Moriarty P, Burke C, McCrossin D, et al. Balamuthia mandrillaris encephalitis: survival of a child with severe meningoencephalitis and review of the literature. J Pediatric Infect Dis Soc. 2014;3(1):e4–9.

12. Reed RP, Cooke-Yarborough CM, Jaquiery AL, et al. Fatal granulomatous amoebic encephalitis caused by Balamuthia mandrillaris. Med J Aust. 1997;167(2):82–4.
13. Krasaelap A, Prechawit S, Chansaenroj J, et al. Fatal Balamuthia amebic encephalitis in a healthy child: a case report with review of survival cases. Korean J Parasitol. 2013;51(3):335–41.
14. Kodet R, Nohýnková E, Tichý M, et al. Amebic encephalitis caused by Balamuthia mandrillaris in a Czech child: description of the first case from Europe. Pathol Res Pract. 1998;194(6):423–9.
15. Tavares M, Correia da Costa JM, Carpenter S, et al. Diagnosis of first case of Balamuthia amoebic encephalitis in Portugal by immunofluorescence and PCR. J Clin Microbiol. 2006;44(7):2660-3.
16. Sarica TK, Cekınmez M, et al. A rare but fatal case of granulomatous amebic encephalitis with brain abscess: the first case reported from Turkey. Turk Neurosurg. 2009;19(3):256–9.
17. Tello-Zavala MC, Bravo-Oro A, Falcón-Escobedo R. Central nervous system infection in an immunocompetent Mexican child. Pediatr Infect Dis J. 2014;33(9):991, 995–6.
18. Riestra-Castaneda JM, Riestra-Castaneda R, Gonzalez-Garrido AA, Pena Moreno P, Martinez AJ, Visvesvara GS, Jardon Careaga F, Oropeza de Alba JL, Gonzalez Cornejo S. Granulomatous amebic encephalitis due to Balamuthia mandrillaris (Leptomyxiidae): report of four cases from Mexico. Am J Trop Med Hyg. 1997;56(6):603–7.
19. Cuevas M, Smoje G, Jofré L, et al. Meningoencefalitis granulomatosa por Balamuthia mandrillaris: Reporte de un caso y revisión de la literatura. Rev Chil Infect. 2006;23:234–9.
20. Tarauto AL, Monges J, Acefe JC, et al. Leptomyxid amoeba encephalitis: report of the first case in Argentina. Trans Royal Soc Trop Med Hyg. 1991;85:77.
21. Martinez AJ, Guerra E, Garcia-Tamayo J, et al. Granulomatous amebic encephalitis: a review and report of a spontaneous case from Venezuela. Acta Neuropathol. 1994;87:430–4.
22. Silva-Vergara ML, Da Cunha Colombo ER, Vissotto E, et al. Disseminated Balamuthia mandrillaris Amoeba infection in an AIDS patient from Brazil. Am J Trop Med Hyg. 2007;77(6):1096–8.
23. Bodi I, Dutt N, Hampton T, et al. Fatal granulomatous amoebic meningoencephalitis due to Balamuthia mandrillaris. Pathol Res Pract. 2008;204(12):925–8.
24. Farnon EC, Kokko KE, Budge PJ, et al. Transmission of Balamuthia mandrillaris by organ transplantation. Clin Infect Dis. 2016;63(7):878–88.
25. Guarner J, Bartlett J, Shieh WJ, et al. Histopathologic spectrum and immunohistochemical diagnosis of amebic meningoencephalitis. Mod Pathol. 2007;20(12):1230–7.
26. Booton GC, Carmichael JR, Visvesvara GS, et al. Genotyping of Balamuthia mandrillaris based on nuclear 18S and mitochondrial 16S rRNA genes. Am J Trop Med Hyg. 2003;68(1):65–9.
27. Kalyatanda G, Rand K, Lindner MS, et al. Rapid, noninvasive diagnosis of *Balamuthia mandrillaris* encephalitis by a plasma-based next-generation sequencing test. Open Forum Infect Dis. 2020;7(7):ofaa189.
28. Gomes TS, Vaccaro L, Magnet A, et al. Presence and interaction of free-living amoebae and amoeba-resisting bacteria in water from drinking water treatment plants. Sci Total Environ. 2020;719:137080.
29. Yamanouchi K, Arima H, Sakamoto Y, et al. First report of the isolation of Balamuthia mandrillaris in the northern region of Japan. Parasitol Res. 2018;117(9):2895–900.
30. Cabello-Vílchez AM, Reyes-Batlle M, Montalbán-Sandoval E, et al. The isolation of Balamuthia mandrillaris from environmental sources from Peru. Parasitol Res. 2014;113(7):2509–13.
31. Recavarren-Arce S, Velarde C, Gotuzzo E, et al. Amoeba angeitic lesions of the central nervous system in Balamuthia mandrilaris amoebiasis. Hum Pathol. 1999;30(3):269–73.
32. Jayasekera S, Matin A, Sissons J, et al. Balamuthia mandrillaris stimulates interleukin-6 release in primary human brain microvascular endothelial cells via a phosphatidylinositol 3-kinase-dependent pathway. Microbes Infect. 2005;7(13):1345–51.

33. Martínez DY, Seas C, Bravo F, et al. Successful treatment of Balamuthia mandrillaris amoebic infection with extensive neurological and cutaneous involvement. Clin Infect Dis. 2010;51(2):e7–11.
34. Gallo RC. The discovery of the first human retrovirus: HTLV-1 and HTLV-2. Retrovirology. 2005;2:17.
35. Sweet RD. A pattern of eczema in Jamaica. Br J Dermatol. 1966;78(Feb (2)):93–100.
36. LaGrenade L, Hanchard B, Fletcher V, et al. Infective dermatitis of Jamaican children: a marker for HTLV-I infection. Lancet. 1990;336(Dec(8727)):1345–7.
37. Gessain A, Cassar O. Epidemiological aspects and world distribution of HTLV-1 infection. Front Microbiol. 2012;3:388.
38. Tous Romero F, Pinilla-Martín B, Palencia Pérez SI. Dermatitis infectiva asociada a HTLV-1: dermatosis a tener en cuenta en pacientes de zonas endémicas. Aten Primaria. 2020:S0212-6567(20)30024-X.
39. Salomon M, Maquera L, Del Solar M, et al. Dermatitis infectiva asociada a HTLV-1 en adulto. Folia Dermatológica. 2001;12(1):41–3
40. Di Martino OB, Riveros R, et al. Infective dermatitis in an adult patient with HTLV-1. Am J Dermatopathol. 2015;37(12):944–8.
41. Bittencourt AL, Oliveira Mde F, Ferraz N, et al. Adult-onset infective dermatitis associated with HTLV-I. clinical and immunopathological aspects of two cases. Eur J Dermatol. 2006;16(1):62–6. PMID: 16436345.
42. Maragno L, Casseb J, Fukumori LM, et al. Human T-cell lymphotropic virus type 1 infective dermatitis emerging in adulthood. Int J Dermatol. 2009;48(7):723–30.
43. Hlela C, Bittencourt A. Infective dermatitis associated with HTLV-1 mimics common eczemas in children and may be a prelude to severe systemic diseases. Dermatol Clin. 2014;32(2):237–48.
44. McGill NK, Vyas J, Shimauchi T, et al. HTLV-1-associated infective dermatitis: updates on the pathogenesis. Exp Dermatol. 2012;21(11):815–21. https://doi.org/10.1111/exd.12007. PMID: 23163646.
45. Bravo FG. Infective dermatitis: a purely cutaneous manifestation of HTLV-1 infection. Semin Diagn Pathol. 2020;37(2):92–7.
46. Bittencourt AL, Barbosa HS, Vieira MD, et al. Adult T-cell leukemia/lymphoma (ATL) presenting in the skin: clinical, histological and immunohistochemical features of 52 cases. Acta Oncol. 2009;48(4):598–604.
47. Bravo F, Gontijo B. Gnathostomiasis: an emerging infectious disease relevant to all dermatologists. An Bras Dermatol. 2018;93(2):172–80.
48. Haddad Junior V, Oliveira ÍF, Bicudo NP, et al. Gnathostomiasis acquired after consumption of raw freshwater fish in the Amazon region: a report of two cases in Brazil. Rev Soc Bras Med Trop. 2020;54:e20200127.
49. Vargas TJ, Kahler S, Dib C, et al. Autochthonous gnathostomiasis. Brazil Emerg Infect Dis. 2012;18(12):2087–9.
50. Schimmel J, Chao L, Luk A, et al. An autochthonous case of gnathostomiasis in the United States. JAAD Case Rep. 2020;6(4):337–8.
51. Clément-Rigolet MC, Danis M, Caumes E. La gnathostomose, une maladie exotique de plus en plus souvent importée dans les pays occidentaux [Gnathostomosis, an exotic disease increasingly imported into Western countries]. Presse Med. 2004;33(21):1527–32.
52. Leroy J, Cornu M, Deleplancque AS, et al. Sushi, ceviche and gnathostomiasis - a case report and review of imported infections. Travel Med Infect Dis. 2017;20:26–30.
53. Roach REJ, van Doorn R, de Bruïne FT, Arend SM, Visser LG. A recurrent migratory swelling. Lancet Infect Dis. 2018;18(9):1045.
54. Rosas R, Marcotti A, Weitzel T, et al. Vulvitis migratoria causada por gnatostomiasis importada. Rev Chil Infectol. 2019;36(5):670–3.
55. Herman JS, Chiodini PL. Gnathostomiasis, another emerging imported disease. Clin Microbiol Rev. 2009;22(3):484–92.

56. Laga AC, Lezcano C, Ramos C, et al. Cutaneous gnathostomiasis: report of 6 cases with emphasis on histopathological demonstration of the larva. J Am Acad Dermatol. 2013;68(2):301–5.
57. Neumayr A, Ollague J, Bravo F, et al. Cross-reactivity pattern of Asian and American human gnathostomiasis in Western Blot assays using crude antigens prepared from Gnathostoma spinigerum and Gnathostoma binucleatum third-stage larvae. Am J Trop Med Hyg. 2016;95:413–6.
58. Ollague Loaiza Wenceslao, Monografía del colegio Ibero Latino Americano de Dermatología, Gnathostomiasis, nueva enfermedad en Ecuador y América del sur. IESS. Guayaquil-Ecuador. 1985.
59. Diaz JH. Gnathostomiasis: an emerging infection of raw fish consumers in Gnathostoma nematode-endemic and nonendemic countries. J Travel Med. 2015;22(5):318–24.
60. Osorio-Velásquez B, García-Zuluaga LM, López-Bueno I, et al. Paederus dermatitis - a bibliometric analysis of an emerging disease in travelers. Infez Med. 2020;28(1):130–2.
61. Pierce JW, Rittman B, Raybould JE. Case report: Paederus dermatitis in the returning traveler. Am J Trop Med Hyg. 2018;98(5):1523–5.
62. Davidson SA, Norton SA, Carder MC, et al. Outbreak of dermatitis linearis caused by Paederus ilsae and Paederus iliensis (Coleoptera: Staphylinidae) at a military base in Iraq. US Army Med Dep J. 2009:6–15. PMID: 20084733.
63. Huang C, Liu Y, Yang J. An outbreak of 268 cases of Paederus dermatitis in a toy-building factory in Central China. Int J Dermatol. 2009;48:128–31.
64. Cressey BD, Paniz-Mondolfi AE, Rodríguez-Morales AJ, et al. Dermatitis linearis: vesicating dermatosis caused by paederus species (coleoptera: staphylinidae). Case series and review. Wilderness Environ Med. 2013;24(2):124–31.
65. Alva-Davalos V, Laguna-Torres VA, Huaman A, et al. Epidemic dermatitis by Paederus irritans in Piura, Perú at 1999, related to El Niño phenomenon. Rev Soc Bras Med Trop. 2002;35(1):23–8.
66. https://web.archive.org/web/20070128130446/http://edition.cnn.com/EARTH/9801/26/kenya.beetle.ap/index.html
67. Borroni G, Brazzelli V, Rosso R, et al. Paederus fuscipes dermatitis. A histopathological study. Am J Dermatopathol. 1991;13(5):467–74.

Skin Adverse Reactions from New Cancer Immunotherapy

Katrin Kerl, Helmut Kerl, and Lucie Heinzerling

Abbreviations

AGEP	Acute generalized exanthematous pustulosis
BSA	Body surface area
CTCAE	Common terminology criteria for adverse events
CTLA-4	Cytotoxic T-lymphocyte-associated protein 4
DRESS	Drug reaction with eosinophils and systemic symptoms
ICIs	Immune checkpoint inhibitors
IRAE	Immune-related adverse event
Mab	Monoclonal antibodies
MAH	Melanoma-associated hypopigmentation
PD-1	Programmed cell death protein 1
PD-L1	Programmed cell death-ligand 1
SCAR	Severe cutaneous adverse reaction
SJS	Stevens–Johnson syndrome
TEN	Toxic epidermal necrolysis

Introduction

The management of cancer patients has significantly changed since the approval of novel classes of immuno-oncology therapeutics. Substantial antitumor activity and response rates up to 58%, with improved overall survival, have been achieved in patients with metastatic melanoma with immune checkpoint inhibitors (ICIs), in

K. Kerl (✉) · L. Heinzerling
Department of Dermatology, Ludwig-Maximilian University Hospital of Munich, Munich, Germany

Department of Dermatology, Medical University Munich, Munich, Germany

H. Kerl
Department of Dermatology, University of Graz, Medical School, Graz, Austria

Department of Dermatology, Medical University Graz, Graz, Austria

F. Rongioletti, B. R. Smoller (eds.), *New and Emerging Entities in Dermatology and Dermatopathology*, https://doi.org/10.1007/978-3-030-80027-7_25

Table 1 Immune checkpoint inhibitors (ICIs)

Pembrolizumab – Keytruda® (anti-PD-1 Mab)
Nivolumab – Opdivo® (anti-PD-1 Mab)
Cemiplimab – Libtayo® (anti-PD-1 Mab)
Avelumab – Bavencio® (anti-PD-L1 Mab)
Atezolizumab – Tecentriq® (anti-PD-L1 Mab)
Durvalumab – Imfinzi® (anti-PD-L1 Mab)
Ipilimumab – Yervoy® (anti-CTLA-4 Mab)
Tremelimumab (anti-CTLA-4 Mab)

particular with anti-programmed cell death protein 1 (PD-1)/anti-programmed cell death-ligand 1 (PD-L1), anti-cytotoxic T-lymphocyte-associated protein 4 (CTLA-4), and their combination [1]. Besides melanoma, ICIs are effective in patients with non-small cell lung cancer, Merkel cell carcinoma, Hodgkin lymphoma, and advanced cutaneous squamous cell carcinoma and several other tumor entities, and a number of them have been approved for the different entities (Table 1).

ICIs, which target specific immune cells rather than destroying the cancer cells, are associated with a broad spectrum of side effects known as immune-related adverse events. These side effects developed in up to 85% of patients after treatment with monotherapy of anti-PD-1 or anti-CTLA4 and up to 96% with combination immunotherapy [2]. Severe side effects developed in 17–21% of patients receiving anti-PD-1 monotherapy [3, 4], 20–28% of those receiving ipilimumab [3, 4], 45% of those receiving ipilimumab (1 mg/kg) plus pembrolizumab [5], and 59% of those receiving approved combination therapy with ipilimumab (3 mg/kg) and nivolumab [2]. The activation of the host immune system can involve nearly all body organs presenting as skin manifestations, gastrointestinal symptoms (colitis and diarrhea) or pneumonitis, hepatitis, thyroiditis, hypophysitis, uveitis, polyarthritis, central nervous, and cardiac complications among many other toxicities [6–8]. In addition, many patients experience fatigue, decreased appetite, and nausea.

The spectrum of IRAE is similar between anti-PD1/anti-PD-L1 and anti-CTLA4 antibodies, but the frequency of specific side effects varies. While thyroid dysfunction and arthralgias are more frequent with nivolumab and pembrolizumab, colitis and hypophysitis are more commonly observed with ipilimumab [2]. For combination therapy, more than one organ system is involved in about one-third of patients [9, 10].

Interestingly, the occurrence of IRAEs has been implicated as a positive prognostic sign [11]. Clearly, patients with metastatic melanoma who stopped ICI therapy due to toxicity do not have a worse outcome [12].

Any checkpoint inhibitor therapy can induce long-lasting side effects, which might not resolve and also potentially be fatal [13]. Especially endocrine side effects are associated with life-long hormone substitution, neurological side effects often induce permanent sequelae, and skin side effects like leucotrichia can permanently stigmatize patients.

Dermatologic Toxicities Induced By Immune Checkpoint Blockade Therapies

The side effect profile of checkpoint inhibitors that may impact the skin is very broad. Dermatological toxicities are the most frequently observed ICI-induced IRAEs with an incidence of 46–62% of patients [2]. Cutaneous adverse events are usually mild to moderate; severe to life-threatening generalized reactions occur in 2–6% of patients with clinicopathological presentations such as DRESS, TEN, or bullous pemphigoid. The majority of events are reversible after systemic use of glucocorticoids (methylprednisolone or equivalents). Skin reactions occur for the most part within the first 6 weeks after the start of the ICI treatment but may be observed delayed, even after termination of the therapy. It has been noted that the profile of the various cutaneous reactions is very similar for both inhibitors [14].

Maculopapular Eruptions

Clinical Features

A pruritic, in many instances a morbilliform exanthem with erythematous macules and papules, symmetrically distributed on trunk and extremities, with a tendency to converge, represents the most frequent IRAE to ICIs. It can be observed in 49–68% of patients treated with anti-CTLA-4 vs 20% of patients receiving anti-PD-1 /PD-L1 [11]. The eruption occurs within the first 6 weeks after the initiation of treatment.

Histopathological Features

The histopathological features of checkpoint inhibitor-related maculopapular exanthema are summarized in Table 2; they are indistinguishable from "standard" maculopapular reactions to more conventional drugs.

Table 2 Histopathology of maculopapular eruptions

Superficial (and deep) perivascular and interstitial inflammatory cell infiltrate. Predominance of CD4-positive lymphocytes, presence of eosinophils and/or neutrophils, and rarely plasma cells
Edema of the papillary dermis
Subtle basal layer vacuolar changes, mild spongiosis, and few (if any) necrotic keratinocytes
Epidermotropism of few lymphocytes and neutrophils

Note: Infiltrate may be devoid of eosinophils

Lichenoid Reactions

Clinical Features

Lichenoid reactions represent one of the most common types of cutaneous IRAEs, which are especially associated with anti-PD-1/PD-L1 agents. The onset of the lichenoid reactions is delayed and typically observed 6–12 weeks after start of therapy [15].

The clinical presentation features a maculopapular eruption or resembles lichen planus (Fig. 1a). When compared with idiopathic lichen planus, the lesions are usually more generalized with involvement of trunk and extremities. Oral manifestations present as a white reticulated or erosive plaques and can limit food intake, which calls for special attention in oncologic patients since body weight represents an independent prognostic factor in some cancer entities.

Histopathological Features

Histopathology (Fig. 1b) is characterized by patchy parakeratosis and focal hypergranulosis with a band-like mixed-cell infiltrate along the dermoepidermal junction associated with vacuolar alteration. Necrotic keratinocytes are present (lichenoid–cytotoxic reaction). The infiltrate contains lymphocytes, eosinophils, some plasma cells, and CD163 positive histiocytes. The immunohistological demonstration of an increased expression of PD-L1 on keratinocytes has been implicated in the

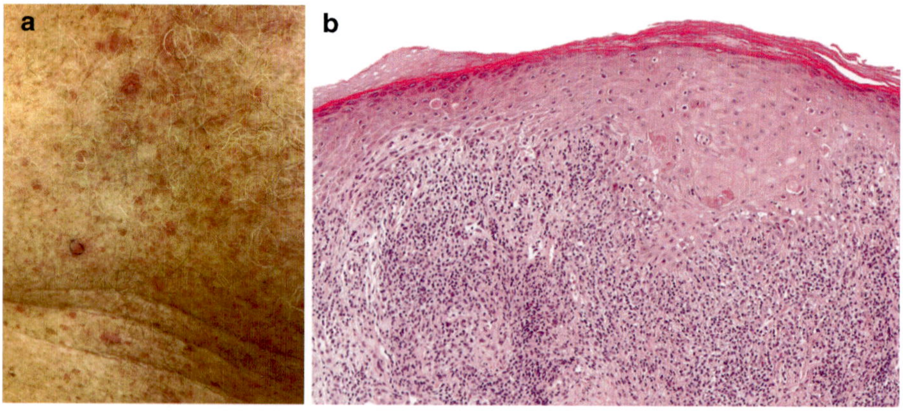

Fig. 1 *Lichenoid drug reaction* (**a**) Induced by ipilimumab and nivolumab in a patient with metastatic melanoma presenting as an exanthema with flat-topped papules on the trunk. (**b**) Histopathology shows typical features of lichen planus with acanthosis and hypergranulosis of the epidermis, apoptotic keratinocytes, and a band-like lymphocytic infiltrate at the dermoepidermal junction

pathogenesis [16]. Special features of ICI-induced lichenoid eruptions are suprabasal/subepidermal clefting simulating paraneoplastic pemphigus [17] and the combination of more than one pattern in a single specimen such as lichenoid and spongiotic pattern or spongiotic and interface dermatitis.

Psoriasis–Psoriasiform Reactions

Clinical Features

ICI can contribute to the development of psoriasiform reactions with all clinical variations including plaque type (most frequent), palmoplantar, guttate, and pustular psoriasis or psoriatic arthritis. T-cell activation and increase of chemokines induced by the checkpoint blockade may induce these however not very frequently. The lesions can appear early, after 3 weeks of treatment start [11], but may occur delayed, after several months of therapy. The exacerbation of psoriasis (similar to an immune reconstitution syndrome) has also been described. In these cases, it can be hard to judge whether it is the natural cause of disease or triggered by the immunotherapy.

Histopathological Features

The histopathological features of psoriasiform reactions are similar to those observed in non-drug-induced psoriasis vulgaris/pustulosa. Helpful clues for the distinction between classic psoriasis vs drug-related psoriasis are fewer necrotic keratinocytes, more pronounced spongiosis, and eosinophils within the inflammatory infiltrate in the latter [18].

Bullous Eruptions

Clinical Features

Most patients with bullous reactions induced by checkpoint inhibitors present with the clinical features of bullous pemphigoid showing localized or generalized tense blisters of different sizes and shapes, erosions, and crusts. Initial stages are characterized by pruritic erythematous macules, papules, urticarial plaques, and eczema-like lesions. Mucosal surfaces may also be affected (in 10–30%). Compared with other IRAEs, bullous pemphigoid-like eruptions may develop (or persist) several months after termination of the immunotherapy [15]. However, rapid manifestations after treatment begin are also documented [19].

Histopathological Features

The histopathological aspects are basically indistinguishable from idiopathic (spontaneously) occurring bullous pemphigoid revealing subepidermal blisters and moderate to dense inflammatory infiltrates with lymphocytes, neutrophils, and numerous eosinophils (Fig. 2). A few necrotic keratinocytes and vacuolar alteration near the margin of the blister favor the diagnosis of a drug-induced pemphigoid. Direct immunofluorescence microscopy on salt-split skin shows deposition of IgG on the roof side of the blister.

Vitiligo/Melanoma-Associated Hypopigmentation (MAH)

Clinical Features

Vitiligo or more specifically melanoma-associated hypopigmentation (MAH) can be observed in melanoma patients independently of the mode of therapy and is associated with a better prognosis. Clinically, MAH and vitiligo have shared and discriminative features. Autoimmune diseases are more frequent and haplotype HLA-A2 twice as common in vitiligo compared with MAH patients. MAH is less progressive compared with classical vitiligo; however, it was more often associated with other acquired leukodermas [20]. In melanoma patients treated with ICIs, an incidence of up to 25% of patients with anti-PD1/PD-L1 therapy and up to 11% with anti-CTLA-4 therapy has been reported, respectively. The period from treatment initiation to the appearance of the depigmentations can range from 6 to

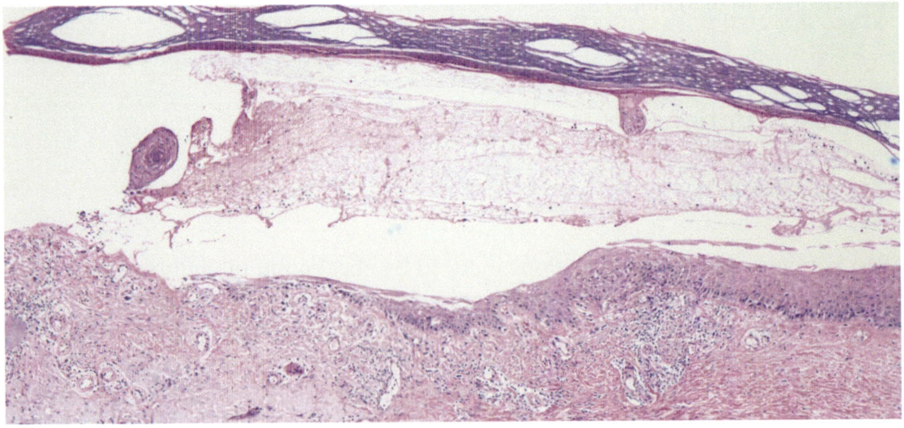

Fig. 2 *Bullous pemphigoid*. After treatment with nivolumab for metastatic melanoma. Skin biopsy shows a subepidermal blister with reepithelialization and a sparse superficial lymphocytic infiltrate with some eosinophils

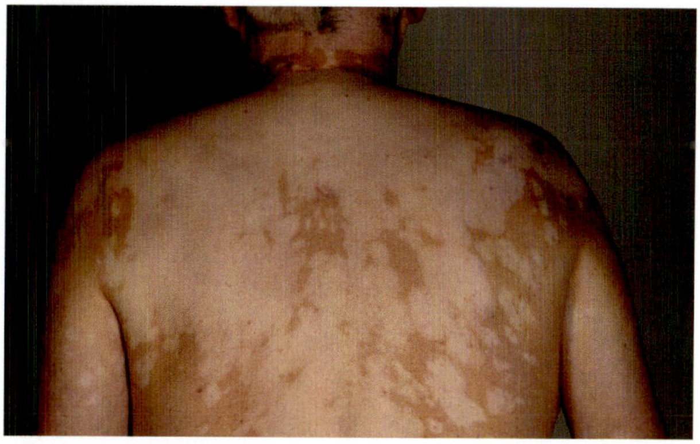

Fig. 3 *Melanoma-associated hypopigmentation* induced by spartalizumab (anti-PD-1-Mab currently in clinical trials; *courtesy PD Dr. T. Maul, Zurich*)

36 weeks [15]. It is not uncommon that the lesions persist after discontinuation of the therapy. MAH correlates with a favorable overall survival [11, 19].

Patients present clinically milk- to chalk-white macules evolving into larger patches of various sizes and often convex borders. The lesions are often symmetrically distributed and most commonly located on sun-exposed areas (Fig. 3).

Histopathological Features

Histological findings are characterized by a decrease (or rarely complete loss) of both melanocytes and melanin. T-cell activation induced by the immunotherapy results apparently in the destruction of melanocytes.

Severe Cutaneous Adverse Reactions

Clinical Features

The prototypic examples of severe cutaneous adverse reactions (=SCARs) are acute generalized exanthematous pustulosis (AGEP), drug reaction with eosinophils and systemic symptoms (DRESS), Stevens–Johnson syndrome (SJS), and toxic epidermal necrolysis (TEN) [21]. These toxicities, which are potentially life-threatening, have rarely been described with the use of immune checkpoint blockade. The interval from start of ICI therapy to the onset of SCARs varies from a few days to 20 weeks [11].

The early clinical findings of TEN are characterized by dusky red macules with a tendency to coalescence. Within a short time span, erosions and blisters with widespread detachment of the epidermis can be observed (Fig. 4). The Nikolsky

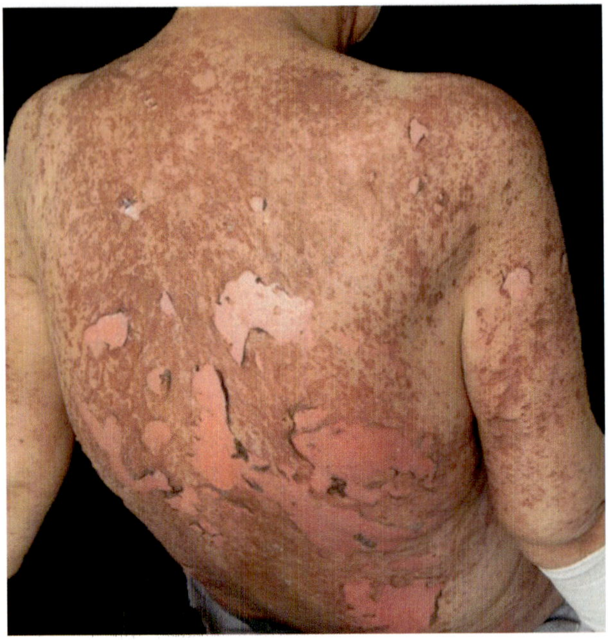

Fig. 4 Platinum-based chemotherapy + pembrolizumab-induced *toxic epidermal necrolysis* in a patient with advanced pulmonary carcinoma. Exanthema with a grayish hue and widespread skin detachment

sign, with separation of the superficial epithelial layers from the basal layer produced by rubbing or gentle pressure, is positive. An erosive mucositis and conjunctivitis are frequently present.

Histopathological Features

Histopathology reveals in the early stages scattered individual keratinocytes, slight vacuolar alteration, and a scarce superficial infiltrate of mainly CD8-positive lymphocytes. The characteristic features of fully developed lesions are subepidermal splitting with a necrotic but otherwise complete epidermis forming the blister roof. It has been demonstrated that both lymphocytes and keratinocytes near the dermo-epidermal junction show an increased expression of PD-L1, probably leading to the targeting and apoptosis of cells by activated cytotoxic T cells [22].

Pruritus

Treatment-induced pruritus is very bothersome side effect with 15–33% of patients being affected (ipilimumab 25%, nivolumab 19%, pembrolizumab 15–25%, and ipilimumab plus nivolumab 33%) [23].

Other Significant Cutaneous Reactions to Immune Checkpoint Inhibitors

In addition to the earlier presented skin toxicities, there exists a wide range of other ICI-induced IRAEs, which mimic specific skin diseases; they are listed in Table 3.

Therapy of Cutaneous Side Effects Induced By Immune Checkpoint Blockers

In general, the severity of side effects is graded into different categories (from 1 to 4+) defined by the "Common Terminology Criteria for Adverse Events", version 5.0 [24, 25].

According to algorithms, for IRAEs grade 1, immune checkpoint blocker therapy should be continued with close monitoring. Topical ointments or steroid containing lotion can alleviate the symptoms.

It is recommended to *consider pausing* the immunotherapy for toxicities of grade 2 and to *stop* ICBs for grade 3 (reassess after 1 week). The administration of corticosteroids with initial doses of 0.5–1 mg/kg/day of prednisone or equivalent for grade 2 and high dose corticosteroids (1–2 mg/kg/day of prednisone or methylprednisolone iv 1–2 mg/kg/day) for grade 3 is recommended. Infliximab may be given, if symptoms do not improve. Rechallenging immune therapy may be considered. In grade 4 events, cessation of therapy with checkpoint blockers is indicated and corticosteroids (dosing like in grade 3) administered. In addition, for all grades, treatment with topical corticosteroids can be recommended. However, a more targeted approach based on the type of cutaneous side effect seems more appropriate

Table 3 Other cutaneous reactions to immune checkpoint inhibitors

Papulopustular eruptions (Fig. 5)
Grover's disease
Dermatomyositis/lupus erythematosus
Vasculitis, necrotizing
Eosinophilic fasciitis
Sweet's syndrome
Panniculitis (erythema nodosum like)
Granulomatous skin reactions, sarcoidosis, and granuloma annulare
Alopecia and telogen effluvium
Nail dystrophy [26]
Oral toxicities (xerostomia and lichenoid reactions)

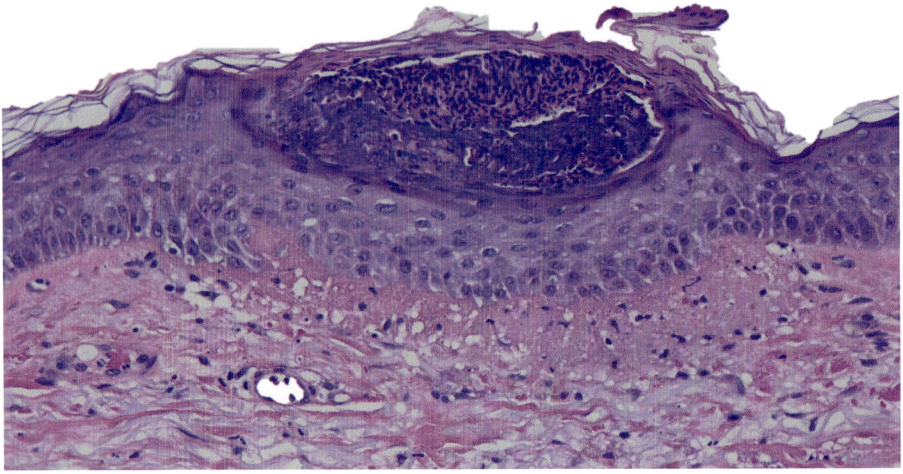

Fig. 5 *Papulopustular eruption* following nivolumab and ipilimumab treatment for metastatic melanoma. Histology reveals a subcorneal pustule

Table 4 Proposed management of cutaneous side effects

Type of cutaneous reaction	Diagnostic procedures	Consequences for immunotherapy	Therapy
Maculopapular rash	Assess other potential culprit drugs	Continue ICIs, if severe delay ICIs	Topical steroids, in severe cases short course of systemic steroids (1 mg/kg body weight), and oral antihistamines in case of pruritus
Psoriasiform reactions	Biopsy, family history? Similar eruptions prior to immunotherapy? Arthritic symptoms	Continue ICIs	Topical steroids/vitamin D analogues/salicylic acid for cutaneous involvement only; NSAIDs for arthritic symptoms, if severe consider low dose steroids or TNF-alpha inhibitors
Bullous eruption	BP180/230, biopsy	Pause ICIs	Systemic steroids
Lichenoid reaction	Biopsy, check mucosae	Pause ICIs	Steroids, retinoids, ECP, and recommendations on nutrition in case of mucosa involvement
MAH	Anti-thyroid antibodies	Continue ICIs	Reassurance of patient of association with better prognosis
TEN	Biopsy	Permanently stop ICIs	Immediate care by dermatologists, steroids, and ivIg

ivIg Intravenous immunoglobulins, *ECP* Extracorporeal photopheresis, *NSAIDs* Nonsteroidal anti-inflammatory drugs

(Table 4) since the mere extent of body surface area (BSA) is unlikely to determine the severity of the reaction [23]. Exanthemas can be managed with topical or systemic steroids even if extensive severe side effects need to be promptly attended to if suspected even if only present in limited body areas. Other rarer side effects like blisters or (erosive) lichenoid papules should be assessed by a dermatologist for optimal treatment, minimal disruption of the quality of life, and potential continuation of the immunotherapy.

The vast majority of cutaneous side effects do not require permanently stopping the immunotherapy. Mostly, these side effects can be well managed.

Conclusions

The management of cancer patients has significantly changed since the approval of novel classes of immuno-oncology therapeutics. Substantial antitumor activity and response rates up to 58%, with improved overall survival, have been achieved in patients with metastatic melanoma with immune checkpoint inhibitors (ICIs), in particular with anti-programmed cell death protein 1 (PD-1)/anti-programmed cell death-ligand 1 (PD-L1), anti-cytotoxic T-lymphocyte-associated protein 4 (CTLA-4), and their combination [1]. However, these classes of immuno-oncology therapeutics have been associated with a broad spectrum of side effects known as immune-related adverse events (IRAE). The spectrum of IRrAE is similar between anti-PD1/anti-PD-L1 and anti-CTLA4 antibodies, but the frequency of specific side effects varies. Interestingly, the occurrence of IRAEs has been implicated as a positive prognostic sign. Clearly, patients with metastatic melanoma who stopped ICI therapy due to toxicity do not have a worse outcome. Investigations to better understand the pathophysiology of IRAE are needed and will help to foresee, prevent, and potentially better treat checkpoint inhibitor induced toxicities to the skin.

References

1. Barrios DM, Do MH, Phillips GS, Postow MA, Akaike T, Nghiem P, Lacouture ME. Immune checkpoint inhibitors to treat cutaneous malignancies. J Am Acad Dermatol. 2020;83(5):1239–53.
2. Heinzerling L, de Toni EN, Schett G, Hundorfean G, Zimmer L. Checkpoint inhibitors: the diagnosis and treatment of side effects. Deutsches Ärzteblatt International I Dtsch Arztebl Int. 2019;116:119–26.
3. Wolchok JD, Chiarion-Sileni V, Gonzalez R, et al. Overall survival with combined nivolumab and ipilimumab in advanced melanoma. N Engl J Med. 2017;377:1345–56.
4. Schachter J, Ribas A, Long GV, et al. Pembrolizumab versus ipilimumab for advanced melanoma: final overall survival results of a multicentre, randomised, open-label phase 3 study (KEYNOTE-006). Lancet. 2017;390:1853–62.
5. Long GV, Atkinson V, Cebon JS, et al. Standard-dose pembrolizumab in combination with reduced-dose ipilimumab for patients with advanced melanoma (KEYNOTE-029): an open-label, phase 1b trial. Lancet Oncol. 2017;18:1202–10.
6. Seidel JA, Otsuka A, Kabashima K. Anti-PD-1 and Anti-CTLA-4 therapies in cancer: mechanisms of action, efficacy, and limitations. Front Oncol. 2018;8:86.
7. Kroschinsky F, Stölzel F, von Bonin S, Beutel G, Kochanek M, Kiehl M, Schellongowski P, Intensive Care in Hematological and Oncological Patients (iCHOP) Collaborative Group. New

drugs, new toxicities: severe side effects of modern targeted and immunotherapy of cancer and their management. Crit Care. 2017;21(1):89.
8. Cousin S, Seneschal J, Italiano A. Toxicity profiles of immunotherapy. Pharmacol Ther. 2018;181:91–100.
9. Shankar B, Zhang J, Naqash AR, Forde PM, Feliciano JL, Marrone KA, Ettinger DS, Hann CL, Brahmer JR, Ricciuti B, Owen D, Toi Y, Walker P, Otterson GA, Patel SH, Sugawara S, Naidoo J. Multisystem immune-related adverse events associated with immune checkpoint inhibitors for treatment of non-small cell lung cancer. JAMA Oncol. 2020;6(12):1952–6.
10. Kim ST, Suarez-Almazor ME. Managing immune dysregulation resulting from immune checkpoint inhibitors: impact of the ASCO guidelines and key take-homes for immunologists. Expert Rev Clin Immunol. 2019;15(3):211–3.
11. Geisler AN, Phillips GS, Barrios DM, Wu J, Leung DYM, Moy AP, Kern JA, Lacouture ME. Immune checkpoint inhibitor-related dermatologic adverse events. J Am Acad Dermatol. 2020;83(5):1255–68.
12. Schadendorf D, Wolchok JD, Hodi FS, Chiarion-Sileni V, Gonzalez R, Rutkowski P, Grob JJ, Cowey CL, Lao CD, Chesney J, Robert C, Grossmann K, McDermott D, Walker D, Bhore R, Larkin J, Postow MA. Efficacy and safety outcomes in patients with advanced melanoma who discontinued treatment with nivolumab and ipilimumab because of adverse events: a pooled analysis of randomized phase II and III trials. J Clin Oncol. 2017;35(34):3807–14.
13. Heinzerling L, Goldinger SM. A review of serious adverse effects under treatment with checkpoint inhibitors. Curr Opin Oncol. 2017;29(2):136–44.
14. Collins LK, Chapman MS, Carter JB, Samie FH. Cutaneous adverse effects of the immune checkpoint inhibitors. Curr Probl Cancer. 2017;41(2):125–8.
15. Simonsen AB, Kaae J, Ellebaek E, Svane IM, Zachariae C. Cutaneous adverse reactions to anti-PD-1 treatment-a systematic review. J Am Acad Dermatol. 2020;83(5):1415–24.
16. Schaberg KB, Novoa RA, Wakelee HA, Kim J, Cheung C, Srinivas S, Kwong BY. Immunohistochemical analysis of lichenoid reactions in patients treated with anti-PD-L1 and anti-PD-1 therapy. J Cutan Pathol. 2016;43(4):339–46.
17. Chou S, Zhao C, Hwang SJE, Fernandez-Penas P. PD-1 inhibitor-associated lichenoid inflammation with incidental suprabasilar acantholysis or vesiculation-report of 4 cases. J Cutan Pathol. 2017;44(10):851–6.
18. Kerl H, Cerroni L, Kokol R, Requena L, Kutzner H, Metze D, Fried I, Stieber W, Wolf IH. Diagnostic cutaneous pathology: clinical-pathological correlation of inflammatory and other non-neoplastic skin diseases. Graz: VHJ; 2018.
19. Sibaud V. Dermatologic reactions to immune checkpoint inhibitors: skin toxicities and immunotherapy. Am J Clin Dermatol. 2018;19(3):345–61.
20. Hartmann A, Bedenk C, Keikavoussi P, Becker JC, Hamm H, Bröcker EB. Vitiligo and melanoma-associated hypopigmentation (MAH): shared and discriminative features. J Dtsch Dermatol Ges. 2008;6(12):1053–9.
21. Kerl K, Kerl H. Severe cutaneous adverse drug reactions. Diagn Histopathol. 2021;27(1):1–5.
22. Vivar KL, Deschaine M, Messina J, Divine JM, Rabionet A, Patel N, Harrington MA, Seminario-Vidal L. Epidermal programmed cell death-ligand 1 expression in TEN associated with nivolumab therapy. J Cutan Pathol. 2017;44(4):381–4.
23. Kähler KC, Hassel JC, Heinzerling L, Loquai C, Thoms KM, Ugurel S, Zimmer L, Gutzmer R, Committee on "Cutaneous Adverse Events" of the German Working Group for Dermatological Oncology (Arbeitsgemeinschaft Dermatologische Onkologie, ADO). Side effect management during immune checkpoint blockade using CTLA-4 and PD-1 antibodies for metastatic melanoma - an update. J Dtsch Dermatol Ges. 2020;18(6):582–609.
24. Brahmer JR, Lacchetti C, Schneider BJ, Atkins MB, Brassil KJ, Caterino JM, Chau I, Ernstoff MS, Gardner JM, Ginex P, Hallmeyer S, Holter Chakrabarty J, Leighl NB, Mammen JS, McDermott DF, Naing A, Nastoupil LJ, Phillips T, Porter LD, Puzanov I, Reichner CA,

Santomasso BD, Seigel C, Spira A, Suarez-Almazor ME, Wang Y, Weber JS, Wolchok JD, Thompson JA, National Comprehensive Cancer Network. Management of immune-related adverse events in patients treated with immune checkpoint inhibitor therapy: American Society of Clinical Oncology Clinical Practice Guideline. J Clin Oncol. 2018;36(17):1714–68.

25. Aggarwal S. Adverse effects of immuno-oncology drugs-awareness, diagnosis, and management: a literature review of immune-mediated adverse events. Indian J Cancer. 2019;56(Supplement):10–22.
26. Lacouture M, Sibaud V. Toxic side effects of targeted therapies and immunotherapies affecting the skin, oral mucosa, hair, and nails. Am J Clin Dermatol. 2018;19(Suppl 1):31–9.

Newly Recognized Variants of Neutrophilic Dermatosis

Gabriel Quintero-Bustos and Marcela Saeb-Lima

Introduction

Neutrophilic dermatoses represent a clinically and histopathological diverse group of disorders characterized by a notorious accumulation of neutrophils in the skin and in rare occasions some internal organs. Not so many years ago, pyoderma gangrenosum and Sweet syndrome, the two classic neutrophilic dermatoses, were included among the autoinflammatory diseases, but since then, an outburst of scientific proposals has emerged to reclassify what we initially thought as secondary components, reactive disorders or variations from other diseases, and that today we acknowledge as previously ignored underlying autoimmune processes that are mediated by neutrophils [1].

In the following lines, we present little-known and rare variants of neutrophilic dermatoses, which have therapeutic implications given their particular clinical and pathophysiological characteristics:

Amicrobial Pustulosis of the Folds Associated with Autoimmune Disorders

Introduction The amicrobial pustulosis of the folds (APF) associated with autoimmune disorders is an infrequent entity described by Crickx et al. in 1991, at the Journées Dermatologiques de Paris. Until today, only approximately 70 cases have been reported [2], of which more than 90% correspond to women living with an autoimmune disease, mainly systemic lupus erythematosus [3]; however, it has also

G. Quintero-Bustos · M. Saeb-Lima (✉)
Pathology Department, National Institute of Medical Sciences and Nutrition Salvador Zubirán, Mexico City, Mexico

F. Rongioletti, B. R. Smoller (eds.), *New and Emerging Entities in Dermatology and Dermatopathology*, https://doi.org/10.1007/978-3-030-80027-7_26

been observed in mixed connective tissue disease [4], myasthenia gravis [5], idiopathic thrombocytopenic purpura [5], Sjögren's syndrome [6], celiac disease [7], rheumatoid arthritis [8], immunoglobulin A nephropathy [9], autoimmune hepatitis [10], and Hashimoto's thyroiditis [11].

Clinical features It is characterized by the recurrent appearance of follicular and non-follicular sterile pustules primarily affecting the scalp, flexures, and periorificial skin [12] (Fig. 1), with a chronic-relapsing clinical course; the list of differential diagnoses covers most subcorneal pustulosis and bacterial and candidal intertrigo. Marzano et al. proposed a set of diagnostic criteria based on the largest description of APF patients with characteristics consistent with skin disease; necessary features include the existence of pustules along one major or minor flexure plus the anogenital area, intraepidermal pustules with a dermal neutrophilic infiltrate, and negative microbial cultures. Minor criteria include autoimmune comorbidities and antinuclear antibody titers of at least 1/160 or positivity in any of the following autoantibodies: anti-ENA, anti-DNA, anti-smooth muscle, anti-mitochondrial, anti-parietal cell, or anti-endomysium. The diagnosis of APF is based on the clinical picture and pathological correlation after excluding possible infectious causes of subcorneal pustules [13].

Histopathological features Findings are similar in almost all cases and demonstrate subcorneal pustules associated with a superficial perivascular and interstitial neutrophilic inflammatory infiltrate; such infiltrate has been found in eccrine glands

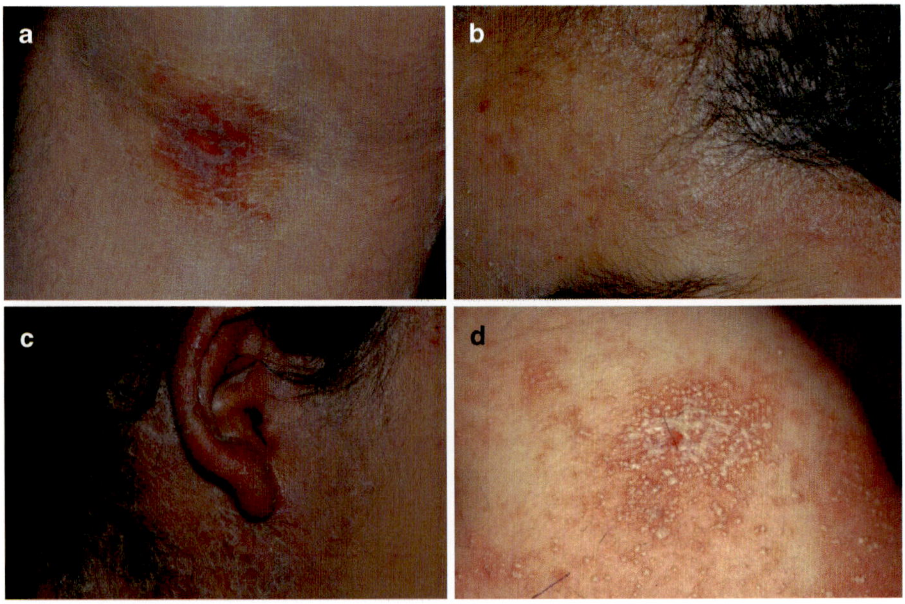

Fig. 1 *Amicrobial pustulosis of the folds* is characterized by eczematous plaques involving folds and periorificial areas (**a**–**c**). Pustules is a frequent finding (**d**)

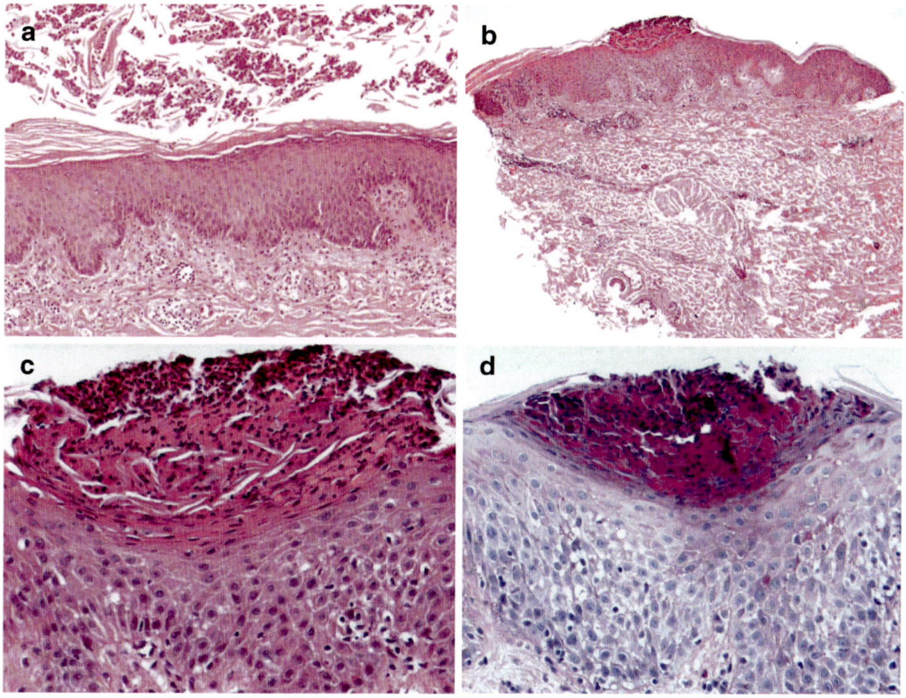

Fig. 2 *Amicrobial pustulosis of the folds*. Subcorneal sterile pustules are characteristic (**a**–**d**). In the dermis, a superficial perivascular lymphocytic infiltrate is accompanied by neutrophils. PAS stain shows no fungi structures

and in subcutaneous cellular tissue and also leukocytoclasia without vasculitis (Fig. 2). It has been described with high expression of Ki67 and involucrin in epidermal keratinocytes [10, 12].

Etiopathogenesis It is still unknown; however, that the overproduction of several cytokines in the systemic milieu of autoimmunity, including interleukin 8, interleukin 1b, tumor necrosis factor, leukotriene B4, CXCL 1/2/3, RANTES, and activated variants of complement C5, has been suggested to play a major role via chemoattraction of neutrophils and dendritic cells to the dermis and epidermis where sterile pustules are formed [14].

Therapy Given the rarity of APF, there are no standard therapeutic regimens. Systemic corticosteroids (0.5 mg/kg/day) represent the most effective treatment; other therapies include dapsone 50–100 mg/day, cyclosporine 3–3.5 mg/kg/day, and steroid-sparing adjunctive therapies, such as colchicine 1 mg/day, hydroxychloroquine 400 mg/day, and methotrexate 15 mg/week [15], although new therapeutic alternatives are emerging such as anakinra and anti-TNF-alpha drugs [16].

Necrotizing Neutrophilic Dermatosis

Introduction Over the last three decades, there have been sporadic case reports of necrosis associated with neutrophilic dermatosis such as pyoderma gangrenosum and Sweet syndrome [17], but it was not until 2012 when Kroshinsky et al. proposed the reclassification of these pathological conditions as a new entity for dermatology [18]. Around 60 cases have been reported to date; in order to integrate the generated information, Sanchez et al. have proposed to unify the neutrophilic dermatoses that morphologically resemble necrotizing fasciitis as *necrotizing neutrophilic dermatosis* (NND) [19].

Clinical features This condition, like many neutrophilic dermatoses, is characterized by pathergy, a nonspecific inflammatory response to skin trauma that typically manifests as erythematous to violaceous papules, plaques, pustules, leading to skin breakdown, and lack of crepitus [20]. The proposed diagnostic criteria include major components such as the previously mentioned clinical characteristics, systemic involvement (shock, fever, and leukemoid reaction), absence of infectious organisms by negative tissue cultures and histopathological tissue stains, compatible histopathological features, and adequate response to treatment; on the other hand, minor diagnostic criteria are previous history of pathergy and the presence of comorbidities (hematologic disorders and malignant neoplasms, inflammatory bowel disease, connective tissue disease, pregnancy, and G-CSF medications) [19].

Histopathological features Findings are sparse diffuse subcutaneous and dermal inflammation with a predominance of neutrophils and associated leukocytoclasia and edema (Fig. 3). The neutrophilic infiltrate and associated necrosis (less than 50% of cases) often extended to the level of fascia or muscle; evidence of vasculitis or an associated atypical or immature myeloid infiltrate is not observed [19].

Differential diagnosis NND presents with significant progression of cutaneous disease with systemic symptoms, which can resemble necrotizing fasciitis both clinically and histopathologically, leading to common misdiagnosis. As opposed to typical Sweet syndrome, in which neutrophilic infiltration primarily involves the dermis and occasionally the subcutaneous fat, NDD is a deeper process involving the fascia and skeletal musculature [21].

Etiopathogenesis Until today, the pathophysiology of the entity has not been completely elucidated. Interestingly, although NND occurs more frequently in patients with myeloproliferative disorders [22, 23], some theories suggest that tumor antigens from myeloproliferative disorders set off a reactive process leading to amplification of pro-inflammatory cytokines, such as IL-1, IL-8, G-CSF, GM-CSF, and IFNϒ [24]. These signaling molecules are typically found in neutrophilic dermatoses and ultimately might have stimulate and trigger a strong and continuous pathergy reaction in multiple cutaneous and soft tissue sites of iatrogenic trauma, with extensive neutrophilic chemotaxis and resultant tissue injury and myonecrosis, mimicking a fatal condition such as necrotizing fasciitis [18], resulting in an aggressive

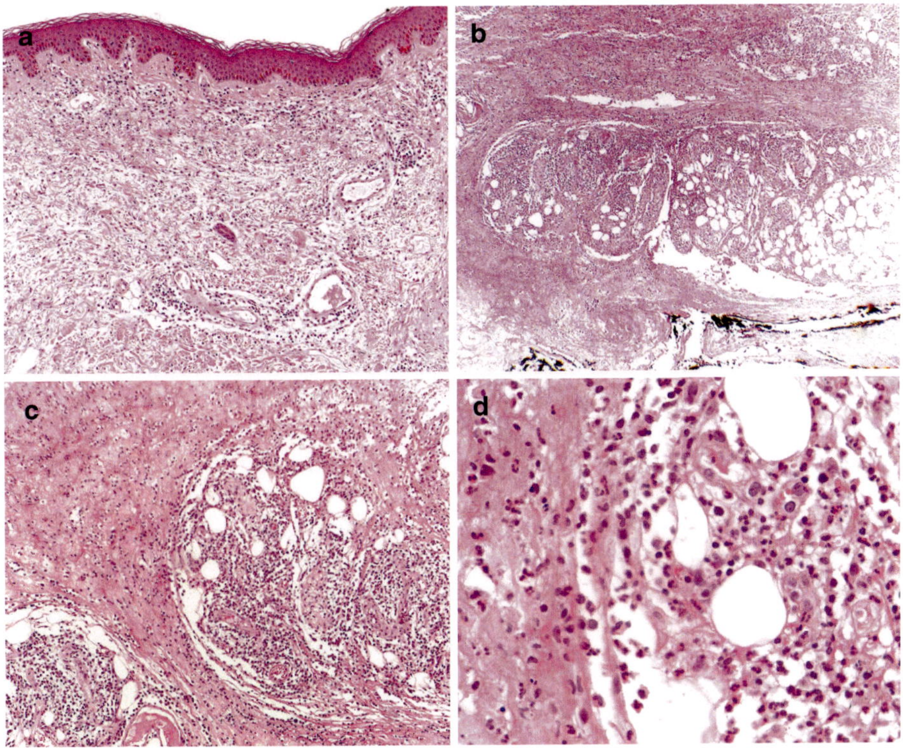

Fig. 3 *Necrotizing neutrophilic dermatosis* shows no involvement of the superficial and deep dermis (**a**, **b**). It is centered in subcutaneous fat and fascia (**c**). The infiltrate is composed mainly of neutrophils with carryorrhexis (**d**)

presentation with extracutaneous involvement such as renal, hepatic, or cardiac dysfunction, with possible progression to multi-organ system failure and death [21, 25].

Therapy Often, misdiagnosis leads to delayed or failed treatment, as the immunosuppression used to treat neutrophilic inflammation may worsen the infection and the surgical procedures that target the infection may exacerbate NDD through pathergy [19]. Immunosuppression can be empirically initiated while waiting for cultures and additional histopathological stains for infection, especially if a critically ill patient does not improve with antimicrobial agents and there is no clear evidence of infection [26]. Concomitant treatment with corticosteroids and antimicrobial agents is an important and potentially lifesaving compromise of therapeutic management [19].

Histiocytoid Autoimmunity-Related Neutrophilic Dermatosis

Introduction Sweet syndrome (SS), also known as acute febrile neutrophilic dermatosis, was described by Dr. Robert Douglas Sweet in 1964 [27]. Clinically, it is characterized by the sudden onset of a cutaneous eruption of painful, erythematous, pseudovesicular plaques and nodules, accompanied by fever, leukocytosis, and neutrophilia. Histologically, the involved skin typically displays a dense, diffuse infiltrate of polymorphonuclear leukocytes associated with papillary dermal edema. The condition may be idiopathic or associated with systemic disease of an inflammatory or neoplastic nature and hematologic malignancies being notable among the latter, either how the autoimmune component plays a crucial role in each one of the clinical scenarios [28]. Forty-one years later, Dr. Requena described what we now recognize as the histiocytic variant of the disease [29].

Clinical features Histiocytoid Sweet syndrome (H-SS) is a rare disease, which occurs with a slight predilection in women (approximately 65% of cases), with a mean age of 50 years, and a wide range that goes from 2 months to 80 years old [29, 30]. The clinical characteristics tend to be the same as those observed in the classic type of Sweet syndrome, with the peculiarities added by the clinical context of the patients, among which we can find hematopoietic neoplasms (36%), myelodysplastic syndromes (27%, ten times more than classical neutrophilic variant [29, 31]), systemic lupus erythematosus, Crohn's disease, pregnancy, renal cell and breast carcinomas, severe respiratory infections such as methicillin-resistant *Staphylococcus aureus*, or none of the above in the idiopathic forms [29, 32].

Histopathological features Histologically, the epidermis is usually spared, but sometimes it can show areas of spongiosis with some exocytosis of inflammatory cells and focal basal layer vacuolar change. The moderate to intense edematous papillary dermis is always involved by a dense, band-like, perivascular, periappendageal, and interstitial inflammatory cell infiltrate, which affects the superficial and mid-dermis, but that in some cases can reach the subcutis (Fig. 4). The mononuclear infiltrate is predominantly composed of histiocytoid cells characterized by pale, vesicular, and variably shaped nuclei and moderate amounts of amphophilic cytoplasm and mild atypia, with mainly elongated nuclei that is curved or serpiginous in the outline, accompanied by an inconspicuous lymphocytic infiltrate in perivascular zones, and neutrophils scattered irregularly among the mononuclear cells [28, 29]. Immunohistochemically, the histiocytoid cells are positive for CD15, CD43, CD68, and CD163, confirming their macrophage/monocytic lineage. In addition, in most instances, the cells also express myeloperoxidase and lysozyme. There is variable staining for CD14, TCL1 oncogene, HLA-DR, BDCA-3, and CD123 [33]. On the other hand, the accompanying lymphoid infiltrate is usually predominantly CD3 positive, with sparse CD20 positive lymphocytes (Fig. 5) [28].

Differential diagnosis The list of clinical differential diagnoses that should always be in consideration includes drug eruptions, Well's syndrome, sarcoidosis, erythema elevatum diutinum, granuloma annulare, erythema multiforme, polymorphous light eruption, and dermatomyositis [28]. On the other hand, histological differential diagnosis of histiocytoid Sweet syndrome includes other cutaneous dermatoses

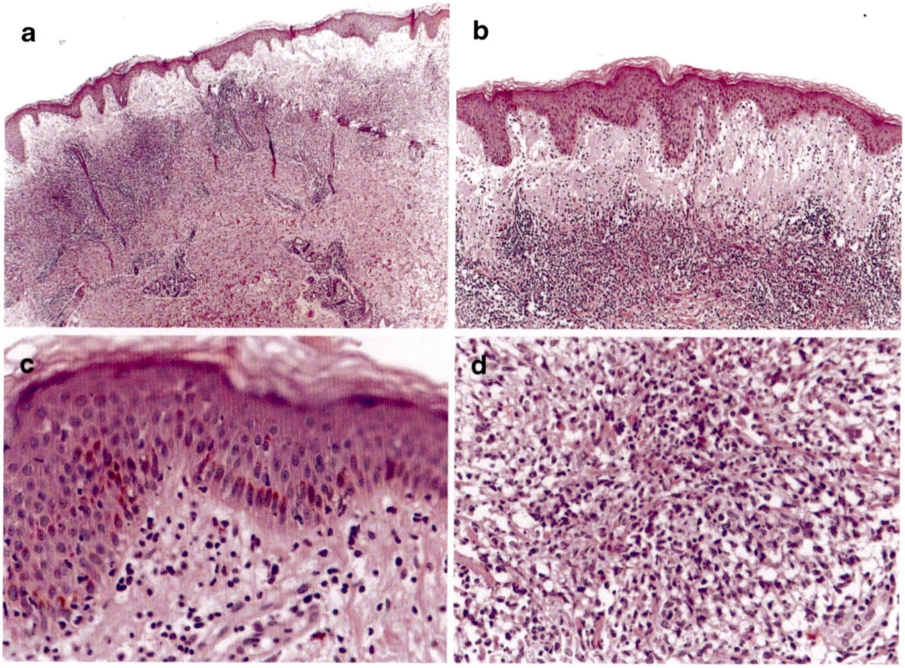

Fig. 4 *Histiocytoid autoimmunity-related neutrophilic dermatosis* shows a superficial and deep nodular neutrophilic infiltrate associated with papillary dermal edema (**a**, **b**). There are vacuolar interface changes caused by the neutrophils with carryorrhexis (**c**). The infiltrate is composed mainly of neutrophils with carryorrhexis associated with macrophages (**d**)

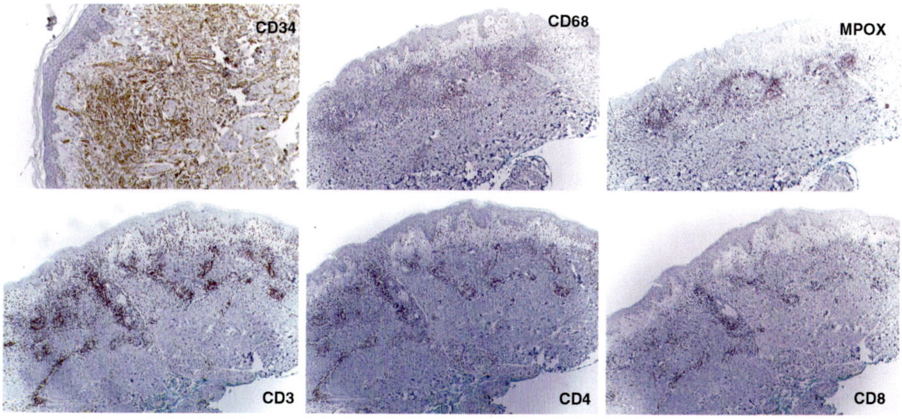

Fig. 5 *Histiocytoid autoimmunity-related neutrophilic dermatosis*. By immunohistochemistry, the infiltrate shows positive reaction for neutrophils with CD34 and MPOX. Associated CD68 macrophages are seen within the infiltrate. Reactive lymphocytes CD3, CD4, and CD8 positive are seen

characterized by the infiltration of abundant histiocytes, including interstitial granuloma annulare, Erdheim–Chester disease, RAS-associated autoimmunne leukoproliferative disease (RALD Cutis), and interstitial granulomatous dermatitis with arthritis. More importantly, in patients with myelodysplastic syndrome, leukemia cutis should always be considered before [34].

Etiopathogenesis The physiopathological significance of histiocytoid Sweet syndrome still remains poorly understood. Fluorescence in situ hybridization assays have shown that the same chromosomal abnormalities present in the associated myeloid malignancies of the patients are also found in the skin-infiltrating neutrophils [35]. Or, as stated by Dr. Goufhi, the disease may also be triggered by an external antigen or induced by a dysregulation of the innate immune system as in autoinflammatory diseases [31].

Therapy In H-SS patients, acute lesions can be treated with high potent topical steroids and/or systemic steroids [28]. There are reports that describe the efficacy of the use of ertacenept and dapsone for refractory cases; however, more studies should corroborate the aforementioned [36, 37].

Erosive Pustular Dermatosis of the Scalp

Introduction Erosive pustular dermatosis of the scalp (EPDS) is an uncommon, pustular, idiopathic, inflammatory disorder that was first described in 1979 by Burton and Pye [38], of which only around 150 cases have been reported in world literature and its actual incidence is unknown due to its rarity; however, its predisposition toward elderly Caucasian women is noteworthy, although it has also been reported in newborns, children, adolescents, young adults, and males to a lesser extent (2:1 ratio) [39–41].

Clinical features Clinically, it is characterized by multiple erythematous large, erosive, and crusted patches with overlying and surrounding pustules and serum exudate involving the bald areas of the scalp with a predominance of the vertex [42], although occasionally it can be observed in other areas such as face and extremities. Due to its extensive chronicity, it is common to observe a pathological cycle of healing and relapse in the same anatomical region, resulting in skin atrophy and the formation of new lesions in the center, or edges, of the initial location; trichoscopic examination shows different patterns that are nonspecific of EPDS, such as follicular keratotic plugging, milky red areas, white patches, hair shaft tortuosity, tapering hair, and the absence of follicular openings [39].

Differential diagnosis EPDS main differential diagnoses to work with include bacterial and fungal infections, skin epithelial tumors, pemphigus foliaceus, pyoderma gangrenosum, factitial damage, and less likely other entities such as pustular psoriasis, cicatricial pemphigoid, pemphigus vulgaris, Darier's disease, chronic mucocutaneous candidiasis, dissecting cellulitis, and the neutrophilic scarring alopecias [43].

Histopathological features Histologically, as characterized by Dr. Starace, we can find different patterns depending on the temporality of the disease: in the early stage, lasting less than 1 year, the epidermis shows laminated orthokeratosis and psoriasiform hyperplasia and the papillary dermis a slight mixed inflammatory infiltrate mainly consisting of neutrophils, lymphocytes, and plasmocytes, with mild fibrosis. Hair follicular density was normal, with terminal, miniaturized anagen follicles and an increased number of catagen follicles. Intermediate-stage patients, lasting 1–2 years, show squamous crusts, parakeratosis, compact orthokeratosis, and psoriasiform hyperplasia of the epidermis. Extensive fibrosis, absence of sebaceous glands, prominent reduced number of terminal, miniaturized anagen follicles, moderate mixed inflammatory infiltrate, fibroplasia around the follicles at the isthmus level, and tufted folliculitis in the papillary and mid dermis were also observed. Some cases, naked hair shafts were evident, with a perifollicular mixed infiltrate containing giant multinucleated cells. Around the erosions, diffuse dermoepidermal cleavages are visible. Late-stage cases, lasting more than 2 years, show laminated, compact orthokeratosis and thin epidermis. "Remainders" or complete absence of follicles and sebaceous glands, with slight mixed inflammatory infiltrate, diffuse and severe fibrosis in the dermis, associated with sclerotic streamers replacing the hair follicles, were evident [44].

Etiopathogenesis Until today, it is still not elucidated; the association between autoimmune diseases and EPDS has been established as it seems to be a common feature in such patients, some of them with a history of long standing rheumatoid arthritis, autoimmune hepatitis, Hashimoto thyroiditis, and Takayasu's arteritis. Impaired immunity and microcirculation may play a role in the pathogenesis of this disease [42]. Some other factors have been taken in consideration, but due to lack of evidence on causality, they can be fully integrated in a pathogenic way that explains the process of disease; among them, some of the most prevalent are immunologic dysregulation and abnormal neutrophil chemotaxis or chemoattractants and cytokine production against epidermal or follicular antigens, actinic keratosis, infections, and mechanical damage [39, 42, 44].

Therapy Because of the rarity and unknown etiology of EPDS, there is no established treatment recommendation; corticosteroids, tacrolimus, and wound dressings appear to be more effective and are considered first-line treatments to promote reepithelialization. High-potency topical corticosteroids are the most frequently used treatment and are established as effective and safe with almost a complete resolution after 1–2 months [42].

Neutrophilic Dermatoses as Adverse Effects of Checkpoint Inhibitors

Introduction In 2018, Dr. Tasuko Honjo and Dr. James Allison were awarded with the Nobel Prize in Physiology or Medicine, for their contribution in understanding one of the major escape mechanisms of cancer cells, by describing the programmed death molecule-1 (PD-1) on T cells and the cytotoxic T-lymphocyte antigen-4 (CTLA-4). Thanks to their discoveries, molecular therapies have been implemented leading to extending the life expectancy of patients with melanoma, for example, by up to 50% [45].

Clinical features Like most therapies, checkpoint inhibitory monoclonal antibodies are not exempted from inducing adverse effects in patients; as such, a wide variety of inflammatory reaction patterns have been observed, such as rash morphologies that include but are not limited to morbilliform, eczematous, psoriasiform, lichenoid, and bullous [46]. Infrequently, other morphologies including Stevens–Johnson syndrome-like, pityriasis rubra pilaris-like, and rashes resembling neutrophilic dermatoses have been reported [47, 48].

Neutrophilic dermatoses secondary to this treatment include Sweet syndrome, pustular eruptions, bullous lupus erythematosus, and pyoderma gangrenosum [49]. There is no epidemiological information available because only few cases have been reported in regard to this association. The onset of neutrophilic dermatoses seems to be relatively delayed, ranging from weeks to months. Interestingly, most of the cases of Sweet syndrome and all cases of pyoderma gangrenosum reported in the literature were induced by ipilimumab (anti-CTLA-4) [49, 50] and less frequently by pembrolizumab (anti-PD1) [51].

Histopathological features The histological changes observed in neutrophilic dermatoses associated with treatment with checkpoint inhibitors are identical to their conventional counterparts.

Etiopathogenesis Some researchers suggest that as a CTLA-4 blocker, ipilimumab promotes T-cell activation and cytokine dysregulation, thus leading to neutrophil homing and accumulation, thereby leading to Sweet syndrome (and potentially other neutrophilic dermatoses). The exact mechanisms by which CTLA-4 and PD-1/L-1 inhibitors may cause neutrophilic dermatoses are unclear [52].

Therapy Active surveillance of dermatological manifestations is important during treatment with checkpoint inhibitors, since they can commonly be confused with skin infections in which treatment must be withdrawn, putting the care of the underlying oncological disease at risk. Most cases of neutrophilic dermatoses are highly sensitive to treatment with systemic steroids and steroid sparing agents like dapsone, colchicine, and tetracyclines with good prognosis overall [51, 53].

Ultimately, further studies are crucial to identify the underlying mechanisms of neutrophilic accumulation secondary to CTLA-4 and PD-1 inhibitors and to investigate which eruptions can be treated through versus which should require complete interruption of a checkpoint inhibitor [46].

Autoimmunity-Related Neutrophilic Dermatosis

Introduction The indisputable relationship between neutrophilic dermatoses and systemic autoimmune diseases has long been recognized; the first to contemplate it was Dr. Bernard Ackerman, who considered it as an altered form of bullous lupus erythematosus [54]; however, in recent years, not more than 70 cases of a disorder distinct from Sweet syndrome or bullous lupus erythematosus (LE) have been described as specifically related to systemic LE under diverse terms, including non-bullous neutrophilic dermatosis, nonbullous neutrophilic LE, and Sweet-like neutrophilic dermatosis [55] characterized by cell-rich Sweet-like neutrophilic reactions and some patients with skin lesions that histologically show paucicellular neutrophilic dermal infiltrates [56].

Clinical features There is few epidemiological information regarding this entity, but by grouping the case reports, as it was done by Dr. Allison, it is evident that, by far, women are the most affected (80%), ranging in age from newborn infants to 70 years old (mean age, 35 years), with not only active SLE but also some other autoimmune diseases such as rheumatoid arthritis and Sjögren's syndrome. The extremities are usually involved in more than 80% of patients, trunk in 60%, and the face or head and neck region in 20% of them [56]. Patients are afflicted with erythematous macules and urticarial papules and plaques bilaterally distributed on the previously described regions (Fig. 6); by the time of diagnosis, lesions have usually been present for a mean of 2 months [55]. In addition to patients with SLE, patients with hydralazine-induced lupus [57] and neonatal lupus may also develop or present with neutrophilic dermatoses [58].

Histopathological features Under the light of the microscope, histological findings are diverse and include from a dense pandermal neutrophilic infiltrate that may form abscesses and is accompanied by scattered plasma cells, histiocytes, and

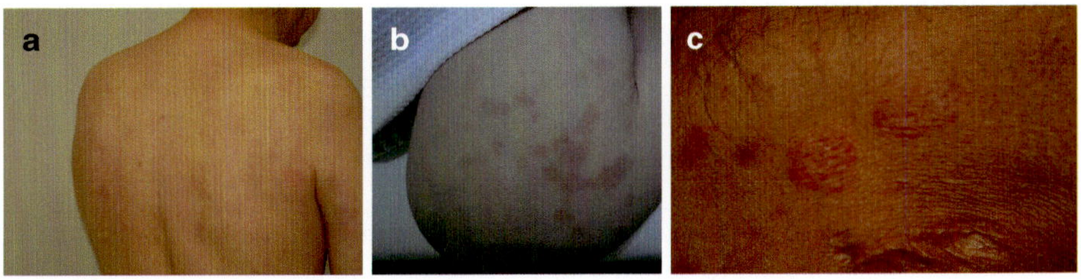

Fig. 6 *Autoimmunity-related neutrophilic dermatosis* is characterized by urticarial plaques in trunk and extremities that persist for more than 24 hours (**a**–**c**)

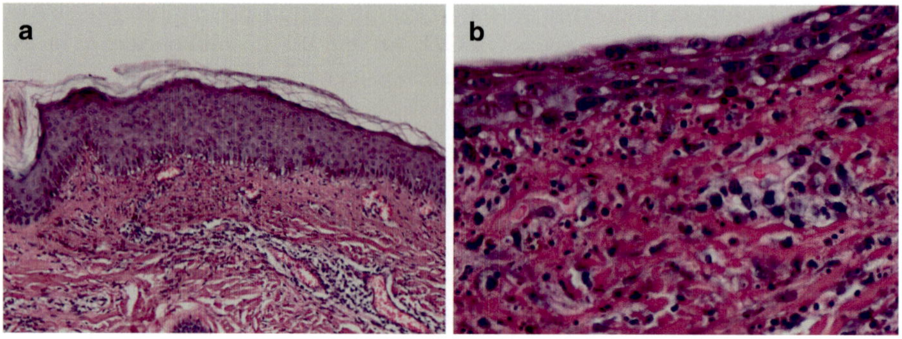

Fig. 7 *Autoimmunity-related neutrophilic dermatosis* is characterized by a vacuolar interface dermatitis with superficial neutrophilic perivascular and interstitial neutrophilic Infiltrate with carryorrhexis and no vasculitis (**a**, **b**)

eosinophils along with not only widely dilated vessels but also interstitial and perivascular neutrophilic infiltrate with leukocytoclasia, vacuolar alteration along the dermal-epidermal junction, and no vasculitis [55]. The histologic differential diagnosis of the lesions described in SLE patients is broad and to some extent depends on the cellularity of the inflammatory infiltrate (Fig. 7).

Differential diagnosis The paucicellular examples are identical to bullous SLE and can be distinguished only by the clinical absence of blisters. The histologic features can also be indistinguishable from dermatitis herpetiformis, and linear IgA disease, also, infections, should always be ruled out. Distinction should be made easily on clinical grounds and with immunofluorescence testing when necessary, in which approximately 50% of the cases present strong or weak IgG, IgM, IgA, and/or C3 granular pattern at the dermal–epidermal junction [56].

Etiopathogenesis Although the pathophysiology of said entity has not been elucidated, it must be similar to the one described in the entities mentioned in the previous paragraphs. Several authors have proposed the role of NETosis and autoantigens in the etiopathogenesis of neutrophilic dermatosis in terms of autoimmune diseases. Neutrophil extracellular traps are associated with a unique form of cell death distinct from apoptosis or necrosis, whereby invading microbes are trapped and killed in extruded extracellular fibers composed of chromatin and granular proteins. It is known that neutrophil extracellular traps can contribute to autoimmunity by exposing autoantigens, inducing IFN-α production, and activating the complement system [59]. Increased neutrophil extracellular trap formation is seen in psoriasis, antineutrophil cytoplasmic antibody-associated vasculitis, antiphospholipid antibody syndrome, rheumatoid arthritis, and systemic lupus erythematosus [60].

Therapy Currently, there is no gold standard of treatment, and it seems that multiple forms of pharmacologic immunosuppression are valuable. Novel therapies are under development in order to use NETs as potential therapeutic targets in the context of SLE, but more studies are needed on the subject.

Conclusions

Neutrophilic dermatoses belong to a group of emerging entities that day after day becomes more complex due to the genetic and pathophysiological characterization of them, and the low number of reported cases, due to the diagnostic difficulty, both clinical and histopathological, which implies recognizing these recently described facet of well-known old diseases, and of course, of newly reported entities.

In the previous pages, we have summarized those neutrophilic dermatoses that have enough clinical, epidemiological, and histopathological information to present a clear picture that can be used in clinical practice; however, there are many others that should take our attention and that are in the process of scientific and medical consolidation, such as those with specific genetic aberrations, like deficiency of IL-36 receptor antagonist, deficiency of IL-1 receptor antagonist, cryopyrin-associated periodic syndromes, C/EBP+-associated autoinflammation and immune impairment of neutrophils, mutations in the MEFV gene, mutations in the ADGRE2 gene, mutations in the NOD2/CARD15 gene, STING-associated vasculopathy with onset in infancy, haploinsufficiency of A20, and among others [61].

We expect a continuous and progressive advance in the consolidation of knowledge of these usually misdiagnosed diseases, which will undoubtedly transcend as relevant clinical and morphological diagnoses that will allow specific treatments to improve the quality of life of patients who suffer from them.

References

1. Kanazawa N. Designation of autoinflammatory skin manifestations with specific genetic backgrounds. Front Immunol. 2020;11:475.
2. Schissler C, Velter C, Lipsker D. Amicrobial pustulosis of the folds: where have we gone 25years after its original description? Ann Dermatol Venereol. 2017;144(3):169–75.
3. Oberlin P, Bagot M, Perrussel M, Leteinturier F, Wechsler J, Revuz J. Amicrobial pustulosis and systemic lupus erythematosus. Ann Dermatol Venereol. 1991;118:824–5.
4. Bénéton N, Wolkenstein P, Bagot M, Cosnes A, Wechsler J, Roujeau JC, et al. Amicrobial pustulosis associated with autoimmune diseases: healing with zinc supplementation. Br J Dermatol. 2000;143:1306–10.
5. Lagrange S, Chosidow O, Piette JC, Wechsler B, Godeau P, Frances C. A peculiar form of amicrobial pustulosis of the folds associated with systemic lupus erythematosus and other auto-immune diseases. Lupus. 1997;6:514–20.
6. Kuyama M, Fujimoto W, Kambara H, Egusa M, Saitoh M, Yamasaki O, et al. Amicrobial pustular dermatosis in two patients with immunological abnormalities. Clin Exp Dermatol. 2002;27:286–9.
7. Marzano AV, Capsoni F, Berti E, et al. Amicrobial pustular dermatosis of cutaneous folds associated with autoimmune disorders: a new entity? Dermatology. 1996;193:88–93.
8. Hoch O, Herbst RA, Gutzmer R, Kiehl P, Kapp A, Weiss J. Amicrobial intertriginous pustulosis in autoimmune disease: a new entity? Hautarzt. 1998;49:634–40.
9. Natsuga K, Sawamura D, Homma E, Nomura T, Abe M, Muramatsu R, et al. Amicrobial pustulosis associated with IgA nephropathy and Sjögren's syndrome. J Am Acad Dermatol. 2007;57:523–6.

10. Méndez-Flores S, Charli-Joseph Y, Saeb-Lima M, OrozcoTopete R, Fernández SM. Amicrobial pustulosis of the folds associated with autoimmune disorders: systemic lupus erythematosus case series and first report on the association with autoimmune hepatitis. Dermatology. 2013;226(1):1–4.
11. Pena-Robichaux V, Hasan A, McHargue C. Amicrobial pustulosis of the folds. J Rheumatol. 2013;40(7):1228–9.
12. Méndez-Flores S, Charli-Joseph Y, Saeb-Lima M, Orozco-Topete R, Fernández SM. Amicrobial pustulosis of the folds associated with autoimmune disorders: systemic lupus erythematosus case series and first report on the association with autoimmune hepatitis. Dermatology. 2013;226(1):1–4.
13. Marzano AV, Ramoni S, Caputo R. Amicrobial pustulosis of the folds: report of 6 cases and a literature review. Dermatology. 2008;216:305–11.
14. Marzano AV, Tavecchio S, Berti E, Gelmetti C, Cugno M. Cytokine and chemokine profile in amicrobial pustulosis of the folds: evidence for autoinflammation. Medicine. 2015;94(50):e2301.
15. Bellinato F, Maurelli M, Colato C, Girolomoni G. Amicrobial pustulosis of the folds: report of three new cases. Indian J Dermatol. 2020;65(4):323–4.
16. Amazan E, Ezzedine K, Mossalayi MD, Taieb A, Boniface K, Seneschal J. Expression of interleukin-1 alpha in amicrobial pustulosis of the skin folds with complete response to anakinra. J Am Acad Dermatol. 2014;71(2):53–6.
17. Attias D, Laor R, Zuckermann E, Naschitz JE, Luria M, Misselevitch I, et al. Acute neutrophilic myositis in Sweet's syndrome: late phase transformation into fibrosing myositis and panniculitis. Hum Pathol. 1995;26:687–90.
18. Kroshinsky D, Alloo A, Rothschild B, Cummins J, Tan J, Montecino R, Hoang MP, Duncan L, Mihm M, Sepehr A. Necrotizing Sweet syndrome: a new variant of neutrophilic dermatosis mimicking necrotizing fasciitis. J Am Acad Dermatol. 2012;67(5):945–54.
19. Sanchez IM, Lowenstein S, Johnson KA, Babik J, Haag C, Keller JJ, Ortega-Loayza AG, Cohen J, McCalmont TH, Demer AM, Mansh MD, Hylwa SA, Liu J, Shinkai K. Clinical features of neutrophilic dermatosis variants resembling necrotizing fasciitis. JAMA Dermatol. 2019;155(1):79–84.
20. Lipof JS, Beck LA, Reddy SC, Southgate RD, Carney-Young K, Hammert WC. Necrotizing Sweet syndrome of the upper extremity after elective hand surgery. J Hand Surg Am. 2018;43(4):389.e1–6.
21. Gowda A, Christensen L, Polly S, Barlev D. Necrotizing neutrophilic dermatosis: a diagnostic challenge with a need for multi-disciplinary recognition, a case report. Ann Med Surg (Lond). 2020;57:299–302.
22. Burton JL. Sweet's syndrome, pyoderma gangrenosum and acute leukaemia. Br J Dermatol. 1980;102:239.
23. Lear JT, Atherton MT, Byrne JP. Neutrophilic dermatoses: pyoderma gangrenosum and Sweet's syndrome. Postgrad Med. 1997;73:65–8.
24. Kinser KN, Panach K, Dominguez AR. Recurrent malignancy-associated atypical neutrophilic dermatosis with noninfectious shock. Am J Med Sci. 2017;354:626–32.
25. Shugarman IL, Schmit JM, Sbicca JA, Wirk B. Easily missed extracutaneous manifestation of malignancy-associated Sweet's syndrome: systemic inflammatory response syndrome. J Clin Oncol. 2011;29(24):e702–5.
26. Gonzalez Santiago TM, Pritt B, Gibson LE, Comfere NI. Diagnosis of deep cutaneous fungal infections: correlation between skin tissue culture and histopathology. J Am Acad Dermatol. 2014;71(2):293–301.
27. Sweet RD. Acute febrile neutrophilic dermatosis. Br J Dermatol. 1964;76:349–56.
28. Chow S, Pasternak S, Green P, Tremaine R, Reardon M, Murray S, Northgrave S, Walsh N. Histiocytoid neutrophilic dermatoses and panniculitides: variations on a theme. Am J Dermatopathol. 2007;29(4):334–41.

29. Requena L, Kutzner H, Palmedo G, Pascual M, Fernández-Herrera J, Fraga J, García-Díez A, Yus ES. Histiocytoid Sweet syndrome: a dermal infiltration of immature neutrophilic granulocytes. Arch Dermatol. 2005;141(7):834–42.
30. Camarillo D, McCalmont TH, Frieden IJ, Gilliam AE. Two pediatric cases of nonbullous histiocytoid neutrophilic dermatitis presenting as a cutaneous manifestation of lupus erythematosus. Arch Dermatol. 2008;144(11):1495–8.
31. Ghoufi L, Ortonne N, Ingen-Housz-Oro S, Barhoumi W, Begon E, Haioun C, Pautas C, Beckerich F, Robin C, Wolkenstein P, Cordonnier C, Chosidow O, Toma A. Histiocytoid Sweet syndrome is more frequently associated with myelodysplastic syndromes than the classical neutrophilic variant: a comparative series of 62 patients. Medicine (Baltimore). 2016;95(15):e3033.
32. Bush JW, Wick MR. Cutaneous histiocytoid Sweet syndrome and its relationship to hematological diseases. J Cutan Pathol. 2016;43(4):394–9.
33. Magro CM, Momtahen S, Nguyen GH, Wang X. Histiocytoid Sweet's syndrome: a localized cutaneous proliferation of macrophages frequently associated with chronic myeloproliferative disease. Eur J Dermatol. 2015;25(4):335–41.
34. Huang CF, Wu BY, Liaw FY, Wang WM, Chiang CP. Histiocytoid Sweet syndrome: report of two cases and review of the literature. Dermatol Sin. 2012;30:71–4.
35. Chavan RN, Cappel MA, Ketterling RP, Wada DA, Rochet NM, Knudson R, Gibson LE. Histiocytoid Sweet syndrome may indicate leukemia cutis: a novel application of fluorescence in situ hybridization. J Am Acad Dermatol. 2014;70(6):1021–7.
36. Watson IT, Haugh I, Gardner AR, Menter MA. Histiocytoid Sweet syndrome successfully treated with etanercept. Proc (Bayl Univ Med Cent). 2018;31:347–9.
37. Spencer B, Nanavati A, Greene J, Butler DF. Dapsone-responsive histiocytoid Sweet's syndrome associated with Crohn's disease. J Am Acad Dermatol. 2008;59(2 Suppl 1):S58–60.
38. Pye RJ, Peachey RD, Burton JL. Erosive pustular dermatosis of the scalp. Br J Dermatol. 1979;100(5):559–66.
39. Tomasini C, Michelerio A. Erosive pustular dermatosis of the scalp: a neutrophilic folliculitis within the spectrum of neutrophilic dermatoses: a clinicopathologic study of 30 cases. J Am Acad Dermatol. 2019;81(2):527–33.
40. Caputo R, Veraldi S. Erosive pustular dermatosis of the scalp. J Am Acad Dermatol. 1993;28(1):96–8.
41. Teng C, Yu J, Taylor J, Rubin AI, Treat JR. Erosive pustular dermatosis of the scalp in an adolescent with near-total hair regrowth: case report and review of the literature. Pediatr Dermatol. 2019;36(5):697–701.
42. Starace M, Alessandrini A, Baraldi C, Piraccini BM. Erosive pustular dermatosis of the scalp: challenges and solutions. Clin Cosmet Investig Dermatol. 2019;12:691–8.
43. Patton D, Lynch PJ, Fung MA, Fazel N. Chronic atrophic erosive dermatosis of the scalp and extremities: a recharacterization of erosive pustular dermatosis. J Am Acad Dermatol. 2007;57(3):421–7.
44. Starace M, Loi C, Bruni F, Alessandrini A, Misciali C, Patrizi A, Piraccini BM. Erosive pustular dermatosis of the scalp: clinical, trichoscopic, and histopathologic features of 20 cases. J Am Acad Dermatol. 2017;76(6):1109–1114.e2.
45. Huang PW, Chang JW. Immune checkpoint inhibitors win the 2018 Nobel Prize. Biom J. 2019;42(5):299–306.
46. Ravi V, Maloney NJ, Worswick S. Neutrophilic dermatoses as adverse effects of checkpoint inhibitors: a review. Dermatol Ther. 2019;32(5):e13074.
47. Coleman E, Ko C, Dai F, Tomayko MM, Kluger H, Leventhal JS. Inflammatory eruptions associated with immune checkpoint inhibitor therapy: a single-institution retrospective analysis with stratification of reactions by toxicity and implications for management. J Am Acad Dermatol. 2019;80(4):990–7.

48. Rudolph BM, Staib F, Von Stebut E, Hainz M, Grabbe S, Loquai C. Neutrophilic disease of the skin and intestines after ipilimumab treatment for malignant melanoma – simultaneous occurrence of pyoderma gangrenosum and colitis. Eur J Dermatol. 2014;24(2):268–9.
49. Apalla Z, Papageorgiou C, Lallas A, Delli F, Fotiadou C, Kemanetzi C, Lazaridou E. Cutaneous adverse events of immune checkpoint inhibitors: a literature review. Dermatol Pract Concept. 2021;11:e2021155.
50. Pintova S, Sidhu H, Friedlander PA, et al. Sweet's syndrome in a patient with metastatic melanoma after ipilimumab. Melanoma Res. 2013;23(6):498–501.
51. Mayer RZ, Ansstas G, Anadkat MJ. Pembrolizumab-induced neutrophilic dermatosis of the dorsal hands. Oncol Case Report J. 2020;3(2):1024.
52. Pintova S, Sidhu H, Friedlander PA, Holcombe RF. Sweet's syndrome in a patient with metastatic melanoma after ipilimumab therapy. Melanoma Res. 2013;23(6):498–501.
53. Muntyanu A, Netchiporouk E, Gerstein W, Gniadecki R, Litvinov IV. Cutaneous immune-related adverse events (irAEs) to immune checkpoint inhibitors: a dermatology perspective on management [Formula: see text]. J Cutan Med Surg. 2021;25(1):59–76.
54. Ackerman AB. Histologic diagnosis of inflammatory skin diseases: an algorithmic method based on pattern analysis. 2nd ed. Baltimore: Williams and Wilkins; 1997. p. 525–42.
55. Saeb-Lima M, Charli-Joseph Y, Rodríguez-Acosta ED, Domínguez-Cherit J. Autoimmunity-related neutrophilic dermatosis: a newly described entity that is not exclusive of systemic lupus erythematosus. Am J Dermatopathol. 2013;35(6):655–60.
56. Larson AR, Granter SR. Systemic lupus erythematosus-associated neutrophilic dermatosis: a review and update. Adv Anat Pathol. 2014;21(4):248–53.
57. Sequeira W, Polisky RB, Alrenga DP. Neutrophilic dermatosis (Sweet's syndrome). Association with a hydralazine-induced lupus syndrome. Am J Med. 1986;81:558–60.
58. Barr KL, O'Connell F, Wesson S, et al. Nonbullous neutrophilic dermatosis: Sweet's syndrome, neonatal lupus erythematosus, or both? Mod Rheumatol. 2009;19:212–5.
59. Barnado A, Crofford LJ, Oates JC. At the bedside: neutrophil extracellular traps (NETs) as targets for biomarkers and therapies in autoimmune diseases. J Leukoc Biol. 2016;99(2):265–78.
60. Villanueva E, Yalavarthi S, Berthier CC, Hodgin JB, Khandpur R, Lin AM, Rubin CJ, Zhao W, Olsen SH, Klinker M, Shealy D, Denny MF, Plumas J, Chaperot L, Kretzler M, Bruce AT, Kaplan MJ. Netting neutrophils induce endothelial damage, infiltrate tissues, andexpose immunostimulatory molecules in systemic lupus erythematosus. J Immunol. 2011;187:538–52.
61. Figueras-Nart I, Mascaró JM Jr, Solanich X, Hernández-Rodríguez J. Dermatologic and dermatopathologic features of monogenic autoinflammatory diseases. Front Immunol. 2019;10:2448.

Cutaneous Reactive Angiomatoses

Franco Rongioletti and Caterina Ferreli

Introduction

Cutaneous reactive angiomatoses include a spectrum of reactive vascular (capillary) proliferations of the skin, involving patients with a variety of underlying systemic diseases. Since the first description of a case of reactive angioendotheliomatosis (RAE) in 1958, a range of histopathological patterns of benign cutaneous vascular proliferations with similar clinical presentations to RAE have been reported leading to a classification of different subtypes including diffuse dermal angiomatosis (DDA), acroangiodermatitis (pseudo-Kaposi sarcoma), reactive intravascular histiocytosis (RIH), glomeruloid RAE, and angiopericytomatosis (angiomatosis with cryoproteins) [1] (Table 1).

RAE is a rare disorder with about 27 anecdotal cases, and only 1 series of 15 cases has been reported till now [2–4]. Historically, it was thought to have benign and malignant forms, but subsequently, the latter has been considered a type of B-cell lymphoma [5]. Glomeruloid reactive angioendotheliomatosis is a subset of RAE with a glomeruloid histological pattern [6].

Diffuse dermal angiomatosis (DDA) is a distinct disorder in the spectrum of RAE with more than 70 cases described so far of which 60% represent the variant DDA of the breast (DDAB) [7, 8].

Acroangiodermatitis (pseudo-Kaposi sarcoma) is the first angiomatosis to be described including two variants: the Mali type also known as acral capillary

F. Rongioletti
Section of Dermatology of the Department of Medical Science and Public Health, University of Cagliari, Cagliari, Italy

Vita-Salute S.Raffaele University, Milan, Italy

C. Ferreli (✉)
Section of Dermatology of the Department of Medical Science and Public Health, University of Cagliari, Cagliari, Italy
e-mail: ferreli@unica.it

F. Rongioletti, B. R. Smoller (eds.), *New and Emerging Entities in Dermatology and Dermatopathology*, https://doi.org/10.1007/978-3-030-80027-7_27

Table 1 Cutaneous reactive angiomatoses: clinical and microscopic features with management

Clinical type	Presentation	Histopathologic features	Main associated conditions	Management
Reactive angioendotheliomatosis (RAE)	Violaceous patches and plaques, occasionally ulcerated and necrotic	*Intravascular* proliferation of endothelial cells (with or without pericytes)	Infections (endocarditis), cholesterol emboli, arteriovenous shunt, antiphospholipid syndrome, renal disease, rheumatoid arthritis, hematological malignancies, hepatitis	Treating the underlying systemic disorder (underlying cause of ischemia) systemic steroids
Diffuse dermal angiomatosis (DDA) Diffuse dermal angiomatosis of the breast (DDAB)	Ulcerated violaceous patches and plaques Painful	Diffuse *extravascular* proliferation of endothelial cells between collagen bundles with development of vascular lumina in reticular dermis	Peripheral vascular diseases, arteriovenous shunt, macromastia, calciphylaxis, anticardiolipin antibodies, overweight, heavy smoking	Revascularization with stent placement, removal of arteriovenous fistula, breast reduction surgery, isotretinoin weight control, smoking cessation
Acroangiodermatitis (pseudo-Kaposi sarcoma)	Coalescent red-brown macules or violaceous papules and plaques (usually on the legs)	*Periluminal* lobular proliferation of endothelial cells (and pericytes) with thick-walled vessels in the papillary dermis	Venous insufficiency, arteriovenous shunt, limb paralysis, amputation stump, thrombophilia syndrome, Klippel-Trénaunay	Treatment of venous hypertension, laser ablation for dilated capillary
Intravascular histiocytosis	Erythematous-violaceous patches and plaques	*Intravascular* proliferation of CD68+ histiocytes inside the lumen with CD31 expression of endothelial cells lining the dilated blood vessels	Monoclonal gammopathy, vascular insufficiency, rheumatoid arthritis, breast carcinoma	Similar to REA and DDA

Table 1 (continued)

Clinical type	Presentation	Histopathologic features	Main associated conditions	Management
Reactive glomeruloid angioendotheliomatosis	Erythemato purpuric patches and ulcerated necrotic plaques	*Intravascular* proliferation of endothelial cells with formation of capillary loops inside the lumen, producing structures reminiscent of renal glomeruli	Cold agglutinins, lymphoma	Similar to REA and DDA
Angiopericytomatosis (angiomatosis with cryoproteins)	Ulcerated necrotic plaques and erythematous patches and papules Painful	*Periluminal* proliferation of pericytes (with or without histiocytes) with or without thrombi	Myeloma, cryoproteinemia	Treating the underlying systemic disorder

angiomatosis (caused by venous stasis) and the Stewart–Bluefarb type (caused by congenital arteriovenous malformation). The condition has also been reported in patients with acquired iatrogenic arteriovenous fistula, paralyzed extremity, suction socket lower limb prosthesis (amputees), hepatitis C, and protein-C deficiency [9].

Intravascular histiocytosis is a rare condition characterized by the presence of histiocytes within the dilated blood vessels of the dermis. It can be primary or secondary to systemic diseases such as rheumatoid arthritis with only six cases reported in the English literature [10]. Actually, intralymphatic histiocytosis in which histiocytes are seen inside the dilated lymphatic vessels is considered a distinct entity [11].

In angiopericytomatosis (angiomatosis with cryoproteins), the proliferating cells are mainly pericytes with only four patients reported in the setting of myeloproliferative disorders [12].

Clinical Features

RAE affects women and men equally (F/M = 1:1.3), and although it has been reported in a wide range of ages, it is most seen in patients with a median age of 60 years. RAE presents with multiple, from 1 to 5 cm in diameter, erythematous–violaceous, livedoid, and purpuric patches and plaques, sometimes with a reticular pattern (Fig. 1a), which may progress toward necrosis and ulceration with a wide distribution, but propensity to involve lower limbs. Symptoms like malaise, fever, chills, and weight loss may associate. RAE has been related to systemic infections

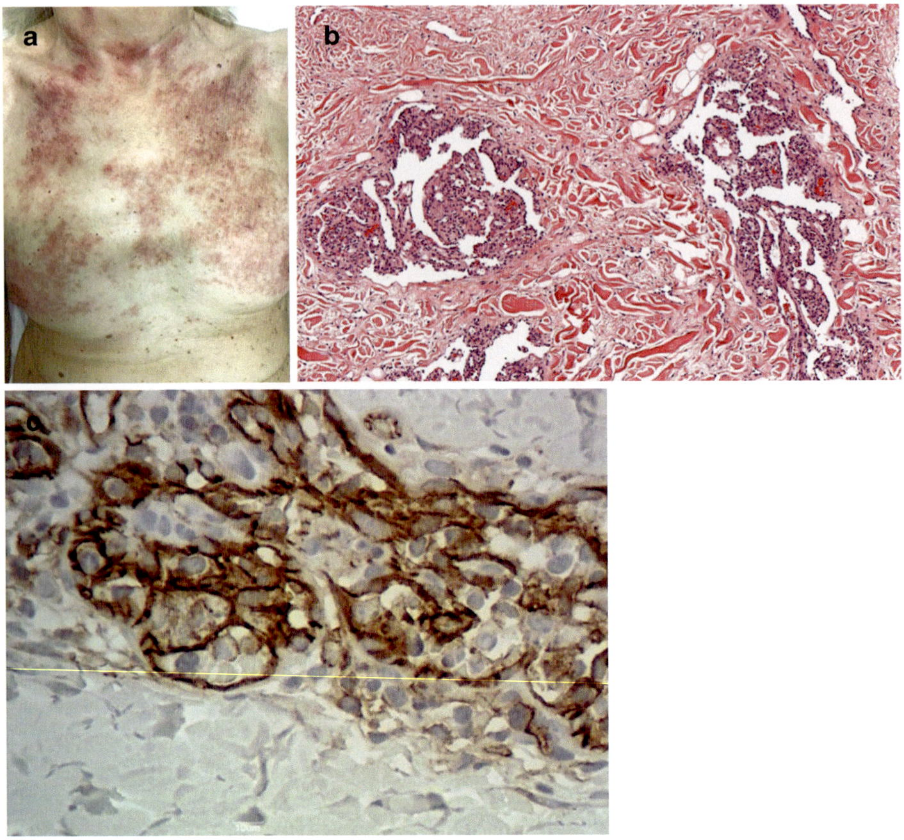

Fig. 1 (a) Reactive angioendotheliomatosis: multiple erythematous, livedoid, and purpuric patches with reticular pattern on the chest. (b) Histopathology of glomeruloid angioendotheliomatosis showing dilated vascular spaces contained a conglomeration of capillaries producing structures reminiscent of renal glomeruli (H&E 40X). (c) The endothelial marker CD31 labels the intravascular capillary proliferation (anti CD31 60X)

like subacute bacterial endocarditis, hepatitis, cholesterol emboli, arteriovenous shunt, antiphospholipid syndrome, chronic lymphatic leukemia, myelodysplastic syndrome, monoclonal gammopathy, renal disease including postrenal transplantation, rheumatoid arthritis, ANCA-vasculitis related to propylthiouracil [1–4, 13, 14]. Similar skin lesions are also reported in glomeruloid RAE that has been associated with cold agglutinin syndrome, non-Hodgkin lymphoma, and monoclonal gammopathy of undetermined significance [15].

In intravascular (intracapillary) histiocytosis, multiple erythematous macules and violaceous patches and plaques develop on the face and upper limbs [10, 11, 16] in association with cardiac disease, cerebrovascular insufficiency, rheumatoid arthritis, infections, hypercoagulable state, and breast carcinoma.

DDA is probably the most common form of cutaneous reactive angiomatosis as the term RAE has been used improperly to describe cases with histological features

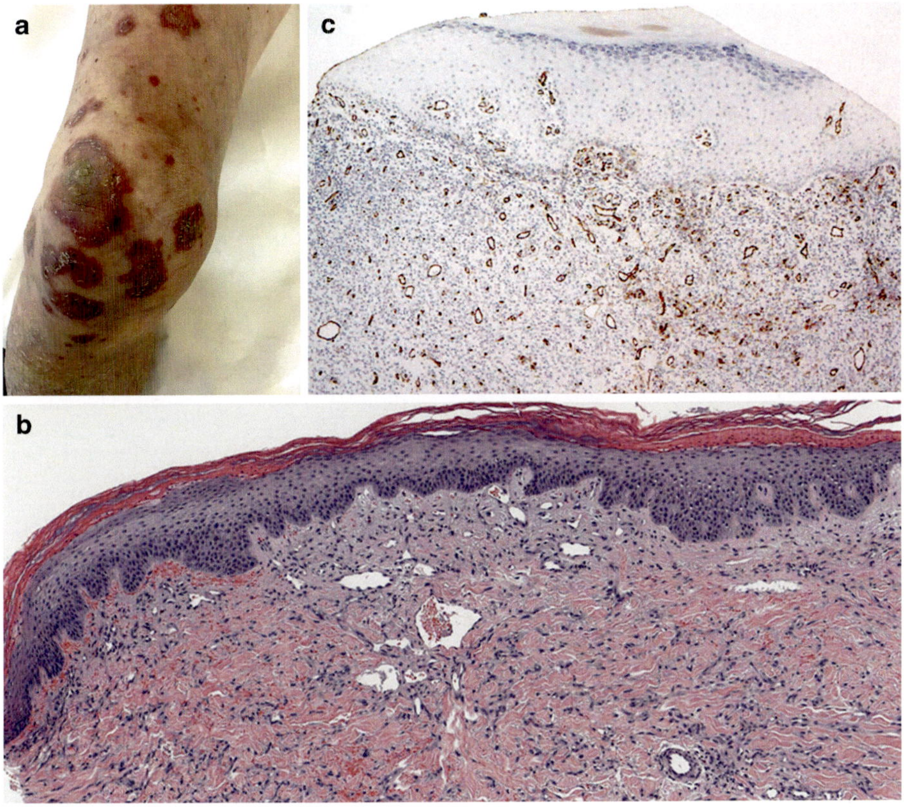

Fig. 2 (**a**) Diffuse dermal angiomatosis: violaceous, purpuric plaques on the lower extremities, partially covered with superficial scale crusts. (**b**) Histopathology showing an interstitial proliferation of endothelial cells and pericytes, forming small caliber or dilated capillaries with minimal or absent intravascular proliferation, in association with extravasated red blood cells. (H&E 10X). (**c**) CD31 positive capillaries and interstitial single cells (anti CD31 10X)

more consistent with DDA. The clinical lesions are indistinguishable from RAE with asymptomatic or painful, violaceous, purpuric, and occasionally ulcerated plaques mainly on the lower extremities or abdomen in patients with peripheral vascular atherosclerotic disease (Fig. 2a). However, any prothrombotic condition that can lead to ischemia can cause DDA as it has also been described on the forearm secondary to iatrogenic arteriovenous fistulas in the setting of chronic hemodialysis or in patients with comorbidities such as hypertension, diabetes, calciphylaxis, obesity, and smoking [17–20]. DDA of the breast is characterized by enlarging, reticulated, and erythematous to purple patches (Fig. 3) with sometimes a tendency to ulcerate occurring exclusively in middle-aged women (mean age 46.6 years), presenting with large pendulous breasts (in five cases there was a history of breast reduction surgery). An association with overweight or frank obesity, smoking, coronary artery disease, hypertension, surgery/trauma, diabetes, calciphylaxis, and antiphospholipid syndrome has also been reported [8, 21].

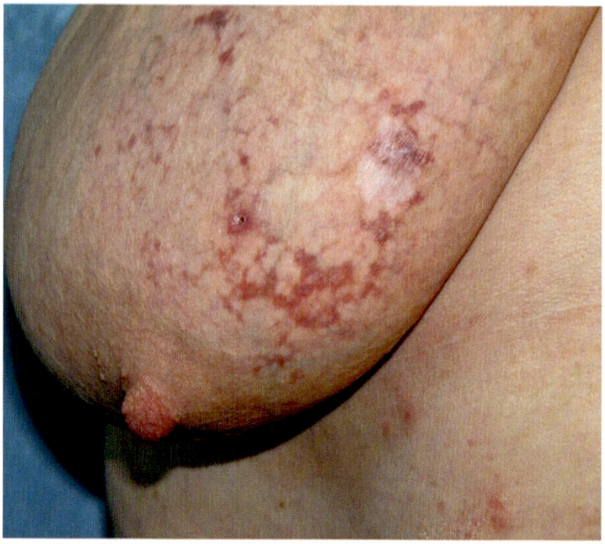

Fig. 3 Diffuse dermal angiomatosis of the breast: reticulated, erythematous to purple patches with small hemorrhagic crust and scar formation

Acroangiodermatitis has a clinical picture characterized by violaceous macules, indurated plaques, or nodules usually bilaterally on the extensor surfaces of lower extremities, mimicking Mediterranean Kaposi disease [22]. Dermoscopy shows many polymorphic vessels with white structureless areas [23].

Finally, angiopericytomatosis (angiomatosis with cryoproteins) presents with widespread, painful erythematous papules and ulcerated plaques, mainly on acral areas [24].

Histopathological Features

Although all cutaneous reactive angiomatoses share a similar clinical presentation, they are characterized by different microscopic patterns of dermal intravascular or extravascular lobular or diffuse hyperplasia of endothelial cells, pericytes, and histiocytes, without significant cellular atypia [1]. Although these angioproliferations can histologically mimic vascular tumors, they are reactive and non-neoplastic. They seem to originate from the sub-occlusion of vascular lumina by different localized or systemic disorders leading to ischemia. The vascular proliferation stops after the inducing hypoxic stimulus has been withdrawn.

Histopathologically, RAE shows a proliferation of epithelioid and spindle-shaped cells in superficial and mid-dermis lining vascular channels, arranged in clusters, and sometimes displaying an intravascular growth pattern. The intravascular cells stain positive for the endothelial cell markers such as CD31 and ERG. A small reactive inflammatory infiltrate and a quote of α-actin-positive pericytes are present. Intravascular thrombi within the proliferation and reactive (fasciitis-like) dermal alterations may also be found. Vascular deposits of amyloid due to an associated monoclonal gammopathy have been anecdotally described [25]. In addition to the skin, RAE has been described only in the intestine without cutaneous involvement [26].

Glomeruloid RAE differs from true RAE due to the presence of dilated vascular spaces that contained a conglomeration of capillaries filled with red blood cells closely producing structures reminiscent of renal glomeruli (Fig. 1b). These capillaries are lined by a flat endothelium with scanty cytoplasm and plump cells with abundant pale cytoplasm, clear vacuoles, or eosinophilic globules that are PAS positive. In lesional skin, the glomeruloid proliferation of endothelial cells is associated with an increased epidermal expression of vascular endothelial growth factor (VEGF), a potent angiogenic mediator [27]. CD31 immunostain highlights the intracapillary proliferation (Fig. 1c).

DDA shows a different pattern including the presence of diffuse extracapillary proliferation of endothelial cells and few pericytes that insinuate themselves between the collagen bundles forming small caliber vessels within the superficial layers of the papillary and reticular dermis, with only minimal or absent intravascular proliferation (Fig. 2b) [11]. Scattered extravasated erythrocytes with hemosiderin are present in the stroma. The cells are positive for CD31 (Fig. 2c), CD34, and ERG immunostains [28].

In acroangiodermatitis, the proliferation of endothelial cells leads to the formation of new thick-walled vessels, often in a lobular arrangement, in the papillary dermis. The vessels are usually surrounded by pericytes. Extravasation of red blood cells, hemosiderin pigment deposition, dermal fibrosis, and a perivascular, superficial infiltrate consisting of lymphocytes, histiocytes, and eosinophils are additional findings. Small luminal thrombi may be seen [29]. Immunohistochemistry for human herpesvirus-8 (HHV-8) is negative allowing a differentiation from Kaposi sarcoma.

Conversely, intravascular (intracapillary) histiocytosis displays intravascular proliferation of CD68- and CD163-positive medium-sized and large-sized cells determining luminal occlusion. Immunostaining shows strong CD31 expression of endothelial cells lining the dilated blood vessels involved in intravascular proliferation. Fibrin thrombi, extravasated erythrocytes, and a mild inflammatory infiltrate of lymphocytes are additional features [2]. D2–40/podoplanin or other antigens that characterize lymphatic differentiation of endothelia are negative [30, 31].

Histopathological picture of angiopericytomatosis exhibit rounded aggregates of capillaries with periluminal proliferation of pericytes and intraluminal thrombi in the papillary and reticular dermis. Immunohistochemical studies confirm that the vessels outlined by the endothelial cells lining the lumina are surrounded and compressed by muscle-specific actin-positive pericytes [24].

Workup

Due to its potential association with localized or life-threatening systemic prothrombotic conditions, systemic infections, autoimmune diseases, and lymphoproliferative disorders, it appears crucial to perform exhaustive investigations when a diagnosis of RAE, DDA, or other cutaneous reactive angiomatoses is made [1, 4].

Differential Diagnosis

Clinically, cutaneous reactive angiomatoses may mimic vasculopathic/vasculitic lesions and vascular tumors. In particular, RAE should be distinguished from all the vascular tumors showing a lobular or intravascular pattern of growth such as glomeruloid hemangioma, tufted angioma, Kaposi's sarcoma, Dabska tumor (malignant endovascular papillary endothelioma), and angiosarcoma. Clinical pathologic correlation is helpful to avoid misdiagnosis [1, 32, 33]. Acroangiodermatitis and DDA should be distinguished from Kaposi sarcoma, a human herpes virus 8–related plurifocal vascular proliferation. A challenging differential diagnosis of RAE is with intravascular lymphoma. The marked atypia of intraluminal cells and immunohistochemistry findings of common leukocyte antigen and B- or T-cell markers play in favor of the latter [5].

Intravascular histiocytosis has to be differentiated from the more frequently reported "intralymphatic histiocytosis." Recent data support the concept that intravascular histiocytosis belongs to the group of RAE, while intralymphatic histiocytosis is a distinct clinical and histologic entity characterized by the accumulation of CD68+ histiocytes within dilated lymphatic vessels (D240/podoplanin + vessels) instead of CD31+ vessels.

Etiopathogenesis

The etiopathogenesis of cutaneous reactive angiomatoses has not been fully clarified. They are commonly associated with underlying systemic diseases capable of producing vascular inflammation and (sub)occlusion, followed by local hypoxia, reactive cellular hyperplasia, and neovascularization. The different histopathological subtypes are sequential stages of this regenerative process of revascularization (Fig. 4). In fact, the occlusive process is followed by the recruitment of histiocytes along with the hyperplasia of the endothelial cells and pericytes. The histiocytes are involved in the organization and the resorption of the microthrombi, and their proliferation produces a histologic pattern of intravascular histiocytosis. The endothelial cells, on the contrary, are involved in the subsequent recanalization of the thrombotic vessels or in the formation of new vessels to restore an adequate blood

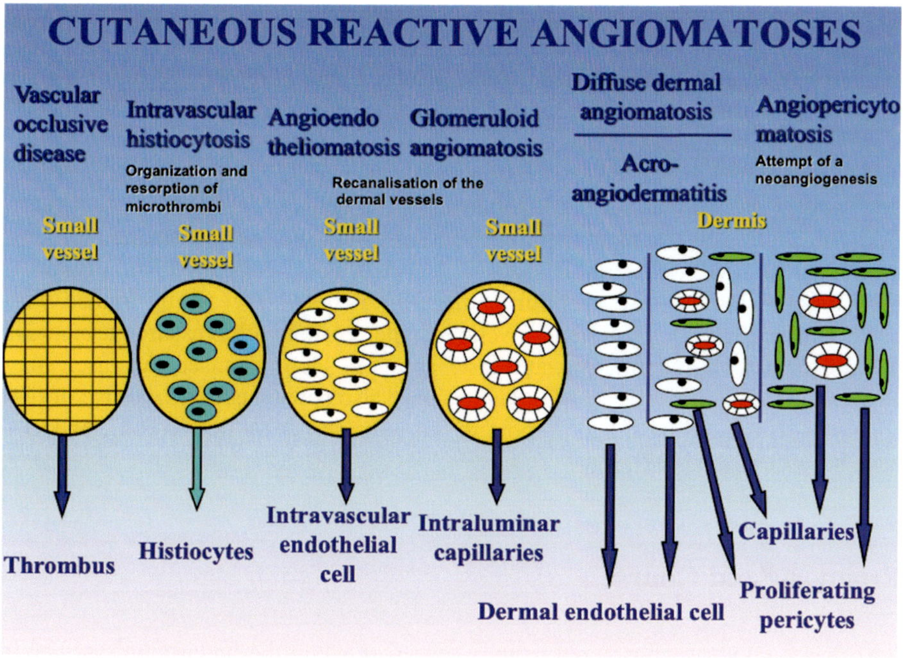

Fig. 4 Pathogenetic hypothesis explaining the different histopathological patterns of cutaneous reactive angiomatoses as sequential stages of a regenerative process of revascularization. (From Rongioletti and Rebora [1])

circulation under the stimulus of vascular endothelial growth factor induced by ischemia. The former condition produces an intravascular growth pattern that is histologically seen as RAE or glomeruloid RAE. In the latter, the extravascular hyperplasia of endothelial cells gives rise to a histologic picture of diffuse dermal angiomatosis. When the extravascular endothelial hyperplasia forms true small capillary loops, then we have the microscopic picture of acroangiodermatitis. The pericytes also are involved in neoangiogenesis in an attempt to restore the integrity of the normal vessel walls. When the hyperplasia of pericytes becomes prominent, the histologic pattern of angiopericytomatosis is produced. The spectrum of lesions, seen mainly on histological grounds, is dependent on the time of the biopsy and on the severity of the underlying pathologic condition [1].

Therapy

The management consists of treating the underlying systemic disorder and consequently the underlying cause of ischemia in all cutaneous reactive angiomatoses [1, 4, 7]. Antibiotics for occult infections and systemic steroids for their suppressive effect on neoangiogenesis have also been used in those rare cases in which no apparent underlying pathology has been found [34]. Revascularization with stent placement, removal of an arteriovenous fistula, or other forms of revascularization should be considered for DDA [35]. Reported medical therapies for DDA include isotretinoin, especially for DDA of the breast due to its antiangiogenesis effect [36]. Taking into consideration the strong association with large pendulous breasts, breast reduction surgery in women with macromastia is an option for DDA of the breast. Additional anecdotal medical therapies such as pentoxifylline, aspirin, and nifedipine have been tried with variable success. A case of RAE associated with monoclonal gammopathy and a severe kidney disease has been successfully treated with lenalidomide [3, 7, 8]. Treatment of venous hypertension with pressure garments is helpful for acroangiodermatitis, and laser ablation, such as pulsed-dye laser, may clear some individual lesions. Skin lesions may also spontaneously improve or disappear. Recurrences have been reported, but only one death due to RAE or DDA have been described [37].

Prognosis and Course

RAE has a good prognosis and usually regresses when the underlying disease, if revealed, is successfully treated. The prognosis depends on the underlying condition. In DDA, after bypass surgery, skin lesions (even ulcerative) demonstrate rapid improvement, with subsequent total healing or mild residual scarring, within a time span of weeks to months.

Conclusions

A spectrum of cutaneous vascular (capillary) proliferations has been described or better characterized in the last few years under the unifying term of *cutaneous reactive angiomatoses*. Clinically, they all have a similar clinical presentation with multiple, erythematous–violaceous and purpuric patches and plaques, sometimes evolving toward necrosis and ulceration with a wide distribution but involving preferentially the limbs. They are commonly associated with underlying systemic diseases capable of producing vascular inflammation and (sub)occlusion followed by local hypoxia, reactive cellular hyperplasia, and neovascularization under the stimulus of vascular endothelial growth factor (VEGF). The different histopathological subtypes represent sequential stages of this regenerative process. Thus, all patients with cutaneous reactive angiomatoses should undergo thorough investigation to rule out the possibility of associated systemic diseases or localized conditions with vascular occlusive involvement. The reestablishment of a relatively normal vascular homeostasis in the skin determine the spontaneous improvement or clearing of all lesions of cutaneous reactive angiomatoses.

References

1. Rongioletti F, Rebora A. Cutaneous reactive angiomatoses: patterns and classification of reactive vascular proliferation. J Am Acad Dermatol. 2003;49(5):887–96.
2. Vacharathit V, Billings SD, Kirksey L. Resolution of reactive angioendotheliomatosis in an arteriovenous fistula with innominate vein angioplasty. J Vasc Access. 2018;19(1):94–7.
3. Di Filippo Y, Cardot-Leccia N, Long-Mira E, Andreani M, Richez V, Lacour JP, Passeron T, Montaudié H. Reactive angioendotheliomatosis revealing a glomerulopathy secondary to a monoclonal gammopathy successfully treated with lenalidomide. J Eur Acad Dermatol Venereol. 2020.
4. McMenamin ME, Fletcher CD. Reactive angioendotheliomatosis (a study of 15 cases demonstrating a wide clinicopathologic spectrum). Am J Surg Pathol. 2002;26:685–97.
5. Wick MR, Rocamora A. Reactive and malignant angioendotheliomatosis (a discriminant clinicopathologic study). J Cutan Pathol. 1988;15:260–71.
6. Porras-Luque JI, Fernández-Herrera J, Daudén E, Fraga J, Fernández-Villalta MJ, García-Díez A. Cutaneous necrosis by cold agglutinins associated with glomeruloid reactive angioendotheliomatosis. Br J Dermatol. 1998;139(6):1068–72.
7. Touloei K, Tongdee E, Smirnov B, Nousari C. Diffuse dermal angiomatosis. Cutis. 2019;103(3):181–4.
8. Ferreli C, Atzori L, Caputo V, Rongioletti F. Diffuse dermal angiomatosis of the breast: an emerging entity in the setting of cutaneous reactive angiomatoses. Clin Dermatol. 2021;39:271–7.
9. Chea EP, Rutt VL, Levin J, McClain R, Purcell SM. Acroangiodermatitis of Mali and Stewart-Bluefarb syndrome. Cutis. 2019 Jun;103(6):336–9.
10. Demirkesen C, Kran T, Leblebici C, Yücelten D, Aksu AE, Mat C. Intravascular/intralymphatic histiocytosis: a report of 3 cases. Am J Dermatopathol. 2015;37(10):783–9.
11. Mazloom SE, Stallings A, Kyei A. Differentiating intralymphatic histiocytosis, intravascular histiocytosis, and subtypes of reactive angioendotheliomatosis: review of clinical and histologic features of all cases reported to date. Am J Dermatopathol. 2017;39(1):33–9.
12. LeBoit PE, Solomon AR, Santa Cruz DJ, Wick MR. Angiomatosis with luminal cryoprotein deposition. J Am Acad Dermatol. 1992;27:969–73.
13. Creamer D, Black MM, Calonje E. Reactive angioendotheliomatosis in association with the antiphospholipid syndrome. Br J Dermatol. 2000;42:903–6.
14. Singer C, Mallon D, Auguston B, Lam M, Foster R. Reactive angioendotheliomatosis presenting as livedo racemosa secondary to propylthiouracil. Pathology. 2020;52(4):494–6.
15. Chen XF, Ong NWR, Tang PY, Pang SM, Sittampalam K. Glomeruloid haemangioma pattern in reactive angioendotheliomatosis leading to the diagnosis of POEMS syndrome. Pathology. 2020:S0031-3025(20)30927–2.
16. Abuawad YG, Diniz TACB, Kakizaki P, Valente NYS. Intravascular histiocytosis: case report of a rare disease probably associated with silicone breast implant. An Bras Dermatol. 2020;95(3):347–50.
17. Ferreli C, Atzori L, Pinna AL, Pau M, Aste N, Ricotti C, Rongioletti F. Diffuse dermal angiomatosis: a clinical mimicker of vasculitis associated with calciphylaxis and monoclonal gammopathy. G Ital Dermatol Venereol. 2015;150(1):115–21.
18. Diaz E, Vanhaecke C, Sanchez J, Durlach A, Gusdorf L, Viguier M. Multifocal diffuse dermal angiomatosis: a reflection of high cardiovascular risk. Acta Derm Venereol. 2020;100(14):adv00202.
19. Frizzell MR, Shah S, Parekh P. Diffuse dermal angiomatosis localized to abdominal striae. Proc (Bayl Univ Med Cent). 2020;33(3):419–21.
20. O'Connor HM, Wu Q, Lauzon SD, Forcucci JA. Diffuse dermal angiomatosis associated with calciphylaxis: a 5-year retrospective institutional review. J Cutan Pathol. 2020;47(1):27–30.
21. Reusche R, Winocour S, Degnim A, Lemaine V. Diffuse dermal angiomatosis of the breast: a series of 22 cases from a single institution. Gland Surg. 2015;4(6):554–60.

22. Samad A, Dodds S. Acroangiodermatitis: review of the literature and report of a case associated with symmetrical foot ulcers. Eur J Vasc Endovasc Surg. 2002;24(6):558–60.
23. Dabas G, De D, Handa S, Chatterjee D. Dermoscopic features in two cases of acroangiodermatitis. Australas J Dermatol. 2018;59(4):e290–1.
24. Rongioletti F, Gambini C, Smoller BR, Parodi A, Rebora A. Angiopericytomatosis and subcutaneous thrombophlebitis in multiple myeloma. Br J Dermatol. 2002;147:1037–40.
25. Ortonne N, Vignon-Pennamen MD, Majdalani G, Pinquier L, Janin A. Reactive angioendotheliomatosis secondary to dermal amyloid angiopathy. Am J Dermatopathol. 2001;23(4):315–9.
26. Ogawa K, Tada T, Takeuchi Y, Suenaga M, Suzuki S, Shirai T. Reactive angioendotheliomatosis of the intestine. Am J Surg Pathol. 2004;28(2):257–61.
27. Eming SA, Sacher C, Eich D, Kuhn A, Krieg T. Increased expression of VEGF in glomeruloid reactive angioendotheliomatosis. Dermatology. 2003;207(4):398–401.
28. Galambos J, Meuli-Simmen C, Schmid R, Steinmann LS, Kempf W. Diffuse dermal angiomatosis of the breast: a distinct entity in the spectrum of cutaneous reactive angiomatoses - clinicopathologic study of two cases and comprehensive review of the literature. Case Rep Dermatol. 2017;9(3):194–205.
29. Pietkiewicz P, Bowszyc-Dmochowska M, Gornowicz-Porowska J, Majewski P, Marszałek A, Dmochowski M. Acroangiodermatitis in a leg amputee using a suction-socket prosthesis: clinical, histological as well as HHV-8 and CD34 immunohistochemical study. Pol J Pathol. 2013;64(2):153–6.
30. Vilas Boas P, Cerroni L, Requena L. Intravascular cutaneous disorders. A clinicopathologic review. Am J Dermatopathol. 2021;43:119–136.
31. Aung PP, Ballester LY, Goldberg LJ, Bhawan J. Incidental simultaneous finding of intravascular histiocytosis and reactive angioendotheliomatosis: a case report. Am J Dermatopathol. 2015;37(5):401–4.
32. Rongioletti F, Gambini C, Lerza R. Glomeruloid hemangioma. A cutaneous marker of POEMS syndrome. Am J Dermatopathol. 1994;16:175–8.
33. Argani P, Athanaian E. Malignant endovascular papillary angioendoteliona (Dabska tumor) arising within a deep intramuscular hemangioma. Arch Pathol Lab Med. 1997;121:992–5.
34. Sriphojanart T, Vachiramon V. Diffuse dermal angiomatosis: a clue to the diagnosis of atherosclerotic vascular disease. Case Rep Dermatol. 2015;7(2):100–6.
35. Sheikh AB, Javed N, Stoltze K. Diffuse dermal angiomatosis manifestation of underlying severe peripheral vascular disease. Eur J Case Rep Intern Med. 2020;7(9):001755.
36. McLaughlin ER, Morris R, Weiss SW, Arbiser JL. Diffuse dermal angiomatosis of the breast (response to isotretinoin). J Am Acad Dermatol. 2001;45:462–5.
37. Kirkland CR, Hawayek LH, Mutasim DF. Atherosclerosis-induced diffuse dermal angiomatosis with fatal outcome. Arch Dermatol. 2010;146:684–5.

Skin Manifestations of Immunoglobulin G4-Related Disease

Roula Katerji and Bruce R. Smoller

Introduction

Immunoglobulin G4-related disease (IgG4-RD) formerly known as IgG4-related systemic disease is a chronic inflammatory condition and immune-mediated disease characterized by tissue infiltration by IgG4+ secreting polyclonal plasma cells and elevated serum levels of IgG4 [1]. The disease most commonly affects middle-aged to elderly males; however, it has also been reported in children [2]. The disease has an estimated incidence of 0.28–1.08/100.000 population and 336–1300 new cases yearly [3].

The term IgG4-RD started to evolve with Mikulicz's disease (MD), which was first described in 1892, as an enlargement of lacrimal and salivary glands and is characterized by a good response to glucocorticoids, leading to the recovery of gland function. For some time, MD was considered as part of Sjögren's disease, but recently, it is classified to be a part of IgG4-RD [4]. The first reported case of IgG4-RD was described in 2001 by Hamano et al. presenting a case of autoimmune sclerosing pancreatitis in a patient with elevated IgG4 serum levels that responded to corticosteroids [5]. However, it wasn't until 2003 when the systemic nature of the disease has been fully described. Other terms have been used to describe IgG4-RD such as IgG4-related sclerosing disease, systemic IgG4 plasmacytic syndrome, and IgG4-related multiorgan lymphoproliferative syndrome [6].

R. Katerji (✉) · B. R. Smoller
Department of Pathology and Laboratory Medicine, University of Rochester School of Medicine and Dentistry, Rochester, NY, USA
e-mail: roula_katerji@urmc.rochester.edu

F. Rongioletti, B. R. Smoller (eds.), *New and Emerging Entities in Dermatology and Dermatopathology*, https://doi.org/10.1007/978-3-030-80027-7_28

Clinical Features

IgG4-RD is a systemic disease that might affect almost any organ, with the pancreas being the most commonly affected, causing autoimmune pancreatitis [7]. Other commonly affected organs are lacrimal glands as MD and inflammatory pseudotumor of the orbit and salivary glands involvement as sclerosing sialadenitis also known as (Küttner's tumor) [8]. IgG4-RS can also affect retroperitoneal organs and the aorta causing chronic periaortitis [9], the lung as IgG4-related lung disease or pneumonitis [10], and lymph nodes causing lymphadenopathy [11].

The skin is not different, and it can certainly be involved by IgG4-RD; however, the cutaneous manifestations of IgG4-RD have not been as widely studied as those in other organs. Skin involvement can be divided into primary and secondary: primary if the skin is involved first by the disease and presents as an isolated skin lesion without systemic involvement and secondary if there is a systemic disease with cutaneous involvement afterward. Secondary IgG4-RSD is more common than primary [12]. Clinically, cutaneous IgG4-RD presents as tumefactive lesions, swelling of red-brown pruritic subcutaneous nodules, plaques, masses, or inflammatory pseudotumors. The most common location is the head and neck, particularly the periauricular region (see Fig. 1 clinical picture of IgG4-RSD) and less commonly upper and lower extremities [13].

The disease has a relapsing-remitting course, and the majority of patients are asymptomatic in the early stages of the disease. Symptoms vary depending on the organ involved. Weight loss and lymphadenopathy (most commonly mediastinal) are common presentations of the disease [14]. Patients might also present with an atopic disease, serum hypergammaglobulinemia (particularly elevation of IgE and IgG levels), hypocomplementemia, and serum eosinophilia [15]. Increased C-reactive protein (CRP) level is observed in around 20% of patients with IgG4-RD. Notably, some patients have nonspecific elevation of antinuclear antibodies (ANA) and rheumatoid factors (RF).

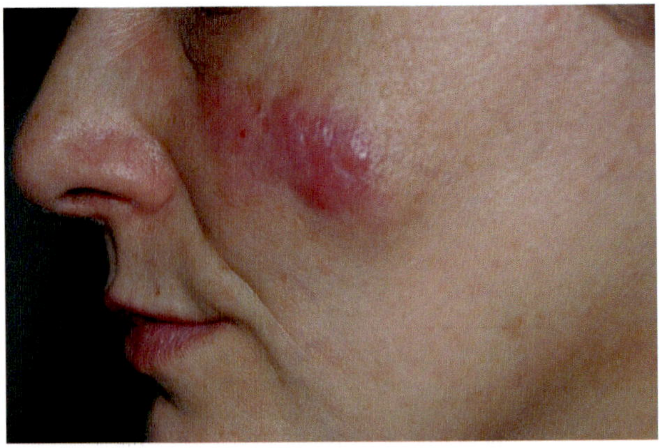

Fig. 1 A clinical picture of IgG4-RSD in a middle-aged woman who presented with an erythematous nodule on the left cheek. (Picture courtesy of F. Rongioletti)

One study estimated the skin involvement by IgG4-RD to be 6% [16]; in our opinion, this percentage is not quite accurate. We think that the cutaneous involvement might be underestimated for the following two reasons: first, not surprisingly, some cases are misdiagnosed as other diseases such as plasma cell infiltration, plasmacytosis, or reactive fibrosis with inflammation, and second, systemic IgG4-RD might be associated with nonspecific cutaneous manifestations, like "rash" or "pruritic lesions"; however, a skin biopsy is not necessarily always performed. Since most patients get better after corticosteroid therapy, this might be indirect evidence of cutaneous involvement without definitive pathological proof [17, 18].

Histologic Features of IgG4-RSD

IgG4-RSD causes various histologic manifestations. Tokura et al. [19] classified IgG4-RSD into primary and secondary IgG4-RSD. The primary form is described as having a massive plasma cell infiltrate causing a mass-forming lesion that can be further subtyped into the following three categories: [1] cutaneous plasmacytosis, [2] pseudolymphoma and angiolymphoid hyperplasia with eosinophilia, and [3] Mikulicz's disease. The secondary form represents lesions without mass formation and consists of the following four categories: [1] psoriasis-like lesions, [2] unspecified maculopapular or erythematous lesions, [3] hypergammaglobulinemia purpura and urticarial vasculitis, and [4] ischemic digit.

It remains debatable as to whether the plasmacytosis and angiolymphoid hyperplasia with eosinophilia represent manifestations of IgG4-RSD or if they represent distinct entities closely related to IgG4-RD.

Other rare cutaneous manifestations reported in the literature are generalized pustular psoriasis reported in two cases: one associated with Mikulicz's disease and the second associated with IgG4-related kidney disease that presented as multiple red erythematous pustules [20]. Another rare presentation is septal panniculitis and polyarthritis nodosa without granulomas, with negative immune deposition. This case was that of a 7-year-old patient who developed renal IgG4-RD with extensive areas of fibrosis in the kidney 4 years after the onset of his skin lesions [21]. Sato et al. presented ten patients with IgG4-RSD. The majority of patients demonstrated a nodular dermatitis pattern and less commonly demonstrated a subcutaneous nodular pattern of lymphoplasmacytic infiltrate with variable amount of fibrosis [22]. Interestingly, association of exposure to zinc and manganese with developing nodules on the skin without any systemic involvement in an IgG4-RSD in an adult male patient has been recently reported [23].

Histopathological Features

Patients with a presumptive diagnosis of IgG4-RSD typically get a biopsy or resection for a diagnosis. Histopathologically, the epidermis is usually spared but might show psoriasiform hyperplasia. The main pathologic features are seen in the dermis, showing an abundant superficial and deep lymphoplasmacytic infiltrate surrounding periadnexal and perivascular tissue [22] (Fig. 2a, b, and c). The plasma cells are polyclonal and can be highlighted by CD138 (Fig. 2d), and the lymphocytes are predominantly CD4+ T cells having a small to medium size, intermixed with eosinophils and histiocytes. Fibrosis and obliterative phlebitis—the typical histopathological features that are commonly seen in systemic IgG4-RD—are not typically seen in IgG4-RSD [16]. The number of positive IgG4+ plasma cells differs from organ to organ, and the consensus statement suggests more than 200 positive IgG4+ plasma cells per HPF in IgG4-RSD [24, 25] (Fig. 3a and b).

Although the diagnosis requires serum IgG4 elevation (higher than 135 mg/dl), it is not entirely specific. There are many systemic diseases manifest with elevated

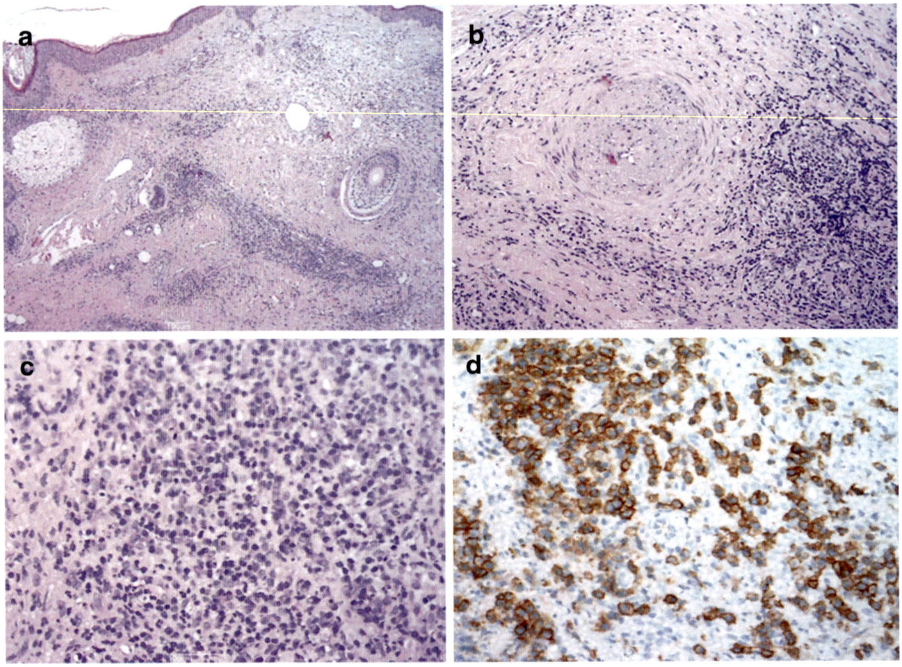

Fig. 2 Skin biopsy specimen from the nodule showing an uninvolved epidermis, there is a dense superficial and deep lymphoplasmacytic infiltrate surrounding the blood vessels and the adnexa with areas of fibrosis in the dermis (**a**, 2× objective). Obliteration of a deep venule at the dermoepidermal junction with a lymphoplasmacytic infiltrates and scattered eosinophils (**b**, 10× objective). The infiltrate is made predominantly of mature plasma cells (**c**, 20× objective). Immunohistochemical stains for CD138 highlight the plasma cells (**d**, 20× objective). (Picture courtesy of F. Rongioletti)

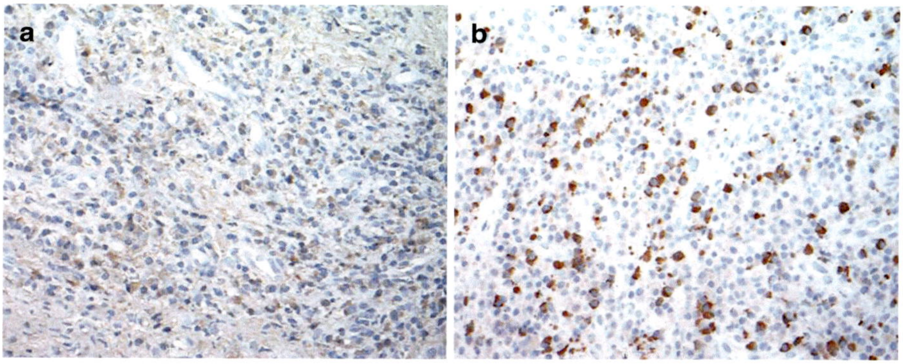

Fig. 3 Immunohistochemical stains for IgG+ (**a**, 20× objective). Immunohistochemical stains for IgG4+ (**b**, 20× objective) with IgG4+/IgG >40%. (Picture courtesy of F. Rongioletti)

serum IgG4 levels including autoimmune diseases, infections, Castleman disease, and cystic fibrosis [26], in addition to cutaneous diseases like pemphigus vulgaris, atopic dermatitis, and bullous pemphigoid [27]. Similarly, the ratio of IgG4+/IgG+ >40% is required for the diagnosis, but other diseases such as pemphigus show a similarly high ratio in more than 40% of cases [28].

The histologic features of IgG4-RSD are not entirely specific; nevertheless, the diagnosis should be considered in any eruption containing polytypic and abundant plasma cells and eosinophilic infiltrate, especially when there is lacrimal or salivary gland involvement.

Workup

Clinical history and thorough physical examination with lab testing, imaging, and most importantly histologic examination remain the most accurate method of diagnosing IgG4-RD. A full skin examination looking for any nodules or masses is essential. As we discussed earlier, H&E sections typically show an increase in polytypic plasma cells with eosinophils and histiocytes. Immunohistochemical stains for IgG and IgG4 show an increase in IgG4+ cells of >200/HPF with IgG4+/IgG+ ratio of >40%. Flow cytometry is helpful to exclude a clonal proliferation of plasma cells and to rule out hematolymphoid malignancies, and it might also demonstrate increased plasmablasts (immature precursors of plasma cells). Plasmablasts are increased in the serum of affected individuals, with a plasmablast value of over 2000/ml having a sensitivity of 87% and specificity of 91%, respectively, for a diagnosis of IgG4-RD. Also, plasmablast count is suggested as a useful biomarker for the diagnosis of IgG4-RD even in patients with normal serum IgG4 concentrations; it is also a useful biomarker for disease activity and for assessing response to treatment [29, 30]. Imaging studies such as computed tomography or magnetic resonance imaging to evaluate for the presence of systemic disease involvement, checking for any visceral masses or fibrosis, is recommended if clinically indicated. Overall, we cannot emphasize enough the importance of a vigorous workup to ensure that malignancy or infection is not the underlying cause of fibro-inflammatory organ involvement.

Diagnostic Criteria

The diagnostic approach is complex and depends on a combination of clinical, laboratory, and histopathological findings. In 2011, two IgG4-RD study groups in Japan established comprehensive diagnostic criteria for IgG4-RD. The criteria and the number of IgG4+ plasma cells are site-dependent, and the consensus for diagnosing IgG4-RD is the presence of the following main criteria:

1. Clinical examination showing diffuse or localized swelling or masses.
2. Hematological examination showing elevation of serum IgG4 > 135 mg/dL.
3. Histopathologic examination showing:
   (a) Lymphoplasmacytic infiltration and fibrosis.
   (b) More than 40% of IgG+ plasma cells are IgG4+ and having more than 10 cells per HPF of the biopsy specimen [3].

By fulfilling all three criteria, the diagnosis of IgG4-RD is definite; by having criteria [1] and [3], the diagnosis is probable; and by fulfilling [1] and [2], the diagnosis is possible [3].

Another international symposium of IgG4-related disease was held in Boston in 2012, and the proposed criteria for diagnosis were the following:

1. Dense lymphoplasmacytic infiltrate
2. Storiform fibrosis
3. Obliterative phlebitis

Other histological features that were suggested that are commonly seen are phlebitis without obliteration and increased eosinophils. A confident diagnosis requires the presence of two of three major histological features [24]. This consortium essentially makes the diagnosis based upon histologic H&E sections. It is worth pointing out that even if there are high IgG4+ cells on tissue sections without fulfilling the criteria on H&E, the diagnosis of IgG4-RD should not be made. These authors also emphasized that the number of IgG4+ cells differs from organ to organ ranging from 10 to 200 cells/HPF [24].

Differential Diagnosis

Kimura Disease (Eosinophilic Granuloma) and Angiolymphoid Hyperplasia with Eosinophilia (Epithelioid Hemangioma)

Kimura disease is a rare benign chronic inflammatory disorder of unknown etiology that most commonly presents as painless lymphadenopathy or as a pruritic subcutaneous mass in the head and neck area, particularly around the ear or the parotid gland. Commonly, there is elevated serum IgE and eosinophilia. Similar to IgG4-RSD, the disease is most commonly present in middle-aged Asian males. The etiology of Kimura disease is still unknown with a suggestion of associated EBV infection, but the association has not been widely detected or accepted [31]. Histologically, it is composed of reactive lymphoid follicles, with florid eosinophils forming eosinophilic abscesses. Recurrence is common in up to 75% of patients [32]. Treatment includes surgical resection and steroid therapy, with an overall excellent prognosis [33].

Angiolymphoid hyperplasia with eosinophilia (ALHE) is an uncommon vasoproliferative condition that presents as single or multiple painful, pruritic red-brown papules and nodules in the head and neck, slightly more common in females [34]. An example of ALHE in a middle aged male patient presented as a mass in the axilla is shown in Fig. 4. There is an increase in serum IL-5, which may explain the

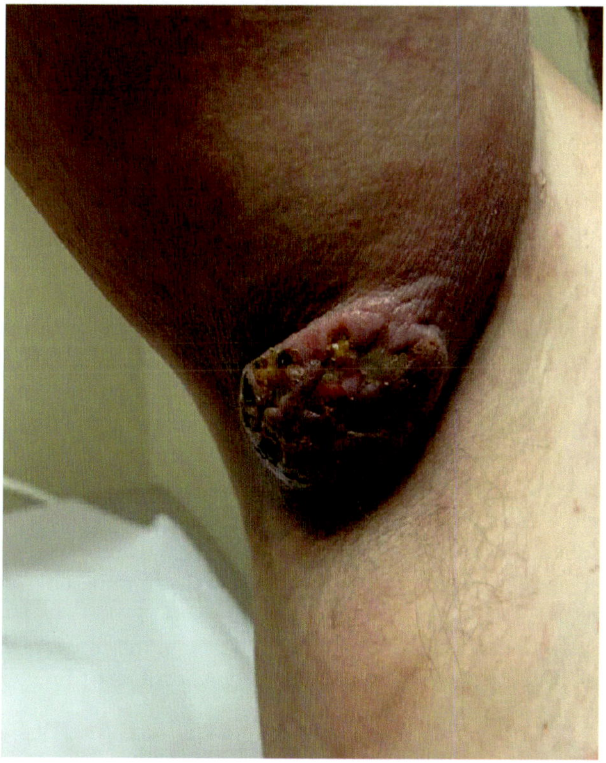

Fig. 4 A clinical picture of angiolymphoid hyperplasia with eosinophilia in the skin in a middle-aged male patient in the right axilla presented as a mass with ulceration and oozing surfaces, developed over few months, the patient denied any weight loss, night sweat or lymphadenopathy

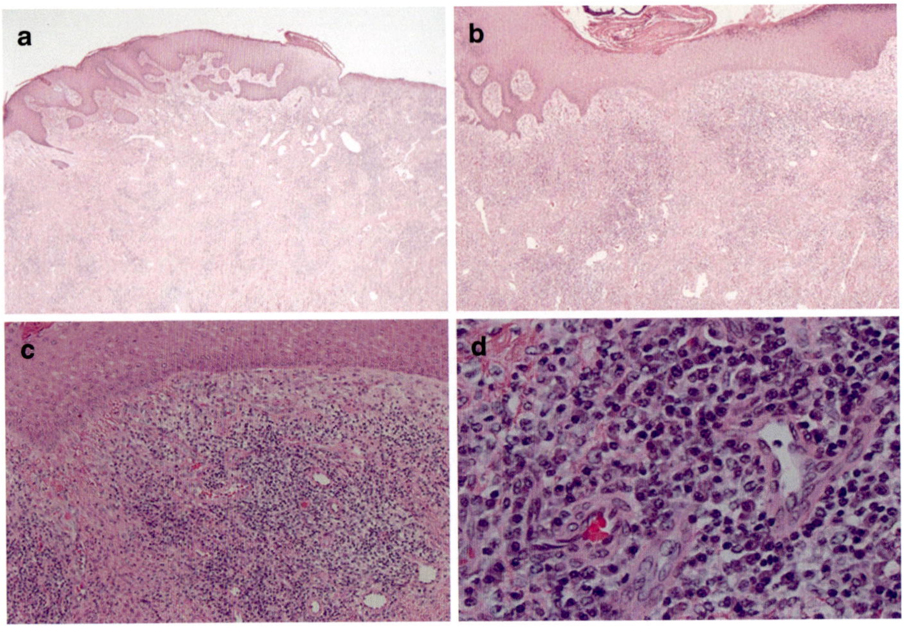

Fig. 5 An excisional biopsy shows the epidermis appears uninvolved, with dense lymphoplasmacytic infiltrate in the dermis without ulceration and minimal fibrosis (**a**, 2× objective) (**b**, 4× objective), respectively. The dense infiltration is surrounding the blood vessels and is composed of mature plasma cells and lymphocytes with scattered eosinophils (**c**, 20× objective) (**d**, 40× objective), respectively

eosinophilia. It has been reported in association with pregnancy [35], HIV [36], and nephrotic syndrome [37]. Histologically, it presents as a proliferation of thin- and thick-walled blood vessels lined by plump endothelial cells, with a dense inflammatory infiltrate composed of plasma cells, and abundant eosinophils, predominantly in the dermis (Fig. 5). Normal mitotic figures might be seen in a background of myxoid stroma [38]. An increase in IgG4+ cells in ALHE can be seen, but usually not abundant. Immunohistochemical stains are helpful to highlight the plasma cells (Fig. 6a and b), IgG+ cells (Fig. 6c and d), and IgG4+ cells (Fig. 6e and f). The overall prognosis is good, but the lesion might be hard to eradicate and recurs in approximately 10% of patients [39]. Treatment is usually excision, topical corticosteroids, anti-IL-5 antibody, and laser therapy.

Although both diseases have similarities, they are different entities as ALHE is more superficial, whereas Kimura disease tends to involve deep lymph nodes and subcutaneous tissue. Kimura disease is usually associated with elevated serum eosinophilia and elevated IgE, which are not commonly seen in patients with ALHE [40].

Both diseases have a close clinical and histological resemblance to IgG4-RD and might be considered as being in the spectrum of IgG4-RD.

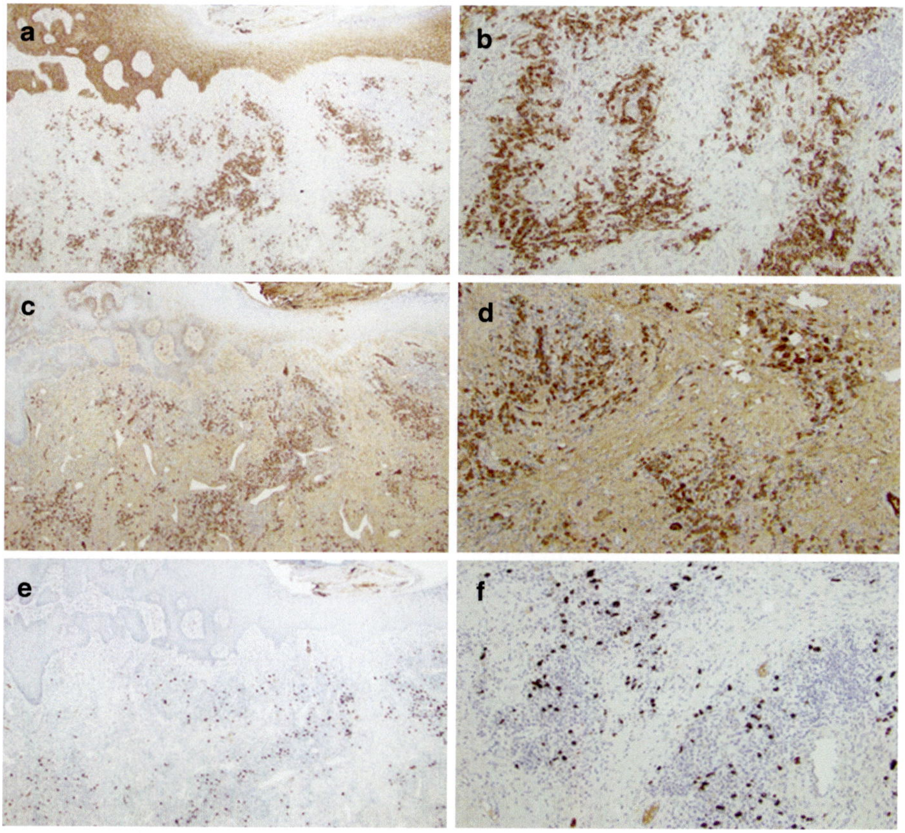

Fig. 6 Immunohistochemical stains for CD138 highlighting the plasma cells (**a**, 4× objective) (**b**, 10× objective), respectively; immunohistochemical stains for IgG+ (**c**, 4× objective) (**d**, 10× objective), respectively; immunohistochemical stains for IgG4+ (**e**, 4× objective) (**f**, 10× objective), respectively, showing that there is a subset of plasma cells express IgG4+ but they do not exceed 200 cells in HPF nor express more than 40% of the IgG+ cells

Eosinophilic Angiocentric Fibrosis

Eosinophilic angiocentric fibrosis is a rare, indolent lesion that affects the mucosa of the upper respiratory tract, sinonasal cavity, and orbit. A previous history of allergy, surgery, or trauma in the same location is common. It affects males and females equally and presents as a tan-white submucosal mass. Histologic examination shows a perivascular eosinophilic vasculitis with variable numbers of other inflammatory cells such as plasma cells and lymphocytes. There are zones of "onion-skinning" fibrosis, and an increased IgG4+/IgG+ ratio and high serum IgG4 levels are common [41]. The disease shares many features with IgG4-RD and is considered by many authors to represent IgG4-RD in the nasal and paranasal sinuses [42]. Surgical excision is the first-line treatment, with some success reported from using corticosteroids.

Granuloma Faciale and Erythema Elevatum Diutinum

Granuloma faciale (GF) is an uncommon, benign inflammatory skin disease with unknown pathogenesis [43]. It presents with well-defined red-brown to violaceous papules, nodules, and plaques, most commonly seen in middle-aged males as a solitary lesion. The histologic changes consist of small vessel vasculitis, concentric fibrosis, and an inflammatory cell infiltrate of plasma cells, eosinophils, and lymphocytes separated from the overlying uninvolved epidermis by a *grenz* zone [44]. The infiltrate is often prominent, and there is overlap with entities such as acute febrile neutrophilic dermatoses and arthropod bite reaction.

Erythema elevatum diutinum (EED) is closely related to GF and presents as plaques, papules, or nodules in ill patients on the dorsum of the joints. It appears as a leukocytoclastic vasculitis with storiform fibrosis. There is a debate whether GF and EED should be considered as variants of IgG4-RD, and several studies support the idea since GF and EED have an elevation of IgG4+ plasma cells with high IgG4/IgG ratios in a subset (24%) of cases [45]. At the same time, the criteria for diagnosis were not always fulfilled [46]. Also, there is a lack of systemic involvement, which is commonly seen in IgG4-RSD.

Multicentric Castleman Disease (MCD)

Castleman disease is a rare distinctive lymphoepithelial disease characterized by lymphoid hyperplasia, most commonly in the mediastinum of middle-aged people. There are three general histologic patterns: hyaline vascular type, plasma cell-rich variant, and mixed hyaline vascular plasma cell type. Based on clinical presentation, Castleman disease has been divided into unicentric and multicentric forms. The multicentric or systemic form presents with generalized lymphadenopathy [47]. Two main etiologies have been proposed, immune dysregulation and viral infection of herpes virus (HHV-8).

MCD patients present with systemic symptoms and laboratory abnormalities with fever, erythematous plaques, and nodules, high CRP, and elevated interleukin −6 [48, 49]. The usual treatment for MCD is rituximab, with an overall poor prognosis.

The pathologic findings in MCD show sheets of regressive follicles, polytypic plasma cells with vascular proliferation [50]. There is extensive fibrosis, eosinophilia, possible elevation of IgG4, and IgG4+/IgG+ plasma cell ratio in the affected tissue.

Cutaneous involvement by Castleman disease is uncommon and includes features of vasculitis, erythroderma, and nodules composed of ill-defined lymphoid follicles in the deep dermis and subcutaneous tissue. There is increased vascular proliferation and fibrosis in an "onion-skinning" appearance, with interfollicular zones composed of lymphocytes and plasma cells.

IgG4-RSD is in the differential diagnosis, but IgG4- RSD has normal or slightly elevated IL-6 [48], whereas MCD has high CRP and IL-6. These findings, as well as lymph node involvement rather than pancreas or salivary gland, support Castleman disease rather than IgG4-RSD. Keeping in mind that even if the diagnostic criteria have been fulfilled for IgG4-RD but tissue sections show Castleman disease morphology, the diagnosis is considered Castleman disease [3].

Cutaneous Plasmacytosis

Cutaneous plasmacytosis is a rare skin disorder that presents with multiple red-brown papules and plaques that most commonly affect the trunk and the axilla and less likely the face and limbs. The disease is seen in Asian people and presents with lymphadenopathy [51]. Tissue sections show mild acanthosis and basal cell hyperpigmentation, with non-light chain-restricted superficial and deep perivascular and periadnexal mature plasma cells with lymphocytes, and scattered lymphoid aggregates [52]. Since there is an increase in IgG4-positive plasma cells reported in some cases [53], the possible relationship in pathogenesis between the two diseases has been raised; however, cutaneous plasmacytosis lacks systemic involvement and does not respond to corticosteroids. Besides, the ratio of IgG4/IgG plasma cells is usually <40% [54]. Treatment with psoralen and ultraviolet A therapy (PUVA) has been used with good response.

Other DD and Mimicker of IgG4-RSD

There is a broad spectrum of other diseases with clinicopathologic features that resembles this condition such as cutaneous marginal zone lymphoma, primary cutaneous plasmacytoma, Sjögren's disease, granulomatosis with polyangiitis, sarcoidosis, systemic lupus erythematosus, and Henoch–Schönlein purpura.

Etiopathogenesis

The pathogenesis of IgG4-RD remains uncertain, but there is evidence that the disease is autoimmune in nature, with a role for both B and T lymphocytes. The role of T lymphocytes has been widely studied since the discovery of the disease. T helper 2 cells, T regulatory cells, and T follicular helper cells have all been proposed to play a central role in the disease. Recently, CD4+ cytotoxic T lymphocytes (CD4 + CTLs) appear to play a major role in understanding the IgG4-RD physiology. It was shown that there is clonal expansion of CD4 + CTLs detected using next-generation sequencing. These cells are thought to be the main drivers of the fibrosis seen in IgG4-RD. The expansion of this cell population was found in the lesion and also in the peripheral blood of affected individuals [55]. These T cells produce granzyme B and perforin and IL-4-IL-5 causing eosinophilia and transforming growth factor-beta (TGF-B) and interferon-gamma (IFNγ), all of which are potentially important mediators of fibrosis and eosinophilia [56]. Interestingly, CD4+ CTLs appear to be increased in the peripheral blood during disease activity and taper down following treatment with rituximab-inducing remission [57]. It has recently been discovered that there is a significant increase in circulating PD-1 + CXCR5− and CXCL13, which are ligands for CXCR5 in affected patients. This study postulated its potential role of initiation of the inflammation [58]. Notably, IgG4 is less pathogenic than other subclasses of IgG because of its low ability to activate complement or bind to FCY receptors. Recent research suggests that peripheral eosinophilia seems to play a role in the duration of symptoms, the number of organs involved, and recurrence rates [59].

Therapy

The main goal of treatment is to reduce the inflammatory response and induce clinical remission. Having no randomized controlled study on the treatment of IgG4-RSD, the best optimal treatment is unknown. Generally, all symptomatic patients require treatment because regression without treatment is not observed. Glucocorticosteroids are considered first-line therapy. These patients typically follow an indolent course with a good response. For relapsed patients, mycophenolate mofetil, azathioprine, or methotrexate can be used alternatively. Other treatment options include rituximab (anti CD20) that has also shown a prompt clinical response in IgG4-RD patients [60]. Thalidomide could be considered as a therapeutic option in IgG4-RD with a good response [61]. The response to the previous treatments supports the autoimmune nature of the disease. In cases with massive fibrosis, surgical resection is recommended.

Prognosis and Course

The disease has a relapsing-remitting course; the majority of patients relapse especially after discontinuation of the therapy, which was seen in approximately one-third of patients treated with rituximab. The disease might recur with a risk for non-Hodgkin lymphomas and other epithelial malignancies [62].

Conclusion

IgG4- RSD is a newly emerging and increasingly recognized autoimmune fibro-inflammatory disease. The diagnosis of IgG4-RSD is challenging, and a high index of suspicion in conjunction with clinical correlation is essential. The disease should be considered in middle-aged Asian males presenting with papules and nodules in the head and neck area. Careful interpretation of the IgG4+ plasma cells correlating clinical, serological, and histological findings is essential to reach the appropriate diagnosis and avoid misinterpretation. An excisional biopsy is generally recommended to be able to examine more tissue and to rule out mimickers.

In this book chapter, we talked about the cutaneous and pathological manifestation of IgG4-RSD in addition to highlighting the most common differential diagnosis. Since IgG4-RSD is rare, a thorough clinical and histological investigation from dermatologists and dermatopathologists is required to reach the diagnosis.

References

1. Kubo K, Yamamoto K. IgG4-related disease. Int J Rheum Dis. 2016;19(8):747–62.
2. Ibrahim SH, Zhang L, Freese DK. A 3-year-old with immunoglobulin G4-associated cholangitis. J Pediatr Gastroenterol Nutr. 2011;53(1):109–11.
3. Umehara H, Okazaki K, Masaki Y, et al. Comprehensive diagnostic criteria for IgG4-related disease (IgG4-RD), 2011. Mod Rheumatol. 2012;22(1):21–30.
4. Himi T, Takano K, Yamamoto M, Naishiro Y, Takahashi H. A novel concept of Mikulicz's disease as IgG4-related disease. Auris Nasus Larynx. 2012;39(1):9–17.
5. Hamano H, Kawa S, Horiuchi A, et al. High serum IgG4 concentrations in patients with sclerosing pancreatitis. N Engl J Med. 2001;344(10):732–8.
6. Masaki Y, Dong L, Kurose N, et al. Proposal for a new clinical entity, IgG4-positive multiorgan lymphoproliferative syndrome: analysis of 64 cases of IgG4-related disorders. Ann Rheum Dis. 2009;68(8):1310–5.
7. Kamisawa T, Chari ST, Lerch MM, Kim MH, Gress TM, Shimosegawa T. Recent advances in autoimmune pancreatitis: type 1 and type 2. Gut. 2013;62(9):1373–80.
8. Geyer JT, Ferry JA, Harris NL, et al. Chronic sclerosing sialadenitis (Kuttner tumor) is an IgG4-associated disease. Am J Surg Pathol. 2010;34(2):202–10.
9. Inoue D, Zen Y, Abo H, et al. Immunoglobulin G4-related periaortitis and periarteritis: CT findings in 17 patients. Radiology. 2011;261(2):625–33.
10. Matsui S, Hebisawa A, Sakai F, et al. Immunoglobulin G4-related lung disease: clinicoradiological and pathological features. Respirology (Carlton, Vic). 2013;18(3):480–7.
11. Wick MR, O'Malley DP. Lymphadenopathy associated with IgG4-related disease: diagnosis & differential diagnosis. Semin Diagn Pathol. 2018;35(1):61–6.
12. Bennett AE, Fenske NA, Rodriguez-Waitkus P, Messina JL. IgG4-related skin disease may have distinct systemic manifestations: a systematic review. Int J Dermatol. 2016;55(11):1184–95.
13. Charrow A, Imadojemu S, Stephen S, Ogunleye T, Takeshita J, Lipoff JB. Cutaneous manifestations of IgG4-related disease (RD): a systematic review. J Am Acad Dermatol. 2016;75(1):197–202.
14. Sato Y, Notohara K, Kojima M, Takata K, Masaki Y, Yoshino T. IgG4-related disease: historical overview and pathology of hematological disorders. Pathol Int. 2010;60(4):247–58.

15. Della Torre E, Mattoo H, Mahajan VS, Carruthers M, Pillai S, Stone JH. Prevalence of atopy, eosinophilia, and IgE elevation in IgG4-related disease. Allergy. 2014;69(2):269–72.
16. Yamada K, Hamaguchi Y, Saeki T, et al. Investigations of IgG4-related disease involving the skin. Mod Rheumatol. 2013;23(5):986–93.
17. Wang KC, Liao HT, Tsai CY. IgG4-related disease coexisting with autoimmune haemolytic anaemia. BMJ Case Reports. 2018;2018:bcr2018224814.
18. Sulieman I, Mahfouz A, AlKuwari E, et al. IgG4-related disease mimicking pancreatic cancer: case report and review of the literature. Int J Surg Case Rep. 2018;50:100–5.
19. Tokura Y, Yagi H, Yanaguchi H, et al. IgG4-related skin disease. Br J Dermatol. 2014;171(5):959–67.
20. Miyazawa H, Fujita Y, Iwata H, et al. Two cases of generalized pustular psoriasis complicated by IgG4-related disease. Br J Dermatol. 2018;179(2):537–9.
21. Nastri MMF, Novak GV, Sallum AEM, Campos LMA, Teixeira RAP, Silva CA. Immunoglobulin G4-related disease with recurrent uveitis and kidney tumor mimicking childhood polyarteritis nodosa: a rare case report. Acta Reumatologica Portuguesa. 2018;43(3):226–9.
22. Sato Y, Takeuchi M, Takata K, et al. Clinicopathologic analysis of IgG4-related skin disease. Mod Pathol. 2013;26(4):523–32.
23. Kondo M, Yamamoto S, Goto H, Nara Y. Nodules behind the ears: IgG4-related skin disease. Br J Dermatol. 2016;175(5):1056–8.
24. Deshpande V, Zen Y, Chan JKC, et al. Consensus statement on the pathology of IgG4-related disease. Mod Pathol. 2012;25(9):1181–92.
25. Takayama R, Ueno T, Saeki H. Immunoglobulin G4-related disease and its skin manifestations. J Dermatol. 2017;44(3):288–96.
26. Clerc A, Reynaud Q, Durupt S, et al. Elevated IgG4 serum levels in patients with cystic fibrosis. PLoS One. 2017;12(9):e0181888.
27. Funakoshi T, Lunardon L, Ellebrecht CT, Nagler AR, O'Leary CE, Payne AS. Enrichment of total serum IgG4 in patients with pemphigus. Br J Dermatol. 2012;167(6):1245–53.
28. Lehman JS, Smyrk TC, Pittelkow MR. Increased immunoglobulin (Ig) G4–positive plasma cell density and IgG4/IgG ratio are not specific for IgG4-related disease in the skin. Am J Clin Pathol. 2014;141(2):234–8.
29. Stone JH, Brito-Zeron P, Bosch X, Ramos-Casals M. Diagnostic approach to the complexity of IgG4-related disease. Mayo Clin Proc. 2015;90(7):927–39.
30. Wallace ZS, Mattoo H, Carruthers M, et al. Plasmablasts as a biomarker for IgG4-related disease, independent of serum IgG4 concentrations. Ann Rheum Dis. 2015;74(1):190–5.
31. Pitak-Arnnop P, Bellefqih S, Chaine A, Dhanuthai K, Bertrand JC, Bertolus C. Head and neck lesions of Kimura's disease: exclusion of human herpesvirus-8 and Epstein-Barr virus by in situ hybridisation and polymerase chain reaction. An immunohistochemical study. J Craniomaxillofac Surg. 2010;38(4):266–70.
32. Kim GE, Kim WC, Yang WI, et al. Radiation treatment in patients with recurrent Kimura's disease. Int J Radiat Oncol Biol Phys. 1997;38(3):607–12.
33. Garcia Carretero R, Romero Brugera M, Rebollo-Aparicio N, Vazquez-Gomez O. Eosinophilia and multiple lymphadenopathy: Kimura disease, a rare, but benign condition. BMJ Case Reports. 2016;2016:bcr2015214211.
34. Adler BL, Krausz AE, Minuti A, Silverberg JI, Lev-Tov H. Epidemiology and treatment of angiolymphoid hyperplasia with eosinophilia (ALHE): a systematic review. J Am Acad Dermatol. 2016;74(3):506–12.e11.
35. Zarrin-Khameh N, Spoden JE, Tran RM. Angiolymphoid hyperplasia with eosinophilia associated with pregnancy: a case report and review of the literature. Arch Pathol Lab Med. 2005;129(9):1168–71.
36. D'Offizi G, Ferrara R, Donati P, Bellomo P, Paganelli R. Angiolymphoid hyperplasia with eosinophils in HIV infection. *AIDS (London, England)*. Jul. 1995;9(7):813–4.
37. Altman DA, Griner JM, Lowe L. Angiolymphoid hyperplasia with eosinophilia and nephrotic syndrome. Cutis. 1995;56(6):334–6; quiz 342

38. Mukherjee B, Kadaskar J, Priyadarshini O, Krishnakumar S, Biswas J. Angiolymphoid hyperplasia with eosinophilia of the orbit and adnexa. Ocular Oncol Pathol. 2015;2(1):40–7.
39. Fontana SC, Borgstadt A, Fraga GR, Reeves AR, Andrews BT. Angiolymphoid hyperplasia with eosinophilia within a vascular malformation: case report and review of the literature. Ann Otol Rhinol Laryngol. 2016;125(9):775–8.
40. Marka A, Cowdrey MCE, Carter JB, Lansigan F, Yan S, LeBlanc RE. Angiolymphoid hyperplasia with eosinophilia and Kimura disease overlap, with evidence of diffuse visceral involvement. J Cutan Pathol. 2019;46(2):138–42.
41. Rimmer J, Andrews P, Lund VJ. Eosinophilic angiocentric fibrosis of the nose and sinuses. J Laryngol Otol. 2014;128(12):1071–7.
42. Deshpande V. IgG4 related disease of the head and neck. Head Neck Pathol. 2015;9(1):24–31.
43. Ziemer M, Koehler MJ, Weyers W. Erythema elevatum diutinum - a chronic leukocytoclastic vasculitis microscopically indistinguishable from granuloma faciale? J Cutan Pathol. 2011;38(11):876–83.
44. Ortonne N, Wechsler J, Bagot M, Grosshans E, Cribier B. Granuloma faciale: a clinicopathologic study of 66 patients. J Am Acad Dermatol. 2005;53(6):1002–9.
45. Cesinaro AM, Lonardi S, Facchetti F. Granuloma faciale: a cutaneous lesion sharing features with IgG4-associated sclerosing diseases. Am J Surg Pathol. 2013;37(1):66–73.
46. Kavand S, Lehman JS, Gibson LE. Granuloma Faciale and erythema Elevatum Diutinum in relation to immunoglobulin G4-related disease: an appraisal of 32 cases. Am J Clin Pathol. 2016;145(3):401–6.
47. Wu D, Lim MS, Jaffe ES. Pathology of castleman disease. Hematol Oncol Clin North Am. 2018;32(1):37–52.
48. Takeuchi M, Sato Y, Takata K, et al. Cutaneous multicentric castleman's disease mimicking IgG4-related disease. Pathol Res Pract. 2012;208(12):746–9.
49. Uldrick TS, Polizzotto MN, Yarchoan R. Recent advances in Kaposi sarcoma herpesvirus-associated multicentric Castleman disease. Curr Opin Oncol. 2012;24(5):495–505.
50. Wang HW, Pittaluga S, Jaffe ES. Multicentric castleman disease: where are we now? Semin Diagn Pathol. 2016;33(5):294–306.
51. Uhara H, Saida T, Ikegawa S, et al. Primary cutaneous plasmacytosis: report of three cases and review of the literature. Dermatology. 1994;189(3):251–5.
52. Han XD, Lee SSJ, Tan SH, et al. Cutaneous plasmacytosis: a clinicopathologic study of a series of cases and their treatment outcomes. Am J Dermatopathol. 2018;40(1):36–42.
53. Miyagawa-Hayashino A, Matsumura Y, Kawakami F, et al. High ratio of IgG4-positive plasma cell infiltration in cutaneous plasmacytosis--is this a cutaneous manifestation of IgG4-related disease? Hum Pathol. 2009;40(9):1269–77.
54. Takeoka S, Kamata M, Hau CS, et al. Evaluation of IgG4+ plasma cell infiltration in patients with systemic plasmacytosis and other plasma cell-infiltrating skin diseases. Acta Derm Venereol. 2018;98(5):506–11.
55. Mattoo H, Mahajan VS, Maehara T, et al. Clonal expansion of CD4(+) cytotoxic T lymphocytes in patients with IgG4-related disease. J Allergy Clin Immunol. 2016;138(3):825–38.
56. Koike T. IgG4-related disease: why high IgG4 and fibrosis? Arthritis Res Ther. 2013;15(1):103.
57. Mattoo H, Stone JH, Pillai S. Clonally expanded cytotoxic CD4(+) T cells and the pathogenesis of IgG4-related disease. Autoimmunity. 2017;50(1):19–24.
58. Kamekura R, Yamamoto M, Takano K, et al. Circulating PD-1(+)CXCR5(−)CD4(+) T cells underlying the immunological mechanisms of IgG4-related disease. Rheumatol Adv Pract. 2018;2(2):rky043.
59. Zhang X, Zhang P, Li J, et al. Different clinical patterns of IgG4-RD patients with and without eosinophilia. Sci Rep. 2019;9(1):16483.
60. Perugino CA, Stone JH. Treatment of IgG4-related disease: current and future approaches. Z Rheumatol. 2016;75(7):681–6. Behandlung IgG4-bedingter Erkrankungen: Aktuelle und zukunftige Vorgehensweisen.

61. Ingen-Housz-Oro S, Ortonne N, Elhai M, Allanore Y, Aucouturier P, Chosidow O. IgG4-related skin disease successfully treated by thalidomide: a report of 2 cases with emphasis on pathological aspects. JAMA Dermatol. 2013;149(6):742–7.
62. Yamamoto M, Takahashi H, Tabeya T, et al. Risk of malignancies in IgG4-related disease. Mod Rheumatol. 2012;22(3):414–8.

Necrolytic Acral Erythema

Tatsiana Pukhalskaya and Bruce R. Smoller

Introduction

NAE was first described in 1996 by El Darouti and El Ela in Egypt, and the first case in the United States was reported in 2000 by V.J. Khanna [1, 2].

This skin condition has a strong association with hepatitis C virus (HCV) and is recognized as one of its early cutaneous markers, although NAE without HCV has also been reported [3–8]. In the United States, the prevalence of NAE among chronic HCV patients is very low [9]. This could be due to the difference of HCV genotypes seen in the United States compared with Egypt [9].

It is best categorized as a psoriasiform disease [1, 9]. This entity belongs to the family of necrolytic erythemas that include necrolytic migratory erythema, acrodermatitis enteropathica, pellagra, and essential fatty acid deficiencies [2, 10, 11]. These conditions are similar clinically and histologically but differ in their etiology. They are known to be linked to altered serum levels of various factors (glucagon, zinc, niacin, biotin, and fatty acids) [11]. NAE has also been associated with reduced amino acid, fatty acid, and zinc levels but differs from other necrolytic erythemas in its predominantly acral distribution and association with HCV [1, 2, 12–14]. It has also been described in a chronically immunosuppressed patient and following hepatitis B vaccination [5]. There is one case report featuring an HIV/HCV coinfected patient with NAE [15].

T. Pukhalskaya (✉) · B. R. Smoller
Department of Pathology and Laboratory Medicine, University of Rochester Medical Center (URMC), Rochester, NY, USA
e-mail: tatsiana_pukhalskaya@urmc.rochester.edu

F. Rongioletti, B. R. Smoller (eds.), *New and Emerging Entities in Dermatology and Dermatopathology*, https://doi.org/10.1007/978-3-030-80027-7_29

The age range of this condition is broad (12–60 years old) with 92% of patients being African in origin [2, 8–10]. This may be due to a reporting bias, with most early cases reported from Egypt. Remission and exacerbation of the disease occur spontaneously [10].

Clinical Features

As emphasized in its name, NAE is characterized by acral distribution with a predilection for the lower extremities, mostly toes, ankle, and the lateral malleolus [10]. Genitalia, buttocks, and the abdomen can also be involved, though much less frequently [10]. Lesions are commonly located on the dorsal surfaces of the extremities, although plantar, palmar, and nail involvement should not exclude this diagnosis [6, 12, 16]. The periorificial area and oral mucosa are usually spared, in contrast to other necrolytic erythemas [12].

The lesions are commonly pruritic and based on their evolution could be grouped into three phases: initial, fully developed, and late stages [10]. The earliest changes on the skin consist of small (2–3 mm) erythematous papules (Fig. 1). They become scaly and develop superficial erosions. With time, the papules increase in size and thickness and show a diminished amount of erythema with increasing hyperpigmentation (Fig. 2a). More chronic lesions appear as erythematous to violaceous plaques with thick scale, erosions and crusting and often have a dark red rim (Fig. 2b) [17]. These lesions may remain unchanged for months.

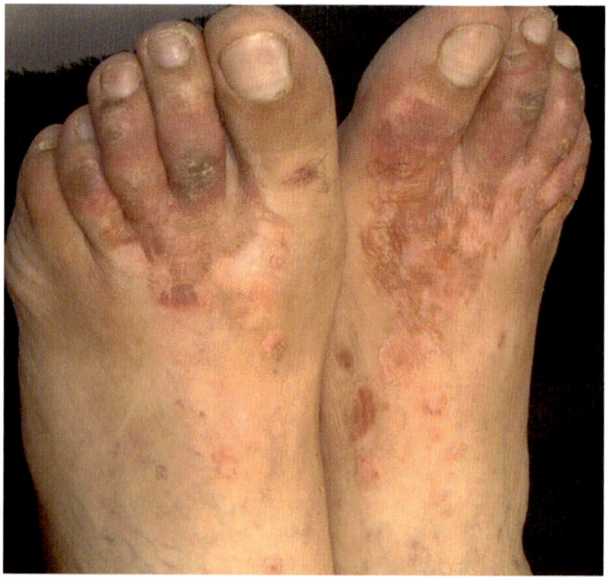

Fig. 1 Clinical picture of NAE showing early stages of the process

Fig. 2 Clinical pictures of NAE showing later stages of the process

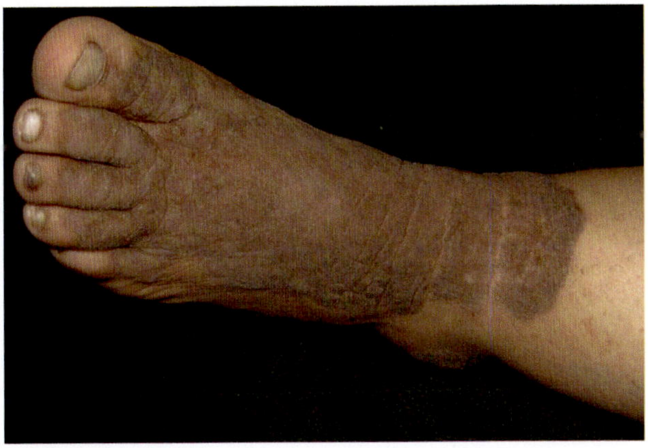

Histopathological Features

Histological examination of early NAE lesions commonly reveals a moderate degree of regular acanthosis with variable spongiosis and inflammation, progressing to a picture resembling nummular eczema or other acute spongiotic processes [8] (Fig. 3a). Associated findings include parakeratosis, focal hypergranulosis, subcorneal pustules, epidermal pallor, vascular ectasia, papillary dermal inflammation, and necrotic keratinocytes in the upper epidermis. The apoptotic keratinocytes can become confluent and lead to cleft formation [17]. In its fully developed form, the disease exhibits psoriasiform hyperplasia and prominent papillomatosis with parakeratosis, subcorneal pustules, epidermal pallor, and necrotic keratinocytes (Fig. 3b–e) [8]. The epidermal pallor is the classic identifying diagnostic feature (Fig. 3b and d). Pigment incontinence is seen in all stages [8]. Interestingly, epidermal spongiosis, reticular degeneration of superficial keratinocytes with dyskeratosis, and vacuolization might be absent, particularly in cases not associated with HCV [6, 16, 18]. Direct immunofluorescence (DIF) occasionally reveals IgG both in the nuclei of keratinocytes and in small vessels of the upper dermis [5]. In the same study, a few scattered C3-positive cytoid bodies were also noted in the dermal–epidermal junction, but this is a nonspecific finding [5].

Workup

Serum analysis may or may not reveal slight elevation of liver function, though no association between severity of hepatic disease and skin findings has been identified [10].

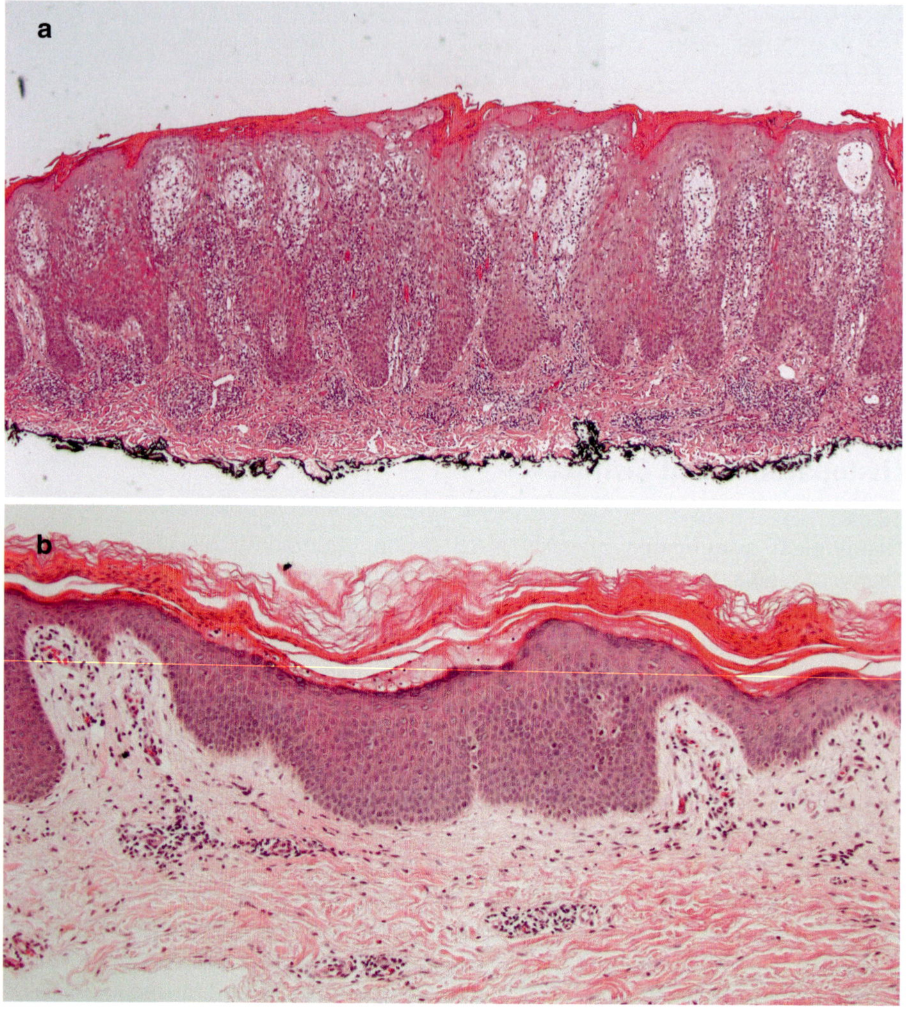

Fig. 3 Histological representation of NAE in different stages of the process

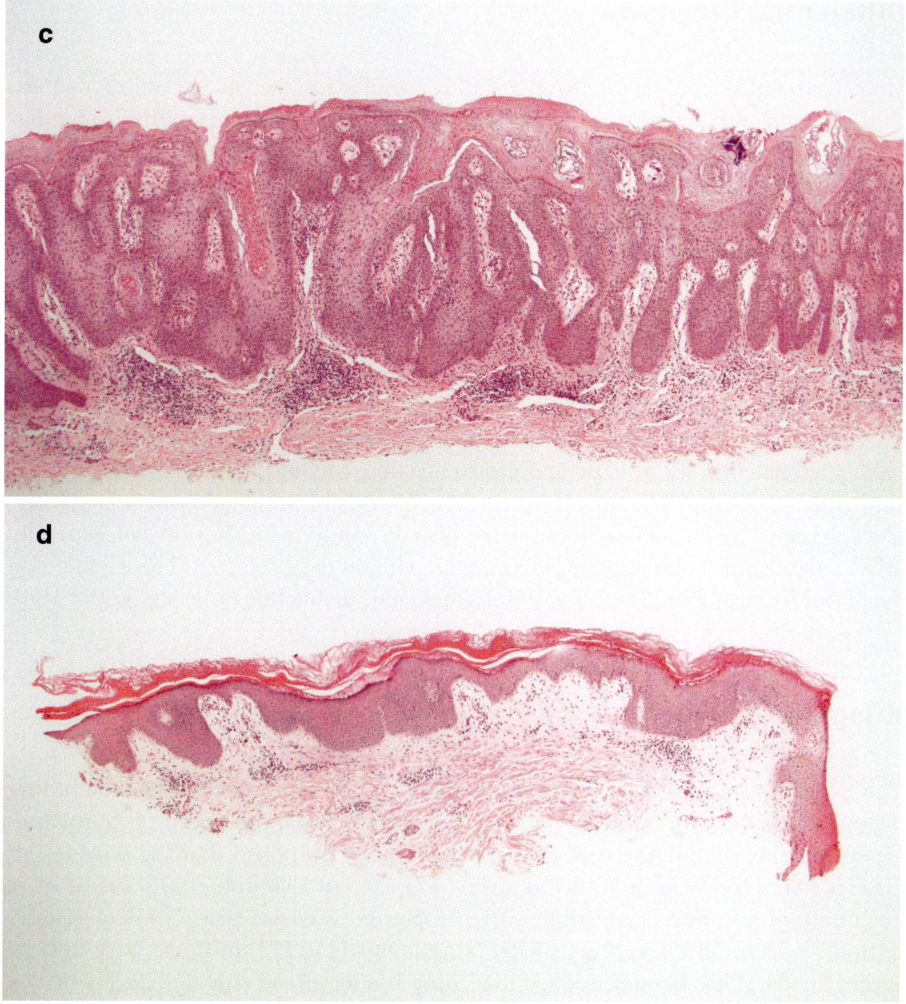

Fig. 3 (continued)

Differential Diagnosis

Since histological findings in NAE are often similar to other necrolytic erythemas, clinical exam and laboratory data are helpful in distinguishing this entity from other necrolytic erythemas [16]. Overall, NAE is most commonly mistaken for psoriasis, but the lack of clinical response to treatment and histology featuring dyskeratotic keratinocytes and epidermal pallor can help in distinguishing between these two entities [5]. Acrodermatitis enteropathica develops in association with systemic zinc deficiency. The eruption typically centers on orifices and has a more eczematous quality with ill-defined borders and more extensive erosion than NAE [10]. Diarrhea and failure to thrive accompany the skin findings. It is also found almost exclusively in a different demographic, most commonly seen in very young children. The rash seen in pellagra has a photodistributed pattern, with early erythema and erosion on the head, neck, upper chest, and distal arms with a characteristically rapid evolution to hyperpigmented patches. Neurologic and gastrointestinal findings are prominent. Another similar disease, necrolytic migratory erythema, arises in conjunction with pancreatic glucagonoma. Its cutaneous findings are also strikingly psoriasiform but generally involve the flexures and may be periorificial, without the strong acral distribution on the dorsal feet and toes. Serologic studies make this distinction quite straightforward.

Etiopathogenesis

The pathophysiology of NAE remains unknown. Several mechanisms including hepatocellular dysfunction, hyperglucagonemia, hypoaminoaciduria, hypoalbuminemia, zinc deficiency, and diabetes have been proposed, but the etiology of NAE appears likely to be multifactorial [17]. It may also potentially result from an immunologic defect of some sort [5]. Serum zinc level in NAE is usually normal, with only few reports of low zinc levels [11, 17]. In those with normal serum levels, it has been proposed that there is a localized zinc deficiency driven by chronic HCV infection [11, 14]. Zinc is antiapoptotic and serves as a cofactor in DNA replication, transcription, translation, and vitamin A metabolism in the liver. Zinc deficiency causes a reduction in serum transport proteins like retinol-binding protein and prealbumin, which impair delivery of nutrients such as vitamin A to tissues [7]. In addition, zinc appears to be primary and essential for the differentiation, proliferation, and survival of the epidermal keratinocytes [19].

The mechanism of HCV effects in relation to NAE is also not completely clear. Simmonds et al. concluded that the clinical picture of NAE depends upon the genotype of HCV [20]. M.A. El-Darouti et al. reported that patients with HCV presenting with leukocytoclastic vasculitis never develop NAE and vice versa. This group of scientists proposes that there are certain factors that influence the type of inflammatory skin reaction occurring in association with HCV infection [21].

Researchers have shown that viral load and not the specific HCV genotype plays a significant role in determining the response of the skin to HCV infection. High levels of HCV viremia significantly favor the development of leukocytoclastic vasculitis and not NAE. This statement could be supported by the lack of viral particles in the skin or vascular endothelium of NAE [21].

Therapy

In one study, topical corticosteroid application resulted in transient improvement in 4 of 19 patients [10]. Of the seven patients treated with systemic corticosteroids, two showed improvement with relapse upon discontinuation [10]. Interferon-α therapy was extremely effective in several patients [2]. Other data report the successful treatment of NAE with interferon in combination with either zinc or ribavirin [2, 12]. However, some reports note the recurrence of the NAE lesions after discontinuation of interferon treatment with relapse of NAE coinciding with worsening of liver disease/HCV viral load recovery [10, 22]. Sole supplementation with zinc is a commonly suggested method of treatment [6, 7, 11, 14, 16, 18]. A clinical response is often noted within several weeks of initiating therapy [2, 11, 12, 22]. The recommended dose is 440 mg/day divided in two doses [2, 13]. It is important to mention that blood levels of zinc prior to therapy have not shown correlation with the response. Zinc supplementation has been effective in patients without a notable systemic deficiency [18]. One case report demonstrated rapid improvement of NAE after discontinuation of oral steroid therapy in a patient without HCV [5]. Oral zinc therapy was ineffective in this patient. There is also a documented resolution of NAE following a liver transplant [9].

Prognosis and Course

Because of its rarity, there is no definite data regarding the prognosis of NAE. The course of the disease is highly variable and depends on the patient's response to the therapy and general state of health and underlying hepatitis.

Conclusions

NAE is a distinct clinical entity with characteristic clinical and histological features. It is a cutaneous marker of HCV infection, although not all cases are associated with HCV. NAE has complex and multifactorial pathophysiology that most likely involves alterations in zinc metabolism. Although normal results do not exclude possibility of NAE, testing for HCV and serum zinc levels is recommended in suspected cases. Treatment of underlying hepatitis and oral zinc therapy might be effective in achieving a sustainable resolution of the lesions, irrespective of zinc levels.

References

1. el Darouti M, Abu el Ela M. Necrolytic acral erythema: a cutaneous marker of viral hepatitis C. Int J Dermatol. 1996;35:252–6.
2. Khanna VJ, Shieh S, Benjamin J, Somach S, Zaim MT, Dorner W Jr, Shill M, Wood GS. Necrolytic acral erythema associated with hepatitis C: effective treatment with interferon alfa and zinc. Arch Dermatol. 2000;136:755–7.
3. Liu A, Erickson CP, Cockerell CJ, Hsu S. Necrolytic acral erythema: a case not associated with hepatitis C infection. Dermatol Online J. 2008;14:10.
4. Nikam BP. Necrolytic acral erythema seronegative for hepatitis C virus--two cases from India treated with oral zinc. Int J Dermatol. 2009;48:1096–9.
5. Wu YH, Tu ME, Lee CS, Lin YC. Necrolytic acral erythema without hepatitis C infection. J Cutan Pathol. 2009;36:355–8.
6. Panda S, Lahiri K. Seronegative necrolytic acral erythema: a distinct clinical subset? Indian J Dermatol. 2010;55:259–61.
7. Das A, Kumar P, Gharami RC. Necrolytic acral erythema in the absence of hepatitis C virus infection. Indian J Dermatol. 2016;61:96–9.
8. Abdallah MA, Ghozzi MY, Monib HA, Hafez AM, Hiatt KM, Smoller BR, Horn TD. Histological study of necrolytic acral erythema. J Ark Med Soc. 2004;100:354–5.
9. Raphael BA, Dorey-Stein ZL, Lott J, Amorosa V, Lo Re V 3rd, Kovarik C. Low prevalence of necrolytic acral erythema in patients with chronic hepatitis C virus infection. J Am Acad Dermatol. 2012;67:962–8.
10. Abdallah MA, Ghozzi MY, Monib HA, Hafez AM, Hiatt KM, Smoller BR, Horn TD. Necrolytic acral erythema: a cutaneous sign of hepatitis C virus infection. J Am Acad Dermatol. 2005;53:247–51.
11. Najarian DJ, Lefkowitz I, Balfour E, Pappert AS, Rao BK. Zinc deficiency associated with necrolytic acral erythema. J Am Acad Dermatol. 2006;55:S108–10.
12. Hivnor CM, Yan AC, Junkins-Hopkins JM, Honig PJ. Necrolytic acral erythema: response to combination therapy with interferon and ribavirin. J Am Acad Dermatol. 2004;50:S121–4.
13. Abdallah MA, Hull C, Horn TD. Necrolytic acral erythema: a patient from the United States successfully treated with oral zinc. Arch Dermatol. 2005;141:85–7.
14. Najarian DJ, Najarian JS, Rao BK, Pappert AS. Hypozincemia and hyperzincuria associated with necrolytic acral erythema. Int J Dermatol. 2008;47:709–11.
15. Oikonomou KG, Sarpel D, Abrams-Downey A, Mubasher A, Dieterich DT. Necrolytic acral erythema in a human immunodeficiency virus/hepatitis C virus coinfected patient: a case report. World J Hepatol. 2019;11:226–33.
16. Bentley D, Andea A, Holzer A, Elewski B. Lack of classic histology should not prevent diagnosis of necrolytic acral erythema. J Am Acad Dermatol. 2009;60:504–7.
17. Nofal AA, Nofal E, Attwa E, El-Assar O, Assaf M. Necrolytic acral erythema: a variant of necrolytic migratory erythema or a distinct entity? Int J Dermatol. 2005;44:916–21.
18. Ghosh A, Aggarwal I, De A, Samanta A, Chatterjee G, Bala S, Biswas P, Chowdhary N. Zinc-responsive acral hyperkeratotic dermatosis-a novel entity or a subset of some wellknown dermatosis? Indian J Dermatol. 2015;60:136–41.
19. Ogawa Y, Kawamura T, Shimada S. Zinc and skin biology. Arch Biochem Biophys. 2016;611:113–9. https://doi.org/10.1016/j.abb.2016.06.003.

20. Simmonds P, Holmes EC, Cha TA, Chan SW, McOmish F, Irvine B, Beall E, Yap PL, Kolberg J, Urdea MS. Classification of hepatitis C virus into six major genotypes and a series of subtypes by phylogenetic analysis of the NS-5 region. J Gen Virol. 1993;74(Pt 11):2391–9.
21. El-Darouti MA, Mashaly HM, El-Nabarawy E, Eissa AM, Abdel-Halim MR, Fawzi MM, El-Eishi NH, Tawfik SO, Zaki NS, Zidan AZ, Fawzi M, Abdelaziz M, Fawzi MM, Shaker OG. Leukocytoclastic vasculitis and necrolytic acral erythema in patients with hepatitis C infection: do viral load and viral genotype play a role? J Am Acad Dermatol. 2010;63:259–65.
22. El-Ghandour TM, Sakr MA, El-Sebai H, El-Gammal TF, El-Sayed MH. Necrolytic acral erythema in Egyptian patients with hepatitis C virus infection. J Gastroenterol Hepatol. 2006;21:1200–6.

Reactive Granulomatous Dermatitis (Interstitial Granulomatous Dermatitis, Palisaded Neutrophilic and Granulomatous Dermatitis, and Variants)

Avrom Caplan, Karolyn A. Wanat, Joseph C. English 3rd, and Misha Rosenbach

Abbreviations

ANA	Antinuclear antibody
ANCA	Antineutrophil cytoplasmic antibody
CCP	Cyclic citrullinated peptide
D-IGD	Drug-induced interstitial granulomatous dermatitis
GA	Granuloma annulare
IFE	Immunofixation
IGD	Interstitial granulomatous dermatitis
IGDR	Interstitial granulomatous drug reaction
PNGD	Palisaded neutrophilic and granulomatous dermatitis
RA	Rheumatoid arthritis
RF	Rheumatoid factor
RGD	Reactive granulomatous dermatitis (RGD)
SFLC	Serum free light chain
SPEP	Serum protein electrophoresis
TNF	Tumor-necrosis factor

A. Caplan
The Ronald O. Perelman Department of Dermatology, NYU Grossman School of Medicine, New York, NY, USA
e-mail: Avrom.caplan@nyulangone.org

K. A. Wanat
Medical College of Wisconsin, Milwaukee, WI, USA
e-mail: kwanat@mcw.edu

J. C. English 3rd
University of Pittsburgh Medical Center, Pittsburgh, PA, USA
e-mail: englishjc@upmc.edu

M. Rosenbach (✉)
Perelman School of Medicine, University of Pennsylvania, Philadelphia, PA, USA
e-mail: Misha.rosenbach@pennmedicine.upenn.edu

F. Rongioletti, B. R. Smoller (eds.), *New and Emerging Entities in Dermatology and Dermatopathology*, https://doi.org/10.1007/978-3-030-80027-7_30

Introduction

First Description

Since the first report of subcutaneous bands in rheumatoid arthritis (RA) in 1965 [2] and necrotizing granulomas associated with systemic diseases in 1977 and 1978 [3, 4], the nomenclature and clinicopathologic descriptions of cutaneous reactive granulomatous processes has expanded, often leading to overlapping descriptions and confusion among clinicians and pathologists. Eventually termed IGD and PNGD, respectively, the question of whether these entities are distinct or whether they represent a disease spectrum has been a source of debate and discussion in the literature [3]. Further complicating the nomenclature of granulomatous processes, the term "interstitial granulomatous drug reaction" was introduced in 1998 to describe granulomatous eruptions with histologic findings distinct from that of drug-induced IGD [4].

Ultimately the concern when seeing a patient with these entities, or a pathology specimen with these features, is what that portends to the patient. With strict definitions and descriptions of each entity, clear differences emerge; however, the substantial overlap in disease association and clinicopathologic descriptions raises the question of whether this is distinction without difference. A reclassification of these entities was proposed in 2015 by Rosenbach and English [1]. They introduced the term "reactive granulomatous dermatitis" in order to highlight the many overlapping findings while still acknowledging distinct clinicopathologic findings within this larger category [1]. The authors termed these variants RGD–IGD type, RGD–PNGD type, and RGD–IGDR type [1]. An overview of the history and nomenclature of reactive granulomatous dermatitis is offered below, before proceeding with a review of epidemiology, clinical and histologic features, workup, and management of each variant of reactive granulomatous dermatitis.

Literature

The earliest acknowledged report of IGD was in 1965 when Dykman and colleagues described two patients with rheumatoid arthritis who developed "elongated subcutaneous granulomas" [2]. Clinically, these were linear, subcutaneous bands extending from the axilla to the flank with histology showing collagen degeneration, collections of histiocytes and fibroblasts infiltrating the collagen bundles, and areas with surrounding lymphocytes and plasma cells [2]. They termed this "linear subcutaneous bands of rheumatoid arthritis." Additional reports of similar clinicopathologic findings in patients with rheumatoid arthritis and other systemic diseases refer to "linear rheumatoid nodules" [5] and "linear granuloma annulare" [6]. In 1993, Ackerman introduced the term "interstitial granulomatous dermatitis with arthritis" to describe the clinicopathologic features separating this entity from interstitial granuloma annulare (GA) and introduced the "rope sign" as a cardinal clinical clue [7]. Subsequently, reports of "interstitial granulomatous dermatitis with cutaneous cords and arthritis" [8, 9], "interstitial granulomatous dermatitis with arthritis" [10], and, after Ackerman's description in 1993, "Ackerman syndrome" [11–13] were published. As these reports emerged, questions arose as to whether these entities were distinct from what was then termed "Churg–Strauss granulomas" or "cutaneous extravascular necrotizing granulomas" – which both later were consolidated under the spectrum of PNGD [9, 14, 15].

"Churg–Strauss granulomas" and "cutaneous extravascular necrotizing granulomas" were first described at the end of the 1970s and early 1980s [16–19] by Finen and Winkelmann. In a review of 27 patients in 1983, Finan and Winkelmann reported granulomatous lesions occurring in patients with a variety of systemic diseases. Histologic analysis demonstrated basophilic necrosis, vasculitis, and palisading granulomas, at times with vasculitis. They introduced the term "Churg–Strauss granulomas" for these lesions [16]. (Churg–Strauss granuloma and cutaneous extravascular necrotizing granulomas describe the same entity, the latter term used to distinguish these lesions from eruptions reported by Churg and Strauss in association with the systemic vasculitis syndrome that ultimately carried their name before being renamed as eosinophilic granulomatosis with polyangiitis [15, 20, 21].) In 1990, Finan proposed that Churg–Strauss granulomas and reports of "rheumatoid papules" should be considered together as the same reactive process [21] in a comment on a paper by Smith et al. in which they described a "rheumatoid papule" as having features of palisading granulomas and vasculitis.

In 1994, Chu et al. introduced PNGD as an umbrella term. In a report of nine patients with systemic disease and a symmetric papular eruption located mainly on the extremities, Chu et al. describe a spectrum of histologic findings ranging from vasculitis to palisaded neutrophilic and granulomatous infiltrates to late-stage fibrosis [14]. The authors suggest that these findings demonstrate PNGD that occurs along a spectrum to explain why prior reports of similar clinical lesions did not consistently show similar findings on histologic analysis [14]. This grouping was carried forward in a 1996 report using the term cutaneous extravascular necrotizing granuloma (Winkelmann granuloma) [22], after which PNGD emerged as the accepted nomenclature. This term was chosen as an umbrella term in a report of 7 additional cases, in which the authors describe a spectrum of disease findings that included many entities previously described: linear subcutaneous bands, interstitial granulomatous dermatitis with cutaneous cords and arthritis, rheumatoid papules, Churg–Strauss granuloma, superficial ulcerating rheumatoid necrobiosis, necrobiotic granuloma, palisading granuloma cutaneous extravascular necrotizing granuloma, and rheumatoid neutrophilic dermatitis [23].

When reviewing the history of RGD nomenclature and clinicopathologic descriptions, it is clear that confusion exists as to whether IGD and PNGD are distinct conditions or exist along a disease spectrum. Similar confusion exists regarding the classification of drug induced forms of interstitial granulomatous dermatitis. In 1998, Magro and colleagues reported on 20 patients with erythematous to violaceous plaques with additional histologic features of eosinophilia and interface dermatitis that differentiated these eruptions, which they termed IGDR, from IGD caused by medication use [4]. Further differentiating IGDR from IGD, Magro and colleagues also reported lymphoid atypia, present in the dermal infiltrate in many cases and in the basal layer and epidermis in others, mimicking mycosis fungoides [4]. Subsequent reports of drug-induced cases of IGD, which lacked the specific histologic features proposed by Magro as defining features of IGDR, and additional cases of IGDR itself continue to add to the confusion in the literature, and Rosenbach and English proposed grouping these two entities as drug-induced forms of RGD [1].

Epidemiology

The epidemiology of RGD–IGD type and RGD–PNGD type is similar, not surprising given the overlapping associations of each type with similar systemic diseases. Both IGD and PNGD have been reported in patients of all ages, though less commonly in pediatric populations [1, 24–29]. Among both adult and pediatric cases, female patients are affected more frequently in approximately a 3:1 ratio [1, 28, 29], owing to the association of RGD with systemic diseases that have a female predominance. The diseases most commonly reported in association with IGD (or RGD–IGD type) include inflammatory arthritis (rheumatoid and seronegative arthritis) and connective tissues diseases (systemic lupus erythematosus, undifferentiated connective tissue disease). Less commonly reported disease associations include hematologic disorders and solid organ malignancies and medications (leading to interstitial granulomatous drug eruption) [1, 30]. For the IGD type of RGD, inflammatory arthritis appears to be the strongest disease association [30].

PNGD (or RGD–PNGD type) is rarely reported outside of an underlying systemic disorder. Common diseases associated with PNGD include connective tissue diseases (systemic lupus erythematosus, systemic sclerosis, undifferentiated connective tissue disease, and Sjögren's syndrome), vasculitides (antineutrophil cytoplasmic antibody [ANCA]-associated vasculitis, mixed cryoglobulinemia, and erythema elevatum diutinum), inflammatory arthritis (rheumatoid arthritis in particular), lymphoproliferative disorders, and medications [1, 30]. The strongest association appears to be connective tissue disease [30]. Among pediatric patients, systemic lupus erythematosus has been highly associated with RGD [28]. Both IGD-type and PNGD-type RGD have also rarely been reported with a host of other conditions, including infections, celiac disease, sarcoidosis, diabetes, and ulcerative colitis [1].

RGD can be seen in the setting of flares or even stable long-standing systemic disease, but it may also herald a new diagnosis of systemic disorder, including on rare occasions malignancy [14, 23, 28, 31, 32]. Notably case reports and case series do not clearly establish whether RGD implies poorly controlled or flaring underlying disease, but in the authors' experience, these reactive processes are usually a sign of ongoing systemic inflammation, and in many cases, control of the underlying disease results in improvement of the cutaneous eruption.

Please see Table 1 for a list of diseases associated with RGD.

Table 1 Diseases reported in association with reactive granulomatous dermatitis [1]

Disease	Strength of association and RGD type
Connective tissue disease Systemic lupus erythematosus [12, 15, 26, 28, 29, 35, 40, 55–60], undifferentiated connective tissue disease [60–63], systemic sclerosis [29, 41, 64, 65], ANCA-associated vasculitis [15, 22, 25, 66, 67], erythema elevatum diutinum [68], Sjögren's syndrome [29, 41, 69], mixed cryoglobulinemia [8, 70], Takayasu arteritis [22, 71]	Strong association with RGD More frequently associated with RGD–PNGD type
Inflammatory arthritis Rheumatoid arthritis [15, 23, 29, 33, 35, 39, 60, 61, 67, 71–83], seronegative arthritis [33, 84–90], ankylosing spondylitis [91]	Strong association with RGD More frequently associated with RGD–IGD type
Hematologic and lymphoproliferative disorders [14, 15, 23, 28, 29, 31–33, 35, 46, 47, 49–51, 92–102] Including IgA gammopathy, anemia and thrombocytopenia, chronic myelomonocytic leukemia, chronic lymphocytic leukemia, lymphoma, marginal zone lymphoma, multiple myeloma, myelodysplastic syndrome, myelodysplasia with leukemic progression, leukemia, polycythemia vera	Reports exist for both RGD–PNGD and RGD–IGD types
Solid organ malignancies [11, 29, 33, 51, 103, 104] Including breast, colon, endometrial, esophageal, lung, prostate	Weak association, more frequently reported in RGD–IGD type
Other Autoimmune hepatitis [29, 105, 106], autoimmune thyroiditis [29, 35, 69, 107, 108], sarcodisis [37, 109–111], ulcerative colitis [15, 50, 112, 113], celiac disease and type 1 diabetes mellitus [35, 114], Behcet's disease [42], pernicious anemia [29], polymyositis [29], multiple sclerosis [41], uveitis [27], vitiligo [29, 35], chronic inflammatory demyelinating polyneuropathy [115], antiphospholipid antibody syndrome [116], primary biliary cirrhosis [117]	Weak association, reports exist more commonly with RGD–PNGD type, but these are best approached under the umbrella term RGD
Infections Cellulitis (in a patient with SLE) [15, 54]; subacute bacterial endocarditis [15, 29]; hepatitis [70]; streptococcal infection [54]; AIDS [118]; borreliosis [119]; erythema migrans (in a patient with a history of autoimmune thyroiditis) [120]; pulmonary coccidiomycosis [121, 122]; pulmonary silicosis [123]; hand, foot, and, mouth disease [29]; parovirus B19 and human herpesvirus 6 [29]	

(continued)

Table 1 (continued)

Disease	Strength of association and RGD type
Medications[a] Tumor necrosis factor inhibitors [39, 72, 124], allopurinol [125], tocilizumab (in a patient with adult-onset Still's disease and articular involvement [126] and a patient with antisynthetase syndrome [127]), TNF inhibitors [53, 78, 79], Soy [128], angiotensin converting enzyme inhibitors [129], furosemide [129], hydrochlorothiazide [130], programmed death 1 (PD-1[b]) immune checkpoint inhibitors [131, 132], talimogen laherparepvec [133]	More commonly associated with RGD–PNGD type More commonly associated with RGD–IGD type

Adapted from Rosenbach and English [1]. With permission from Elsevier

Abbreviations: *RGD* Reactive granulomatous dermatitis, *PNGD* palisaded neutrophilic and granulomatous dermatitis, *IGD* interstitial granulomatous dermatitis

[a]This table excludes medications more specifically reported with features of IGDR; however, significant overlap exists in the literature

[b]Immune checkpoint inhibitor associated granulomatous eruptions present more commonly as sarcoid-like eruptions

Clinical Features

With strict definitions of RGD subtype, classic presentations are noted for IGD and PNGD that draw distinctions between these entities. Over time, however, the clinical spectrum of RGD has continued to expand, and multiple morphologies have been described, often leading to overlap between the subtypes.

IGD Variant

The initial description of IGD was of linear, subcutaneous cords on the proximal trunk in a patient with rheumatoid arthritis [2]. Subsequent reports of similar lesions led to the term "rope-sign" to describe what was felt to be a classic finding in IGD [1, 7–9, 11, 12, 29, 30, 33, 34]. As the clinical spectrum of IGD has expanded, reports have documented this "classic" sign of IGD in less than 5%–10% of cases [29, 33] (Fig. 1). Additional reports of morphology include papules and plaques [10], plaques and macules at time in an annular array [10, 11, 29, 35], nodules [10, 11], and skin-colored papules [33]. The distribution of lesions is often symmetric on the trunk, proximal inner arms, and proximal thighs [1, 29, 33]. Atypical locations such as involvement of head and neck, umbilicus, or buttock have been reported [1, 29, 36]. IGD is usually asymptomatic though can burn or itch [1, 33, 35].

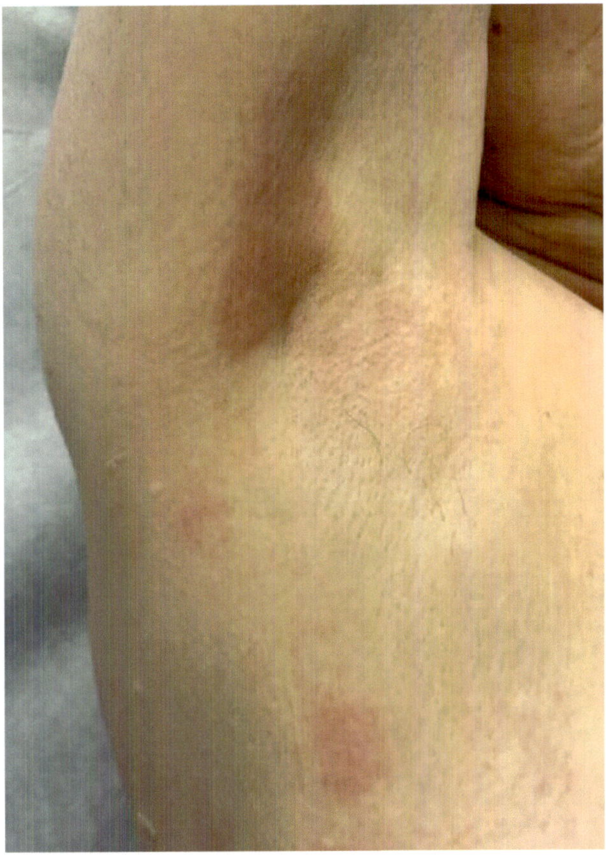

Fig. 1 Reactive granulomatous dermatitis: interstitial granulomatous dermatitis type. Linear erythematous cords or plaques, typically on the trunk or proximal extremities

PNGD Variant

Classically, PNGD presents as erythematous or flesh-colored papules, at times crusted or umbilicated, occurring symmetrically on the elbows and knees [1, 14, 15, 30] (Fig. 2). However, as with IGD, the clinical spectrum of PNGD has expanded since initial reports [30]. Annular or urticarial plaques [23, 29], erythematous nodules [37, 38], violaceous patches and plaques [39], and linear bands have been reported [23, 40]; however, some authors have grouped together IGD with PNGD [14, 21, 23] suggesting that the clinical spectrum includes lesions at different stages of development [1]. Extending beyond the classic location of elbows and knees, PNGD lesion location is also reported to occur symmetrically on the limbs (upper extremities more common) and trunk [1, 23, 29]. Less common locations include the face and scalp [41] and legs [42]. PNGD lesions can be associated with tenderness [29, 37, 38].

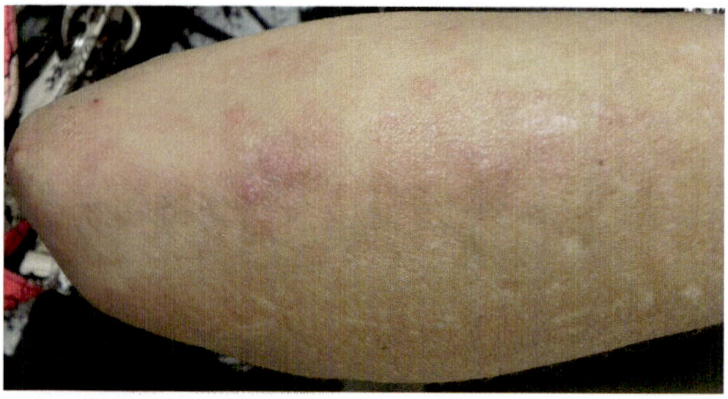

Fig. 2 Reactive granulomatous dermatitis: palisaded neutrophilic and granulomatous dermatitis type. Erythematous papules, sometimes crusted, classically located near the elbows

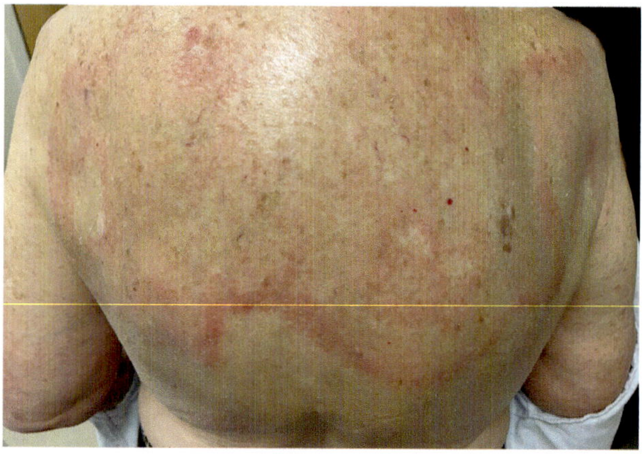

Fig. 3 Reactive granulomatous dermatitis: polycyclic variant (granuloma annulare like). There are erythematous indurated rings and arcuate plaques, often thicker than typical granuloma annulare bands

Granuloma Annulare-like Variant

As noted, there may be both clinical and histological overlap in the presentation of reactive granulomatous cutaneous processes. While less well described than either the IGD-like or PNGD-like variants, the authors have observed a large number of patients presenting with atypical polycyclic plaques, which may clinically resemble granuloma annulare (although these patients typically have broader, thicker rings), but histologically lack mucin and more closely resemble IGD-type changes. Given the suggested overarching term of reactive granulomatous dermatitis, the authors have proposed that these atypical, GA-like polycyclic- thick ringed can also be considered within the spectrum of RGD (Fig. 3). Diffuse plaques of RGD with near erythroderma may also be seen.

IGDR

In the report by Magro et al., IGDR was described in 20 patients with erythematous to violaceous plaques that were annular and located predominantly on the inner arms, proximal thighs, trunk, and intertriginous sites [4]. They reported distinct histologic features (see *Histopathology* section). As with IGD and PNGD, an expanded clinical spectrum has been reported over time, with many publications overlapping IGDR with drug-induced IGD [1]. Given the lack of consensus as to whether drug-induced IGD and IGDR are truly separate entities and in the setting of both eruptions necessitating a thorough review of medication exposures, Rosenbach and English in 2015 argued that these entities should be grouped as drug-induced forms of RGD [1].

Histopathological Features

Histologic patterns and criteria have been described that draw distinctions between IGD, PNGD, and IGDR (the "floating sign" of IGD, vasculitis in PNGD, basal vacuolar degeneration, eosinophilia, and lymphoid atypia in IGDR). However, as with the clinical findings, histologic features of RGD at times overlap and therefore may be best considered as IGD, PNGD, or IGDR variants of RGD associated with similar systemic diseases [43].

IGD Variant

When first termed IGD with arthritis by Ackerman in 1993, the histologic findings felt to be most representative of this entity (and which most differentiated this from interstitial granuloma annulare) included the following: histiocytes distributed in an interstitial, diffuse, or palisading fashion; scant mucin; eosinophils and neutrophils; atypical nuclei and sometimes mitotic figures; rosettes of histiocytes around discrete bundles of degenerated collagen; no multi-nucleate histiocytes; and a bottom-heavy distribution of the granulomatous infiltrate [7]. An additional characteristic finding of IGD is the "floating sign" [1, 33]. This is a visible cleft between histiocyte rosettes and degenerated collagen that is seen in up to 2/3 of patients with IGD patterns on biopsy [33]. Other histologic findings in IGD include predominance of CD68 positive macrophages infiltrating collagen bundles in the mid- and deep dermis and macrophages surrounded by degenerated collagen fibers [33]. With additional reports over time, these patterns came to more specifically characterize IGD and set it apart from both interstitial GA [23] and PNGD, though subsequent authors continue to draw attention to the overlapping spectrum of histologic findings [29] (Fig. 4).

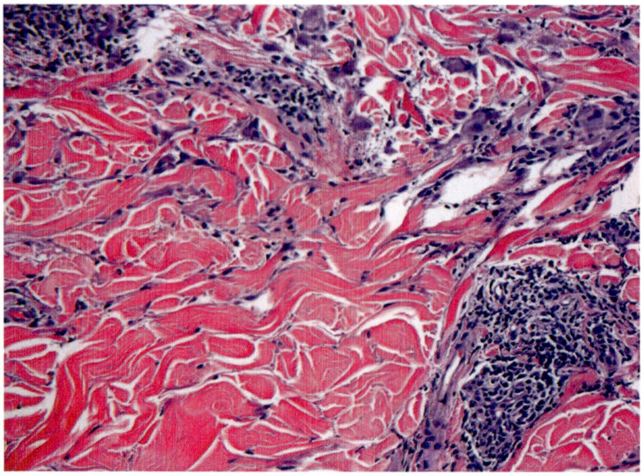

Fig. 4 Reactive granulomatous dermatitis histology: interstitial granulomatous dermatitis predominant features. This specimen shows aggregates of histiocytes forming small granulomas around altered collagen fragments, with scant to absent mucin, characteristic of IGD. Other sections of the biopsy demonstrated more prominent neutrophils with leukocytoclasis (not shown) with some concentration around small vessels, more characteristic of PNGD histology. Some patients may have overlapping features either at one time point, or in specimens taken at multiple timepoints over the course of their disease

PNGD Variant

Histologic findings in PNGD may vary in part depending on the age of the lesion [14]. Early lesions may demonstrate leukocytoclastic vasculitis with dense neutrophilic infiltrates and degenerated collagen, whereas more developed lesions can show palisaded granulomas surrounding leukocytoclastic debris, fibrin, and altered collagen [14]. Late lesions demonstrate dermal fibrosis and scant neutrophilic debris [14]. Additional reports of PNGD reflect these findings and support a histologic evolution of disease [1, 23]. Mucin is rare, helping to distinguish PNGD from GA. As noted above, vasculitis is a prominent finding in PNGD and not IGD. (A single report of vasculitis in IGD fails to include histologic images for evaluation [1, 12, 33]). Similarly, the "floating sign" is described in IGD, but not PNGD. Interface dermatitis and vacuolar degeneration have been rarely reported in cases of RGD without a clear association with medication exposure; yet as discussed below, these histopathological findings, along with eosinophilia or atypical lymphocytosis, should prompt a thorough medication review [29].

Interstitial Granulomatous Drug Reaction

In their report describing IGDR, Magro and colleagues define clinical and key histologic features of this reactive granulomatous process. Histologic features of IGDR include diffuse interstitial histiocytes with granulomas including rare giant cells, surrounding piecemeal fragmentation of collagen, and scant mucin with absent vasculitis. However, unlike the other entities described previously, IGDR should include basal vacuolar degeneration and areas of dyskeratotic keratinocytes and prominent tissue eosinophilia; lymphocyte atypia was also noted [1, 4]. The most commonly implicated medications included angiotensin-converting enzyme inhibitors, lipid-lowering agents, beta-blockers, and calcium-channel blockers [4].

Workup

One of the key drivers behind the suggested unifying term, RGD, is that regardless of subtype, the suggested evaluation for patients with RGD is similar whether addressing IGD, PNGD, or IGDR variants. This evaluation should include a thorough review of patient medications and an evaluation for systemic diseases. These diseases include autoimmune disease, inflammatory arthritis, malignancy, and occult infections [1]. A medication review should include inquiries about supplements and medication classes that in particular have been associated with RGD (calcium channel blockers, beta-blockers, angiotensin-converting enzyme inhibitors, and statins) (Table 2). As granulomatous inflammation can be slow to develop, patients may not realize that even medications they have been on for months may induce RGD and drug cessation trials may require months to observe resolution.

Table 2 Medications associated with interstitial granulomatous drug reaction (IGDR) or drug-induced interstitial granulomatous dermatitis (D-IGD) [1]

Reaction	Drug
Interstitial granulomatous drug reaction	Calcium channel blockers [4], bosutinib (in a patient with chronic myelogenous leukemia) [134], beta-blockers [4], angiotensin converting enzyme (ACE) inhibitors [4, 135, 136], hydrochlorothiazide [130], lipid-lowering agents [4], brompheniramine [4], ranitidine [4], bupropion [4], furosemide [4], sennoside [137], Chinese herbal medication [138], trastuzumab [139], thalidomide [140], allopurinol [141], tocilizumab [126, 127], quetiapine [142], programmed death 1 (PD-1) immune checkpoint inhibitors [131, 132], talimogen laherparepvec [133]
Drug-induced interstitial granulomatous dermatitis	Intranasal desmopressin [143], tumor necrosis factor-inhibitors [53, 78, 79], soy [128], ACE inhibitors [129], furosemide [129], hydrochlorothiazide [130]
Borderline/ indeterminate	Atorvastatin [144], sorafenib [145], anakinra [146], adalimumab [147], gabapentin [148], ganciclovir [149], Chinese herbal medication [150, 151], febuxostat [152], strontium ranelate [153]

Adapted from Rosenbach and English [1]. With permission from Elsevier

If publication included histologic description consistent with true IGDR, classified as IGDR; if publication reported a reaction as IGDR but it lacked features of IGDR as described by Magro and colleagues [4], classified as IGD; if publication reported partial features of IGD/IGDR classified as borderline/indeterminate

Laboratory analysis should include tests for the following:

1. Connective tissue disease testing: Antinuclear antibody testing (ANA), antineutrophil cytoplasmic antibody (ANCA), and additional testing as indicated by symptoms. For example, laboratory testing for antibodies to double-stranded DNA, anti-Ro (SS-A) and anti-La (SS-B) antibodies, topoisomerase-I (Scl-70) antibodies, anticentromere antibodies, or anti-RNA polymerase III antibodies can be checked depending on concerns for systemic lupus erythematosus, Sjögren's syndrome, or systemic sclerosis, respectively.

   Additional testing for autoimmune disease may be considered based on patient signs and systems. For example, patients with abnormal liver biochemical testing and/or who develop nonspecific fatigue, pruritus, or jaundice may require evaluation with anti-smooth muscle antibody or anti-mitochondrial antibody testing or other autoantibody testing for autoimmune hepatitis. Patients with abnormal thyroid screening may require evaluation for autoimmune thyroiditis. Patients may require celiac workup if presenting with signs and symptoms of celiac disease (e.g., diarrhea and weight loss). Importantly, clinicians should keep in mind that many autoimmune diseases have been associated with RGD and patients may present with early or nonspecific symptoms. Close communication with colleagues in various specialties is often necessary to fully evaluate patients in the setting of RGD. As there are continuous new reports added to the literature about rare potential underlying triggers of RGD, clinicians are encouraged to tailor the workup to the individual patient and their signs and symptoms. In recalcitrant cases, a more thorough investigation for underlying triggers or disease associations may be necessary.
2. Testing for arthritis with rheumatoid factor (RF) and cyclic citrullinated peptide (CCP) antibody test should be included for all patients with RGD, especially for those with IGD-type RGD. While RF-negative RA is rare and the presence of RGD is normally a sign of active disease, in select cases where clinical suspicion for inflammatory arthritis remains high but serologic testing is negative, imaging (plain films, MRI, and others) and/or referral to a rheumatologist may be warranted.
3. All patients should be up to date with malignancy screening. For atypical presentations of RGD or for patients who are older (generally 65 and older), extended testing can be considered. Extended testing can include serum protein electrophoresis with immunofixation (SPEP/IFE) and serum free light chain (SFLC) testing, complete blood counts with differentials, and chest radiography to evaluate for lymphadenopathy. Patients with RGD and with atypical manifestations of granulomatous eruptions warrant careful evaluation for potential underlying malignancy [17, 44–52].
4. Additional testing as indicated by symptoms including chest radiography to evaluate for lymphoma or occult infections or other testing including hepatitis, blood cultures, or echocardiography for endocarditis evaluation [30].

Please see Table 3 for a review of testing in RGD.

Table 3 Initial evaluation of patients with RGD [1]

Evaluate for systemic diseases	Autoimmune connective tissue disease evaluation	ANA, ANCA, dsDNA, anti-Ro/La, anti-Scl70, anticentromere Additional evaluation based on patient signs and symptoms Referral to Rheumatology
	Arthritis	RF, CCP Referral to rheumatology Radiography based on patient signs and symptoms
	Malignancy	Age-appropriate cancer screenings CBC with differential SPEP/IFE and SFLC
	Other	Chest radiography Evaluation for occult infection
Evaluate for drug induced RGD	Review patient medications	Review supplements, diet, herbal medications CCBs, BBs, ACE inhibitors, statins If none of these are present, review for less frequently associated medications
Management	General	Skin biopsy Medication cessation trial of at least 3 months duration if indicated Control associated systemic condition
	RGD-specific	Monitoring Topical or intralesional corticosteroids NSAIDs Dapsone Hydroxychloroquine Systemic corticosteroids Additional agents can be considered if needed

Adapted from Rosenbach and English [1]. With permission from Elsevier
Abbreviations: ACE inhibitor angiotensin converting enzyme inhibitor, *ANA* antinuclear antibody, *ANCA* anti-neutrophilic cytoplasmic antibodies, *BB* B-blocker, *CBC* complete blood count, *CCB* calcium channel blocker, *CCP* cyclic citrullinated peptide, *dsDNA* double-stranded DNA, *IFE* immunofixation electrophoresis, *NSAIDs* nonsteroidal anti-inflammatory drugs, *RGD* reactive granulomatous dermatitis, *RF* rheumatoid factor, *SFLC* serum free light chains, *SPEP* serum protein electrophoresis

Differential Diagnosis

The clinical differential diagnosis of IGD and PNGD is largely driven by the particular morphology of the presenting eruption (and possibly by the evolution of disease along a clinical spectrum, as has been suggested primarily with PNGD).

The classic morphology of PNGD with papules and nodules on the elbows may appear similar to papular granuloma annulare or rheumatoid nodules. PNGD may overlap or appear clinically similar to interstitial granuloma annulare. For patients who have atypical clinical or histologic features, a differential diagnosis may include Sweet's syndrome or other neutrophilic dermatoses. Leukemia cutis can be considered in the differential as well based on clinical or atypical histopathological features. Clinical features of IGD may appear similar to patch granuloma annulare, morphea, urticarial vasculitis, sarcoidosis, or cutaneous T-cell lymphoma among other clinical entities. While the "rope sign" of IGD is considered a classic clinical exam finding, this occurs in less than 5%–10% of patients [29, 33], and thrombotic events such as Mondor's disease can closely mimic this. Additionally, other cutaneous reactive granulomatous processes that are not included within the classic framework of RGD presented in this chapter may be considered in the differential diagnosis. Generalized granulomatous dermatitis in the setting of myelodysplasia, generalized-GA-like polymorphic eruptions, and drug reactions such as checkpoint inhibitor-induced granulomatous reactions and BRAF-inhibitor granulomatous eruption may all share some features with RGD and can be considered in the clinical and histologic differential [1] or, alternatively, may suggest that the concept of RGD as an umbrella term be extended to encompass these findings as well.

Etiopathogenesis

The etiopathogenesis of RGD remains unknown; however, as these eruptions occur largely in the setting of a systemic disease or medication, many feel that underlying inflammation results in a systemic immune dysfunction [1]. As the literature alternately draws distinctions or groups these reactive granulomatous processes, a true understanding of the etiopathogenesis remains unclear [1]. IGD may be a result of immune complex deposition in dermal vessels, resulting in inflammation, collagen damage, and granulomatous reactions [1, 35]. PNGD may similarly be a result of immune complex deposition [14, 15]. This may lead to vasculitis, collagen damage, granulomatous inflammation, and fibrosis evolving along a spectrum [14, 29]. Further work is necessary to clarify the etiopathogenesis of RGD; over time, if there are different immune signatures of the RGD subtypes, it may be prudent to revisit the proposed terminology and subdivide these entities based on those findings.

Therapy

The primary treatment strategy for RGD is to identify and manage the underlying systemic disease or identify and remove the medication trigger. Some cases of RGD may spontaneously resolve [29, 33, 41, 43]; therefore, treatment strategies should target symptoms and address control of the underlying disease. RGD can precede, occur simultaneously, or follow a flare or diagnosis of a systemic disease; however, obtaining control of the systemic disease may also control the skin. Depending on the systemic disease, treatment options include colchicine, dapsone, hydroxychloroquine, methotrexate, cyclosporine, corticosteroids, and tumor-necrosis factor (TNF) inhibitors [1]. TNF inhibitors have also been rarely implicated in causing RGD and should be considered as part of an evaluation of potential triggers if patients are already on this class of medication [53]. This class of medication may not be used as initial treatment of RGD alone, although may be indicated for the treatment of the associated underlying disease [1]. Drug cessation trials should be continued for 3 months prior to assessing for response [30].

Prognosis and Course

The prognosis and course of RGD is variable and may depend on removal of drug triggers and identifying and controlling the associated systemic disease. As noted above, some cases of RGD may spontaneously resolve [29, 33, 41, 43]. In pediatric cases, control of the associated disease resulted in resolution of cutaneous findings, whereas recurrence corresponded with decreased disease control [28]. A recent clinicopathologic review of IGD and PNGD evaluated the course of RGD in comparison with histologic findings. Patients with the PNGD histologic reaction pattern tended to have a limited course. This includes patients with biopsies showing neutrophils, karyorrhexis, and/or vasculitis. Lesions with a predominantly lymphocytic infiltrate tended to have a longer course marked by disease flares prior to remission, and patients with the IGD histologic reaction pattern were less likely to self-resolve [29].

Conclusions

IGD, PNGD, and IGDR have significant clinical and histologic overlap. While the particular subtype of RGD may have clinical or therapeutic implications, it may be best to approach these eruptions as representing subtypes within the larger category of reactive granulomatous dermatitis [1]. Importantly, clinicians should remember that granulomatous dermatitis is not a diagnosis but a clinicopathologic description and reaction pattern in the skin. Patients who develop these eruptions require a thorough evaluation for associated conditions, which include autoimmune disease, inflammatory arthritis, infection, malignancy, and medications.

References

1. Rosenbach M, English JC. Reactive granulomatous dermatitis: a review of palisaded neutrophilic and granulomatous dermatitis, interstitial granulomatous dermatitis, interstitial granulomatous drug reaction, and a proposed reclassification. Dermatol Clin. 2015;33(3):373–87.
2. Dykman CJ, Galens GJ, Good AE. Linear subcutaneous bands in rheumatoid arthritis. An unusual form of rheumatoid granuloma. Ann Intern Med. 1965;63:134–40.
3. Hawryluk EB, Izikson L, English JC. Non-infectious granulomatous diseases of the skin and their associated systemic diseases: an evidence-based update to important clinical questions. Am J Clin Dermatol. 2010;11(3):171–81.
4. Magro CM, Crowson AN, Schapiro BL. The interstitial granulomatous drug reaction: a distinctive clinical and pathological entity. J Cutan Pathol. 1998;25(2):72–8.
5. Betlloch I, Moragon M, Jorda E, Jimenez A, Ramon D, Verdeguer JM. Linear rheumatoid nodule. Int J Dermatol. 1988;27(9):645–6.
6. Harpster EF, Mauro T, Barr RJ. Linear granuloma annulare. J Am Acad Dermatol. 1989;21(5 Pt 2):1138–41.
7. Ackerman A. Histologic diagnosis of inflammatory skin diseases: interstitial granulomatous dermatitis with arthritis. In: Ackerman A, Guo Y, Vitale P, editors. Clues to diagnosis in dermatopathology. 1st ed. Chicago: ASCP Press; 1993. p. 309–12.
8. Verneuil L, Dompmartin A, Comoz F, Pasquier CJ, Leroy D. Interstitial granulomatous dermatitis with cutaneous cords and arthritis: a disorder associated with autoantibodies. J Am Acad Dermatol. 2001;45(2):286–91.
9. Gottlieb G, Duve R, Ackerman A. Interstitial granulomatous dermatitis with cutaneous cords and arthritis: linear subcutaneous bands in rheumatoid arthritis revisited. In: Dermatopathology: practical and conceptual. Philadelphia: Hanley & Belfus; 1995. p. 1:3-6.
10. Long D, Thiboutot DM, Majeski JT, Vasily DB, Helm KF. Interstitial granulomatous dermatitis with arthritis. J Am Acad Dermatol. 1996;34(6):957–61.
11. Busquets-Pérez N, Narvaez J, Valverde-García J. Interstitial granulomatous dermatitis with arthritis (Ackerman syndrome). J Rheumatol. 2006;33(6):1207–9.
12. Dubey S, Merry P. Clinical vignette. Interstitial granulomatous dermatitis (Ackerman's syndrome) in SLE presenting with the "rope sign". Rheumatology (Oxford). 2007;46(1):80.
13. Felcht M, Faulhaber J, Göttmann U, Koenen W, Goerdt S, Goebeler M. Interstitial granulomatous dermatitis (Ackerman's syndrome). Eur J Dermatol. 2010;20(5):661–2.
14. Chu P, Connolly MK, LeBoit PE. The histopathologic spectrum of palisaded neutrophilic and granulomatous dermatitis in patients with collagen vascular disease. Arch Dermatol. 1994;130(10):1278–83.
15. Finan MC, Winkelmann RK. The cutaneous extravascular necrotizing granuloma (Churg-Strauss granuloma) and systemic disease: a review of 27 cases. Medicine (Baltimore). 1983;62(3):142–58.
16. Dicken CH, Winkelmann RK. The Churg-Strauss granuloma: cutaneous, necrotizing, palisading granuloma in vasculitis syndromes. Arch Pathol Lab Med. 1978;102(11):576–80.
17. Finan MC, Winkelmann RK. Cutaneous extravascular necrotizing granuloma and lymphocytic lymphoma. Arch Dermatol. 1983;119(5):419–22.
18. Crotty CP, DeRemee RA, Winkelmann RK. Cutaneous clinicopathologic correlation of allergic granulomatosis. J Am Acad Dermatol. 1981;5(5):571–81.
19. Hu CH, O'Loughlin S, Winkelmann RK. Cutaneous manifestations of Wegener granulomatosis. Arch Dermatol. 1977;113(2):175–82.
20. Churg J, Strauss L. Allergic granulomatosis, allergic angiitis, and periarteritis nodosa. Am J Pathol. 1951;27(2):277–301.
21. Finan MC. Rheumatoid papule, cutaneous extravascular necrotizing granuloma, and Churg-Strauss granuloma: are they the same entity? J Am Acad Dermatol. 1990;22(1):142–3.

22. Wilmoth GJ, Perniciaro C. Cutaneous extravascular necrotizing granuloma (Winkelmann granuloma): confirmation of the association with systemic disease. J Am Acad Dermatol. 1996;34(5):753–9.
23. Sangueza OP, Caudell MD, Mengesha YM, Davis LS, Barnes CJ, Griffin JE, et al. Palisaded neutrophilic granulomatous dermatitis in rheumatoid arthritis. J Am Acad Dermatol. 2002;47(2):251–7.
24. Kwon EJ, Hivnor CM, Yan AC, Forbes B, Elenitsas R, Albert D, et al. Interstitial granulomatous lesions as part of the spectrum of presenting cutaneous signs in pediatric sarcoidosis. Pediatr Dermatol. 2007;24(5):517–24.
25. Hunt RD, Hartman RD, Molho-Pessach V, Votava HJ, Schaffer JV. Palisaded neutrophilic and granulomatous dermatitis in an adolescent girl with perinuclear antineutrophil cytoplasmic antibody–positive pauci-immune glomerulonephritis and arthritis. J Am Acad Dermatol. 2012;67(4):e164–6.
26. Germanas JP, Mehrabi D, Carder KR. Palisaded neutrophilic granulomatous dermatitis in a 12-year-old girl with systemic lupus erythematosus. J Am Acad Dermatol. 2006;55(2, Supplement):S60–2.
27. Warycha MA, Fangman W, Kamino H, Schaffer JV. Interstitial granulomatous dermatitis in a child with chronic uveitis. J Am Acad Dermatol. 2008;58(5 Suppl 1):S100–2.
28. Akinshemoyin Vaughn OL, Siegel DH, Chiu YE, DeBord LC, Hogeling M, Hunt RD, et al. Clinical and histologic presentation of pediatric reactive granulomatous dermatitis. Pediatr Dermatol. 2020;37(3):498–503.
29. Rodríguez-Garijo N, Bielsa I, Mascaró JM, Quer A, Idoate MA, Paricio JJ, et al. Reactive granulomatous dermatitis as a histological pattern including manifestations of interstitial granulomatous dermatitis and palisaded neutrophilic and granulomatous dermatitis: a study of 52 patients. J Eur Acad Dermatol Venereol. 2021;35(4):988–94.
30. Imadojemu S, Rosenbach M. Advances in inflammatory granulomatous skin diseases. Dermatol Clin. 2019;37(1):49–64.
31. Pei S, Hinshaw MA. Palisaded neutrophilic granulomatous dermatitis leading to diagnosis of hodgkin lymphoma: report of rare case and literature review of paraneoplastic granulomatous dermatitides. Am J Dermatopathol. 2019;41(11):835–45.
32. Thompson L, Abner S, Malone J, Callen JP. Interstitial granulomatous dermatitis as the initial manifestation of myeloma. JAMA Dermatol. 2015;151(10):1141.
33. Peroni A, Colato C, Schena D, Gisondi P, Girolomoni G. Interstitial granulomatous dermatitis: a distinct entity with characteristic histological and clinical pattern. Br J Dermatol. 2012;166(4):775–83.
34. Altaykan A, Erkin G, Boztepe G, Gököz A. Interstitial granulomatous dermatitis with arthritis. Hum Pathol. 2004;35(7):892–4.
35. Tomasini C, Pippione M. Interstitial granulomatous dermatitis with plaques. J Am Acad Dermatol. 2002;46(6):892–9.
36. Patsatsi A, Kyriakou A, Triantafyllidou E, Sotiriadis D. Interstitial granulomatous dermatitis: another clinical variant. Case Rep Dermatol. 2011;3(3):195–200.
37. Mahmoodi M, Ahmad A, Bansal C, Cusack CA. Palisaded neutrophilic and granulomatous dermatitis in association with sarcoidosis. J Cutan Pathol. 2011;38(4):365–8.
38. Heidary N, Mengden S, Pomeranz MK. Palisaded neutrophilic and granulomatous dermatosis. Dermatol Online J. 2008;14(5):17.
39. Stephenson SR, Campbell SM, Drew GS, Magro CM. Palisaded neutrophilic and granulomatous dermatitis presenting in a patient with rheumatoid arthritis on adalimumab. J Cutan Pathol. 2011;38(8):644–8.
40. Gulati A, Paige D, Yaqoob M, Proby CM, Cerio R, Harwood CA. Palisaded neutrophilic granulomatous dermatitis associated with systemic lupus erythematosus presenting with the burning rope sign. J Am Acad Dermatol. 2009;61(4):711–4.
41. Hantash BM, Chiang D, Kohler S, Fiorentino D. Palisaded neutrophilic and granulomatous dermatitis associated with limited systemic sclerosis. J Am Acad Dermatol. 2008;58(4):661–4.

42. Kim S-K, Park C-K, Park Y-W, Jun J-B, Yoo D-H, Bae S-C. Palisaded neutrophilic granulomatous dermatitis presenting as an unusual skin manifestation in a patient with Behçet's disease. Scand J Rheumatol. 2005;34(4):324–7.
43. Coutinho I, Pereira N, Gouveia M, Cardoso JC, Tellechea O. Interstitial granulomatous dermatitis: A Clinicopathological study. Am J Dermatopathol. 2015;37(8):614–9.
44. Balin SJ, Wetter DA, Kurtin PJ, Letendre L, Pittelkow MR. Myelodysplastic syndrome presenting as generalized granulomatous dermatitis. Arch Dermatol. 2011;147(3):331–5.
45. Vestey JP, Turner M, Biddlestone L, McLaren K, Goulden N, Hunter JA. Disseminated cutaneous granulomatous eruptions associated with myelodysplastic syndrome and acute myeloid leukaemia. Clin Exp Dermatol. 1993;18(6):559–63.
46. Cornejo KM, Lum CA, Izumi AK. A cutaneous interstitial granulomatous dermatitis-like eruption arising in myelodysplasia with leukemic progression. Am J Dermatopathol. 2013;35(2):e26–9.
47. Patsinakidis N, Susok L, Hessam S, Othlinghaus N, Möllenhoff K, Stücker M, et al. Interstitial granulomatous dermatitis associated with myelodysplastic syndrome - complete clearance under therapy with 5-azacytidine. Acta Derm Venereol. 2014;94(6):725–6.
48. Weed J, Ko C, Stahl M, Much M, Witt D, Zeidan AM, et al. Reactive granulomatous dermatitis presenting as subcutaneous nodules and cords in a patient with advanced myelodysplastic syndrome. Ann Hematol. 2017;96(6):1037–9.
49. Swing DC, Sheehan DJ, Sangüeza OP, Woodruff RW. Interstitial granulomatous dermatitis secondary to acute promyelocytic leukemia. Am J Dermatopathol. 2008;30(2):197–9.
50. Aung PP, Bowker B, Masterpol KS, Mahalingam M. Disseminated noninterstitial granulomatous dermatitis as a cutaneous manifestation of the preleukemic state in a patient with myelodysplasia and ulcerative colitis--apropos a case and review of the literature. Am J Dermatopathol. 2014;36(7):e117–20.
51. Schreckenberg C, Asch PH, Sibilia J, Walter S, Lipsker D, Heid E, et al. Interstitial granulomatous dermatitis and paraneoplastic rheumatoid polyarthritis disclosing cancer of the lung. Ann Dermatol Venereol. 1998;125(9):585–8.
52. Katz KA. Disseminated cutaneous granulomatous eruption occurring in the setting of myelodysplasia. Dermatol Online J. 2003;9(4):22.
53. Deng A, Harvey V, Sina B, Strobel D, Badros A, Junkins-Hopkins JM, et al. Interstitial granulomatous dermatitis associated with the use of tumor necrosis factor alpha inhibitors. Arch Dermatol. 2006;142(2):198–202.
54. Misago N, Narisawa Y, Tada Y, Nagasawa K. Palisaded neutrophilic granulomatous dermatitis caused by cellulitis in a patient with systemic lupus erythematosus. Int J Dermatol. 2011;50(12):1583–5.
55. Blaise S, Salameire D, Carpentier PH. Interstitial granulomatous dermatitis: a misdiagnosed cutaneous form of systemic lupus erythematosus? Clin Exp Dermatol. 2008;33(6):712–4.
56. Wong HK, Kaffenberger BH, Zirwas M. A palpable erythematous cord over the trunk in a patient with systemic lupus erythematosus. Interstitial granulomatous dermatitis (IGD). JAMA Dermatol. 2013;149(5):609–14.
57. Marmon S, Robinson M, Meehan SA, Franks AG Jr. Lupus-erythematous-associated interstitial granulomatous dermatitis. Dermatol Online J. 2012;18(12):31.
58. Arévalo M, Moreno M, Gratacós J. Interstitial granulomatous dermatitis associated with lupus: A case report. Reumatol Clin. 2017;13(6):367–8.
59. Jandali B, Uthman I, Abbas O. Interstitial granulomatous dermatitis associated with systemic lupus erythematosus: case report and review of the literature. Lupus. 2016;25(2):209–13.
60. Savoia F, Stinchi C, Gaddoni G, Patrizi A, Odorici G, Tengattini V, Cataleta P, Zago S. The rope sign: a case of interstitial granulomatous dermatitis with arthritis. G Ital Dermatol Venereol. 2016;151(1):102–5.
61. Bremner R, Simpson E, White CR, Morrison L, Deodhar A. Palisaded neutrophilic and granulomatous dermatitis: an unusual cutaneous manifestation of immune-mediated disorders. Semin Arthritis Rheum. 2004;34(3):610–6.

62. Felcht M, Faulhaber J, Göttmann U, Koenen W, Goerdt S, Goebeler M. Interstitial granulomatous dermatitis (Ackerman's syndrome). Eur J Dermatol. 2010;20(5):661–2.
63. Khan M, Kennedy C, Clinch J. Palisaded neutrophilic and granulomatous dermatitis: an unusual combination with mixed connective tissue disease and celiac disease. J Am Acad Dermatol. 2014;70(5, Supplement 1):AB147.
64. Sawamura S, Kajihara I, Ihn H. A case of scleroderma associated with interstitial neutrophilic granulomatous reaction. Australas J Dermatol. 2019;60(4):e338–40.
65. Jung KH, Jeong S, Kwon SR, Lim MJ, Gwon J, Shin J, Park W. Palisaded neutrophilic granulomatous dermatitis in a patient with systemic sclerosis-rheumatoid arthritis overlap syndrome. Ann Dermatol. 2017;29(6):804–6.
66. Akagawa M, Hattori Y, Mizutani Y, Shu E, Miyazaki T, Seishima M. Palisaded neutrophilic and granulomatous dermatitis in a patient with granulomatosis with Polyangiitis. Case Rep Dermatol. 2020;12(1):52–6.
67. Ragab G, Hegazy MT, Ali M, Abdel-Halim MRE, Puéchal X. Three patterns of cutaneous involvement in granulomatosis with Polyangiitis. J Adv Res. 2020;24:311–5.
68. Muscardin LM, Cota C, Amorosi B, Ferraro C. Erythema elevatum diutinum in the spectrum of palisaded neutrophilic granulomatous dermatitis: description of a case with rheumatoid arthritis. J Eur Acad Dermatol Venereol. 2007;21(1):104–5.
69. Corrà A, Quintarelli L, Verdelli A, Portelli F, Massi D, Caproni M. Granulomatous dermatitis and systemic disease: an association to consider. Biomed Res Int. 2020;2020:3281380.
70. Rato M, Gil F, Monteiro AF, Aranha J, Tavares E. Interstitial granulomatous dermatitis in a patient with chronic hepatitis C and mixed cryoglobulinemia. Dermatol Online J. 2018;24(1):13030/qt3x33s9m7.
71. Perniciaro C, Winkelmann RK. Cutaneous extravascular necrotizing granuloma in a patient with Takayasu's aortitis. Arch Dermatol. 1986;122(2):201–4.
72. Collaris EJ, van Marion AM, Frank J, Poblete-Gutiérrez P. Cutaneous granulomas in rheumatoid arthritis. Int J Dermatol. 2007;46(Suppl 3):33–5.
73. Kalen JE, Shokeen D, Ramos-Caro F, Motaparthi K. Palisaded neutrophilic granulomatous dermatitis: Spectrum of histologic findings in a single patient. JAAD Case Rep. 2017;3(5):425–8.
74. Worsnop FS, Ostlere L. Interstitial granulomatous dermatitis with arthritis presenting with the rope sign. Clin Exp Dermatol. 2013;38(5):564–5.
75. Zoli A, Massi G, Pinnelli M, Lo Cuccio CD, Castri F, Ferraccioli G. Interstitial granulomatous dermatitis in rheumatoid arthritis responsive to etanercept. Clin Rheumatol. 2010;29(1):99–101.
76. Leloup P, Aubert H, Causse S, Le Goff B, Barbarot S. Ustekinumab therapy for severe interstitial granulomatous dermatitis with arthritis. JAMA Dermatol. 2013;149(5):626–7.
77. Comte C, Guillot B, Durand L, Picot E, Dereure O. Dermatite granulomateuse interstitielle avec arthrites: quatre cas [Interstitial granulomatous dermatitis with arthritis: four cases]. Ann Dermatol Venereol. 2008;135(1):38–43.
78. Levine SD, Robinson M, Honda K, Nedorost S. Interstitial granulomatous dermatitis in a patient with rheumatoid arthritis on etanercept. Cutis. 2009;83(1):50.
79. Hu S, Cohen D, Murphy G, Mody E, Qureshi AA. Interstitial granulomatous dermatitis in a patient with rheumatoid arthritis on etanercept. Cutis. 2008;81(4):336–8.
80. Takahashi H, Satoh K, Takagi A, Ishida-Yamamoto A, Iizuka H. Interstitial granulomatous dermatitis associated with rheumatoid arthritis. J Dermatol. 2017;44(6):e130–1.
81. Kim YS, Lee JH, Lee JY, Park YM. Interstitial granulomatous dermatitis associated with rheumatoid arthritis. Ann Dermatol. 2016;28(3):395–7.
82. Veronez IS, Dantas FL, Valente NY, Kakizaki P, Yasuda TH, Cunha TA. Interstitial granulomatous dermatitis: rare cutaneous manifestation of rheumatoid arthritis. An Bras Dermatol. 2015;90(3):391–3.
83. Kern M, Shiver MB, Addis KM, Gardner JM. Palisaded neutrophilic and granulomatous dermatitis/interstitial granulomatous dermatitis overlap: A striking clinical and histologic pre-

sentation with "burning rope sign" and subsequent Mirror-image contralateral recurrence. Am J Dermatopathol. 2017;39(9):e141–6.
84. Jabbari A, Cheung W, Kamino H, Soter NA. Interstitial granulomatous dermatitis with arthritis. Dermatol Online J. 2009;15(8):22.
85. Lucas A, Bañuls J, Mataix J, Pérez-Crespo M, Jiménez MJ, Botella R, Betlloch I. Localized acquired cutis laxa secondary to interstitial granulomatous dermatitis. Clin Exp Dermatol. 2009;34(5):e102–5.
86. Aloi F, Tomasini C, Pippione M. Interstitial granulomatous dermatitis with plaques. Am J Dermatopathol. 1999;21(4):320–3.
87. Chen DL, Chong AH, Green J, Orchard D, Williams R, Clemens L. A novel case of polyfibromatosis and interstitial granulomatous dermatitis with arthritis. J Am Acad Dermatol. 2006;55(2 Suppl):S32–7.
88. Wollina U, Schönlebe J, Unger L, Weigel K, Köstler E, Nüsslein H. Interstitial granulomatous dermatitis with plaques and arthritis. Clin Rheumatol. 2003;22(4–5):347–9.
89. Ucelli JLR, Rudolph FSB, Obadia DL, Dionello CDF. Interstitial granulomatous dermatitis with arthritis. An Bras Dermatol. 2017;92(3):434–6.
90. Hussain K, Thomas L, Shaikh NA, Ahmed Abdul Hamid B. Ackerman syndrome: a rare cause of arthritis with dermatitis. BMJ Case Rep. 2015;2015:bcr2014207054.
91. de Unamuno BB, Rabasco AG, Sánchez RB, de Miquel VA. Palisaded neutrophilic and granulomatous dermatitis associated with ankylosing spondylitis. Am J Dermatopathol. 2013;35(8):847–50.
92. Calonje JE, Greaves MW. Cutaneous extravascular necrotizing granuloma (Churg-Strauss) as a paraneoplastic manifestation of non-Hodgkin's B-cell lymphoma. J R Soc Med. 1993;86(9):549–50.
93. Michailidou D, Voulgarelis M, Pikazis D. Exacerbation of interstitial granulomatous dermatitis with arthritis by anakinra in a patient with diffuse large B-cell lymphoma. Clin Exp Rheumatol. 2014;32(2):259–61.
94. Choi MJ, Shin D, Kim YC, Oh SH, Kim M. Interstitial granulomatous dermatitis with arthritis accompanied by anaplastic large cell lymphoma. J Dermatol. 2014;41(4):363–4.
95. Yoneta K, Fujimoto N, Teramura K, Takayama S, Tanaka T. Disseminated granulomatous skin lesions associated with myelodysplastic syndrome treated successfully with tranilast: a case report and review of the literature. Eur J Dermatol. 2016;26(4):398–400.
96. Cases-Merida S, Lorente-Lavirgen A, Pérez-Gil A. Interstitial granulomatous dermatitis due to a rare myeloproliferative neoplasia. Indian J Dermatol. 2018;63(3):264–7.
97. Corneli P, di Meo N, Zalaudek I, Chiarelli C, Signoretto D, Zacchi A, Colli C. Interstitial granulomatous dermatitis as primary manifestation of marginal zone lymphoma. Int J Dermatol. 2020;59:e412–e41.
98. Lozano-Masdemont B, Baniandrés-Rodríguez O, Parra-Blanco V, Suárez-Fernández R. Granulomatous dermatitis as a cutaneous manifestation of hematologic disorders: the first case associated with polycythemia vera and a new case associated with myelodysplasia. Actas Dermosifiliogr. 2016;107(5):e27–32.
99. Riaz IB, Kamal MU, Segal RJ, Anwer F. First reported association of chronic lymphocytic leukaemia and interstitial granulomatous dermatitis. BMJ Case Rep. 2016;2016:bcr2016215108.
100. Federmann B, Bonzheim I, Yazdi AS, Schmidt J, Fend F, Metzler G. Generalized palisaded neutrophilic and granulomatous dermatitis-a cutaneous manifestation of chronic myelomonocytic leukemia? A clinical, histopathological, and molecular study of 3 cases. Hum Pathol. 2017;64:198–206.
101. Kyriakou A, Patsatsi A, Papadopoulos V, Kioumi A, Efstratiou I, Lazaridou E. A case of palisaded neutrophilic granulomatous dermatitis with subsequent development of chronic myelomonocytic leukemia. Clin Case Rep. 2019;7(4):695–8.
102. Deen J, Banney L, Perry-Keene J. Palisading neutrophilic and granulomatous dermatitis as a presentation of Hodgkin lymphoma: A case and review. J Cutan Pathol. 2018;45(2):167–70.

103. Kim SM, Cho SH, Lee JD, Kim HS. Interstitial granulomatous dermatitis in a patient with prostate Cancer. Ann Dermatol. 2017;29(3):337–40.
104. Moyano Almagro B, López Navarro N, Contreras Steyls M, Gallego Dominguez E, Herrera Acosta E, Herrera CE. Interstitial granulomatous dermatitis and arthritis revealing oesophageal carcinoma. Clin Exp Dermatol. 2013;38(5):501–3.
105. Szepetiuk G, Lesuisse M, Piérard GE, Quatresooz P, Piérard-Franchimont C. Autoimmunity-related granulomatous dermatitis in association with hepatitis. Case Rep Dermatol. 2012;4(1):80–4.
106. Lee KJ, Lee ES, Lee DY, Jang KT. Interstitial granulomatous dermatitis associated with autoimmune hepatitis. J Eur Acad Dermatol Venereol. 2007;21(5):684–5.
107. Antunes J, Pacheco D, Travassos AR, Soares-Almeida LM, Filipe P, Sacramento-Marques M. Autoimmune thyroiditis presenting as interstitial granulomatous dermatitis. An Bras Dermatol. 2012;87(5):748–51.
108. Sakaizawa K, Hasegawa J, Kawachi S, Takata M, Saida T, Ikegawa S. Interstitial granulomatous dermatitis with plaques. Eur J Dermatol. 2008;18(5):600–1.
109. Gordon EA, Schmidt AN, Boyd AS. Palisaded neutrophilic and granulomatous dermatitis: a presenting sign of sarcoidosis? J Am Acad Dermatol. 2011;65(3):664–5.
110. Miyagawa F, Yamaoka K, Miyamoto S, Ogawa K, Asada H. Case of systemic sarcoidosis involving skin lesions that exhibited histological evidence of interstitial granulomatous dermatitis accompanied by widespread thrombophlebitis. J Dermatol. 2021;48:e159–60.
111. Paštar Z, Radoš J, Pavić I, Kovačević S, Vukasović A, Milavec-Puretić V, Lipozenčić J. Palisaded neutrophilic and granulomatous dermatitis in association with subcutaneous nodular and systemic sarcoidosis. Acta Dermatovenerol Croat. 2013;21(4):245–9.
112. Asahina A, Fujita H, Fukunaga Y, Kenmochi Y, Ikenaka T, Mitomi H. Early lesion of palisaded neutrophilic granulomatous dermatitis in ulcerative colitis. Eur J Dermatol. 2007;17(3):234–7.
113. Stiff KM, Cohen PR. Palisaded granulomatous dermatitis associated with ulcerative colitis: A comprehensive literature review. Cureus. 2017;9(1):e958.
114. Biswas A, Chittari K, Gey van Pittius D, Stephens M, Tan BB. Palisaded neutrophilic and granulomatous dermatitis in a child with type I diabetes mellitus and coeliac disease. Br J Dermatol. 2008;159(2):488–9.
115. Walling HW, Swick BL. Interstitial granulomatous dermatitis associated with chronic inflammatory demyelinating polyneuropathy. Cutis. 2012;90(1):30–2.
116. Lee HW, Chang SE, Lee MW, Choi JH, Moon KC, Koh JK. Interstitial granulomatous dermatitis with plaques associated with antiphospholipid syndrome. Br J Dermatol. 2005;152(4):814–6.
117. Wang Y, Wu Y, Zheng Z, Bai Y, Cui Y. Interstitial granulomatous dermatitis associated with primary biliary cirrhosis. J Dermatol. 2018;45(1):112–3.
118. Golden BD, Wong DC, Dicostanzo D, Solomon G. Rheumatoid papules in a patient with acquired immune deficiency syndrome and symmetric polyarthritis. J Rheumatol. 1996;23(4):760–2.
119. di Meo N, Stinco G, Trevisan G. Interstitial granulomatous dermatitis due to borreliosis. Indian J Dermatol Venereol Leprol. 2015;81(3):327.
120. Badin DJ, O'Hern K, Simmons BJ, Mann JA, Momtahen S. Localized reactive granulomatous dermatitis secondary to erythema migrans. JAAD Case Rep. 2020;6(12):1236–8.
121. DiCaudo DJ, Connolly SM. Interstitial granulomatous dermatitis associated with pulmonary coccidioidomycosis. J Am Acad Dermatol. 2001;45(6):840–5.
122. Mangold AR, DiCaudo DJ, Blair JE, Sekulic A. Chronic interstitial granulomatous dermatitis in coccidioidomycosis. Br J Dermatol. 2016;174(4):881–4.
123. Kroesen S, Itin PH, Hasler P. Arthritis and interstitial granulomatous dermatitis (Ackerman syndrome) with pulmonary silicosis. Semin Arthritis Rheum. 2003;32(5):334–40.
124. Singh M, Comfere N. Images in clinical medicine. Palisaded neutrophilic and granulomatous dermatitis. N Engl J Med. 2012;366(22):e33.

125. Gordon K, Miteva M, Torchia D, Romanelli P. Allopurinol-induced palisaded neutrophilic and granulomatous dermatiti. Cutan Ocul Toxicol. 2012;31(4):338–40.
126. Altemir A, Iglesias-Sancho M, Sola-Casas MLÁ, Novoa-Lamazares L, Fernández-Figueras M, Salleras-Redonnet M. Interstitial granulomatous dermatitis following tocilizumab, a paradoxical reaction? Dermatol Ther. 2020;33(6):e14207.
127. de Perosanz LD, Saceda Corralo D, Ortega Quijano D, Carrillo Gijón R. Interstitial granulomatous dermatitis and tocilizumab: is this treatment useful for this skin condition? Actas Dermosifiliogr. 2020;111(4):343–5.
128. Dyson SW, Hirsch A, Jaworsky C. Interstitial granulomatous dermatitis secondary to soy. Am Acad Dermatol. 2004;51(2 Suppl):S105–7.
129. Perrin C, Lacour JP, Castanet J, Michiels JF. Interstitial granulomatous drug reaction with a histological pattern of interstitial granulomatous dermatitis. Am J Dermatopathol. 2001;23(4):295–8.
130. Grose E, Ramien M. Interstitial granulomatous drug reaction related to hydrochlorothiazide. Dermatol Online J. 2019;25(7):13030/qt1gs433hj.
131. Trinidad C, Nelson KC, Glitza Oliva IC, Torres-Cabala CA, Nagarajan P, Tetzlaff MT, Ivan D, Hwu WJ, Prieto VG, Curry JL, Aung PP. Dermatologic toxicity from immune checkpoint blockade therapy with an interstitial granulomatous pattern. J Cutan Pathol. 2018;45(7):504–7.
132. Singh P, Wolfe SP, Alloo A, Gottesman SP. Interstitial granulomatous dermatitis and granulomatous arteritis in the setting of PD-1 inhibitor therapy for metastatic melanoma. J Cutan Pathol. 2020;47(1):65–9.
133. Frauchiger AL, Brüggen MC, Goldinger SM, Dummer R. Interstitial granulomatous dermatitis during talimogen laherparepvec treatment. Melanoma Res. 2017;27(4):400–1.
134. Aria AB, Chen L, Huen AO. A case report of bosutinib-induced interstitial granulomatous drug reaction in a patient with chronic myelogenous leukemia: a case report. SAGE Open Med Case Rep. 2018;10:6.
135. Siami K, Wilkerson M, Clark SH, et al. An indurated plaque on the ankle of a 74-year-old woman. Arch Pathol Lab Med. 2004;128:e129–30.
136. Chen YC, Hsiao CH, Tsai TF. Interstitial granulomatous drug reaction presenting as erythroderma: remission after discontinuation of enalapril maleate. Br J Dermatol. 2008;158:1143–4.
137. Fujita Y, Shimizu T, Shimizu H. A case of interstitial granulomatous drug reaction due to sennoside. Br J Dermatol. 2004;150:1035–7.
138. Lee HW, Yun WJ, Lee MW, et al. Interstitial granulomatous drug reaction caused by Chinese herbal medication. J Am Acad Dermatol. 2005;52:712–3.
139. Martin G, Cañueto J, Santos-Briz A, et al. Interstitial granulomatous dermatitis with arthritis associated with trastuzumab. J Eur Acad Dermatol Venereol. 2010;24:493–501.
140. Yazgano KD, Tambay E, Mete O, et al. Interstitial granulomatous drug reaction due to thalidomide. J Eur Acad Dermatol Venereol. 2009;23:490–3.
141. Kim MS, Lee JH, Park K, et al. Allopurinol-induced DRESS syndrome with a histologic pattern consistent with interstitial granulomatous drug reaction. Am J Dermatopathol. 2014;36:193–5.
142. Tan ES, Robson A, Lai-Cheong JE, Wain EM. Interstitial granulomatous drug reaction induced by quetiapine. Clin Exp Dermatol. 2016;41(2):210–1.
143. Maione V, Stinco G, Orsaria M, Errichetti E. Interstitial granulomatous drug reaction after intranasal desmopressin administration. Indian J Dermatol. 2016;61(1):125.
144. Hernandez N, Pen Ate Y, Borrego L. Generalized erythematous-violaceous plaques in a patient with a history of dyslipidemia. Int J Dermatol. 2013;52:393–4.
145. Martinez-Moran C, Nájera L, Ruiz-Casado AI, et al. Interstitial granulomatous drug reaction to sorafenib. Arch Dermatol. 2011;147:1118–9.
146. Regula CG, Hennessy J, Clarke LE, et al. Interstitial granulomatous drug reaction to anakinra. J Am Acad Dermatol. 2008;59:S25–7.
147. Martorell-Calatayud A, Balmer N, Cardona LF, et al. Interstitial granulomatous drug reaction to adalimumab. Am J Dermatopathol. 2010;32:408–9.

148. Georgesen C, McDonough P, Cruz P. Interstitial granulomatous dermatitis associated with gabapentin. Dermatitis. 2014;25(6):374–5.
149. Marcollo Pini A, Kerl K, Kamarachev J, et al. Interstitial granulomatous drug reaction following intravenous ganciclovir. Br J Dermatol. 2008;158:1391–2.
150. Lee MW, Choi J, Sung KJ, et al. Interstitial and granulomatous drug reaction presenting as erythema nodosum-like lesions. Acta Derm Venereol. 2002;82:473–4.
151. Du XF, Yin XP, Zhang GL, Shi HJ, Shao MH. Interstitial granulomatous drug reaction to a Chinese herb extract. Eur J Dermatol. 2012;22(3):419–20.
152. Atzori L, Luca P, Pinna AL. Interstitial granulomatous drug reaction due to febuxostat. Indian J Dermatol Venereol Leprol. 2014;80:182–4.
153. Groves C, McMenamin ME, Casey M, et al. Interstitial granulomatous reaction to strontium ranelate. Arch Dermatol. 2008;144:268–9.

Chronic Atypical Neutrophilic Dermatosis with Lipodystrophy and Elevated Temperature (CANDLE) and Proteasome-Associated Autoinflammatory Syndrome (PRAAS)

Alberto Fernández, Isabel Colmenero, and Antonio Torrelo

Introduction

Chronic atypical neutrophilic dermatosis with lipodystrophy and elevated temperature (CANDLE) is an autosomal recessive disorder characterized by episodic fevers, characteristic skin lesions, and lipodystrophy. CANDLE was first described in 2010 [1] and was subsequently known to be caused by mutations in the genes that encode certain subunits of the proteasome and immunoproteasome [2, 3]. Proteasome dysfunction leads to an accumulation of intracellular waste proteins and overproduction of type 1 interferons (INFs) that cause tissue damage [4, 5]. PSMB8 is the most frequently mutated gene, which encodes the β5i subunit of the immunoproteasome. Other conditions that share similar clinical features with CANDLE are also described, with mutations in genes other than PSMB8; the term PRAAS (proteasome associated autoinflammatory syndrome) has been proposed to encompass these syndromes [6].

Clinical Features

Patients with CANDLE syndrome generally do not have a family history of the disease. Consanguinity has been reported in several families and two siblings affected in one family [1, 7, 8].

The symptoms start in the first months of life, usually within the first weeks [1, 9]. The most common presenting sign is periodic fever (> 38.3 °C) or temperature

A. Fernández · I. Colmenero · A. Torrelo (✉)
Departments of Dermatology and Pathology, Hospital Infantil Universitario Niño Jesús, Madrid, Spain
e-mail: atorrelo@aedv.es

F. Rongioletti, B. R. Smoller (eds.), *New and Emerging Entities in Dermatology and Dermatopathology*, https://doi.org/10.1007/978-3-030-80027-7_31

elevations. These appear daily or almost daily. Fever, along with annular skin plaques and periorbital edema, is the most characteristic presenting triad of the disease. Lipodystrophy begins later in life, with facial involvement during the first two years of life, but takes some years to be fully developed.

Skin Manifestations

The most characteristic skin feature of CANDLE is the presence of annular plaques, sometimes reported as papules or nodules (Fig. 1a, b). These lesions start during the first months of life and consist of erythematous or purpuric, edematous plaques, often with an annular shape with raised borders and a flat, purpuric center. They are usually widespread but favor the face, trunk, and limbs. They appear in crops coinciding with attacks of fever and resolve within days or weeks leaving purpuric macules or post-inflammatory hyperpigmentation. These residual macules can overlap with new crops of active plaques. The annular plaques tend to be less conspicuous with the passing of years [1].

Periorbital violaceous edema is another characteristic early sign of CANDLE. It usually develops during the first months of life and persists for years, fading as the patients reach puberty or adulthood. It is commonly reported as puffy eyelids. Perioral edema and lip swelling are also common features, although approximately only half of the patients present this manifestation.

There have been other skin manifestations irregularly described in the literature. Acral perniosis-like lesions are present in the neonatal period and can be the first skin sign of the disease. Other features include edema, ecchymoses, and hemorrhagic blisters on the palms. These acral lesions are more common during early infancy and do not recur with age [1, 10].

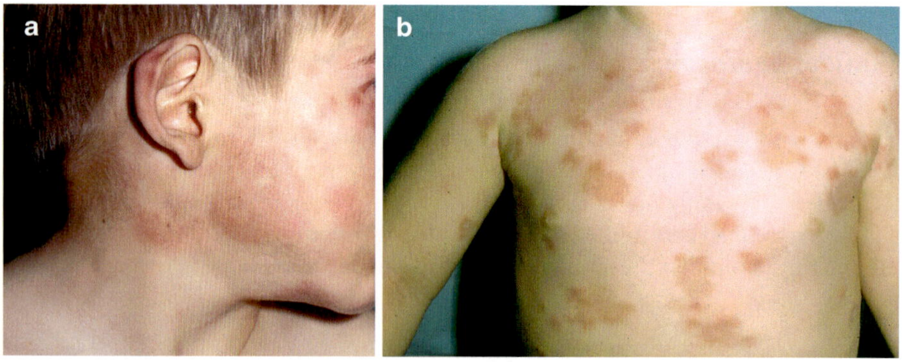

Fig. 1 (**a**) Annular, purpuric plaques on the cheeks of a child with CANDLE; note ear deformity from chondritis and periocular edema. (**b**) Annular plaques on the trunk and upper limbs of an infant with CANDLE

Other possible skin features of CANDLE are hypertrichosis and acanthosis nigricans, both probably related to fat loss and alterations of the carbohydrate metabolism. Diabetes mellitus has been reported in association with CANDLE [1, 2, 10].

Oral manifestations include gingival bleeding at probing, microdontia, and alveolar bone loss [11, 12].

General Examination

Patients with CANDLE present growth delay, with height and weight centiles below the tenth and often below the third [1, 7–9, 13]. However, the presence of mental retardation is unusual [1].

Lipodystrophy is a key manifestation of CANDLE [1, 2, 14]. The cause of lipodystrophy is not well known, but it can be related to chronic inflammation involving the fatty tissue [15, 16]. Alternatively, increased expression of proinflammatory cytokines in adipose tissue and reduced secretion of adiponectin and leptin may be involved [17, 18].

The first area to exhibit fat loss is the face and more specifically the cheeks. The loss of subcutaneous fat of the cheeks, together with periorbital and perioral violaceous edema, confers CANDLE patients a unique phenotype. In adulthood, the eyelids and the lips are retracted, causing a false proptosis and exposure of the teeth. These features confer an unmistakable appearance [19]. Other less characteristic facial traits include a broad forehead, epicanthal folds, and broad philtrum [13].

Fat loss progresses through the years, affecting the limbs, predominantly the upper ones, with demarcation of the muscle lines. Patients also show a prominent abdomen that may be related to increased visceral fat, which remains the main fat storage capability of the patient [1, 10]. An increased distance between nipples is also typical in CANDLE [1].

Upon physical examination, hepatomegaly, splenomegaly, and generalized lymphadenopathy are very common. These findings are thought to be in relation to the generalized state of inflammation and loss of fat tissue.

Musculoskeletal Signs

Arthralgias are very common in children with CANDLE, but patients do not show radiologic features of arthritis. Some joint swelling can appear in the interphalangeal joints and knees, but the absence of overt arthritis distinguishes CANDLE from rheumatoid arthritis or juvenile idiopathic arthritis [1, 7–9]. With time, hyperextensibility of interphalangeal joints can occur, and during adulthood, most patients will develop variable degrees of joint contractures on the hands and feet, which are often disabling [19].

Other

As CANDLE is a systemic autoinflammatory disease, any organ could potentially be involved. The eye is a commonly affected organ, showing a wide range of manifestations such as conjunctivitis, epiescleritis, posterior uveitis, corneal edema, leukoma, microaneurysms, and retinal hemorrhage [1, 13, 20].

Other complications documented in the literature are generalized tonic-clonic attacks, acute sterile aseptic meningitis, meningoencephalitis, chondritis, myositis, epididymitis, parotitis, pneumonitis, nephritis, carditis, and otitis. Some of these complications have been reported to be fatal [1]. Basal ganglia and frontotemporoparietal lobe deep/subcortical white matter calcifications can be seen under radiologic studies and are possibly due to chronic or recurrent meningoencephalitis [1, 8].

Autoimmune diseases such as autoimmune hemolytic anemia or autoimmune hepatitis can occur [1, 13], provided that type 1 IFNs promote survival and proinflammatory properties of transitional B cells [21]. Antinuclear autoantibodies may also be present in CANDLE patients [2, 9, 13, 20].

Laboratory Investigations

There is no characteristic laboratory finding for CANDLE. Elevated acute phase reactants (ESR above 40 mm/h, CRP higher than 70 mg/L, and thrombocytosis) are present in nearly every patient. Most patients develop anemia, generally mild to moderate and hypochromic due to chronic inflammation, although the development of autoimmune hemolytic anemia is also possible in CANDLE patients. Leukopenia and leukocytosis with neutrophilia have both been reported [1, 9, 10, 20]. Liver enzymes are usually moderately elevated but not higher than three times the upper normality level. Mild triglyceride elevation can also be present [1, 8]. Less frequently, elevated muscle enzymes (CPK and aldolase) reveal chronic muscle involvement [1]. Studies for autoimmunity are usually negative, but finding increased levels of antinuclear antibodies or cytoplasmic antineutrophil antibodies is not uncommon; these are usually detected at low titers and with no clinical relevance [2, 13]. Serum levels of immunoglobulins are regularly normal. Bone marrow and lymph node biopsies have been inconspicuous, revealing only reactive changes. Other laboratory and imaging anomalies observed during acute inflammatory attacks are dependent on the organs affected by inflammation.

Histopathological Features

The histological features of the skin lesions in CANDLE are very characteristic and may permit a diagnosis even in the early stages of the disease [1, 5]. The papillary and reticular dermis contains a perivascular and interstitial infiltrate of varying

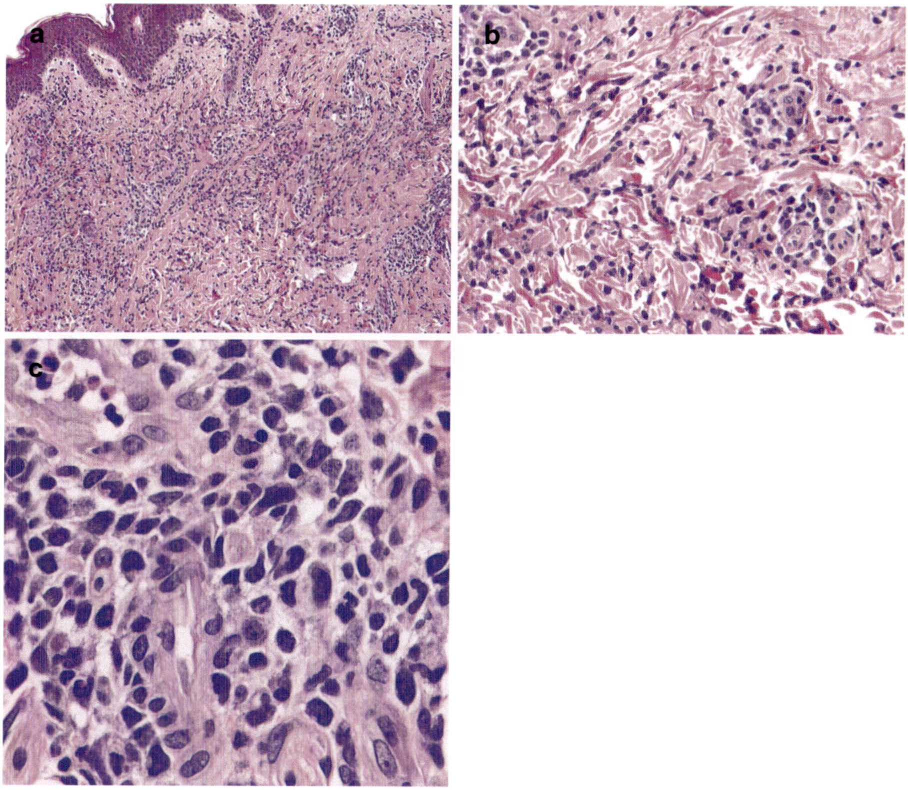

Fig. 2 (**a**) Dense, dermal, interstitial, and periadnexal infiltrate involving the whole dermis. (**b**) The infiltrate is composed of mononuclear cells showing bizarre, irregular nuclei; leukocytoclasia is present in scattered areas. (**c**) High-power view showing nuclei with atypical features. (H&E stain; original magnification: **a**, 10×; **b**, 40×; **c**, 100×)

intensity, extending to the subcutaneous fat as lobular panniculitis (Fig. 2a). The infiltrate is predominantly composed of mononuclear cells, many of which have large, irregularly shaped nuclei; the atypical appearance of the infiltrate may lead to a diagnosis of skin malignancy (Fig. 2b, c).

The infiltrate also contains mature neutrophils, some eosinophils, and a few mature lymphocytes. Leukocytoclasia is often seen, without fibrinoid necrosis of the vessels [1, 5]. Immunohistochemistry shows that the infiltrate is mixed, with an important presence of myeloid cells (positive for myeloperoxidase) and a prominent cell population of macrophages (positive for CD163 and CD68/PMG1) [5]. CD123-positive plasmacytoid dendritic cells are also seen in clusters [5].

Etiopathogenesis

The proteasome is a multiprotein structure present in all eukaryotic cells. It is involved in the removal of waste intracellular proteins, marked through ubiquitination [22]. The immunoproteasome, however, is constitutively expressed in hematopoietic cells and can be induced in other cells by proinflammatory cytokines, mostly IFN1. Its function is the degradation of foreign and waste proteins [23].

The proteasome and its inducible counterpart, the immunoproteasome, contain a catalytic subunit 20S formed by four heptameric rings. The two outer rings are composed of seven α subunits, and the two inner rings are composed of seven β subunits. Of these, only β1, β2, and β5 retain proteolytic activity and are responsible for caspase-like, trypsin-like, and chymotrypsin-like activities, respectively.

In eukaryotic cells, assembly of the proteasome starts with the formation of the outer α ring, in a process aided by the intervention of two chaperone heterodimers, PAC 1/ 2 and PAC 3 /4. Once the α ring is assembled, each of the β subunits is then added to it in a specific order (β2, β3, β4, β5, β6, β1, and β7) to form a half-proteasome. The incorporation of β7 is closely followed by the dimerization of the two half-proteasomes to complete the 20S subunit. The incorporation of β subunits to the α ring and the dimerization of the half-proteasome need the action of the proteasome maturation protein (POMP), which is then degraded by the own proteasome [24]. The 20S catalytic subunit can then bind to a 19S regulatory subunit and the interferon (IFN)-inducible activator PA28 to form the 26S hybrid proteasome.

Patients with CANDLE/PRAAS have been identified to bear mutations in PSMA genes, encoding for α subunits, PSMB genes encoding for β subunits of the proteasome, PSMG genes encoding for the chaperone proteins, or POMP [25]. Interestingly, when a gain-of-function mutation in POMP is present, patients show a distinct phenotype associated with autoimmunity and primary immunodeficiency (read below).

Four types of PRAAS are considered:

- PRAAS 1 is caused by homozygous mutations in the PSMB8 gene on chromosome 6p21 [1, 2] or by a heterozygous mutation in the PSMB8 gene and a heterozygous mutation in the PSMA3 gene on chromosome 14q23 or in the PSMB4 gene on chromosome 1q21 [3]. These genes encode for the β5i subunit of the immunoproteasome, the α7 subunit of the proteasome, and the β7 subunit of the proteasome, respectively. As the β5i subunit is responsible for the chymotrypsin-like activity, PRAAS 1 patients, especially those with homozygous forms, show decreased chymotrypsin-like activity. In addition, they also show impaired proteasome assembly. PSMB8 is the most reported mutated gene in CANDLE/PRAAS.
- PRAAS 2 is caused by a heterozygous mutation in the POMP gene on chromosome 13q12. POMP insufficiency causes proteasome precursor accumulation, reduced mature proteasome formation, and reduced overall proteasome activity [3]. An entity called POMP-related autoinflammation and immune dysregulation

(PRAID) was reported in two unrelated patients by Poli et al. in 2018 [26]. They presented since the first weeks of life with erythematous papules and plaques with central ulceration that progressed to necrosis and scarring affecting the face, trunk, and extremities. A biopsy of the lesions showed a neutrophilic infiltrate with vascular fibrinoid necrosis in one of the patients. They also had high antibody titers and severe infections since early infancy. Lipodystrophy was not reported as a feature, although patients were followed for just 3 years and future development of lipodystrophy could not be ruled out. In these cases, the cause was a heterozygous gain of function in POMP. Although PRAID and PRAAS patients show some similar clinical features, they differ in the ulcerated aspect of the lesions, the presence of autoimmunity, and severe immunodeficiency.

- PRAAS 3 is caused by homozygous mutations in the PSMB4 gene on chromosome 1q21 or by a heterozygous mutation in the PSMB4 gene and a heterozygous mutation in the PSMB9 gene on chromosome 6p21. These genes encode for β7 subunit of the proteasome and the β1i subunit of the immunoproteasome, respectively. These patients have proteasome assembly severely impaired, and patients with the digenic form also show decreased levels of caspase-like activity [2, 3].
- PRAAS 4 is caused by a homozygous mutation in the PSMG2 gene on chromosome 18p11. This gene encodes for the chaperone protein PAC2. The patient in the initial case had decreased levels of PAC1/PAC2 and a marked reduction in assembled proteasome complexes even when compared with other PRAAS patients, although she had similar decreased proteolytic activity [27].

Recently, a case of a patient with a homozygous mutation in the PSMB10 gene on chromosome 16q22 was reported. This gene encodes for the β2i subunit of the immunoproteasome and had not been previously reported. The patient showed only decreased levels of trypsin-like activity [28].

Proteasome-immunoproteasome dysfunction leads to an accumulation of intracellular waste proteins that cannot be effectively removed, with subsequent cellular stress [29] that acts as a vicious cycle. This leads to increased production of type 1 IFN and the recruitment of inflammatory cells that ultimately produce the tissue damage [4].

Differential Diagnosis

In 2010, Garg et al. [19] reported three adult patients with a disease they named JMP (joint contractures, muscle atrophy, microcytic anemia, and panniculitis-induced lipodystrophy syndrome). The authors emphasized the lipodystrophic features that were related to panniculitis and the joint features, but did not mention the skin manifestations of the disease. Fever was also not reported as a feature of this disease.

Nakajo in 1939 and Nishimura in 1950 reported two cases under the names "secondary hypertrophic osteoperiostosis with pernio" – a syndrome with nodular erythema, elongated and thickened fingers, and emaciation – and "hereditary lipo muscular atrophy with joint contracture, skin eruptions, and hyper-γ-globulinemia." The eponym "Nakajo–Nishimura syndrome" was proposed by the Japanese authors [30]. Overall, patients described started in early infancy with a pernio-like rash, periodic high fever, nodular erythema-like eruptions, and myositis. Lipoatrophy and joint contractures occurred progressively in life, mainly on the upper part of the body, leading to a very characteristic facial appearance. Kitamura et al. renamed the condition as Japanese autoinflammatory syndrome with lipodystrophy (JASL). Patients developed lipodystrophy in their upper bodies and nodular erythema. Patients also had hand deformities in addition to spiking fevers, and basal ganglia calcification was found in two related patients [31].

The term PRAAS (proteasome-associated autoinflammatory syndrome) has been used to encompass these syndromes and CANDLE [6]. JMP and Nakajo–Nishimura syndromes show an autosomal recessive pattern of inheritance with mutations in PSMB8, whereas CANDLE patients have shown additional related mutations (see above). All conditions share clinical features such as periodic fevers, skin eruptions, lipodystrophy, and myositis with onset during early infancy and are most likely part of the same disease spectrum.

The main differential diagnosis of PRAAS patients is cryopyrin-associated periodic syndromes (CAPS). CAPS is a disease spectrum that comprises the familial cold autoinflammatory syndrome (FCAS), Muckle–Wells syndrome (MWS), and neonatal-onset multisystem inflammatory disorder (NOMID), also known as chronic infantile neurologic, cutaneous, and articular (CINCA) syndrome [32]. A gain-of-function mutation in NLRP3 in CAPS patients leads to activation of the cryopyrin inflammasome, resulting in the inappropriate release of inflammatory cytokines including IL-1β [33].

CAPS show periodic fevers that can be associated with skin lesions such as an urticaria-like rash, macules, or papules, and musculoskeletal symptoms like arthralgia/arthritis/myalgia. Triggering by cold exposure is a diagnostic criterion. Other diagnostic criteria are sensorineural hearing loss, chronic aseptic meningitis, and skeletal abnormalities (epiphyseal overgrowth/frontal bossing). Normal IL-1β and the absence of response to IL-1 inhibitors such as anakinra observed in CANDLE further distinguish PRAAS from CAPS [34].

TNF receptor-associated periodic syndrome (TRAPS) and mevalonate kinase deficiency (MKD) are other syndromes that show periodic fevers with skin manifestations and can also be considered in the differential diagnosis [35].

Familial lipodystrophy syndromes can be distinguished by the absence of fever and elevated acute-phase reactant [6]. Other differential diagnoses include monogenic interferonopathies [20], Sweet's syndrome, and leukemia cutis.

Prognosis

Prognosis is variable. Most patients reach adulthood with variable degrees of disability, although a minority of patients can die at an early age due to acute attacks of inflammation affecting important organs of the body. Three patients described as JASL lived over 47 years of age and died of respiratory or cardiac problems [31]. The advances in the treatment of the disease, especially the use of JAK inhibitors, may allow for the longer survival of these patients with lower degrees of disability [36].

Regular clinical follow-up is mandatory. A protocol has not been established, but attention must be paid to identify inflammatory attacks as early as possible. Regular skin, eye, and joint exams are recommended. Endocrinologist consultation is mandatory for diet and metabolic control because of lipodystrophy. Basic laboratory follow-up must include CBC (with special attention to anemia, leukocytosis with an increased neutrophil count, and thrombocytosis), ESR, CRP, serum liver enzymes, muscle enzymes, and metabolic profile (including glucose, triglyceride, and cholesterol levels). Ultrasound may help detect enlarged liver, spleen, or lymph nodes. Specific tests for organ involvement must be considered in patients with abnormal clinical examination [25].

Therapy

Oral corticosteroids have been used as the first line of treatment, especially during flares, with doses ranging from 1 to 2 mg/kg; however, the moderate success of the treatment in controlling the disease and the necessity to maintain high doses for long periods of time discourage the use of glucocorticoids for maintenance treatment. Methotrexate can provide some improvement and has been considered first-line therapy as a GC sparing agent. NSAIDs may provide partial control of fevers. Dapsone and colchicine have been ineffective. Cyclosporine, azathioprine, or intravenous immunoglobulins have achieved minimal improvements, if any. Anti-TNF drugs such as etanercept have not been helpful and have even been the cause of disease exacerbations [1]. Acute attacks may also need organ-specific therapy.

Lately, there has been growing evidence about the efficacy of the JAK 1/2 inhibitor baricitinib as a treatment for CANDLE. As kinases JAK 1 and TYK2 are the ones bound to the IFN1 receptor, blocking these could lead to the inhibition of the IFN 1-activated JAK/STAT signaling pathway. Boyadzhiev et al. [10] treated a young patient with baricitinib for 1 year and 6 months, who after a few months of treatment showed no fever, no skin manifestations, and significant recovery in growth, allowing the discontinuation of systemic GCs with no serious adverse effects.

Sanchez et al. studied 12 patients followed for at least 6 months, with a mean follow-up period of 1.7 years [37]. The mean Autoinflammatory Diary Score (ADS) decreased from 1.3 at baseline to 0.3 at the time of their last visit. The mean use of GCs decreased by 73%. Seventeen adverse effects were seen in four patients, mainly upper respiratory tract infections. One patient abandoned the study due to lack of efficacy and development of avascular necrosis. The mean dose of baricitinib at last patient visit was 8.5 mg/day. In a longer follow-up period, eight out of ten patients achieved a reduction of >0.5 points in the ADS with a mean decrease from 1.3 to 0.25. Five out of ten patients achieved remission with no disease symptoms despite discontinuation of corticosteroids [36]. All patients had at least one adverse effect, upper respiratory tract infection being the most common, although only one patient had to abandon treatment due to the development of BK viremia and kidney injury.

In children, the average half-life reported for baricitinib is shorter than in adults, so it can be dosed into four times a day, especially for children under 20 kg. The decrease in interferon activity correlates with the serum levels of the drug [38].

Ruxolitinib, a JAK inhibitor selectively targeting JAK 1/2, has also been used in an 8-year-old patient, resulting in marked improvement and corticosteroid discontinuation in 14 months. Although there is a lack of evidence, JAK inhibitors could potentially be used as a treatment for CANDLE/PRAAS.

References

1. Torrelo A, Patel S, Colmenero I, Gurbindo D, Lendínez F, Hernández A, et al. Chronic atypical neutrophilic dermatosis with lipodystrophy and elevated temperature (CANDLE) syndrome. J Am Acad Dermatol. 2010;62:489–95.
2. Liu Y, Ramot Y, Torrelo A, Paller AS, Si N, Babay S, et al. Mutations in proteasome subunit β type 8 cause chronic atypical neutrophilic dermatosis with lipodystrophy and elevated temperature with evidence of genetic and phenotypic heterogeneity. Arthritis Rheum. 2012;64:895–907.
3. Brehm A, Liu Y, Sheikh A, Marrero B, Omoyinmi E, Zhou Q, et al. Additive loss-of-function proteasome subunit mutations in CANDLE/PRAAS patients promote type I IFN production. J Clin Invest. 2015;125:4196–211.
4. Crow YJ. Type I interferonopathies: Mendelian type I interferon up- regulation. Curr Opin Immunol. 2015;32:7–12.
5. Torrelo A, Colmenero I, Requena L, Paller AS, Ramot Y, Richard Lee CC, et al. Histologic and immunohistochemical features of the skin lesions in CANDLE syndrome. Am J Dermatopathol. 2015;37:517–22.
6. McDermott A, Jacks J, Kessler M, Emanuel PD, Gao L. Proteasome-associated autoinflammatory syndromes: advances in pathogeneses, clinical presentations, diagnosis, and management. Int J Dermatol. 2015;54:121–9.
7. Cavalcante MP, Brunelli JB, Miranda CC, Novak GV, Malle L, Aikawa NE, et al. CANDLE syndrome: chronic atypical neutrophilic dermatosis with lipodystrophy and elevated temperature-a rare case with a novel mutation. Eur J Pediatr. 2016;175:735–40.
8. Wang H, Das L, Tan Hung Tiong J, Vasanwala RF, Arkachaisri T. CANDLE syndrome: an extended clinical spectrum. Rheumatology (Oxford). 2014;53:2119–20.

9. Ramot Y, Czarnowicki T, Maly A, Navon-Elkan P, Zlotogorski A. Chronic atypical neutrophilic dermatosis with lipodystrophy and elevated temperature syndrome: a case report. Pediatr Dermatol. 2011;28:538–41.
10. Boyadzhiev M, Marinov L, Boyadzhiev V, Iotova V, Aksentijevich I, Hambleton S. Disease course and treatment effects of a JAK inhibitor in a patient with CANDLE syndrome. Pediatr Rheumatol Online J. 2019;17:19.
11. Roberts T, Stephen L, Scott C, Pasquale TD, Naser-Eldin A, Chetty M, et al. CANDLE syndrome: orofacial manifestations and dental implications. Head Face Med. 2015;11:38.
12. McKenna GJ, Ziada HM. Periodontal manifestations of chronic atypical neutrophilic dermatosis with lipodystrophy and elevated temperature (CANDLE) syndrome in an 11-year-old patient. Clin Adv Periodontics. 2015;5:153–8.
13. Yamazaki-Nakashimada MA, Santos-Chávez EE, de Jesus AA, Rivas-Larrauri F, Guzmán-Martínez MN, Goldbach-Mansky R, et al. Systemic autoimmunity in a patient with CANDLE syndrome. J Investig Allergol Clin Immunol. 2019;29:75–6.
14. Tüfekçi O, Bengoa Ş, Karapinar TH, Ataseven EB, Irken G, Ören H. CANDLE syndrome: a recently described autoinflammatory syndrome. J Pediatr Hematol Oncol. 2015;37:296–9.
15. Bingham A, Mamyrova G, Rother KI, Oral E, Cochran E, Premkumar A, et al. Predictors of acquired lipodystrophy in juvenile-onset dermatomyositis and a gradient of severity. Medicine (Baltimore). 2008;87:70–86.
16. Torrelo A, España A, Boixeda P, Ledo A. Partial lipodystrophy and dermatomyositis. Arch Dermatol. 1991;127:1846–7.
17. Brown TT. Approach to the human immunodeficiency virus-infected patient with lipodystrophy. J Clin Endocrinol Metab. 2008;93:2937–45.
18. Mallewa JE, Wilkins E, Vilar J, Mallewa M, Doran D, Back D, et al. HIV-associated lipodystrophy: a review of underlying mechanisms and therapeutic options. J Antimicrob Chemother. 2008;62:648–60.
19. Garg A, Hernandez MD, Sousa AB, Subramanyam L, Martínez de Villarreal L, dos Santos HG, et al. An autosomal recessive syndrome of joint contrac-tures, muscular atrophy, microcytic anemia, and panniculitis-associated lipodystrophy. J Clin Endocrinol Metab. 2010;95:58–63.
20. Al-Mayouf SM, AlSaleem A, AlMutairi N, AlSonbul A, Alzaid T, Alazami AM, et al. Monogenic interferonopathies: phenotypic and genotypic findings of CANDLE syndrome and its overlap with C1q deficient SLE. Int J Rheum Dis. 2018;21:208–13.
21. Liu M, Guo Q, Wu C, Sterlin D, Goswami S, Zhang Y, et al. Type I interferons promote the survival and proinflammatory properties of transitional B cells in systemic lupus erythematosus patients. Cell Mol Immunol. 2019;16:367–9.
22. Gomes AV. Genetics of proteasome diseases. Scientifica (Cairo). 2013;2013:637629.
23. Limanaqi F, Biagioni F, Gaglione A, Busceti CL, Fornai F. A sentinel in the crosstalk between the nervous and immune system: the (immuno)-proteasome. Front Immunol. 2019;10:628.
24. Budenholzer L, Cheng CL, Li Y, Hochstrasser M. Proteasome structure and assembly. J Mol Biol. 2017;429:3500–24.
25. Torrelo A. CANDLE syndrome as a paradigm of proteasome-related autoinflammation. Front Immunol. 2017;8:927.
26. Poli MC, Ebstein F, Nicholas SK, de Guzman MM, Forbes LR, Chinn IK, et al. Heterozygous truncating variants in POMP escape nonsense-mediated decay and cause a unique immune dysregulatory syndrome. Am J Hum Genet. 2018;102:1126–42.
27. De Jesus AA, Brehm A, VanTries R, Pillet P, Parentelli AS, Sanchez GAM, et al. Novel Proteasome Assembly Chaperone mutations in PSMG2/PAC2, cause the autoinflammatory interferonopathy, CANDLE/PRAAS4. J Allergy Clin Immunol. 2019;143:1939–43.
28. Sarrabay G, Méchin D, Salhi A, Boursier G, Rittore C, Crow Y, et al. PSMB10, the last immunoproteasome gene missing for PRAAS. J Allergy Clin Immunol. 2020;145:1015–7.
29. Seifert U, Bialy LP, Ebstein F, Bech-Otschir D, Voigt A, Schröter F, et al. Immunoproteasomes preserve protein homeostasis upon interferon-induced oxidative stress. Cell. 2010;142:613–24.

30. Kanazawa N. Nakajo-Nishimura syndrome: an autoinflammatory disorder showing pernio-like rashes and progressive partial lipodystrophy. Allergol Int. 2012;61:197–206.
31. Kitamura A, Maekawa Y, Uehara H, Izumi K, Kawachi I, Nishizawa M, et al. A mutation in the immunoproteasome subunit PSMB8 causes autoinflam-mation and lipodystrophy in humans. J Clin Invest. 2012;121:4150–60.
32. Kuemmerle-Deschner JB. CAPS--pathogenesis, presentation and treatment of an autoinflammatory disease. Semin Immunopathol. 2015;37:377–85.
33. Booshehri LM, Hoffman HM. CAPS and NLRP3. J Clin Immunol. 2019;39:277–86.
34. Kuemmerle-Deschner OS, Tyrrell PN, Kone-Paut I, Goldbach-Mansky R, Lachmann H, et al. Diagnostic criteria for CRYOPYRIN-Associated Periodic Syndrome (CAPS). Ann Rheum Dis. 2017;76:942–7.
35. Lachmann HJ. Periodic fever syndromes. Best Pract Res Clin Rheumatol. 2017;31:596–609.
36. Sanchez GAM, Reinhardt A, Ramsey S, Wittkowski H, Hashkes PJ, Berkun Y, et al. JAK1/2 inhibition with baricitinib in the treatment of autoinflammatory interferonopathies. J Clin Invest. 2018;128:3041–52.
37. Sanchez GAM, Reinhardt A, Brogan P, Berkun Y, Zlotogorski A, Brown D, et al. Preliminary response to Janus kinase inhibition with baricitinib in chronic atypical neutrophilic dermatosis with lipodystrophy and elevated temperatures (CANDLE). Pediatr Rheumatol. 2015;13(Suppl 1):O314.
38. Kim H, Brooks KM, Tang CC, Wakim P, Blake M, Brooks SR, et al. Pharmacokinetics, pharmacodynamics, and proposed dosing of the oral JAK1 and JAK2 inhibitor baricitinib in pediatric and young adult CANDLE and SAVI patients. Clin Pharmacol Ther. 2018;104:364–73.

Spiny Keratoderma

Tatsiana Pukhalskaya and Bruce R. Smoller

Introduction

The entity was first described in 1871 by Brown, who called it punctate keratoderma [1]. Since then, in large part due to its rarity, it acquired many different names, i.e., filiform hyperkeratosis, hyperkeratotic spicules, parakeratotic horns, follicular hyperkeratosis, multiple minute digitate hyperkeratosis, minute aggregate keratosis, punctate porokeratotic keratoderma, and music box spine keratotic plugs. Spiny keratoderma (SK) is the most recent name.

The disorder has been reported in all races and the age of onset ranges from 12 to 50 [2]. Several different forms are known including familial, sporadic, postinflammatory, and paraneoplastic. Around one-quarter of these patients with spiny keratoderma demonstrates a family predisposition [3].

Spiny keratoderma can arise with chronic renal failure, Darier's disease, hypovitaminosis A, Crohn's disease, polycystic kidney disease, and liver cysts [4]. It is also frequently found to accompany diabetes mellitus, suggesting that spiny keratoderma may be a function and manifestation of metabolic impairment [5–7]. Some case reports note an increase in spines with manual labor [1, 8].

Interesting is an association with various malignancies. This condition has been linked to lymphoma, multiple myeloma, myelofibrosis, and breast, renal, rectal, bronchial, and gingival carcinoma, and nodular malignant melanoma [9–16]. It also appears that certain malignant conditions are associated with particular patterns of

T. Pukhalskaya (✉)
Department of Pathology and Laboratory Medicine, University of Rochester Medical Center (URMC), Rochester, NY, USA
e-mail: tatsiana_pukhalskaya@urmc.rochester.edu

B. R. Smoller
Department of Pathology and Laboratory Medicine, University of Rochester School of Medicine and Dentistry, Rochester, NY, USA

F. Rongioletti, B. R. Smoller (eds.), *New and Emerging Entities in Dermatology and Dermatopathology*, https://doi.org/10.1007/978-3-030-80027-7_32

SK [10, 17]. Those with visceral malignancies tend to have a more peripheral distribution of skin lesions, while those with multiple myeloma and monoclonal gammopathy display more central distribution of the lesions [10–13, 18]. The finding of monoclonal immunoglobulin deposition within the epidermis and at the dermo-epidermal junction of these lesions has been shown [17, 19].

Clinical, Histopathological Features, and Workup

This skin condition manifests as numerous small spines of keratin on the palms and soles, usually sparing the dorsal surfaces, or disseminated over the trunk (Fig. 1) [16]. Rarely, lesions are found on the lateral surfaces of the fingers or arranged in a linear pattern [16, 20]. In most cases, these lesions have a nonfollicular distribution, but some are found in association with underlying follicules [19, 21]. The asymptomatic spiny keratotic projections are approximately 1–2 mm in size and are firmly attached to the underlying epidermis. Wood's light examination may reveal white fluorescence of punctate hyperkeratoses, resembling stars under the moonlight [22].

The name "punctate porokeratoses" arose due to the histological look of SK. The "spine" represents a cornoid lamella, i.e., a column of hyperkeratosis; however, variations in the histology may occur with columns of parakeratosis or orthokeratosis arising in individual cases. The column can be easily distinguished from the neighboring keratin as it stains poorly with eosin, is separated by fissures, and demonstrates a difference in birefringence color under polarized light (Fig. 2a–c) [3]. No dermal inflammation is present.

Electron microscopy of the SK lesions reveals keratinization of the spines without significant formation of keratohyalin granules but the presence of large keratohyalin-like masses in the upper dermis [3]. Many bundles of densely aggregated or laterally accreted tonofilaments merge into these keratohyalin-like masses. These structures are often attached to desmosomes. The marginal band formation is poor to absent in the upper epidermal layers of the spine and even in completely

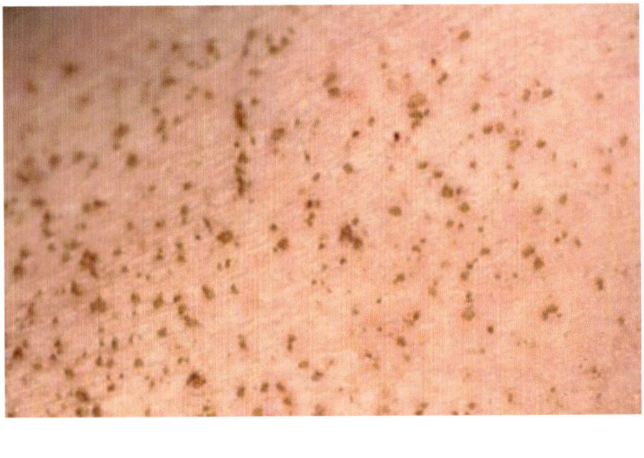

Fig. 1 Clinical illustration of spiny keratoderma. (Courtesy of Dr. Pietro Donati, Rome, Italy)

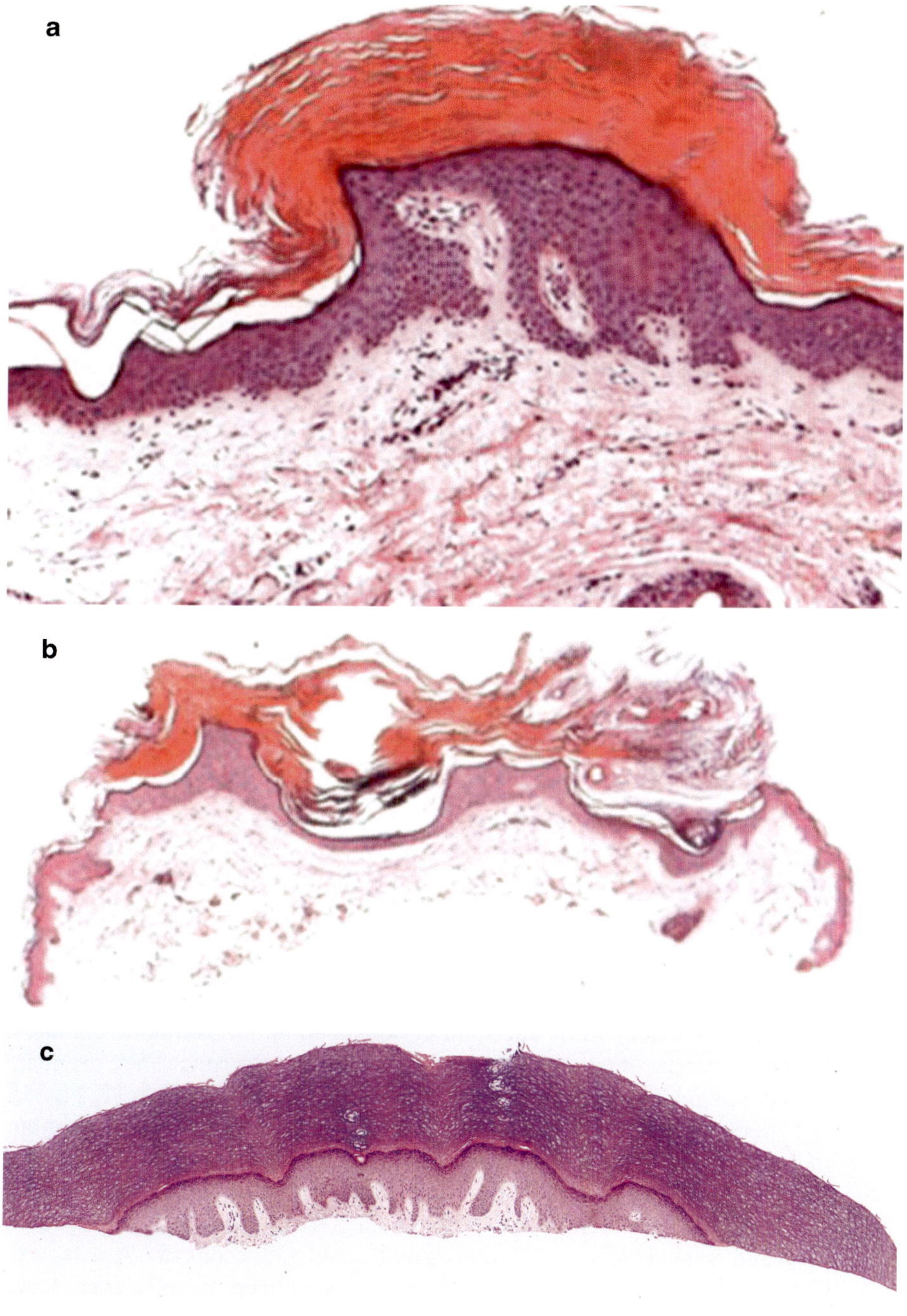

Fig. 2 **(a–c)** Histological presentation of spiny keratoderma on biopsies from three different patients designated as a, b, and c. There are noticeable columns of hyperkeratosis in a form of little "spines." (Courtesy of Pietro Donati, Rome, Italy (2a&2b) and Dr. Timothy H. McCalmont, Departments of Pathology and Dermatology, UCSF (2c))

keratinized cells. This data supports the theory of ectopic hair formation since normal cortical hair cells at the same level of keratinization don't form the marginal band. Immunofluorescent studies were performed in one study and were negative [16].

Differential Diagnosis

The differential diagnosis of palmoplantar hyperkeratosis can be extensive. Since the filiform appearance is typical, clinical inspection can often distinguish spiny keratoderma from entities such as verrucae, nevoid basal cell carcinoma lesions, and pitted keratolysis [23]. Overall, the main distinction is between spiny keratoderma and other palmoplantar keratodermas. The latter is a heterogeneous group and includes multiple similar entities and several rare genodermatoses in which palmoplantar keratoderma is a major feature. Clinically, this group is characterized by diffuse or localized hyperkeratosis of the palms and soles, sometimes accompanied by other ectodermal abnormalities (i.e., large ears, hypopigmented hair, alopecia, and frontal skull bossing), genetic impairments, and other features. Histologically, these entities might present with psoriasiform hyperplasia, hypogranulosis, alternating parakeratosis, and orthohyperkeratosis and have completely nonspecific combination of features. Spiny keratoderma can be distinguished from the rest upon clinical presentation and characteristic histological features previously described in this chapter.

Etiopathogenesis

It is thought that SK involves enhanced epidermal proliferation of the basal layer under the columnar hyperkeratosis [24, 25]. In fact, analysis of keratotic plugs has identified them to express keratins 6 and 16, which are typically present in hyperproliferative epidermal cells [25]. The spines correspond to orthokeratotic columns, located over the eccrine ducts, follicles, or interadnexal epidermis. They originate from the center of epidermal invaginations, which lack the granular layer [2, 24, 25].

One of the theories postulates that SK is a form of an ectopic hair formation, albeit abortive. It is possible that palmar/plantar skin of affected patients acquires a generalized potential for hair keratin production and, upon stimulation, can actually produce hair keratin [3]. Other theories propose that SK might be caused by repeated trauma or result from epidermal hyperplasia associated with coenzyme A reductase inhibitors [26]. Disruption of cholesterol synthesis may disrupt lamellar bodies and cause hyperproliferation [26].

Therapy

In one case report, palms were treated with topical 0.002% tacalcitol ointment. It dramatically improved the keratotic spicule lesions within 3 months, and a diminished keratotic column with normal appearance of the granular layer was seen at that time [15]. Five percent 5-fluorouracil cream and 12% ammonium lactate have been reported to provide a relatively good response [26, 27]. A combination of 0.05% tretinoin cream and ammonium lactate 12% lotion twice daily as well brought some improvement in one report [4]. In addition, mechanical debridement has been used to physically destroy the lesions.

Prognosis and Course

Prognosis of spiny keratoderma is vague due to its rarity and connections to multiple systemic conditions and malignancies. Paraneoplastic association is unclear since SK often begins years before any cancer appears and persists after the cancer is treated [28]. There is only one case yet reported in the literature where spines completely regressed after treatment of the underlying malignancy [29].

Conclusions

Spiny keratoderma is an extremely rare benign skin disorder. It might manifest in either a familial or acquired form. It is continuously reported in association with various systemic diseases, dysregulations, and malignancies. A thorough evaluation of family and personal history, appropriate cancer screenings, and regular medical examinations are critical to rule out the possibility of underlying problems. Topical treatment, surgical debridement, or control of underlying systemic disease might be successful to provide symptomatic relief. Patient education and counseling are highly recommended to alleviate possible psychological impact and social embarrassment spiny keratoderma might bring.

References

1. Brown FC. Punctate keratoderma. Arch Dermatol. 1971;104:682–3.
2. Sakas EL, Gentry RH. Porokeratosis punctata palmaris et plantaris (punctate porokeratosis). Case report and literature review. J Am Acad Dermatol. 1985;13:908–12.
3. Hashimoto K, Toi Y, Horton S, Sun TT. Spiny keratoderma–a demonstration of hair keratin and hair type keratinization. J Cutan Pathol. 1999;26:25–30.

4. Anderson D, Cohen DE, Lee HS, Thellman C. Spiny keratoderma in association with autosomal dominant polycystic kidney disease with liver cysts. J Am Acad Dermatol. 1996;34:935–6.
5. Nakamura Y, Muto M. Spiny keratoderma of the palms in an insulin-treated diabetic patient. Int J Dermatol. 2013;52:1460–1.
6. Chee SN, Ge L, Agar N, Lowe P. Spiny keratoderma: case series and review. Int J Dermatol. 2017;56:915–9.
7. Adegbayibi A, Doherty V, Biswas A. Multiple keratotic papules on the palm and fingers. Spiny keratoderma. Am J Dermatopathol. 2015;37:620–58.
8. McGovern TW, Gentry RH. Spiny keratoderma: case report, classification, and treatment of music box spine dermatoses. Cutis. 1994;54:389–94.
9. Campbell EH, Becknell C. Spiny keratoderma exposes underlying renal cell carcinoma. JAAD Case Rep. 2018;4:382–3.
10. Kaddu S, Soyer HP, Kerl H. Palmar filiform hyperkeratosis: a new paraneoplastic syndrome? J Am Acad Dermatol. 1995;33:337–40.
11. Hillion B, Le Bozec P, Moulonguet-Michau I, Blanchet-Bardon C, Petit A, Stephan J, Civatte J. Filiform palmoplantar hyperkeratosis and cancer of the breast. Ann Dermatol Venereol. 1990;117:834–6.
12. Beylot C, Taieb A, Bioulac P, Doutre MS, Foix P. Filiform palmoplantar hyperkeratosis and visceral neoplasia. Ann Dermatol Venereol. 1982;109:747–8.
13. Fegueux S, Bilet S, Crickx B, Perron J, Grossin M, Belaich S. Filiform palmar hyperkeratosis and rectosigmoid cancer. Ann Dermatol Venereol. 1988;115:1145–6.
14. Nazzaro P, Argentieri R, Balus L, Bassetti F, Fazio M, Giacalone B, Ponno R. Paraneoplastic syndrome with papulo-keratosic lesions of the extremities and diffuse spinulose pilar keratosis. Ann Dermatol Syphiligr (Paris). 1974;101:411–3.
15. Yukawa M, Satoh T, Higuchi T, Yokozeki H. Spiny keratoderma of the palms successfully treated with topical tacalcitol. Acta Derm Venereol. 2007;87:172–4.
16. Mehta RK, Mallett RB, Green C, Rytina E. Palmar filiform hyperkeratosis (FH) associated with underlying pathology? Clin Exp Dermatol. 2002;27:216–9.
17. Paul C, Fermand JP, Flageul B, Caux F, Duterque M, Dubertret L, Aractingi S. Hyperkeratotic spicules and monoclonal gammopathy. J Am Acad Dermatol. 1995;33:346–51.
18. Bernacchi E, Bianchi B, Amato L, Giorgini S, Fabbri P, Tavoni A, Bombardieri S. Xerosis in primary Sjogren syndrome: immunohistochemical and functional investigations. J Dermatol Sci. 2005;39:53–5.
19. Bork K, Bockers M, Pfeifle J. Pathogenesis of paraneoplastic follicular hyperkeratotic spicules in multiple myeloma. Follicular and epidermal accumulation of IgG dysprotein and cryoglobulin. Arch Dermatol. 1990;126:509–13.
20. Friedman SJ, Herman PS, Pittelkow MR, Su WP. Punctuate porokeratotic keratoderma. Arch Dermatol. 1988;124:1678–82.
21. Lukitsch O, Gebhardt KP, Kovary PM. Follicular hyperkeratosis and cryocrystalglobulinemia syndrome. Occurrence in a patient with multiple myeloma. Arch Dermatol. 1985;121:795–8.
22. Erkek E, Atasoy P. Fluorescence of hereditary type II punctate porokeratotic keratoderma (spiny keratoderma) with a Wood's light: stars under the moonlight. J Am Acad Dermatol. 2007;57:S63–4.
23. Torres G, Behshad R, Han A, Castrovinci AJ, Gilliam AC. "I forgot to shave my hands": a case of spiny keratoderma. J Am Acad Dermatol. 2008;58:344–8.
24. Bianchi L, Orlandi A, Iraci S, Spagnoli LG, Nini G. Punctate porokeratotic keratoderma--its occurrence with internal neoplasia. Clin Exp Dermatol. 1994;19:139–41.
25. Kondo S, Shimoura T, Hozumi Y, Aso K. Punctate porokeratotic keratoderma: some pathogenetic analyses of hyperproliferation and parakeratosis. Acta Derm Venereol. 1990;70:478–82.
26. Horton SL, Hashimoto K, Toi Y, Miner JE, Mehregan D, Fligiel A, Savoy LB, Aronson P. Spiny keratoderma: a common under-reported dermatosis. J Dermatol. 1998;25:353–61.

27. Osman Y, Daly TJ, Don PC. Spiny keratoderma of the palms and soles. J Am Acad Dermatol. 1992;26:879–81.
28. Salmon-Ehr V, Armingaud P, Cambie-Vanderschelden MP, Rault S, Kalis B. Spiny keratoderma. J Am Acad Dermatol. 1997;36:656.
29. Rosina P, Papagrigoraki A. Palmar filiform hyperkeratosis. Int J Dermatol. 2012;51:1483–4.

Vasculitis/Vasculopathy Syndrome Induced by Cocaine–Levamisole

Catherine G. Chung and Mary Gail Mercurio

Introduction

Levamisole is a pharmacologic agent first produced in 1966 as an antihelminthic agent and approved for human use for the treatment of rheumatoid arthritis, ulcerative colitis, nephrotic syndrome, and as an adjuvant in chemotherapeutic treatment of colorectal cancer [1–4]. Due to its unfavorable side effect profile, however, levamisole was withdrawn from the US market in 1999 and is currently commercially available only for veterinary purposes as an antiparasitic agent [1, 5]. Severe neutropenia was observed as an idiosyncratic reaction in up to 20% of patients receiving levamisole for rheumatoid arthritis [6–11]. In 1978, an occlusive necrotizing vasculitis was reported in a patient with rheumatoid arthritis treated with levamisole and presenting with a livedoid rash [12]; similar findings were subsequently noted children treated with levamisole for nephrotic syndrome presenting with skin necrosis in association with antinuclear antibodies (ANA) and antineutrophil cytoplasmic antibodies (ANCA) [13–17]. Common side effects associated with levamisole therapy included nausea, vomiting, headache, fatigue, fever, diarrhea, myalgia, and rash [3, 18–21].

Levamisole was first identified in cocaine in the United States in 2003 and was reported by the Drug Enforcement Agency (DEA) in 69% of all seized cocaine in 2009; more recent reports estimate over 80% of cocaine is laced with levamisole [18, 22–24]. The rationale behind the addition of levamisole to cocaine is not entirely known, but is believed to be multifactorial including being an inexpensive

C. G. Chung
The Ohio State University Wexner Medical Center, Columbus, OH, USA
e-mail: Catherine.Chung@osumc.edu

M. G. Mercurio (✉)
University of Rochester Medical Center, Rochester, NY, USA
e-mail: MaryGail_Mercurio@urmc.rochester.edu

F. Rongioletti, B. R. Smoller (eds.), *New and Emerging Entities in Dermatology and Dermatopathology*, https://doi.org/10.1007/978-3-030-80027-7_33

bulking agent, widely available through veterinary sources, and having similar physical properties to cocaine so its presence is not recognizable. Additionally, levamisole may enhance the effects of cocaine by potentiation of nicotinic and dopaminergic effects [1, 11, 23, 25, 26]. In 2009, a series of agranulocytosis occurring in association with levamisole-laced cocaine was reported [27], followed in 2010 by multiple reports of a distinct syndrome of necrotic facial lesions, retiform purpura, neutropenia, and ANCA positivity in patients with recent cocaine use [28–30].

Clinical Features

Cocaine-associated levamisole-induced vasculitis/vasculopathy (LIV) was first reported in 2010 in several patients presenting with a syndrome of facial lesions, retiform purpura, neutropenia, and various antibodies in the setting of cocaine abuse. Characteristic skin lesions consist of purpuric and necrotic plaques involving the face, often prominently involving the earlobes and malar cheeks (Fig. 1 a–c) [28–30]. The extremities (especially lower) are also frequent sites of involvement, often with retiform plaques, with relative sparing of the trunk (Fig. 2) [31–33]. Skin lesions occur 1–4 days after initial exposure to levamisole-adulterated cocaine and recur with reexposure [18, 34]. Less commonly and more recently, pyoderma gangrenosum of the upper and lower extremities has been recognized as a complication of exposure to levamisole (Fig. 3) [35]. Rare presentations with erythema elevatum diutinum-like lesions [36], eyelid necrosis with cicatricial ectropion [37], and inflammatory orbitopathy [38] have also been reported. Constitutional symptoms including generalized malaise, arthralgia, and myalgia may be present. Renal, pulmonary, and neurologic systems may also be affected, including acute kidney injury with hematuria and/or proteinuria, pulmonary hemorrhage and hypertension, and multifocal inflammatory leukoencephalopathy [39, 40]. A case of systemic cocaine-associated LIV in the absence of cutaneous lesions has been reported [41].

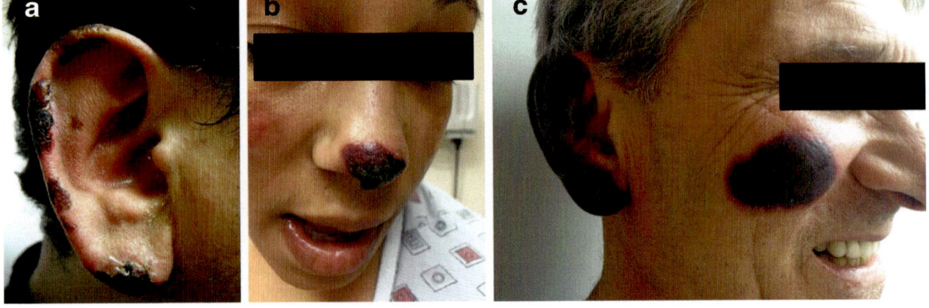

Fig. 1 Cocaine-associated levamisole-induced vasculitis/vasculopathy. Characteristic purpura of the face including ears (**a**, **c**), nose (**b**), and malar cheeks (**c**)

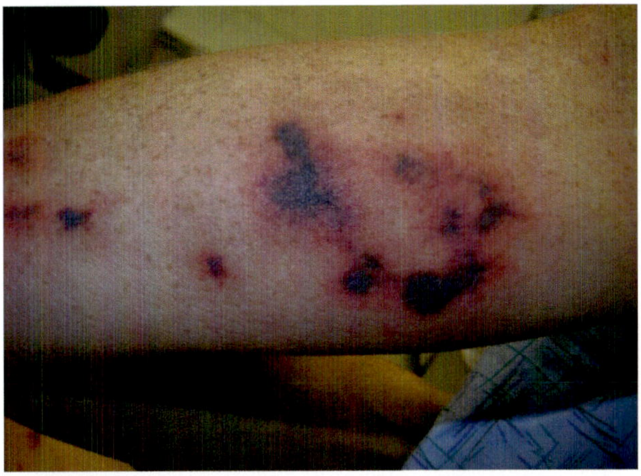

Fig. 2 Cocaine-associated levamisole-induced vasculitis/vasculopathy. Retiform purpura involving the upper extremity

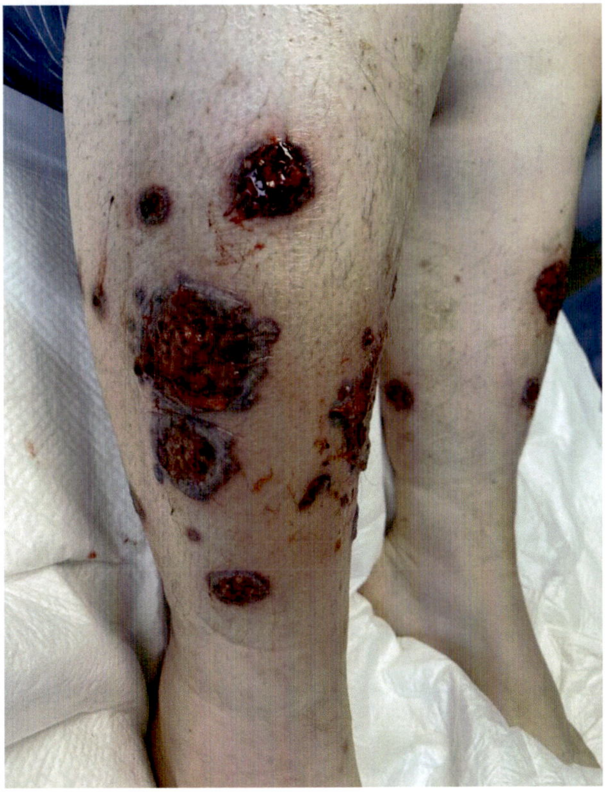

Fig. 3 Pyoderma gangrenosum occurring in the setting of levamisole-adulterated cocaine use. (Photo courtesy of Ritesh V. Agnihothri)

Multiple laboratory abnormalities are frequently encountered with cocaine-associated LIV, most notably elevated ANCA levels in 85–100% of cases that typically consists of elevated p-ANCA without substantial antibodies against myeloperoxidase (MPO), the usual antigenic target of p-ANCA. Instead, p-ANCA in LIV is directed against human neutrophil elastase (HNE), lactoferrin, and cathepsin [32, 42–44]. Titers are typically unusually high, with ranges of 1:40–1:2560 reported in a large case series [42]. In some cases of cocaine-associated LIV, elevated p-ANCA may be associated with anti-PR3 antibodies (typically associated with c-ANCA) and is believed to be secondary to cross-reactivity of antibodies against homologous epitopes on PR3 and HNE [43, 44]. Most cases of cocaine-associated LIV also demonstrate elevation in anti-phospholipid antibodies, including anti-cardiolipin antibody and/or lupus coagulant. Elevations in ANA and anti-dsDNA are also frequently present [32, 43]. Approximately one-third of cases are characterized by leukopenia, half of which have been associated with severe neutropenia with absolute neutrophil count (ANC) <1000. Thrombocytopenia may also occur [42, 43, 45]. Urine toxicology detects the presence of cocaine; detection of levamisole in urine by gas chromatography/mass spectrometry is frequently negative due to the short half-life of levamisole [39, 46–50]. Hair testing has therefore been suggested as a more reliable sample source for confirmation of the presence of levamisole [51, 52].

Histopathological Features

Histopathology from cutaneous specimens of cocaine-associated LIV demonstrates necrotizing small-vessel vasculitis of both superficial and deep dermal vessels with or without the presence of intravascular thrombi (Fig. 4). Involvement of the subcutis may occur, and medium-sized vessel involvement has been reported. In addition to prominent vascular and perivascular neutrophils, eosinophils may be present and

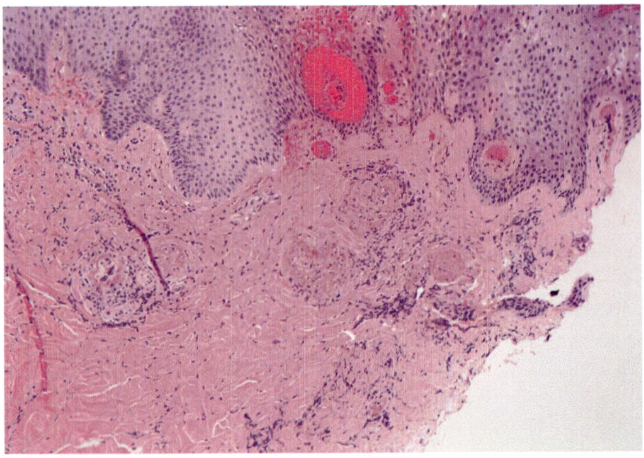

Fig. 4 Levamisole-induced vasculitis/vasculopathy. Small vessels demonstrate necrotizing leukocytoclastic vasculitis with intravascular fibrin thrombi (hematoxylin and eosin, 100×)

numerous. Direct immunofluorescence findings are consistent with immune complex-mediated vasculitis, including granular deposition of IgM, C3, and fibrin in dermal vessels [31, 34, 43, 53].

In patients with renal injury, histopathology most frequently demonstrates focal necrotizing and crescentic pauci-immune glomerulonephritis, although membranous nephropathy and immune complex glomerulonephritis have also been reported [32, 42, 43, 45, 54–56].

Pathogenesis

Although the complete mechanisms by which cocaine-associated LIV syndrome occurs are not fully known, a large part of the clinical spectrum likely occurs due to the formation of neutrophil extracellular traps (NET), a process also known as NETosis. NETosis is a unique process of programmed cell death in which activated neutrophils release NETs containing dsDNA, histones, and granule contents including MPO, PR3, elastase, cathepsin G, and lactoferrin. Levamisole may trigger NETosis, which may both generate and be induced by ANCAs and subsequently cause direct endothelial damage and inflammation via activation of the alternative complement pathway. NETs are also a major component of thromboemboli and activate the coagulation cascade [40, 57–63]. In contrast, the process by which severe neutropenia/agranulocytosis occurs is not certain, but is believed to be idiosyncratic secondary to immune-mediated destruction of neutrophils [40, 64, 65].

Differential Diagnosis

The main clinical considerations in the differential diagnosis of cocaine-associated LIV are those of idiopathic and drug-induced ANCA-associated vasculitis (AAV) but includes a broad spectrum of disease that may present with skin necrosis, retiform purpura, systemic symptoms, and laboratory abnormalities including autoimmune connective tissue disease, anti-phospholipid antibody syndrome, polyarteritis nodosa, cryoglobulinemia, intravascular infections, disseminated intravascular coagulation, and warfarin necrosis [18, 30, 34, 53].

Of note, cocaine in the absence of levamisole may induce cocaine-induced midline destructive lesions (CIMDL), an AAV clinically and histopathologically identical to granulomatosis with polyangiitis (GPA). While idiopathic GPA is associated with elevation in c-ANCA against PR3, CIMDL is most commonly associated with elevated p-ANCA against HNE, a similar profile to that seen in LIV [13, 18, 53, 66–71]. Laboratory findings are also helpful in differentiating LIV from idiopathic AAV, as the latter presents with lower ANCA titers compared with those seen in LIV and with specific antibodies to one neutrophilic target rather than several [43].

Prognosis

Cocaine-associated LIV carries an overall favorable prognosis, with complete resolution of cutaneous lesions 1–3 weeks after discontinuation of cocaine use. Extensive necrotizing skin lesions requiring nasal and extremity amputation however have been reported [72, 73]. Neutropenia typically recovers 5–10 days after cocaine cessation with normalization of antibody titers over 2–14 months [11, 27, 28, 33, 46, 50, 53, 74–76]. Rare deaths have been reported in the setting of cocaine-associated LIV, typically attributed to cardiac, pulmonary, or brain pathology [3, 22, 75, 77–79].

Therapy

While standard therapy for cocaine-associated LIV has not been established due to its relatively low prevalence, the mainstay of treatment is discontinuation of cocaine use. Clinical findings recur with reexposure to levamisole. Of those patients requiring treatment, most received systemic steroids, azathioprine, chloroquine, methotrexate, cyclophosphamide, rituximab, acetyl salicylic acid, colchicine, and anticoagulation have also been reported [11, 30, 32, 42, 45, 80–82]. A refractory case of cocaine-associated LIV was successfully treated with aspirin, prednisone, and vardenafil [83].

References

1. Brunt TM, van den Berg J, Pennings E, Venhuis B. Adverse effects of levamisole in cocaine users: a review and risk assessment. Arch Toxicol. 2017;91(6):2303–13.
2. Wolford A, McDonald TS, Eng H, Hansel S, Chen Y, Bauman J, et al. Immune-mediated agranulocytosis caused by the cocaine adulterant levamisole: a case for reactive metabolite(s) involvement. Drug Metab Dispos. 2012;40(6):1067–75.
3. Solomon N, Hayes J. Levamisole: a high performance cutting agent. Acad Forensic Pathol. 2017;7(3):469–76.
4. Le Garff E, Tournel G, Becquart C, Cottencin O, Dupin N, Delaporte E, et al. Extensive necrotic purpura in levamisole-adulterated cocaine abuse – a case report. J Forensic Sci. 2016;61(6):1681–5.
5. Bertol E, Mari F, Di Milia MG, Politi L, Furlanetto S, Karch SB. Determination of aminorex in human urine samples by GC-MS after use of levamisole. J Pharm Biomed Anal. 2011;55(5):1186–9.
6. Espinoza LR, Dorval G, Osterland CK. Levamisole-induced adverse reactions and histocompatibility testing in malignant melanoma. Tissue Antigens. 1979;236–7.
7. Mielants H, Veys EM. B27 and agranulocytosis and rheumatoid arthritis patients treated with levamisole. Clin Endocrinol Metab. 1979.
8. Symoens J, Veys E, Mielants M, Pinals R. Adverse reactions to levamisole. Cancer Treat Rep. 1978.
9. Hodinka L, Meretey K, Zahumenszky Z, Bozsoky S. Levamisole: clinical and immunological experiences in one year levamisole treatment of rheumatoid arthritis patients; opportunities

of immune modulation in the base therapy of rheumatoid arthritis. Rheumatol Balneol Allergol. 1979.
10. Drew SI, Carter BM, Nathanson DS, Terasaki PI. Levamisole-associated neutropenia and autoimmune granulocytotoxins. Ann Rheum Dis. 1980.
11. Khan TA, Cuchacovich R, Espinoza LR, Lata S, Patel NJ, Garcia-Valladares I, et al. Vasculopathy, hematological, and immune abnormalities associated with levamisole-contaminated cocaine use. Semin Arthritis Rheum. 2011;
12. Scheinberg MA, Bezerra JB, Almeida FA, Silveira LA. Cutaneous necrotising vasculitis induced by levamisole. Br Med J. 1978;1(6110):408.
13. Menni S, Pistritto G, Gianotti R, Ghio L, Edefonti A. Ear lobe bilateral necrosis by levamisole-induced occlusive vasculitis in a pediatric patient. Pediatr Dermatol. 1997.
14. Barbano G, Ginevri F, Ghiggeri GM, Gusmano R. Disseminated autoimmune disease during levamisole treatment of nephrotic syndrome. Pediatr Nephrol. 1999.
15. Rongioletti F, Ghio L, Ginevri F, Bleidl D, Rinaldi S, Edefonti A, et al. Purpura of the ears: a distinctive vasculopathy with circulating autoantibodies complicating long-term treatment with levamisole in children. Br J Dermatol. 1999.
16. Powell J, Grech H, Holder J. A boy with cutaneous necrosis occurring during treatment with levamisole. Clin Exp Dermatol. 2002.
17. Laux-End R, Inaebnit D, Gerber HA, Bianchetti MG. Vasculitis associated with levamisole and circulating autoantibodies [3]. Arch Dis Child. 1996.
18. Larocque A, Hoffman RS. Levamisole in cocaine: unexpected news from an old acquaintance. Clin Toxicol. 2012;50(4):231–41.
19. Segal AW, Levi AJ, Loewi G. Levamisole in the treatment of Crohn's disease. Lancet. 1977.
20. Pinals RS, Robertson F, Blechman WJ. A double-blind comparison of high and low doses of levamisole in rheumatoid arthritis. J Rheumatol. 1981.
21. Parkinson DR, Jerry LM, Shibata HR, Lewis MG, Cano PO, Capek A, et al. Complications of cancer immunotherapy with levamisole. Lancet. 1977.
22. Centers for Disease Control and Prevention (CDC). Agranulocytosis associated with cocaine use - four states, March 2008-November 2009. MMWR Morb Mortal Wkly Rep. 2009.
23. Tallarida CS, Egan E, Alejo GD, Raffa R, Tallarida RJ, Rawls SM. Levamisole and cocaine synergism: a prevalent adulterant enhances cocaine's action in vivo. Neuropharmacology. 2014.
24. Tallarida CS, Tallarida RJ, Rawls SM. Levamisole enhances the rewarding and locomotor-activating effects of cocaine in rats. Drug Alcohol Depend. 2015.
25. Fucci N. Unusual adulterants in cocaine seizured on Italian clandestine market. Forensic Sci Int. 2007.
26. Raymon LP, Isenschmid DS. The possible role of levamisole in illicit cocaine preparations. J Anal Toxicol. 2009.
27. Zhu NY, Legatt DF, Turner AR. Agranulocytosis after consumption of cocaine adulterated with levamisole. Ann Intern Med. 2009.
28. Waller JM, Feramisco JD, Alberta-Wszolek L, McCalmont TH, Fox LP. Cocaine-associated retiform purpura and neutropenia: is levamisole the culprit? J Am Acad Dermatol. 2010.
29. Bradford M, Rosenberg B, Moreno J, Dumyati G. Bilateral necrosis of earlobes and cheeks: another complication of cocaine contaminated with levamisole. Ann Intern Med. 2010.
30. Chung C, Tumeh PC, Birnbaum R, Tan BH, Sharp L, McCoy E, et al. Characteristic purpura of the ears, vasculitis, and neutropenia - a potential public health epidemic associated with levamisole-adulterated cocaine. J Am Acad Dermatol. 2011;65(4):722–5.
31. Arora NP. Cutaneous vasculopathy and neutropenia associated with levamisole- adulterated cocaine. Am J Med Sci. 2013.
32. Graf J, Lynch K, Yeh CL, Tarter L, Richman N, Nguyen T, et al. Purpura, cutaneous necrosis, and antineutrophil cytoplasmic antibodies associated with levamisole-adulterated cocaine. Arthritis Rheum. 2011.
33. Walsh NMG, Green PJ, Burlingame RW, Pasternak S, Hanly JG. Cocaine-related retiform purpura: evidence to incriminate the adulterant, levamisole. J Cutan Pathol. 2010.

34. Fernandez Armenteros JM, Veà Jódar A, Matas Nadal C, Cortés Pinto CP, Soria Gili X, Martí Laborda RM, et al. Severe and recurrent levamisole-induced cutaneous vasculopathy. J Cutan Pathol. 2018.
35. Jeong HS, Layher H, Cao L, Vandergriff T, Dominguez AR. Pyoderma gangrenosum (PG) associated with levamisole-adulterated cocaine: clinical, serologic, and histopathologic findings in a cohort of patients. J Am Acad Dermatol. 2016;74(5):892–8.
36. Dewan AK, Pinard J, Jadeja S, Granter S, Merola JF. Erythema elevatum diutinum-like vasculitis secondary to cocaine adulterated with levamisole. Clin Exp Dermatol. 2018;43(4):494–6.
37. Ramesh S, Sobti D, Mancini R. Eyelid necrosis and secondary cicatrical ectropion secondary to levamisole-associated vasculitis. Ophthal Plast Reconstr Surg. 2017;33(3S):S38–40.
38. Muniz Castro HM, Do TH, Bhattacharjee MB, Adesina OOO, Richani K. A unique presentation of levamisole-induced antineutrophil-cytoplasmic-antibody-positive vasculitis presenting as inflammatory orbitopathy. Ophthal Plast Reconstr Surg. 2020;36(4):e96–100.
39. Lee KC, Ladizinski B, Federman DG. Complications associated with use of levamisole-contaminated cocaine: an emerging public health challenge. Mayo Clin Proc. 2012;87(6):581–6.
40. Cascio MJ, Jen KY. Cocaine/levamisole-associated autoimmune syndrome: a disease of neutrophil-mediated autoimmunity. Curr Opin Hematol. 2018;25(1):29–36.
41. Baptiste GG, Alexopoulos AS, Masud T, Bonsall JM. Systemic levamisole-induced vasculitis in a cocaine user without cutaneous findings: a consideration in diagnosis. Case Rep Med. 2015;2015:10–3.
42. Muñoz-Vahos CH, Herrera-Uribe S, Arbeláez-Cortés Á, Jaramillo-Arroyave D, González-Naranjo LA, Vásquez-Duque G, et al. Clinical profile of levamisole-adulterated cocaine-induced vasculitis/vasculopathy: a 30-case series. J Clin Rheumatol. 2019.
43. Nolan AL, Jen KY. Pathologic manifestations of levamisole-adulterated cocaine exposure. Diagn Pathol. 2015;10(1):4–9.
44. Graf J. Rheumatic manifestations of cocaine use. Curr Opin Rheumatol. 2013.
45. McGrath MM, Isakova T, Rennke HG, Mottola AM, Laliberte KA, Niles JL. Contaminated cocaine and antineutrophil cytoplasmic antibody-associated disease. Clin J Am Soc Nephrol. 2011.
46. Lee KC, Culpepper K, Kessler M. Levamisole-induced thrombosis: literature review and pertinent laboratory findings. J Am Acad Dermatol. 2011.
47. Jenkins J, Babu K, Hsu-Hung E, Robinson-Bostom L, Kroumpouzos G. ANCA-positive necrotizing vasculitis and thrombotic vasculopathy induced by levamisole-adulterated cocaine: a distinctive clinicopathologic presentation. J Am Acad Dermatol. 2011.
48. Mouzakis J, Somboonwit C, Lakshmi S, Rumbak M, Sinnott J, Cherpelis B, et al. Levamisole induced necrosis of the skin and neutropenia following intranasal cocaine use: a newly recognized syndrome. J Drugs Dermatol. 2011.
49. Herms B, Kaplon M, Baumann M. Agranulocytosis in cocaine users in Ohio: suspected levamisole taint. Leuk Res. 2011.
50. Buchanan JA, Oyer RJ, Patel NR, Jacquet GA, Bornikova L, Thienelt C, et al. A confirmed case of agranulocytosis after use of cocaine contaminated with levamisole. J Med Toxicol. 2010.
51. Lazareth H, Peytavin G, Polivka L, Dupin N. The hairy-print for levamisole-induced vasculitis. BMJ Case Rep. 2012;1:2–4.
52. Van Der Veer T, Pennings E, Tervaert JWC, Korswagen LA. Levamisole-contaminated cocaine: a hairy affair. BMJ Case Rep. 2015;2015:10–2.
53. Crowe DR, Kim PS, Mutasim DF. Clinical, histopathologic, and immunofluorescence findings in levamisole/cocaine-induced thrombotic vasculitis. Int J Dermatol. 2014;53(5):635–7.
54. Díaz HÁ, Callejo AIM, Rodríguez JFG, Pazos LR, Buela IG, Barrera AMB. ANCA-positive vasculitis induced by levamisole-adulterated cocaine and nephrotic syndrome: the kidney as an unusual target. Am J Case Rep. 2013;14:557–61.
55. Collister D, Sathianathan C, Ryz K, Karpinski M, Bernstein K, Gibson IW. ANCA associated vasculitis secondary to levamisole-adultered cocaine with associated membranous nephropathy: a case series. Am J Nephrol. 2017;45(3):209–16.

56. Garg L, Gupta S, Swami A, Zhang P. Levamisole/cocaine induced systemic vasculitis and immune complex glomerulonephritis. Case Rep Nephrol. 2015;2015:1–5.
57. Jin Q, Kant S, Alhariri J, Geetha D. Levamisole adulterated cocaine associated ANCA vasculitis: review of literature and update on pathogenesis. J Community Hosp Intern Med Perspect. 2018;8(6):339–44.
58. Pieterse E, van der Vlag J. Cracking the pathogenesis of cocaine-induced vasculitis. Rheumatol (United Kingdom). 2017;56(4):503–5.
59. Lood C, Hughes GC. Neutrophil extracellular traps as a potential source of autoantigen in cocaine-associated auto immunity. Rheumatol (United Kingdom). 2017.
60. Sangaletti S, Tripodo C, Chiodoni C, Guarnotta C, Cappetti B, Casalini P, et al. Neutrophil extracellular traps mediate transfer of cytoplasmic neutrophil antigens to myeloid dendritic cells toward ANCA induction and associated autoimmunity. Blood. 2012.
61. Rao AN. Do neutrophil extracellular traps contribute to the heightened risk of thrombosis in inflammatory diseases? World J Cardiol. 2015.
62. Kambas K, Chrysanthopoulou A, Vassilopoulos D, Apostolidou E, Skendros P, Girod A, et al. Tissue factor expression in neutrophil extracellular traps and neutrophil derived microparticles in antineutrophil cytoplasmic antibody associated vasculitis may promote thromboinflammation and the thrombophilic state associated with the disease. Ann Rheum Dis. 2014.
63. Jorch SK, Kubes P. An emerging role for neutrophil extracellular traps in noninfectious disease. Nat Med. 2017.
64. Mielants H, Veys EM. Adverse reactions to levamisole in the treatment of rheumatoid arthritis. Acta Rhumatol. 1980.
65. Hellmann A, Goldman JM. Effect of levamisole on granulopoiesis in agar culture. Biomed Express. 1980.
66. Rachapalli SM, Kiely PDW. Cocaine-induced midline destructive lesions mimicking ENT-limited Wegener's granulomatosis. Scand J Rheumatol. 2008.
67. Wiesner O, Russell KA, Lee AS, Jenne DE, Trimarchi M, Gregorini G, et al. Antineutrophil cytoplasmic antibodies reacting with human neutrophil elastase as a diagnostic marker for cocaine-induced midline destructive lesions but not autoimmune vasculitis. Arthritis Rheum. 2004.
68. Csernok E, Lamprecht P, Gross WL. Clinical and immunological features of drug-induced and infection-induced proteinase 3-antineutrophil cytoplasmic antibodies and myeloperoxidase-antineutrophil cytoplasmic antibodies and vasculitis. Curr Opin Rheumatol. 2010.
69. Gao Y, Zhao MH. Review article: drug-induced anti-neutrophil cytoplasmic antibody-associated vasculitis. Nephrology. 2009.
70. Carrasco MD. Cutaneous vasculitis associated with propylthiouracil therapy. Arch Intern Med. 1987.
71. Neynaber S, Mistry-Burchardi N, Rust C, Samtleben W, Burgdorf WHC, Seitz MA, et al. PR3-ANCA-positive necrotizing multi-organ vasculitis following cocaine abuse. Acta Derm Venereol. 2008.
72. Baltarowich L, Schlichting A, Leder C, Ormsby A. Skin necrosis associated with exposure to cocaine contaminated with levamisole: an emerging phenomenon. Clin Toxicol. 2011;49(6):524–5.
73. Ching JA, Smith DJ. Levamisole-induced necrosis of skin, soft tissue, and bone: case report and review of literature. J Burn Care Res. 2012.
74. Wiens MO, Son WK, Ross C, Hayden M, Carleton B. Cocaine adulterant linked to neutropenia. CMAJ. 2010.
75. Czuchlewski DR, Brackney M, Ewers C, Manna J, Fekrazad MH, Martinez A, et al. Clinicopathologic features of agranulocytosis in the setting of levamisole-tainted cocaine. Am J Clin Pathol. 2010.
76. Buchanan JA, Vogel JA, Eberhardt AM. Levamisole-induced occlusive necrotizing vasculitis of the ears after use of cocaine contaminated with levamisole. J Med Toxicol. 2011.

77. Indorato F, Romano G, Barbera N. Levamisole-adulterated cocaine: two fatal case reports and evaluation of possible cocaine toxicity potentiation. Forensic Sci Int. 2016.
78. Matthews AR, Oladapo O, Morgan BW. A cocaine death with concomitant adulterant-induced toxicity. Clin Toxicol. 2009;47(7):761.
79. Knowles L, Buxton JA, Skuridina N, Achebe I, LeGatt D, Fan S, et al. Levamisole tainted cocaine causing severe neutropenia in Alberta and British Columbia. Harm Reduct J. 2009.
80. Ullrich K, Koval R, Koval E, Bapoje S, Hirsh JM. Five consecutive cases of a cutaneous vasculopathy in users of levamisole-adulterated cocaine. J Clin Rheumatol. 2011.
81. Gross RL, Brucker J, Bahce-Altuntas A, Abadi MA, Lipoff J, Kotlyar D, et al. A novel cutaneous vasculitis syndrome induced by levamisole-contaminated cocaine. Clin Rheumatol. 2011;30(10):1385–92.
82. Poon SH, Baliog CR, Sams RN, Robinson-Bostom L, Telang GH, Reginato AM. Syndrome of cocaine-levamisole-induced cutaneous vasculitis and immune-mediated leukopenia. Semin Arthritis Rheum. 2011;
83. Mandrell J, Kranc CL. Prednisone and vardenafil hydrochloride for refractory levamisole-induced vasculitis. Cutis. 2016;98(2):E15–9.

Lymphocytic Thrombophilic Arteritis (Macular Lymphocytic Arteritis)

Maxime Battistella and Bernard Cribier

Introduction

Lymphocytic thrombophilic arteritis (LTA), macular lymphocytic arteritis (MLA), is a clinicopathologic entity first described by Fein et al. in 2003 under the name macular arteritis (MA), as a new peculiar and indolent vasculitis [1]. They described three patients with minimally symptomatic hyperpigmented macules on the extremities, without palpable purpura or erythematous nodules, whose histology demonstrated a medium-sized vessel arteritis with lymphocytic infiltrate. Later, the same team made the name evolve to macular lymphocytic arteritis (MLA) [2]. In parallel, in 2008, Lee et al. described five females with similar clinicopathologic features and proposed the name of lymphocytic thrombophilic arteritis (LTA) describing the presence of both vascular thrombosis and lymphocytic arterial inflammation [3]. Later studies used the terms LTA or MLA to describe a spectrum of disease with similar histology and similar appearing clinical pictures [4]. A debate also exists on whether LTA/MLA is an indolent form of cutaneous polyarteritis nodosa (cPAN), adding complexity to the understanding of the entity [4–7]. Finally, recent works suggested to use LTA as a unifying naming, rather than MLA, as non-macular cases have been reported [8].

M. Battistella (✉)
Pathology Department, Hôpital Saint-Louis, AP-HP, Université de Paris, INSERM U976, Paris, France
e-mail: maxime.battistella@aphp.fr

B. Cribier
Dermatology and Dermatopathology, Clinique Dermatologique, Hôpitaux Universitaires de Strasbourg, Strasbourg, France

F. Rongioletti, B. R. Smoller (eds.), *New and Emerging Entities in Dermatology and Dermatopathology*, https://doi.org/10.1007/978-3-030-80027-7_34

Clinical Features

Less than 100 cases of LTA (MLA) have been reported to date in the literature. The vast majority of patients are females, with a median age of about 40 years (range, 6–73 years) [8]. Children with the condition have been very rarely reported [9, 10]. The disease occurs in patients of various ethnic descent, including 30% of Black and 20% of Asian patients [8]. LTA is commonly an indolent disease with sometimes long duration before diagnosis. The most common clinical presentation includes bilateral erythematous to brown hyperpigmented macules or livedoid patches, involving the lower extremities (almost 100% of patients), the upper extremities (around 50% of patients), and much less frequently the trunk (Figs. 1 and 2). Lesions can include petechiae and poikilodermatous patches. Small punctate ulcers have been described [8]. Skin lesions may rarely be palpable (papules) [4], appear as a non-blanching erythematous annular eruption [10, 11], or be unilateral [12].

All patients present with subtle or no symptoms. When present, symptoms include pruritus, pain/tenderness, numbness, or extremity weakness.

Histopathological Features

LTA/MLA lesions are characterized by a lymphocyte-predominant medium-sized vessel arteritis near the deep dermal subcutaneous junction with scant or no neutrophils (Fig. 3) [2–5]. Involved arteries are typically infiltrated by lymphocytes and

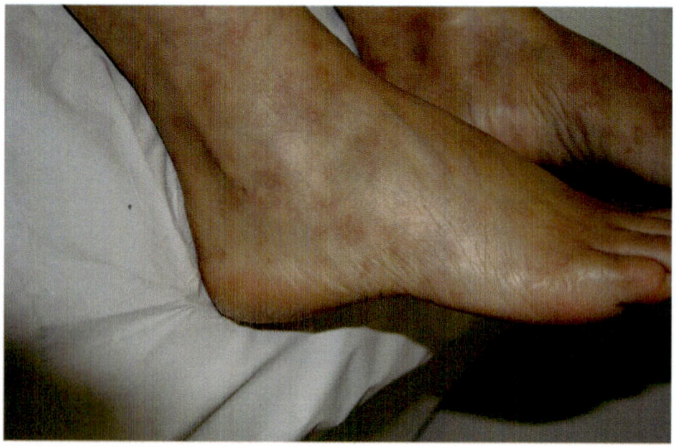

Fig. 1 Lymphocytic thrombophilic arteritis: Erythematous and brown macules on the feet

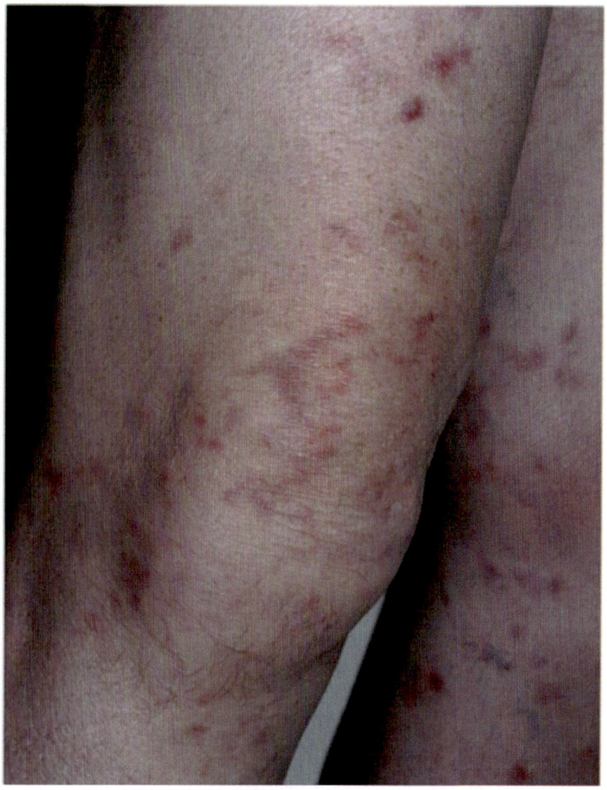

Fig. 2 Lymphocytic thrombophilic arteritis: Livedoid erythematous macules on the legs and thigh, with the presence of slightly palpable lesions

display a concentric intimal hyalinized fibrin ring, with respect to the internal elastic lamina (Fig. 4) [13]. The intimal fibrin deposits may involve a part or the totality of the intima circumference. Inflammation is confined to the vicinity of the vessel and the immediate surrounding panniculus. Lumina of arteries are narrowed by the thick intimal fibrin deposit and may be occluded by a luminal thrombosis.

Etiopathogenesis

Laboratory investigations are heterogeneous in the literature, and few data are available regarding the pathogenesis of the disease. Initial workup is often unremarkable. Elevated erythrocyte sedimentation rate and the presence of anticentromere or antinuclear antibody, lupus anticoagulant, and anti-Ro/SSA have been reported in some cases [8]. Anti-beta2 GP1 antibodies have been detected in some cases with luminal thrombosis [3, 14, 15]. However, no typical reproducible laboratory findings are known to date.

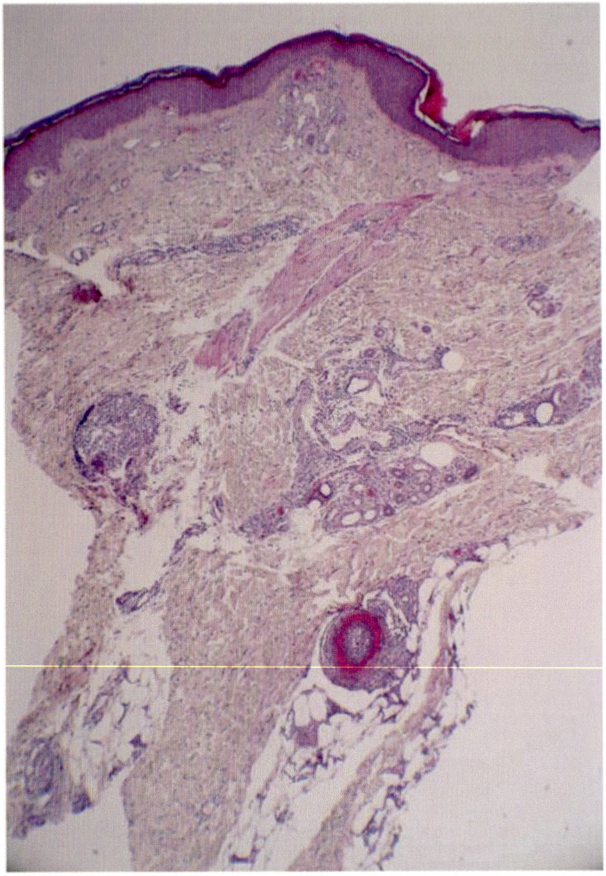

Fig. 3 Lymphocytic thrombophilic arteritis: Inflammation and necrosis of a medium-sized artery of the dermal subcutaneous junction (Haematoxylin and eosin staining; x10 magnification)

In 2017, Magro et al. described a consistent C5b-9 deposition on the endothelium and intima of involved vessel, an upregulated type I interferon microenvironment and marked upregulation of the inducible interferon gamma 16 protein, in ten patients [16]. Anecdotally, one case has been described with concurrent HIV and VHB infection [15], two cases with minocycline use [17, 18], and one case in a patient with rheumatoid arthritis [19]. No strong association is reported to other disease.

Altogether, LTA (MLA) probably lies somewhere between an inflammatory vasculitis mediated by lymphocytes and thrombotic vasculopathy restricted to the skin, and further studies elucidating pathophysiology are needed.

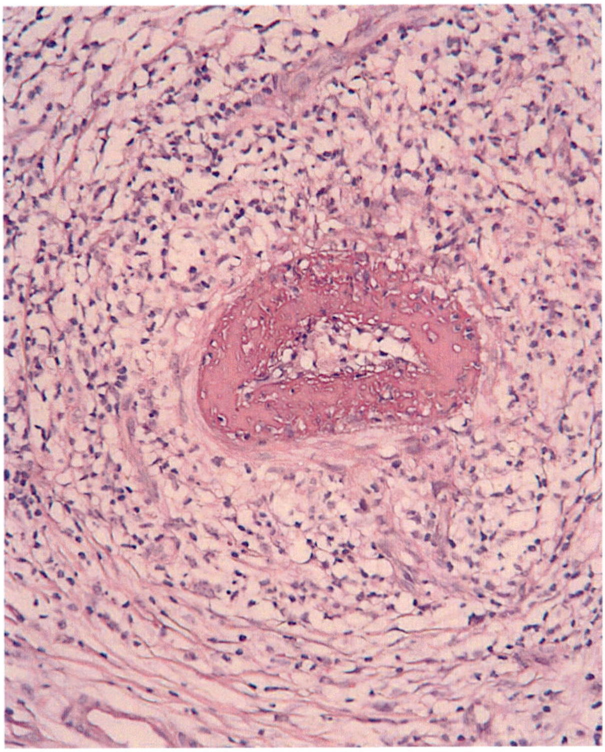

Fig. 4 Lymphocytic thrombophilic arteritis: Concentric hyaline fibrin ring in the intima of the involved artery, with respect to the internal elastic lamina. The lumen is partly occluded, and the vessel wall and periarterial tissue contain a lymphocytic inflammatory infiltrate, with no neutrophils (hematoxylin and eosin staining; ×200 magnification)

Differential Diagnosis

Clinically, LTA (MLA) may mimic pigmented purpuric dermatosis, but histology will easily discriminate both conditions [9]. When LTA (MLA) presents as a chronic persistent widespread blanchable livedo racemosa, Sneddon syndrome may also be evocated [20]. Again, histological features will discriminate both diseases, as Sneddon syndrome involves small vessel of the subcutis and appears as a fibrous endarteritis obliterans with few or no inflammation. Sneddon syndrome does not involve medium-sized vessels and lacks the typical intimal hyalinized fibrin deposits of LTA (MLA).

Far more complex is the differential diagnosis with cPAN. Since the initial description of LTA (MLA), there has been continuous debate regarding its classification as a distinct disease or as an indolent latent form of cPAN [4–8, 15].

cPAN is a neutrophilic-mediated medium-sized necrotizing arteritis of the deep dermal/subcutaneous tissue, characterized clinically by nodules, ulceration, and livedo reticularis. In some cases, lesions may be macular, but evolution to brown/pigmented macules is not a classical feature. cPAN is often associated with pain/tenderness, arthralgias, neuropathy, and less frequently fever [6, 8]. Histopathological features of cPAN vary according to the dynamics of the inflammatory process. In the acute stage, there is transmural fibrinoid necrosis with disruption of the internal elastic lamina and a neutrophil-rich inflammatory infiltrate. Thrombosis may occur. Later on, cPAN lesions evolve to a reparative/healing stage where neutrophils decrease and fibrous endarteritis is seen [21, 22]. Cases of cPAN with histopathological features consistent with LTA (MLA) have been reported [6, 21]. Therefore, it appears possible that the reparative stage of cPAN mimic LTA (MLA) histopathologically [8]. In this context, careful clinicopathologic correlation and clinical follow-up is mandatory to classify a patient as having LTA (MLA) or cPAN.

Prognosis

LTA (MLA) is typically a nonprogressive indolent but chronic and persistent disease. In almost all cases, there is no progression to systemic vasculitis, even after long follow-up [8, 23]. In one case only, bilateral focal testicular infarcts were described [24]. Peripheral neuropathy has been documented in very few patients [8, 24]. Importantly, no serious ischemic systemic manifestations have been reported to date, especially no central nervous system involvement.

As LTA (MLA) histopathological features have been described in cPAN and because LTA (MLA) has thrombotic features with possible circulating prothrombotic factors, a close follow-up of the patients is recommended. Performing a new skin biopsy seems necessary in case of new types of skin lesions, such as nodule or ulceration, to rule out proper cPAN.

Therapy

Because of the benign indolent but persistent course of LTA (MLA), treatment can be symptom driven, and treatment efficacy is particularly difficult to assess from literature data [8]. Treatments have been largely unsuccessful in providing long-term clinical remission. A variety of immune modulating treatment have been used, of which two patients had durable symptom regression while on dapsone and one patient demonstrated resolution with low-dose prednisone, methotrexate, and colchicine [8]. In one study, three patients had clinical response to aspirin and pentoxifylline, including a patient with relapse and remission upon cessation and readministration of therapy [11].

For patients with asymptomatic lesions, an expectant management may be appropriate. Oral and topical steroids do not seem helpful. Anticoagulation or antiplatelet treatments do not provide consistent responses. Altogether, due to the limited number of patients reported and to the diversity of treatment regimen used with inconsistent treatment response, caution must be taken in speculating treatment efficacy in LTA (MLA) [8].

References

1. Fein H, Sheth AP, Mutasim DF. Cutaneous arteritis presenting with hyperpigmented macules: macular arteritis. J Am Acad Dermatol. 2003;49:519–22.
2. Saleh Z, Mutasim DF. Macular lymphocytic arteritis: a unique benign cutaneous arteritis, mediated by lymphocytes and appearing as macules. J Cutan Pathol. 2009;36:1269–74.
3. Lee JS, Kossard S, McGrath MA. Lymphocytic thrombophilic arteritis: a newly described medium-sized vessel arteritis of the skin. Arch Dermatol. 2008;144:1175–82.
4. Macarenco RS, Galan A, Simoni PM, Macarenco AC, Tintle SJ, Rose R, Halasz CL, Carlson JA. Cutaneous lymphocytic thrombophilic (macular) arteritis: a distinct entity or an indolent (reparative) stage of cutaneous polyarteritis nodosa? Report of 2 cases of cutaneous arteritis and review of the literature. Am J Dermatopathol. 2013;35:213–9.
5. Al-Daraji W, Gregory AN, Carlson JA. "Macular arteritis": a latent form of cutaneous polyarteritis nodosa? Am J Dermatopathol. 2008;30:145–9.
6. Buffière-Morgado A, Battistella M, Vignon-Pennamen MD, de Masson A, Rybojad M, Petit A, Cordoliani F, Begon E, Flageul B, Mahr A, Bagot M, Bouaziz JD. Relationship between cutaneous polyarteritis nodosa (cPAN) and macular lymphocytic arteritis (MLA): blinded histologic assessment of 35 cPAN cases. J Am Acad Dermatol. 2015;73:1013:20.
7. Kelly RI, Wee E, Balta S, Williams RA. Lymphocytic thrombophilic arteritis and cutaneous polyarteritis nodosa: clinicopathologic comparison with blinded histologic assessment. J Am Acad Dermatol. 2020;83:501–8.
8. Vakili S, Zampella JG, Kwatra SG, Blanck J, Loss M. Lymphocytic thrombopilic arteritis: a review. J Clin Rheumatol. 2019;25:147–52.
9. Buckthal-McCuin J, Mutasim DF. Macular arteritis mimicking pigmented purpuric dermatosis in a 6 year-old Caucasian girl. Pediatr Dermatol. 2009;26:93–5.
10. Juan-Carpena G, Palazon-Cabanes JC, Silva-Ortega S, Blanes-Martinez M, Betlloch-Mas I. Atypical pediatric presentation of lymphocytic thrombophilic arteritis: diagnostic difficulties and recent nosological clarification. Pediatr Dermatol. 2020 Oct 21; https://doi.org/10.1111/pde.14412.
11. Kelly RI, Wee E, Tancharoen C, Tam MM, Balta S, Williams RA. Three cases of lymphocytic arteritis presenting with an annular eruption. Australas J Dermatol. 2018;59:e127–32.
12. Arana-Guajardo A, Mendoza-Rodriguez C, Miranda-Maldonado I. Unilateral macular lymphocytic arteritis. J Rheumatol. 2016;43:1763–4.
13. Morruzzi C, Cribier B, Lipsker D. Macular arteritis. Ann Dermatol Venereol. 2010;137:460–3.
14. Garcia C, Dandurand M, Roger P, Joujoux JM, Meunier L, Stoebner PE. Macular lymphocytic arteritis: three cases questioning its classification as primary lymphocytic vasculitis. Dermatology. 2014;228:103–6.
15. Kolivras A, Thompson C, Metx T, André J. Macular arteritis associated with concurrent HIV and hepatitis B infections: a case report and evidence for a disease spectrum association with cutaneous polyarteritis nodosa. J Cutan Pathol. 2015;42:416–9.
16. Magro CM, Saab J. Lymphocytic thrombophilic arteritis: a distinct inflammatory type I interferon and C5b-9 mediated subcutaneous endovasculitis. Ann Diagn Pathol. 2017;31:23–9.

17. Kassardjian M, Horowitz D, Shitabata PK, Clark LE. Lymphocytic thrombophilic arteritis induced by minocycline. J Clin Aesthet Dermatol. 2012;5:38–43.
18. Tan CWX, Koh MJA. Lymphocytic thrombophilic arteritis : a possible association with minocycline. Pediatr Dermatol. 2017;34:e160–3.
19. Munehiro A, Yoneda K, Koura A, Nakai K, Kubota Y. Macular lymphocytic arteritis in a patient with rheumatoid arthritis. Eur J Dermatol. 2012;22:427–8.
20. Ting S, Kelly RI. Three cases of Sneddon syndrome: a comparison with lymphocytic thrombophilic arteritis. Australas J Dermatol. 2020.
21. Morimoto A, Chen KR. Reappraisal of histopathology of cutaneous polyarteritis nodosa. J Cutan Pathol. 2016;43:1131–8.
22. Ishibashi M, Chen KR. A morphological study of evolution of cutaneous polyarteritis nodosa. Am J Dermatopathol. 2008;30:319–26.
23. Morita TCAB, Tres GFS, Criado PR. Is macular lymphocytic arteritis limited to the skin ? Long-term follow-up of seven patients. An Bras Dermatol. 2020;95:32–9.
24. Wee E, Nikpour M, Balta S, Williams RA, Kelly RI. Lymphocytic thrombophilic arteritis complicated by systemic involvement. Australas J Dermatol. 2018;59:223–5.

Dermal Hyperneury

Zlatko Marušić and Eduardo Calonje

Introduction

The first detailed description of dermal hyperneury (DN) can probably be attributed to Winkelmann and Carney [1]. In their 1982 study on cutaneous neuropathology in multiple endocrine neoplasia 2B syndrome (MEN 2B), the authors noted that the dermal nerve fascicles in patients with MEN 2B were 1.5–4 times larger than in normal controls. A similar finding (hypertrophic nerves in a number of cutaneous biopsies) was noted by Starink et al. in a study of 21 Cowden syndrome patients [2], while multiple mucocutaneous neuromas have been note in PTEN hamartoma tumour syndrome [3]. DN has also been associated with neurofibromatosis type 2 [4] and MEN 2A syndrome [5].

Outside syndromic association, DN mostly presents in the form of solitary lesions; however, a series of multiple skin lesions with no syndromic association has been reported by Ieremia et al. [6]. Incidental dermal hyperneury may be rarely seen in skin biopsies with different pathologies including basal cell carcinoma and dermatofibroma. It has also been described exceptionally in lichen simplex chronicus/ nodular prurigo and notalgia paresthetica.

Z. Marušić
Clinical Department of Pathology and Cytology, University Hospital Centre Zagreb, Zagreb, Croatia

E. Calonje (✉)
Dermatopathology Department, St John's Institute of Dermatology, St Thomas' Hospital, London, UK
e-mail: jaime.calonje@kcl.ac.uk

F. Rongioletti, B. R. Smoller (eds.), *New and Emerging Entities in Dermatology and Dermatopathology*, https://doi.org/10.1007/978-3-030-80027-7_35

Clinical Features

MEN2B patients present with pathognomonic early onset periorificial mucocutaneous neuromas of the eyelids, lips, and tongue [7]. Less frequently, the mucocutaneous neuromas can be found in cutaneous sites. These clinically characteristic, somewhat cobblestone-shaped lesions show a certain degree of histopathological overlap with DN, as discussed later. As mentioned previously, the enlarged dermal nerve fascicles of DN that can be appreciated on histology in MEN 2B patients produce no visible clinical lesions. DN in other syndromes presents mostly as skin-coloured papules or nodules on the trunk or the extremities [4, 5].

The multiple non-syndromic lesions described by Ieremia et al. in four patients (3F, 1M, median age 58) [6] were pink or skin-coloured papules with occasional indentation that involved the trunk and the limbs, with no scalp or face predilection (Fig. 1a, b). Many of the lesions were longstanding and none of the patients reported pruritus or pain.

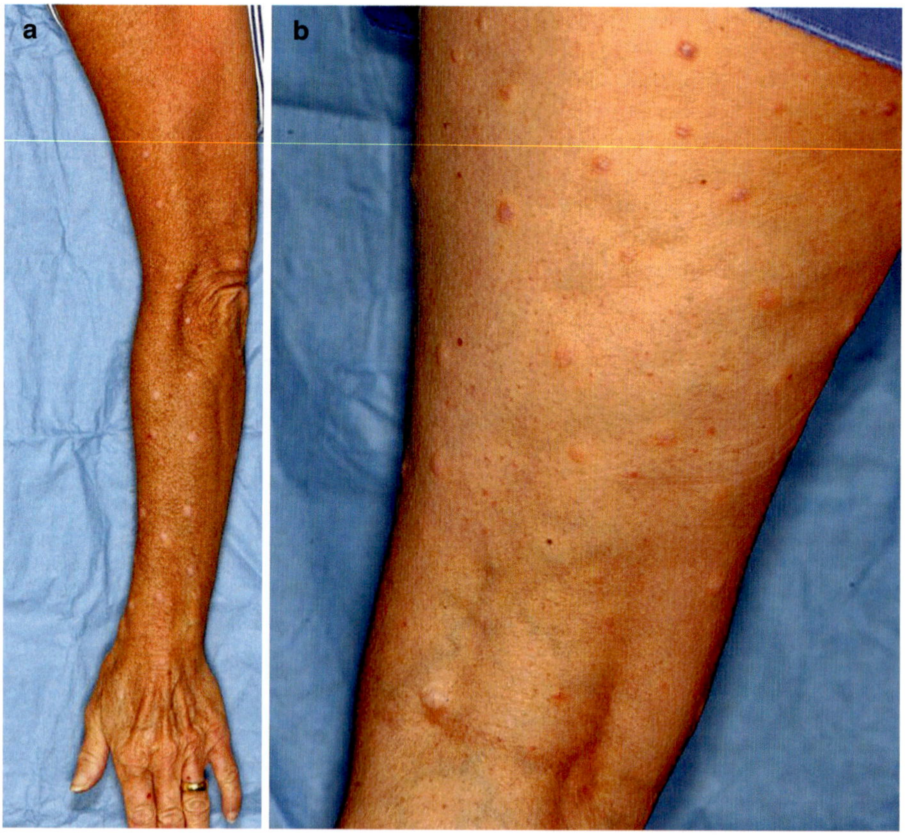

Fig. 1 Clinical presentation of dermal hyperneury as multiple pink (**a**) and skin-coloured (**b**) papules

Histopathological Features

Dermal hyperneury is characterized by an exaggerated size and prominence of dermal nerve fibres, even though there is no well-defined consensus on histologic quantitative parameters. The nerves focally exhibit a tortuous course with a variably prominent perineurium and are characteristically seen closely beneath the epidermis, usually within one higher-power field (100×) [1] (Fig. 2a, b). Sometimes, there

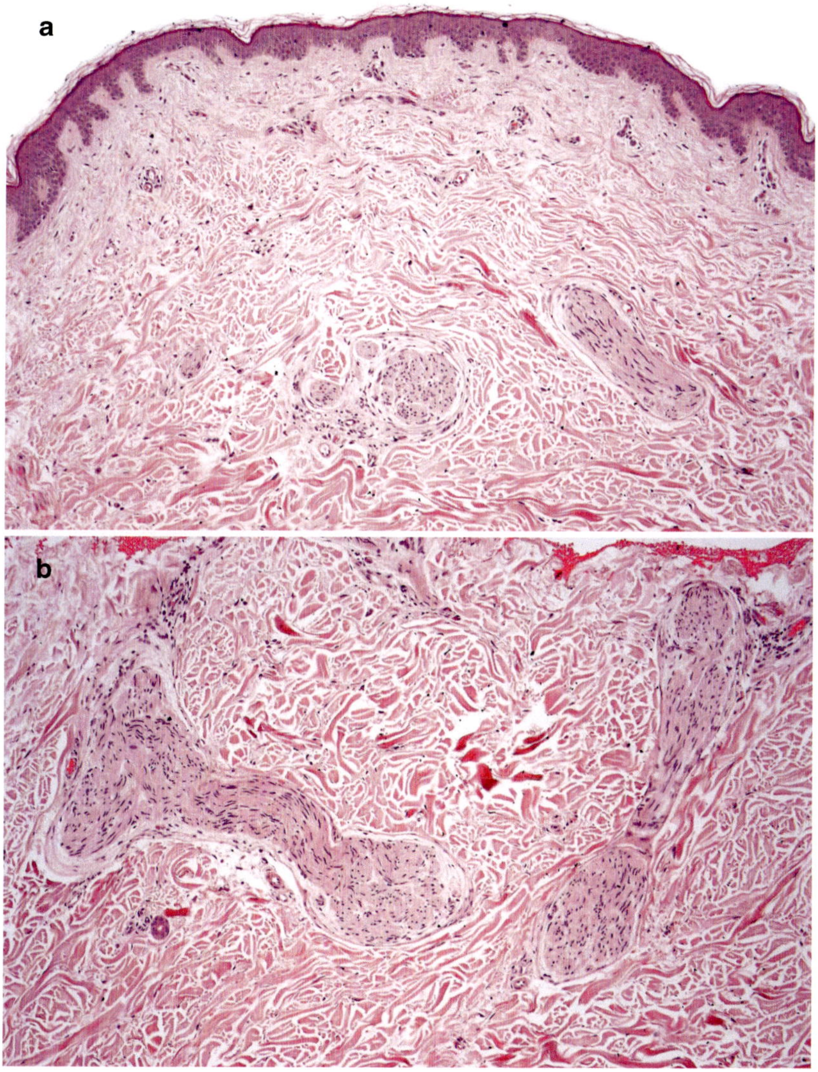

Fig. 2 (**a**) Histology (haematoxylin and eosin) of dermal hyperneury showing increased number of nerve fascicles or trunks at the dermal level; (**b**) well-formed nerves with a focal tortuous course and perineurium of variable thickness

can be a degree of internal architectural disorganization similar to neuroma, focal mucinous change within the nerve fascicles, or an associated inflammatory infiltrate composed of lymphocytes, histiocytes and occasional plasma cells [6]. The immunohistochemical profile is typical for normal nerve tissue (S-100 positive, surrounded by EMA-positive perineurium). None of the reported multiple idiopathic lesions showed loss of PTEN or amplification of RET by immunohistochemistry or clinical features of the associated syndromes [6].

Neuromas associated with MEN 2B and other syndromes consist of two patterns: one pattern resembles solitary circumscribed neuroma, a well-delineated dermal tumour containing numerous fascicles of Schwann cells and axons, while the other one is more diffuse and showing more overlap with DN. According to Winkelmann and Carney [1], the main difference between mucocutaneous neuromas and enlarged dermal nerve fascicles of DN in MEN 2B patients is the bulk of the lesion and the fact that the former are not associated with a clinically visible lesion.

Workup

The paramount question in diagnostic workup is whether DN is syndrome-related, given that all of the syndromes mentioned above are linked to genetic mutations that substantially increase the risk of malignancy over the course of patients' life. MEN 2B is linked with medullary thyroid carcinoma and phaeochromocytoma, while MEN 2A includes the former and also parathyroid tumours. Cowden syndrome carries an increased risk for breast, thyroid and visceral malignancies, while neurofibromatosis may carry an increased risk for malignant peripheral nerve sheath tumours.

DN in combination with multiple mucocutaneous neuromas or obvious cutaneous lesions associated with one of the above-described syndromes should prompt a syndrome workup. A solitary DN lesion or lesion accompanying some other diagnosis such as basal cell carcinoma, actinic keratosis [6], dermatofibroma (personal observation, E.C.), nodular prurigo [8] or notalgia paresthetica [9] should point to sporadic aetiology, while multiple lesions can be either syndromic or idiopathic, as demonstrated by Ieremia et al. Confirmation of syndromic association may require genetic testing, especially in children, such as the RET gene variation testing for MEN 2 syndrome [10]. Neurofibromatosis type 2 (NF2) [11] and Cowden syndrome [12] typically require a set of clinical criteria for the diagnosis.

Differential Diagnosis

Mucocutaneous neuromas share a certain degree of overlap with DN within their spectrum as mentioned previously and are encountered within identical syndromes. Epithelial sheath neuroma (ESN) [13] is the other main differential diagnosis, and it

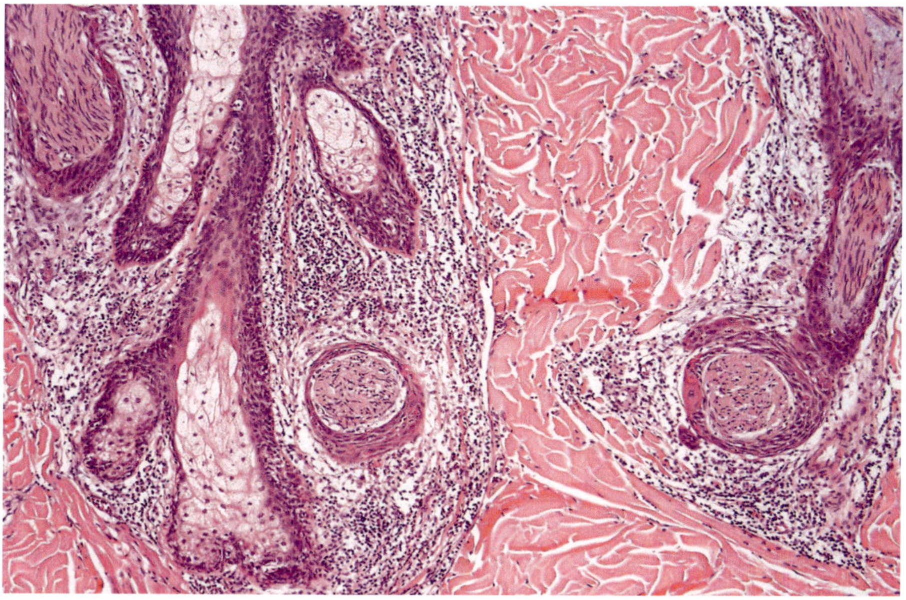

Fig. 3 Epithelial sheath neuroma showing nerve fascicles encased by a squamoid-appearing and thickened perineurium

may represent a variant of dermal hyperneury exhibiting putatively metaplastic epithelial elements. It is a non-syndromic entity morphologically similar to DN, as it features large and prominent nerve fascicles in the superficial dermis. It also shows a characteristic perineural thickening, resembling squamous epithelium. The squamoid epithelial collar surrounding the nerve fascicles may be as thick and prominent as to simulate perineural infiltration by squamous cell carcinoma (Fig. 3). Both DN and ESN are benign, but as DN may be syndrome-related, the differential diagnosis is not unimportant. Distinction is allowed by the fact that DN does not exhibit the characteristic squamoid perineural collar, even though perineurium might be thickened.

Etiopathogenesis

Non-syndromic DN is idiopathic. It has been closely associated with nodular prurigo and lichen simplex chronicus, which has been overemphasized in the authors' view and the view of others [14]. In the authors' experience, it is occasionally encountered next to other cutaneous lesions (basal cell carcinoma, actinic keratosis and dermatofibroma), but the simultaneous occurrence is likely coincidental. None of the reported multiple idiopathic lesions showed loss of PTEN or amplification of RET by immunohistochemistry [6].

Syndromic DN is most notably associated with MEN 2B and MEN 2A, both of which are associated with alterations in the *RET* gene. *RET* is a proto-oncogene with tyrosine kinase function whose loss of function mutations are associated with the development of Hirschsprung's disease, whereas gain of function mutations are found in the MEN syndromes [15]. DN occurrence in *RET*-driven syndromes is putatively associated with the gene function inciting neuronal development. *PTEN*, a tumour suppressor gene, is known to suppress growth of certain tissues. Its inhibition in knockout mice is known to result in a dramatic regrowth of axons following injuries [16], and therefore, its inactivation in Cowden syndrome might result in neuronal stimulation. Neurofibromin in NF2 is known to stimulate development of neural tissue, hence the association with neurofibromas, and among others, DN.

Therapy

Solitary or pauci-focal lesions can be excised, while syndromic lesions need cancer surveillance, as previously discussed. While multiple lesions might be somewhat physically disfiguring, they are usually asymptomatic and, thus, multiple excisions are impractical in most such cases.

Prognosis and Course

As mentioned previously, DN lesions are indolent, long-standing and typically do not produce pain or pruritus. It is not known whether spontaneous regression or regression following any putative therapy can occur. The syndromes associated with DN follow the course described in respective textbooks.

Conclusions

Dermal hyperneury is a cutaneous nerve hypertrophy, which occurs within several syndromes, such as MEN 2B, MEN 2A, Cowden syndrome and NF 2. Solitary or multiple non-syndromic DN lesions have also been described. Malignancy surveillance is very important in syndromic settings. The ability to distinguish between syndromic and non-syndromic settings relies upon an awareness of DN as an entity and the knowledge of its main clinicopathologic features. Suspicion of a hereditary cancer syndrome should prompt pertinent diagnostic workup, including genetic testing, especially in paediatric patients.

References

1. Winkelman RK, Carney A. Cutaneous neuropathology in multiple endocrine neoplasia type 2b. J Invest Dermatol. 1982;79:307–12.
2. Starink TM, van der Veen JP, Arwert F, et al. The Cowden syndrome: a clinical and genetic study in 21 patients. Clin Genet. 1986;29:222–33.
3. Schaffer JV, Kamino H, Witkiewicz A, et al. Mucocutaneous neuromas: an underrecognized manifestation of PTEN hamartoma-tumor syndrome. Arch Dermatol. 2006;142:625–32.
4. Rhee DY, Chung WK, Chang SE, Lee MW, Choi JH, Moon KC. A case of cutaneous nerve hypertrophy: association with multiple endocrine neoplasia type 2 or neurofibromatosis type 2? J Cutan Pathol. 2008;35:1156–8.
5. Alegria-Landa V, Alegría-Landa V, Jo-Velasco M, Robledo M, Requena L. Dermal hyperneury and multiple sclerotic fibromas in multiple endocrine neoplasia type 2A syndrome. J Am Acad Dermatol. 2017;153:1298–301.
6. Ieremia E, Marušić Z, Mudaliar V, et al. Expanding the clinical spectrum of dermal hyperneury: report of nine new cases and a review of the literature. Histopathology. 2019;75:738–45.
7. Marušić Z, Korša L, Calonje E. Dermal hyperneury. Clin Dermatol 2021;39(2):291–94.
8. Harris B, Harris K, Penneys NS. Demonstration by S100 protein staining of increased numbers of nerves in the papillary dermis of patients with prurigo nodularis. J Am Acad Dermatol. 1992;26:56–8.
9. Inaloz HS, Kirtak N, Erguven HG, Karakok M, Inaloz SS. Notalgia paresthetica with a significant increase in the number of intradermal nerves. J Dermatol. 2002;29:739–43.
10. Norton JA, Krampitz G, Jensen RT. Multiple endocrine neoplasia: genetics and clinical management. Surg Oncol Clin N Am. 2015;24:795–832.
11. Evans DGR, Baser ME, O'Reilly B, et al. Management of the patient and family with neurofibromatosis 2: a consensus conference statement. Br J Neurosurg. 2005;19:5–12.
12. Pilarski R, Burt R, Kohlman W, Pho L, Shannon KM, Swisher E. Cowden syndrome and the PTEN hamartoma tumor syndrome: systematic review and revised diagnostic criteria. J Natl Cancer Inst. 2013;105:1607–16.
13. Requena L, Grosshans E, Kutzner H, et al. Epithelial sheath neuroma: a new entity. Am J Surg Pathol. 2000;24:190–6.
14. Lindley RP, Payne CM. Neural hyperplasia is not a diagnostic prerequisite in nodular prurigo. A controlled morphometric microscopic study of 26 biopsy specimens. J Cutan Pathol. 1989;16:14–8.
15. Takahashi M, Kawai K, Asai N. Roles of the *RET* proto-oncogene in cancer and development. JMA J. 2020;3:175–81.
16. Du K, Zheng S, Zhang Q, et al. Pten deletion promotes regrowth of corticospinal tract axons 1 year after spinal cord injury. J Neurosci. 2015;35:9754–63.

Emergent Cutaneous T-Cell Pseudolymphomas

Christina Mitteldorf and Werner Kempf

Introduction

Cutaneous pseudolymphomas (C-PSL) can be defined as an excessive immune response, which mimics clinically and/or histologically a malignant lymphoma [1]. Reasons for the development of C-PSL include the persistence or the delayed elimination of the antigen(s), insufficient control by regulators of the immune response due to genetic predisposition, or immunodeficiency. The spectrum of infections leading to PSL includes viral infections (herpes simplex and varicella zoster virus and molluscum virus), bacterial infections (*Borrelia* sp.and *Treponema pallidum*), parasitic infections (e.g., leishmaniasis), infestations, and in some cases exacerbated by immunodeficiency (e.g., lues maligna in HIV and CD8 papular eruption in HIV).

Although the classification according to the causative agent allows a logically coherent and easily comprehensible approach, it is only of limited help in practical diagnostic work, since the same PSL pattern can be caused by different pathogens and in addition a distinct pathogen can cause different PSL patterns. Moreover, the pathogen can often only be detected with special techniques, so that the definite diagnosis is only possible with delay.

Clinically and histologically, C-PSL is divided into four major groups, which have recently outlined in details elsewhere [1]. The nodular form (N-PSL)

C. Mitteldorf (✉)
University Medical Center Göttingen, Department of Dermatology, Venereology and Allergology, Göttingen, Germany
e-mail: christina.mitteldorf@med.uni-goettingen.de

W. Kempf
Kempf und Pfaltz Histologische Diagnostik, Zürich, Switzerland

Department of Dermatology, University Hospital Zürich, Zürich, Switzerland
e-mail: werner.kempf@kempf-pfaltz.ch

F. Rongioletti, B. R. Smoller (eds.), *New and Emerging Entities in Dermatology and Dermatopathology*, https://doi.org/10.1007/978-3-030-80027-7_36

resembles cutaneous lymphomas clinically and histologically as it is clinically characterized by a nodular lesion, which cannot be distinguished from a nodular form of cutaneous T- or B-cell lymphoma. Histologically, N-PSL shows a dense nodular infiltrate often extending throughout all dermal layers and the superficial parts of the subcutaneous fat tissue. In some cases, a significant number of CD30-positive enlarged and atypically appearing cells are admixed, which resemble cutaneous CD30-lymphoproliferative disorders, particularly lymphomatoid papulosis (LYP). Those lesions can be considered as CD30+ pseudolymphoma. Another pattern of C-PSL shows clinically and/or histologically features of mycosis fungoides (MF) and is hence referred to as pseudo-MF. In this chapter, we focus on the emerging and still expanding spectrum of cutaneous T-cell pseudolymphomas due to infections.

Clinical Features

The spectrum depends upon the causative agent and individual immunologic response mechanism. It encompasses solitary, localized or generalized patches, plaques, or nodules and can therefore perfectly resemble MF or other cutaneous T-cell lymphomas (CTCLs). Helpful are subtle clinical aspects (e.g., blisters) and the patients' history (e.g., no response to topical steroids and UV light), unusual localization or distribution (e.g., unilateral distribution), and travel history.

Histopathological Features

Infiltrates, which resemble MF (so called "pseudo-MF"), present with a superficial band-like and/or deep periadnexal and perivascular infiltrate of small or medium-sized lymphocytes (Fig. 1a, b). Some larger T-lymphocytes can be also admixed but most often in a low number. The most common reason to suspect MF is a band-like arrangement of at least four lymphocytes in the junctional zone ("lining-up"). Nuclear atypia can also occur in reactive infiltrates and is not a reliable criterion to differentiate from a CTCL. If one finds Pautrier's microabscesses (collections of at least three neoplastic lymphocytes), they are a helpful diagnostic criterion for MF, but they have to be differentiated from intraepidermal collections of Langerhans cells (the so-called pseudo-Pautrier's microabscesses).

The infiltrate consists predominantly of CD3-positive T-lymphocytes, and most of the cases show an equal CD4/CD8 ratio in regard to the entire infiltrate. However, intraepidermal lymphocytes (especially in cases with lining up) can show a clear CD8 predominance, which might lead to the misdiagnosis of CD8+ MF. In contrast, in most MF cases, the CD8/CD4-ratio shift is also found in the dermal part, whereas in reactive infiltrates, the ratio is more equal or shows even a slight CD4 predominance [2]. A variable number of CD30+ cells can be intermingled, which results in overlapping features to CD30+ cutaneous PSL. In CD30-positive PSLs, the infiltrate is often wedge shaped and usually eosinophils are found. A high number of CD30+ cells are found in reactive infiltrates caused by molluscum contagiosum, *Parapoxvirus* infections, and scabies. A loss of T-cell markers (e.g., CD2 and CD7) has also been described in C-PSL and is not restricted to CTCLs [3]. In general, in reactive infiltrates, the composition is more mixed and concerns more often higher numbers of histiocytes and B-lymphocytes. As reactive infiltrates in infectious diseases can rarely show clonal T-cell receptor rearrangements, these results should be only interpreted together with the histology and the clinical context.

Workup

Patients' history and clinical presentation. Skin biopsy, clonality analysis, and detection of the suspected agent (e.g., serology, immunohistochemistry, and PCR).

Differential Diagnosis

Mycosis fungoides, subcutaneous panniculitis-like T-cell lymphoma (SPLTCL), CD30-positive lymphoproliferative disorders and rarely other T-cell lymphomas.

Etiopathogenesis

Viral (including alpha herpes viruses, molluscum contagiosum, and *Parapoxvirus*), bacterial (especially spirochetal) infections, and infestation (e.g., scabies) are the most relevant infections, which might simulate cutaneous T-cell lymphomas.

Borrelia species can induce not only B-cell pseudolymphomas but also two different types of T-cell pseudolymphomas (pseudo-MF and simulator of SPLTCL) [4, 5]. Clinically, some patients present a classical acrodermatitis chronica atrophicans, and others show disseminated lichenoid patches, thin plaques, or indurated erythema. Histologically, pseudo-MF type is characterized by a superficial band-like (Fig. 1a) or diffuse lymphohistiocytic infiltrate; eosinophils can be also found. The lymphocytes show an epidermotropism, often combined with a mild vacuolar interface dermatitis (Fig. 1b). Plasma cells can be admixed, but they are less common than generally expected [4]. T-cell receptor analysis and the detection of *Borrelia sp.* by PCR can be helpful. However, these results do not offer absolute diagnostic certainty.

The SPLTCL-like type shows a lobular histiocytic-rich panniculitis with medium-sized atypical lymphocytes, eosinophils, and plasma cells [5]. The lymphocytes express CD8 and show a rimming around the adipocytes, which might lead to the misdiagnosis of SPLTCL [5].

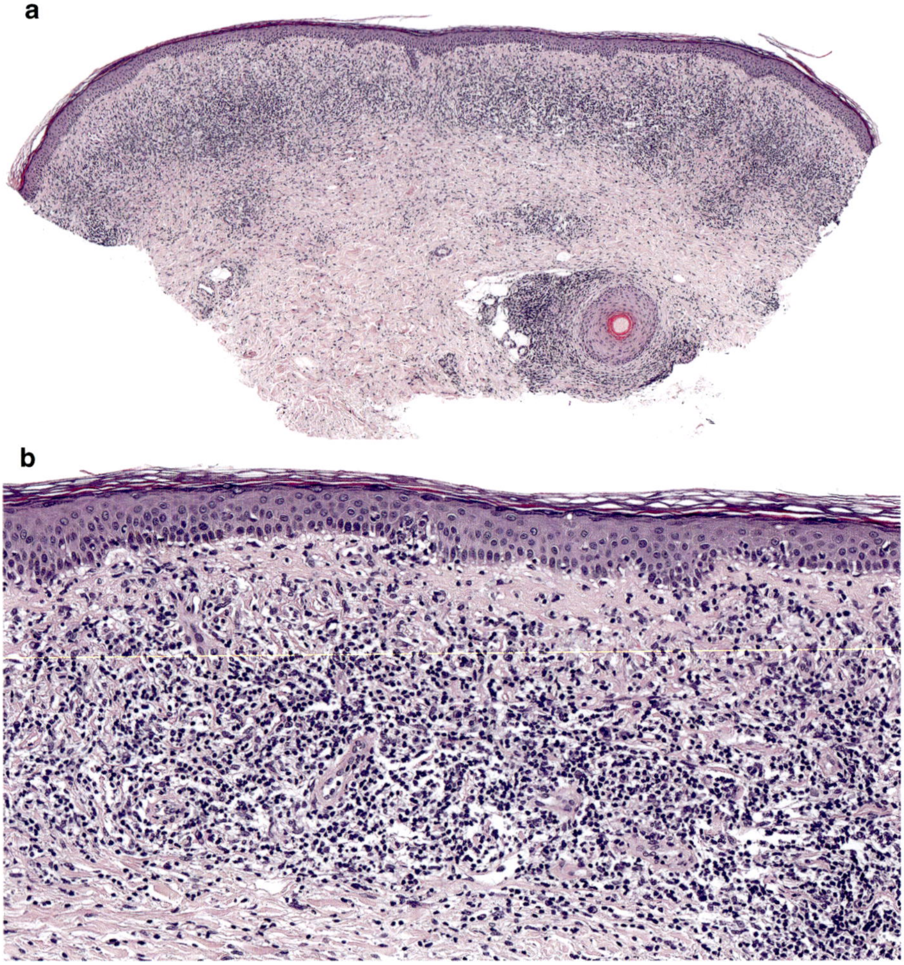

Fig. 1 *Borrelia*-induced T-cell pseudolymphoma and pseudo-MF type (**a**), superficial band-like or diffuse lymphohistiocytic infiltrate (hematoxylin and eosin, magnification ×5) and (**b**) mild vacuolar interface dermatitis with band-like infiltrate (hematoxylin and eosin, magnification ×100)

Cutaneous leishmaniasis can rarely present as a T-cell-rich variant with epidermotropism. If amastigotes cannot be found by conventional histology or special stains (Giemsa) [6, 7], the diagnosis cannot be confirmed by histology alone, and a provisory diagnosis of C-PSL is made. In these cases, PCR diagnostic is critical and should be performed in all presumed idiopathic cPSL in countries where Leishmaniasis is endemic [6].

If *herpes simplex virus (HSV)* and *varicella zoster virus (VZV)* present with atypical superficial and deep perivascular/periadnexal lymphohistiocytic infiltrates (Fig. 2a) without pathognomonic epithelial herpes virus-related alterations, they can be easily misinterpreted as cutaneous lymphomas [8–11]. In some cases, a lining up of CD8+ lymphocytes can occur (Fig. 2b). The T cells can be slightly enlarged with atypical chromatin dense nuclei. The presence of plasma cells, papillary edema, a careful CPC, and the patients' history are important clues for a herpes virus infection [8–11]. It is important to realize that immunohistochemical stains for

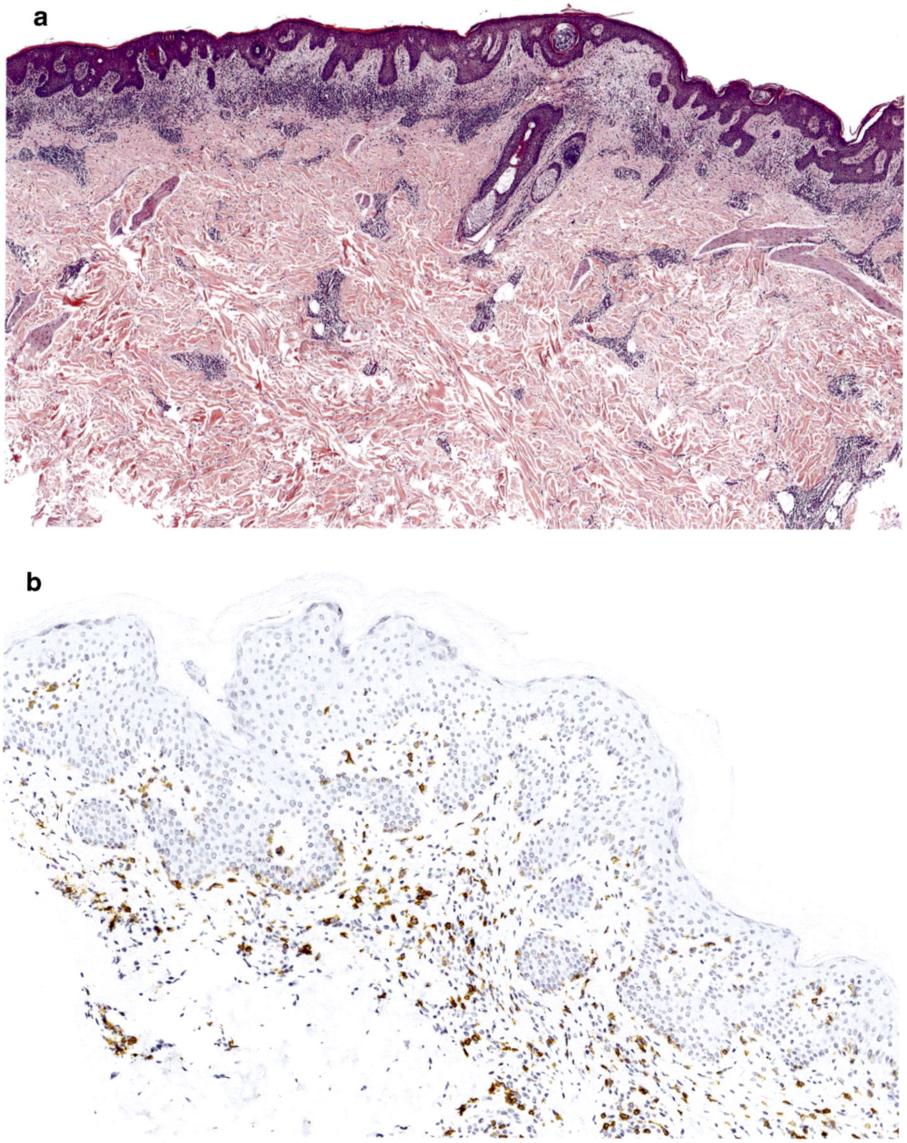

Fig. 2 Herpes simplex virus induced T-cell pseudolymphoma. (**a**) The epidermis is slightly acanthotic. Superficial band-like and deep perivascular lymphohistiocytic infiltrate (hematoxylin and eosin, magnification ×25). (**b**) Lining up of CD8+ lymphocytes (magnification ×130)

viral antigens and viral DNA by PCR are only diagnostic if infected cells/virus DNA are presented on the slide at the time of biopsy. The biopsy, however, is often not taken in the acute stage of the disease [8].

An infection with *Treponema pallidum* can simulate cutaneous T- and B-cell lymphomas [12–14]. The clinical and histologic spectrum of syphilis is broad and also related to the immunity and the disease stage. Secondary syphilis can show superficial or deep lymphohistiocytic infiltrates with exocytosis of lymphocytes in the epidermis. The epidermis is often psoriasiform and commonly combined with an interface dermatitis [15]. Plasma cells can only be detected in 2/3 of the cases [15]. *Treponema pallidum* can be identified by Warthin–Starry or immunohistochemical stains. In forms containing a low number of pathogens, a syphilis serology is needed to make the diagnosis. A coinfection with HIV might lead to a strong CD8 predominance and is a pitfall for misinterpretation of cutaneous lymphoma [16].

Several infections have been reported to harbor CD30+ lymphocytes in their infiltrate (Table 1). The number of CD30-positive cells is highly variable, and there are overlapping features of CD30+ PSLs and other T-cell PSLs.

We highlight three infections, which are common and typically contain a high number of CD30-positive lymphocytes.

Parapoxvirus-associated disorders (*Milker's nodule* and *Orf disease*) can present with superficial and deep T-cell infiltrate with numerous admixed CD30+ cells, eosinophils, and plasma cells. The epidermis is often acanthotic, and there is a papillary edema [17].

Molluscum contagiosum (MC) can have an intensive T-cell-rich infiltrate containing large and pleomorphic lymphocytes (Fig. 3a) with CD30 expression (Fig. 3b). If the diagnostic histological features of MC (epidermal invagination with molluscum bodies) are absent, they can be easily misinterpreted as CD30+ lymphoproliferative disorder, especially LYP [18, 19]. The infiltrate is most commonly positive for CD4 [19, 20], but CD8 [18] predominance has also been reported. The CD30 component is highly variable and ranges from a few scattered CD30+ lymphocytes to cohesive sheets [18, 20, 21].

An infestation by *Sarcoptes scabiei* can show a significant number of CD30 positive lymphocytes in early and especially in late stage, the so-called post-scabietic nodules. The T-cell-rich infiltrate is superficial or deep perivascular (Fig. 4a), with

Table 1 Infectious diseases and infestations with CD30 expression

Molluscum contagiosum
Herpes simplex virus/herpes zoster virus
Milker's nodule
Orf disease
Verruca vulgaris
Mycotic infections
Mycobacteriosis
Lues
Leishmania
Scabies

a

b

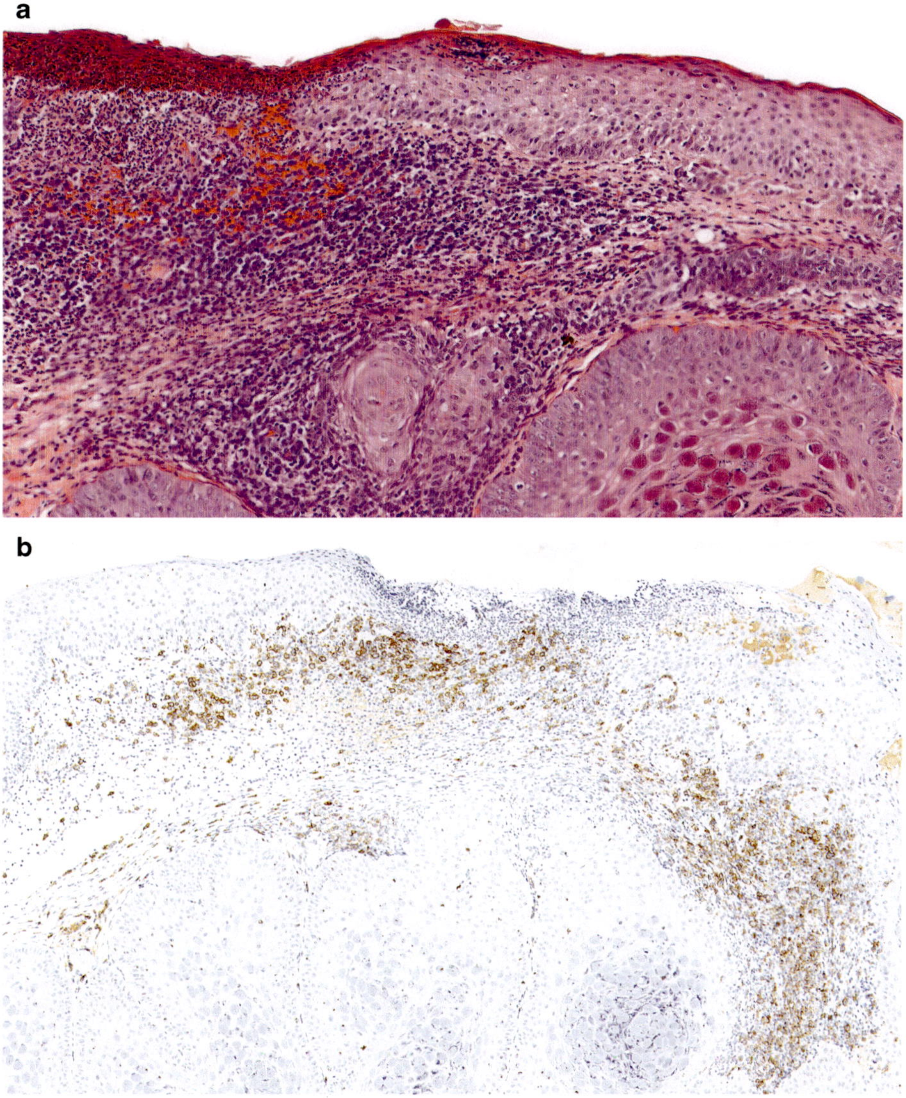

Fig. 3 CD30-positive T-cell pseudolymphoma in Molluscum contagiosum. (**a**) Superficial infiltrate of large lymphocytes. At the base of the picture, part of epidermal invagination with molluscum bodies was seen (hematoxylin and eosin, magnification ×200). (**b**) Dense lymphocytic infiltrates with numerous CD30-positive lymphocytes (magnification ×100)

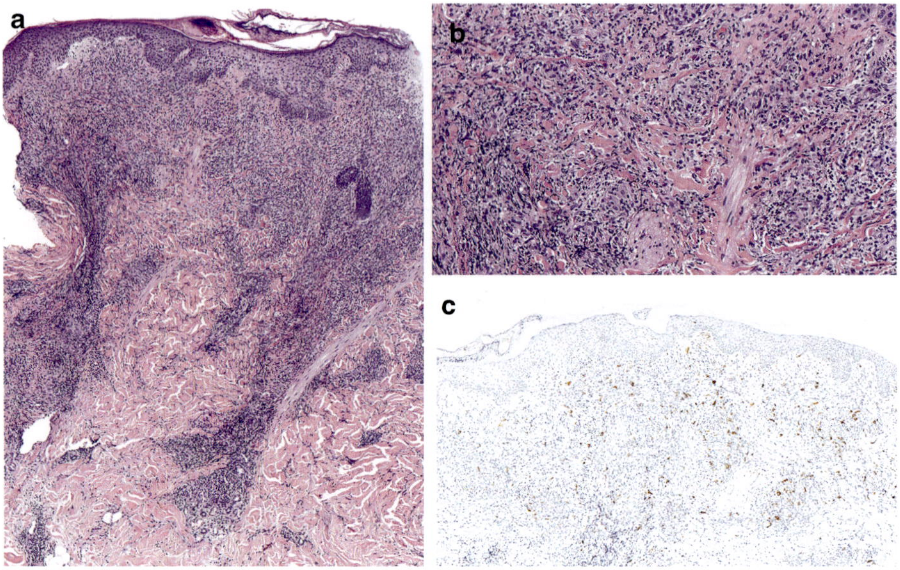

Fig. 4 CD30-positive T-cell pseudolymphoma in *Sarcoptes scabiei* infestation. (**a**) Superficial and deep perivascular infiltrate (hematoxylin and eosin, magnification × 25). (**b**) Pleomorphic lymphocytic infiltrates with numerous eosinophils (hematoxylin and eosin, magnification ×70). (**c**) Admixed CD30+ lymphocytes (magnification ×200)

papillary edema and usually many eosinophils (Fig. 4b). The number of CD30+ lymphocytes (Fig. 4c) can be high (up to 72%) [22].

Therapy

Treatment of the causative infectious agent.

Prognosis and Course

The clinical course is indolent, and the prognosis is good. In most of the cases, the skin lesions heal, after the causative agent is removed.

Conclusion

A broad spectrum of infectious diseases can mimic mycosis fungoides (MF) or other CTCLs, especially on histological grounds. The detection of the agent and a careful clinicopathological correlation are essential to avoid misdiagnosis.

Conflict of Interest The authors have nothing to disclose.
FundingNone

References

1. Mitteldorf C, Kempf W. Cutaneous pseudolymphoma-a review on the spectrum and a proposal for a new classification. J Cutan Pathol. 2020;47(1):76–97.
2. Fujimoto M, Basko-Plluska JL, Petronic-Rosic V, Shea CR. Early morphea simulating patch-stage mycosis fungoides. Am J Dermatopathol. 2015;37(5):409–12.
3. Magro CM, Daniels BH, Crowson AN. Drug induced pseudolymphoma. Semin Diagn Pathol. 2018;35(4):247–59.
4. Kempf W, Kazakov DV, Hubscher E, Tinguely M. Cutaneous borreliosis with a T-cell-rich infiltrate and simultaneous involvement by B-cell chronic lymphocytic leukemia with t(14;18)(q32;q21). Am J Dermatopathol. 2015;37(9):715–8.
5. Kempf W, Kazakov DV, Kutzner H. Lobular panniculitis due to Borrelia burgdorferi infection mimicking subcutaneous panniculitis-like T-cell lymphoma. Am J Dermatopathol. 2013;35(2):e30–3.
6. Tomasini C, Moneghini L, Barbui AM. Chronic amastigote-negative cutaneous leishmaniasis: a clinical, histopathologic and molecular study of 27 cases with emphasis on atypical and pseudolymphomatous presentations. J Cutan Pathol. 2017;44(6):530–7.
7. Boer A, Blodorn-Schlicht N, Wiebels D, Steinkraus V, Falk TM. Unusual histopathological features of cutaneous leishmaniasis identified by polymerase chain reaction specific for Leishmania on paraffin-embedded skin biopsies. Br J Dermatol. 2006;155(4):815–9.
8. Boer A, Herder N, Blodorn-Schlicht N, Falk T. Herpes incognito most commonly is herpes zoster and its histopathologic pattern is distinctive! Am J Dermatopathol. 2006;28(2):181–6.
9. Lewin JM, Farley-Loftus R, Pomeranz MK. Herpes simplex virus-associated pseudolymphoma. Cutis. 2013;92(6):E1–2.
10. Sbidian E, Battistella M, Legoff J, Lafaurie M, Bezier M, Agbalika F, et al. Recalcitrant pseudotumoral anogenital herpes simplex virus type 2 in HIV-infected patients: evidence for predominant B-lymphoplasmocytic infiltration and immunomodulators as effective therapeutic strategy. Clin Infect Dis. 2013;57(11):1648–55.
11. Mitteldorf C, Geissinger E, Pleimes M, Schon MP, Kempf W. T-cell pseudolymphoma in recurrent herpes simplex virus infection. J Cutan Pathol. 2019;46(10):717–22.
12. Hodak E, David M, Rothem A, Bialowance M, Sandbank M. Nodular secondary syphilis mimicking cutaneous lymphoreticular process. J Am Acad Dermatol. 1987;17(5 Pt 2):914–7.
13. Erfurt C, Lueftl M, Simon M Jr, Schuler G, Schultz ES. Late syphilis mimicking a pseudolymphoma of the skin. Eur J Dermatol. 2006;16(4):431–4.
14. Moon HS, Park K, Lee JH, Son SJ. A nodular syphilid presenting as a pseudolymphoma: mimicking a cutaneous marginal zone B-cell lymphoma. Am J Dermatopathol. 2009;31(8):846–8.
15. Flamm A, Parikh K, Xie Q, Kwon EJ, Elston DM. Histologic features of secondary syphilis: a multicenter retrospective review. J Am Acad Dermatol. 2015;73(6):1025–30.
16. Mitteldorf C, Plumbaum H, Zutt M, Schon MP, Kaune KM. CD8-positive pseudolymphoma in lues maligna and human immunodeficiency virus with monoclonal T-cell receptor-beta rearrangement. J Cutan Pathol. 2019;46(3):204–10.
17. Rose C, Starostik P, Brocker EB. Infection with parapoxvirus induces CD30-positive cutaneous infiltrates in humans. J Cutan Pathol. 1999;26(10):520–2.
18. Guitart J, Hurt MA. Pleomorphic T-cell infiltrate associated with molluscum contagiosum. Am J Dermatopathol. 1999;21(2):178–80.
19. Moreno-Ramirez D, Garcia-Escudero A, Rios-Martin JJ, Herrera-Saval A, Camacho F. Cutaneous pseudolymphoma in association with molluscum contagiosum in an elderly patient. J Cutan Pathol. 2003;30(7):473–5.

20. Kempf W. CD30+ lymphoproliferative disorders: histopathology, differential diagnosis, new variants, and simulators. J Cutan Pathol. 2006;33 Suppl 1:58–70.
21. Baykal C, Buyukbabani N, Seckin D, Polat Ekinci A, Yilmaz Z, Kempf W. Cutaneous atypical papular CD8+ lymphoproliferative disorder at acral sites in a renal transplant patient. Clin Exp Dermatol. 2017;42(8):902–5.
22. Gallardo F, Barranco C, Toll A, Pujol RM. CD30 antigen expression in cutaneous inflammatory infiltrates of scabies: a dynamic immunophenotypic pattern that should be distinguished from lymphomatoid papulosis. J Cutan Pathol. 2002;29(6):368–73.

Index

F. Rongioletti, B. R. Smoller (eds.), *New and Emerging Entities in Dermatology and Dermatopathology*, https://doi.org/10.1007/978-3-030-80027-7

M

N

R

W

X

GPSR Compliance

The European Union's (EU) General Product Safety Regulation (GPSR) is a set of rules that requires consumer products to be safe and our obligations to ensure this.

If you have any concerns about our products, you can contact us on ProductSafety@springernature.com

In case Publisher is established outside the EU, the EU authorized representative is:

Springer Nature Customer Service Center GmbH
Europaplatz 3
69115 Heidelberg, Germany

Batch number: 10756373

Printed by Printforce, the Netherlands